MAYO CLINIC
COMPLETE BOOK OF PREGNANCY & BABY'S FIRST YEAR

Other Mayo Clinic titles
Published by
William Morrow and Company, Inc., New York

Mayo Clinic Family Health Book, David E. Larson, M.D., Editor-in-Chief, 1990

Mayo Clinic Heart Book, Michael D. McGoon, M.D., Editor-in-Chief, 1993

Mayo Clinic Interactive CD-ROM Discs
Published by IVI Publishing, Eden Prairie, MN

Mayo Clinic Family Health Book Interactive Edition CD-ROM, 1992
Mayo Clinic — The Total Heart CD-ROM, 1993
Mayo Clinic Family Pharmacist CD-ROM, 1994
AnnaTommy, Mayo Clinic Learning Series CD-ROM, 1994
Mayo Clinic Sports Health and Fitness CD-ROM, 1994

MAYO CLINIC COMPLETE BOOK OF PREGNANCY & BABY'S FIRST YEAR

Robert V. Johnson, M.D.

Editor-in-Chief

William Morrow and Company, Inc.

New York

Mayo Clinic Complete Book of Pregnancy & Baby's First Year provides reliable, practical, comprehensive, easy-to-understand information on all aspects of pregnancy and baby care through age 1. Much of its information comes directly from the experience of Mayo's 1,300 physicians and medical scientists.

Mayo Clinic Complete Book of Pregnancy & Baby's First Year supplements advice of your personal physician, whom you should consult for individual medical problems. No endorsement of any company or product is implied or intended.

Mayo Clinic Complete Book of Pregnancy & Baby's First Year provides comprehensive health information in a single, authoritative source. *Mayo Clinic Health Letter*, a monthly eight-page newsletter, offers the same kind of easy-to-understand, reliable information, with a special focus on timely topics. For information on how this award-winning newsletter can be delivered to your home every month, call 800-333-9037.

Library of Congress Cataloging-in-Publication Data

Mayo Clinic Complete Book of Pregnancy & Baby's First Year/Mayo Foundation for Medical Education and Research.
 p.   cm.
 Includes Index.
 ISBN 0-688-11761-9
 1. Pregnancy. 2. Infants—Care. 3. Childbirth. 4. Parenting.
 I. Mayo Foundation for Medical Education and Research.
 RG525.M382   1994   94-7264
 618.2—dc20   CIP

Printed in the United States of America
First Edition
    5 6 7 8 9 10

Contents

Part One — Pregnancy

Part Two — Childbirth

Part Three — Living With and Understanding Your Baby

Part Four — From Partners to Parents: A Family Is Born

Editorial Staff

Editor-in-Chief	Robert V. Johnson, M.D.
Editorial Director	Sara C. Gilliland
Editor	David E. Swanson
Medical Illustrators	Michael A. King M. Alice McKinney James D. Postier
Photographers	Mary T. Frantz Joseph M. Kane Randy J. Ziegler
Editorial Production	LeAnn M. Stee
Designers	Karen E. Barrie Kathryn K. Shepel

Foreword

As change sweeps over health care, one fact remains certain: Mayo Clinic will continue its 100-year tradition of providing the highest-quality, most cost-effective medical care, blending practice with medical education and research. That's always been our goal. It will not change.

Each year, more than 350,000 individuals seek Mayo health care from our facilities in Rochester, Minnesota; Scottsdale, Arizona; and Jacksonville, Florida. Through the years, we've served the needs of more than 4,000,000 people.

At Mayo, we are committed to helping people stay well. In 1932, one of our founders, Dr. Charles H. Mayo, noted that "the object of all health education is to change the conduct of individual men, women and children by teaching them to care for their bodies well." The words "change the conduct" have special meaning to us because they set the tone for the health information we publish. Our aim is to offer practical information, facts you can use, not just interesting theory.

Mayo Clinic Complete Book of Pregnancy & Baby's First Year upholds our tradition of providing the very best in authoritative, easy-to-understand, practical health information. This is a comprehensive guide to the latest information available on pregnancy and child care through that critical first year of your baby's development. If you plan to start a family, if you're pregnant or if you already have a new baby, this book can guide your thoughts and actions on a host of practical issues that confront every new or prospective parent.

On behalf of the nearly 19,000 health professionals and support personnel who make up Mayo Foundation, thank you for selecting this book. We hope you'll find, in this single comprehensive volume, all of the information that you need as you look ahead to the turning point in your life that having a baby represents.

Robert R. Waller, M.D.
President and Chief Executive Officer
Mayo Foundation

Acknowledgments

Pregnancy is a time of excitement, anticipation and uncertainty. Information from sources such as this book can help satisfy your need for details and reassurances about your own health and the health of your unborn baby. It can also help prepare you for childbirth and the memorable first year. As you might expect, this book covers the health-related issues surrounding pregnancy and your baby's first year. It also covers many of the family adjustment issues you may encounter as you add a new baby to your family.

Expectant and new parents have been an important part of the creation of this book. We began by asking newly pregnant women how a book could satisfy their information needs beyond the traditional resources of medical care providers, family and friends. As the book was written, we included many quotes and stories from parents because we believe that they can best express some of the joys and surprises that accompany new parenthood. We are grateful to the parents who gave us their reactions to and suggestions for many of the chapters.

Ultimately, the combined resources of parents and the collective knowledge and experience of a wide variety of professionals resulted in a book that we believe is authoritative, practical, comprehensive and uniquely designed to meet the concerns of pregnant couples and new parents. A book of this scope requires the teamwork of many individuals. More than 100 Mayo physicians, nurses, nurse-practitioners, parent educators, dietitians, social workers and medical technicians had a "hands-on" role in writing this book. Mayo editors, illustrators, photographers, designers and other publishing support personnel refined, packaged and enhanced the information.

Through words and images, we have created a book that we hope will help you feel prepared for pregnancy, childbirth and the care of your baby.

Special thanks to Paul L. Ogburn, Jr., M.D., Jill A. Swanson, M.D., Helen E. Walker, R.N., C.P.N.P., Roger W. Harms, M.D., Charles S. Field, M.D., John W. Bachman, M.D., John M. Wilkinson, M.D., Cynthia E. Hammersley, R.N., Margaret (Peg) C. Harmon, R.N., and Christine M. Alexander, R.N., for outstanding assistance throughout this project. To my colleagues in Obstetrics, Family Medicine and Pediatrics, this book is a compilation of your knowledge, skill and compassion; thank you for the hours of editing and revising.

Obstetrics
Diana R. Danilenko-Dixon, M.D.
Mary Palmquist Evans, M.D.
Charles S. Field, M.D.
Roger W. Harms, M.D.
Robert H. Heise, M.D.
John A. Jefferies, M.D.
Keith L. Johansen, M.D.
Bruce W. Johnston, M.D.
Thomas M. Kastner, M.D.
Paul L. Ogburn, Jr., M.D.
Karl C. Podratz, M.D.
Kirk J. Ramin, M.D.
Jo T. Van Winter, M.D.

Family Medicine
David C. Agerter, M.D.
John W. Bachman, M.D.
Gregory A. Bartel, M.D.
Harvey D. Cassidy, M.D.
Laurie J. Daum, M.D.
Bradley C. Eichhorst, M.D.
Robert G. Fish, M.D.
Walter B. Franz III, M.D.
Michele A. Hanson, M.D.
Thomas R. Harman, M.D.
Margaret S. Houston, M.D.
Robert E. Nesse, M.D.
Lynda C. Sisson, M.D.
Susan L. Wickes, M.D.
John M. Wilkinson, M.D.
Floyd B. Willis, M.D.

Pediatrics
Garth F. Asay, M.D.
William J. Barbaresi, M.D.
Daniel D. Broughton, M.D.
Michelle C. Capizzi, M.D.
Douglas P. Derleth, M.D.
David J. Driscoll, M.D.
Gerald S. Gilchrist, M.D.
Carol Hennessey, R.N., C.P.N.P.
Nancy K. Henry, M.D.
Jay L. Hoecker, M.D.
Roy F. House, Jr., M.D.
Robert M. Jacobson, M.D.
Fredric Kleinberg, M.D.
Katherine M. Konzen, M.D.
Marilyn A. Mellor, M.D.
Bruce Z. Morgenstern, M.D.
Richard D. Olsen, M.D.
Marc C. Patterson, M.D.
Jean Perrault, M.D.
Julia A. Rosekrans, M.D.
Jill A. Swanson, M.D.
Maria G. Valdes, M.D.
Helen E. Walker, R.N., C.P.N.P.

Pediatric Orthopedic Surgery
William J. Shaughnessy, M.D.

Pediatric Surgery
Christopher Moir, M.D.

Pediatric Urologic Surgery
Stephen A. Kramer, M.D.

To my colleagues in Parent Education, who help couples understand and celebrate pregnancy and birth, my deepest thanks for your work on the book. Your perspective was invaluable.

Christine M. Alexander, R.N.
Arla J. Bernard, R.N.
Susan J. Brook, R.N.
Kathryn A. Cossette, R.N.
Anita J. DeAngelis, R.N.

Beverly A. Gerdes
Cynthia E. Hammersley, R.N.
Margaret (Peg) C. Harmon, R.N.
Ann M. Lansing, R.N.
Patricia J. Nyland, R.N.

Thank you to all the nurses and respiratory therapists in the Saint Marys Hospital Newborn Intensive Care Unit and Rochester Methodist Hospital Special Care Nursery, especially:

Renae K. Hendrickson, R.N.

Ann E. Teske, R.N.

Thank you to all the obstetrics nurses at Rochester Methodist Hospital Perinatal Center, especially:

Virginia M. Caspersen, R.N.
Susan K. Crawley, R.N.
Jenifer R. Hoff, R.N.
Linda K. Letts, R.N.
Patricia J. Lowrie, R.N.
Laura J. Lukes, R.N.
Mary C. Madden, R.N.

Linda K. Matti, R.N.
Karen S. Sandberg, R.N.
Jeri M. Sehl, R.N.
Cynthia M. Severson, R.N.
Carol D. Vigeland, R.N.
Becky A. Walkes, R.N.

I would also like to recognize the many other colleagues at Mayo who contributed to ensure the accuracy and comprehensiveness of this book:

Steven I. Altchuler, M.D.
Margaret R. Baker, R.D.
Linda K. Bausman, L.P.N.
Jill A. Beed, J.D.
Uldis Bite, M.D.
Robert J. Breckle
Bonnie M. Brown
Gregory D. Cascino, M.D.
Ricky P. Clay, M.D.
Mary E. Cook, R.N., I.B.C.L.C.
Matthew D. Dacy
Joseph Duffy, M.D.
M.A. (Tony) Enquist
Lisa D. Erickson, M.D.
Patricia J. Erwin
William N. Friedrich, Ph.D.
Pat A. Gallenberg, R.N.
Jean B. Goerss, M.D.
Victoria J. Hagstrom, M.D.
Dorothy M. Haley
Mary L. Halling, L.P.N.
Jo M. Helder, L.P.N.
Francis Helminski, J.D.

Janie L. Holmes, L.P.N.
Daniel L. Hurley, M.D.
Diane M. Huse, R.D.
John Huston III, M.D.
John E. Huxsahl, M.D.
Mary E. Johnson, Chaplain
Pamela S. Karnes, M.D.
Kathryn S. Kleist, L.P.N.
Brenda J. Knutson, R.D.
Stephen L. Kopecky, M.D.
Elizabeth A. Lafleur, R.N., I.B.C.L.C.
Karen E. Larsen
Craig H. Leicht, M.D.
Marilyn R. Lermon, L.P.N.
Alexander R. Lucas, M.D.
Gerard A. Malanga, M.D.
James K. Marttila, Pharm.D.
Lisa R. Mattson, M.D.
Deb K. McCauley, R.N.
Kathleen A. Meyerle, J.D.
Virginia V. Michels, M.D.
Jennifer K. Nelson, R.D.
Carolene M. Neumann, R.N.

Judith A. Ney, M.D.
Kathryn M. Niesen, R.N.
Stephen F. Noll, M.D.
Diane L. Olson, R.D.
Steven J. Ory, M.D.
Kristi L. Pesch
Sheryl M. Peterson
Rose J. Prissel, R.D.
Stephanie M. Quigg
Dawn M. Raadt, L.S.W.
Norman H. Rasmussen, Ed.D.
Paula J. Santrach, M.D.
Doreen J. Severson
Carol Jean Smidt, L.P.N.
Erica R. Smith
Stephen Q. Sponsel
Joyce E. Stenstrom
Paula J. Sullivan, R.N.
Rodney L. Thompson, M.D.
Kathleen A. Van Norman, L.P.N.
Christine K. Voeltz, L.P.N.
Catherine Walsh Vockley, M.S.
Lloyd A. Wells, M.D.

Thank you to the team of medical writers and editors who drafted and patiently revised chapters: Susie Blackmun, Felicia Busch, Jere Daniel, Peggy Eastman, Lindsay E. Edmunds, Harriet Hodgson, Lynn Madsen, Hara Marano, Susan Prosser, Deborah J. Shuman, Robert T. Sorrells, Ruth Taswell, Robin Taylor and Beth A. Watkins.

The staff of Mayo's Section of Publications provided meticulous editing, layout, proofreading and cross-referencing services. Our special thanks to LeAnn M. Stee, editor; Carl F. Anderson, M.D., head of Publications; Mary K. Horsman, editorial assistant; Mary L. Schwager, proofreader; and Roberta J. Schwartz, supervisor.

A talented team of medical illustrators, M. Alice McKinney, Michael A. King and James D. Postier, executed with clarity and sensitivity more than 90 illustrations to enhance the book.

More than 100 photographs, taken by photographers Mary T. Frantz, Joseph M. Kane and Randy J. Ziegler, capture the personal side of pregnancy and baby's first year. Photographs by Mayo photographers David M. Jorgenson and Melissa J. Lushinsky also appear. Thanks also to everyone who helped schedule and process the photographs, especially Marilyn J. Hanson and Mary E. Hedstrom. I am grateful to everyone who served as a photo model, especially those who allowed photographers to document personal, intimate moments.

Marsha Cohen, Parallelogram Graphic Communications, designed the book. Karen E. Barrie, Kathryn K. Shepel and Mary J. Welp, Mayo Visual Information Services, refined the elegant design and implemented the layout with precision. Special thanks also to Ronald R. Ward, R. Michael Belknap, Jon M. Curry and Thomas F. Flood, Mayo Visual Information Services, for their technical expertise and support.

To all the staff of William Morrow and Company, Inc., especially Al Marchioni, Toni Sciarra, Debbie Weiss, Ann Cahn, Susan Halligan, Jeanmarie Houlihan and Tom Nau, thank you for your trust and support.

Special thanks to Arthur Klebanoff, Scott Meredith Literary Agency, for your energy, creativity and good advice.

We are fortunate to have had various non-Mayo professionals who shared their expertise during the development of the book. Thanks to Tutti Sherlock and colleagues at Child Care Resource & Referral, Inc., Peggy O'Toole Martin from Parents Are Important in Rochester, Debra Carlsen, Mary Scanlan and Nancy Hartzler from Children's Home Society of Minnesota, Dr. Walter Larimore, Orlando, Florida, and the staff and families from Kiddie Corner Child Care in Rochester. We are also grateful to other organizations, including La Leche League International, International Lactation Consultant Association, RESOLVE, Inc., Adoptive Families of America, International Adoption Clinic and American Association of Marriage and Family Therapy, for their assistance.

Warmest thanks to the team at Mayo Medical Ventures for their talent, hard work and teamwork. Dr. Lynwood H. Smith, Dr. Richard F. Brubaker, Dr. David E. Larson, Rick F. Colvin and Vicki L. Moore provided leadership and guidance. Support was also provided by members of the Medical/Industry Relations Committee. The efforts of the marketing, customer service and communications staff started long before the book was finished and will continue after its publication: Michael A. Casey, Lindsay A. E. Dingle, Marne J. M. Gade, Christie L. Herman, Scott D. Olson, Louis Porter II and John La Forgia. Joan L. Benjamin, M. Lillian Haapala and Anne L. Nichols provided impeccable secretarial and support services.

Special thanks to Sara C. Gilliland for her wonderful blend of creativity and efficiency and for steady guidance in keeping this large project on track. Thank you to David E. Swanson for outstanding editing and innovative solutions to challenges.

Very special thanks to Janet Johnson—wonderful wife, mother, childbirth educator and tireless editorial assistant. To Brita and Joel, I hope that the joy we have from being your parents is passed on to new parents through the pages of this book.

Robert V. Johnson, M.D.
Editor-in-Chief

Credits

We gratefully acknowledge the photographers who provided the photographs that appear on the following pages:

Pages 38, A4 (top), 401: Gary Bistram, Bistram Photography, Maplewood, MN.

Page 44: Dean Riggott, *Rochester Post-Bulletin*, Rochester, MN.

Pages A1, A2, A3 (top): Lennart Nilsson, *A CHILD IS BORN*, Dell Publishing Company, New York, NY.

Page 574: Morris Evans, Black Hills Photography, Rapid City, SD.

Page 604: Jim Barbour, Jim Barbour Photography, Minnetonka, MN.

Pages 667, 669: Curt Sanders, Sanders Portrait Design, Rochester, MN.

We acknowledge the following sources for material used in this book:

Page 59: "Chromosome abnormalities" is from *Guidelines for Perinatal Care.* Third edition. American Academy of Pediatrics, Elk Grove Village, IL, and American College of Obstetricians and Gynecologists, Washington, DC, 1992, p. 57. By permission of the publishers.

Page 88: The Food Guide Pyramid is modified from the U.S. Department of Agriculture and U.S. Department of Health and Human Services.

Page 264: The chart is modified from Mozingo JN: Pain in labor: a conceptual model for intervention. *JOGN Nursing* 7 no. 4:47-49, 1978. By permission of Harper & Row.

Page 349: "Apgar scores" is from Behrman RE: *Nelson Textbook of Pediatrics.* Fourteenth edition. Philadelphia, WB Saunders Company, 1992, p. 427. By permission of the publisher.

Page 377: "Welcome to Holland." ©1987 by Emily Perl Kingsley. Printed with permission of the author. All rights reserved.

Page 422: The height and weight guidelines are from *Nutrition and Your Health: Dietary Guidelines for Americans*, 1990, U.S. Departments of Agriculture (USDA) and Health and Human Services (USDHHS).

Page 511: The growth chart is modified from Hamill PVV, Drizd TA, Johnson CL, Reed RB, Roche AF, Moore WM: Physical growth: National Center for Health Statistics percentiles. *Am J Clin Nutr* 32:607-629, 1979. By permission of American Society for Clinical Nutrition.

Welcome to the reader

This book will help you better understand pregnancy, birth and your baby's first year. It is meant to enhance, not replace, your relationship with your medical care team. Tell your health care provider that you have been reading this book. Your doctor, nurse-midwife or nurse-practitioner will guide your medical care based on your individual medical needs and your local medical resources.

About language

Throughout this book we have tried to use great care in our explanations; our intent is to avoid misunderstandings. At the same time, it is important that this book be easy to read. You'll notice that we commonly use the term "doctor" or "physician," yet medical care today requires the involvement of an entire team of people with different skills and responsibilities. When discussing primary care issues we have tried to indicate the various people involved in complementary and often interchangeable roles: physician, nurse-practitioner or certified nurse-midwife. If the topic of discussion involved subspecialists, we tried to use the more specific terms: obstetrician, perinatologist, neonatologist or pediatrician.

In a similar way we have tried to use care in using gender-specific terms. Most of the book is written from the viewpoint that "you, the reader" is the pregnant woman or the mother. We definitely wish to encourage the men involved to read the entire book; yet, for the sake of readability we often omit the male references.

We also want all types of families to be comfortable in reading this book. Because the traditional terms "husband" and "wife" may not always apply, we preferred to use the more generally applicable term "partner." We also describe parenthood, motherhood and fatherhood as social and psychological roles, rather than restricting these terms to biological parenting.

Part One

Pregnancy

CHAPTER ONE

You're Planning to Start a Family

This chapter begins at the very beginning, even before pregnancy starts. If you aren't already pregnant but you plan to start a family, this chapter begins with an overview of preparing for pregnancy. If you believe you are pregnant, the section that begins on page 53 covers tests used to confirm pregnancy and includes a calendar that shows key dates during pregnancy. For couples who have so far been unsuccessful in conceiving, there's a section on infertility, beginning on page 8.

Getting ready to have a baby can be similar to planning a wedding. Some couples begin wedding preparations far in advance. Every detail, from choosing the date and guest list to deciding on the wedding dress, flowers and cake, is coordinated and organized. Other couples might prefer to elope or to have a small, private ceremony.

Plans to start a family can range from well orchestrated to spontaneous or unexpected. Whether you feel more comfortable knowing as much as you can and being as prepared as you can or you adopt a more take-it-as-it-comes attitude, it's important to realize that you can't plan or control everything about your pregnancy. Planning a birth is perhaps more like planning an outdoor wedding. On the one hand, you can't control the rain clouds that threaten to postpone the ceremony; on the other hand, you couldn't have ordered the beautiful rainbow that appeared afterward.

This book is not about how to have the "perfect" pregnancy. There is no such thing. There will be high points during the next year that you never imagined would be so good. And there will be surprises along the way, regardless of how prepared you have tried to be.

Preparing for Pregnancy

Before you become pregnant, you can take steps to promote a healthy pregnancy. That's not to say you won't have a healthy pregnancy if you skip these recommendations, but by following them you can feel confident that you're helping to create the best conditions for your baby to grow and develop:

- If you have been taking oral contraceptives, your doctor may recommend using alternative methods of birth control for the first month or two after stopping use of the birth control pills.

- Your doctor may recommend stopping use of certain medications, or changing dosages, before pregnancy.

- Planning a pregnancy can be an excellent incentive to stop smoking. (See page 103 for more information about the hazards of smoking while you're pregnant.)

- Avoiding alcohol while you're trying to become pregnant and during pregnancy prevents exposing your baby to its harmful effects. Drinking excessive amounts of alcohol during pregnancy can cause a serious condition called fetal alcohol syndrome. There is no known safe level of alcohol consumption during pregnancy. (See page 105 for more information about fetal alcohol syndrome.)

- Because elevated maternal body temperature can increase the risk of neural tube defects in the baby, avoid prolonged use of a hot tub during early pregnancy. (See page 110 for more information on precautions about hot tubs.)

- If your doctor considers that you have a higher than normal risk of having a baby with a birth defect, genetic counseling might be recommended. (See page 55 for more information on risks for birth defects.)

Avoid these medications if you're planning to become pregnant

If you are taking these medicines, ask your doctor about possible adjustments or precautions to follow before becoming pregnant:

- Contraceptive medications
- Accutane, a prescription medication to treat acne
- Anticonvulsant/seizure medications
- Prednisone or prednisone-like medications
- Anticoagulant medications, such as warfarin (Coumadin, Panwarfin), that are used to prevent blood clots
- Antithyroid medications, such as propylthiouracil or methimazole, that are used to suppress activity of the thyroid gland
- Tetracycline, an antibiotic that is sometimes used to treat acne
- Medicines used for treatment of cancer

Preconception Medical Care

Your health care. Instead of waiting until you suspect you are pregnant to see your health care provider, you may consider preconception medical care, which is becoming more and more popular. Preconception medical care encourages optimal health for you and your partner at the time your child is conceived. This may be particularly important for women with chronic medical conditions such as diabetes mellitus, asthma or epilepsy. Also, decisions regarding fetal or genetic testing may be easier to make before a pregnancy begins.

A preconception visit is similar to the first prenatal visit (see page 45). However, seeing your health care provider before you become pregnant has a few advantages. For example, a preconception visit allows your health care provider to make sure that you are immune to certain infections, such as rubella, that could cause serious birth defects in a developing baby. If you are not immune, your health care provider may recommend a vaccination at least three months before you try to become pregnant. For women who have some type of ongoing medical condition, such as diabetes, high blood pressure, asthma or lupus, making sure the condition is controlled before pregnancy occurs is an important safeguard for your health and that of your future baby. Pregnancy places extra demands on a woman's body, so even conditions that have remained under control before pregnancy may require special medical management during pregnancy. A preconception visit also allows your health care provider to review any other factors about your health and lifestyle which could improve your chances for a healthy pregnancy.

Sometimes laboratory tests are done at a preconception visit, and others are deferred until you are pregnant. If you need certain tests, such as mammography, that are best deferred during pregnancy, now may be a good time to take care of these concerns.

If you're planning to become pregnant, it's best to discontinue use of birth control pills several months before you conceive. Occasionally, it takes several months for your menstrual periods to return to a regular pattern; until this happens, it's more difficult to pinpoint when ovulation occurs or to estimate your due date.

Although rare, failure of birth control pills can occur. If you become pregnant while you're still taking birth control pills, the hormones in the pills pose no extra risk of a birth defect in your baby. Similarly, spermicides used in vaginal creams and condom lubricants have no significant risks.

Pregnancy in your 30s or 40s

Women in their 30s and 40s sometimes wonder if they've waited too long to have a baby or if their chances of having a healthy baby are reduced. Fertility rates remain relatively stable until the early 30s, and then they decrease to very low levels by the early 40s. A woman's peak fertility is between ages 20 and 24. In women aged 30 to 35, fertility is 15 to 20 percent less than maximum. In women aged 35 to 39, the decrease is 25 to 50 percent. In women 40 to 45, there is a 95 percent decrease in fertility. Factors not related to age, such as smoking, diabetes, infections and endometriosis, also diminish fertility.

The risk of miscarriage increases after age 35, increasing even further after age 40. This increasing risk of pregnancy loss is primarily caused by chromosome abnormalities in the fetus.

Even though achieving pregnancy can be more difficult in an older woman, the overall outcomes are excellent. There are some concerns about higher risks of having a baby with low birth weight, premature labor or a child with chromosome abnormalities such as Down syndrome (see page 58). Older women also have a somewhat higher risk of gestational diabetes (see page 166), preeclampsia (see page 192) and placenta previa (see page 195). In general, however, women in their 30s who start pregnancy in good health are likely to have a healthy, normal pregnancy.

The hormone progesterone is in two newer contraceptive options—Norplant contraceptive implants and Depo-Provera injections. Pregnancy rarely occurs when these methods are used, but if it does occur the risks to the baby appear to be very small. Discuss your risks and options with your doctor.

If you use an intrauterine device (IUD) and become pregnant while it's still in place, an infection could result, possibly leading to miscarriage. However, removal of the IUD while you're pregnant also puts you at risk for a miscarriage. Most often, IUDs are removed. You and your doctor will decide what's best.

Your partner's medical history. If your partner is able to attend the pre-conception visit, he should be prepared to answer some of the same questions you'll be asked about family medical conditions and risk factors for infections or birth defects. Your partner's health and lifestyle are important because they can affect yours. Stopping smoking or making a commitment to a healthier diet is often easier when your partner is included and is supportive.

Are You Pregnant?

Some women experience a few telltale symptoms right away which make them suspect they are pregnant (see page 12). The earliest way to know if you are pregnant is to do a pregnancy test. Four days after fertilization, the fertilized egg begins to produce a hormone called human chorionic gonadotropin (hCG). This hormone can be detected first in the woman's blood and shortly thereafter in the urine.

Many women use home pregnancy tests soon after they miss a menstrual period. The tests detect hCG in a sample of your urine. After a specified length of time, usually less than five minutes, a color change indicates pregnancy.

The accuracy of home pregnancy tests depends on how closely you follow the instructions. If you do a home pregnancy test four to seven days after you'd expect your next period to begin, it will be positive about 95 percent of the time (assuming you are pregnant). It's important to know that home pregnancy tests, particularly when done in the early days of pregnancy, sometimes indicate you are not pregnant when in fact you are. This mistake can occur because levels of hCG are low in early pregnancy and may go undetected. For this reason, test results that indicate you are not pregnant are more often wrong than test results that indicate you are pregnant.

Home pregnancy tests should be considered screening tests. If your test result is negative but you have the symptoms of pregnancy, consult your health care provider. If your result is positive, make plans to see your doctor for confirmation and to begin prenatal care.

Important Dates During Pregnancy

Use this chart to determine milestones during pregnancy. For example: If the first day of your last menstrual period was March 27, your estimated due date is January 1.

If the first day of your last menstrual period is not listed, use the closest listed date and adjust the other dates accordingly. For example, if the first day of your last menstrual period was April 4 (one day past the listed date of April 3), your estimated due date is January 9 (one day past the listed date of January 8).

If the first day of your last menstrual period was:	Conception likely occurred around:	Period of greatest risk for birth defects (3-8 weeks) after conception		End of first trimester (12 weeks)–risk of miscarriage decreases	23 weeks—some preemies can now survive	End of second trimester (27 weeks)	Estimated due date (40 weeks–full term)
		Beginning of organ formation	Major organs have formed				
Jan 2	Jan 16	Feb 6	Mar 13	Mar 27	Jun 12	Jul 10	**Oct 9**
Jan 9	Jan 23	Feb 13	Mar 20	Apr 3	Jun 19	Jul 17	**Oct 16**
Jan 16	Jan 30	Feb 20	Mar 27	Apr 10	Jun 26	Jul 24	**Oct 23**
Jan 23	Feb 6	Feb 27	Apr 3	Apr 17	Jul 3	Jul 31	**Oct 30**
Jan 30	Feb 13	Mar 6	Apr 10	Apr 24	Jul 10	Aug 7	**Nov 6**
Feb 6	Feb 20	Mar 13	Apr 17	May 1	Jul 17	Aug 14	**Nov 13**
Feb 13	Feb 27	Mar 20	Apr 24	May 8	Jul 24	Aug 21	**Nov 20**
Feb 20	Mar 6	Mar 27	May 1	May 15	Jul 31	Aug 28	**Nov 27**
Feb 27	Mar 13	Apr 3	May 8	May 22	Aug 7	Sep 4	**Dec 4**
Mar 6	Mar 20	Apr 10	May 15	May 29	Aug 14	Sep 11	**Dec 11**
Mar 13	Mar 27	Apr 17	May 22	Jun 5	Aug 21	Sep 18	**Dec 18**
Mar 20	Apr 3	Apr 24	May 29	Jun 12	Aug 28	Sep 25	**Dec 25**
Mar 27	Apr 10	May 1	Jun 5	Jun 19	Sep 4	Oct 2	**Jan 1**
Apr 3	Apr 17	May 8	Jun 12	Jun 26	Sep 11	Oct 9	**Jan 8**
Apr 10	Apr 24	May 15	Jun 19	Jul 3	Sep 18	Oct 16	**Jan 15**
Apr 17	May 1	May 22	Jun 26	Jul 10	Sep 25	Oct 23	**Jan 22**
Apr 24	May 8	May 29	Jul 3	Jul 17	Oct 2	Oct 30	**Jan 29**
May 1	May 15	Jun 5	Jul 10	Jul 24	Oct 9	Nov 6	**Feb 5**
May 8	May 22	Jun 12	Jul 17	Jul 31	Oct 16	Nov 13	**Feb 12**
May 15	May 29	Jun 19	Jul 24	Aug 7	Oct 23	Nov 20	**Feb 19**
May 22	Jun 5	Jun 26	Jul 31	Aug 14	Oct 30	Nov 27	**Feb 26**
May 29	Jun 12	Jul 3	Aug 7	Aug 21	Nov 6	Dec 4	**Mar 5**
Jun 5	Jun 19	Jul 10	Aug 14	Aug 28	Nov 13	Dec 11	**Mar 12**
Jun 12	Jun 26	Jul 17	Aug 21	Sep 4	Nov 20	Dec 18	**Mar 19**
Jun 19	Jul 3	Jul 24	Aug 28	Sep 11	Nov 27	Dec 25	**Mar 26**
Jun 26	Jul 10	Jul 31	Sep 4	Sep 18	Dec 4	Jan 1	**Apr 2**
Jul 3	Jul 17	Aug 7	Sep 11	Sep 25	Dec 11	Jan 8	**Apr 9**
Jul 10	Jul 24	Aug 14	Sep 18	Oct 2	Dec 18	Jan 15	**Apr 16**
Jul 17	Jul 31	Aug 21	Sep 25	Oct 9	Dec 25	Jan 22	**Apr 23**
Jul 24	Aug 7	Aug 28	Oct 2	Oct 16	Jan 1	Jan 29	**Apr 30**
Jul 31	Aug 14	Sep 4	Oct 9	Oct 23	Jan 8	Feb 5	**May 7**
Aug 7	Aug 21	Sep 11	Oct 16	Oct 30	Jan 15	Feb 12	**May 14**
Aug 14	Aug 28	Sep 18	Oct 23	Nov 6	Jan 22	Feb 19	**May 21**
Aug 21	Sep 4	Sep 25	Oct 30	Nov 13	Jan 29	Feb 26	**May 28**
Aug 28	Sep 11	Oct 2	Nov 6	Nov 20	Feb 5	Mar 5	**Jun 4**
Sep 4	Sep 18	Oct 9	Nov 13	Nov 27	Feb 12	Mar 12	**Jun 11**
Sep 11	Sep 25	Oct 16	Nov 20	Dec 4	Feb 19	Mar 19	**Jun 18**
Sep 18	Oct 2	Oct 23	Nov 27	Dec 11	Feb 26	Mar 26	**Jun 25**
Sep 25	Oct 9	Oct 30	Dec 4	Dec 18	Mar 5	Apr 2	**Jul 2**
Oct 2	Oct 16	Nov 6	Dec 11	Dec 25	Mar 12	Apr 9	**Jul 9**
Oct 9	Oct 23	Nov 13	Dec 18	Jan 1	Mar 19	Apr 16	**Jul 16**
Oct 16	Oct 30	Nov 20	Dec 25	Jan 8	Mar 26	Apr 23	**Jul 23**
Oct 23	Nov 6	Nov 27	Jan 1	Jan 15	Apr 2	Apr 30	**Jul 30**
Oct 30	Nov 13	Dec 4	Jan 8	Jan 22	Apr 9	May 7	**Aug 6**
Nov 6	Nov 20	Dec 11	Jan 15	Jan 29	Apr 16	May 14	**Aug 13**
Nov 13	Nov 27	Dec 18	Jan 22	Feb 5	Apr 23	May 21	**Aug 20**
Nov 20	Dec 4	Dec 25	Jan 29	Feb 12	Apr 30	May 28	**Aug 27**
Nov 27	Dec 11	Jan 1	Feb 5	Feb 19	May 7	Jun 4	**Sep 3**
Dec 4	Dec 18	Jan 8	Feb 12	Feb 26	May 14	Jun 11	**Sep 10**
Dec 11	Dec 25	Jan 15	Feb 19	Mar 5	May 21	Jun 18	**Sep 17**
Dec 18	Jan 1	Jan 22	Feb 26	Mar 12	May 28	Jun 25	**Sep 24**
Dec 25	Jan 8	Jan 29	Mar 5	Mar 19	Jun 4	Jul 2	**Oct 1**

Infertility

Some people mistakenly assume that infertility means sterility. Perhaps "under-fertility" is a better term. For some couples, it will take longer than they expect to become pregnant. For couples who have frequent sexual intercourse without using any contraception, three out of four become pregnant within six months. About 10 percent do not become pregnant within a year.

The key to improved fertility can be through either or both partners. However, infertility evaluations often begin with the man because it's simpler to perform the tests necessary to evaluate male infertility.

Tests for the Man

For a man to be fertile, several factors are essential. His testicles must produce enough sperm. The sperm must be delivered effectively into a woman's vagina. The sperm must then be able to enter the cervix and move up into the fallopian tube to fertilize the egg. Tests for the man identify whether any of these steps are impeded. The evaluation begins with a complete physical examination and questions concerning illnesses or disabilities, medications and sexual habits.

Tests to analyze the sperm in a semen sample will probably be required. The instructions for collecting and transporting a sample to the laboratory must be followed carefully. For example, the sperm must be analyzed within one to two hours after ejaculation and must be protected against cold temperatures before analysis. Semen samples may be required more than once.

The laboratory will determine whether the number of sperm present in the semen is adequate for fertility. The general health of the sperm is analyzed by looking at the shape, appearance and motility (activity) of the sperm.

Further testing for the male partner depends on his general health and on the results of his physical exam and the sperm analysis.

Tests for the Woman

For a woman to be fertile, her ovaries must release healthy eggs regularly, and the reproductive tract must allow unobstructed passage for the eggs and sperm to meet in the fallopian tubes.

Evaluation begins with a general physical examination, including a pelvic exam. The history will include questions about your general health, illnesses, medications, menstrual cycle and sexual habits.

Specific fertility tests will follow. Your doctor first establishes whether healthy eggs are being released. There are different methods for determining if ovulation is occurring. One common method is using an ovulation predictor kit. You can purchase these kits in drugstores, or your doctor may provide one. The test monitors Lh (luteinizing hormone) in a urine sample. The level of Lh increases one day before ovulation.

Blood tests are also helpful in determining whether levels of hormones are adequate for successful ovulation.

Another useful test is the postcoital test. This test is done two to 16 hours after intercourse, which is timed to coincide with ovulation. The doctor takes a tiny sample of the mucus lining the cervix (the lower portion of the uterus where it meets the vagina). The sample is examined under a microscope to determine how well sperm penetrate and survive.

Endometrial biopsy is a test in which the doctor takes a small sample of tissue from the uterine lining (endometrium) shortly before the beginning of your menstrual period. This procedure helps determine whether and when ovulation is occurring and whether the lining of the uterus is hormonally prepared for pregnancy.

Once one or more of these tests have been performed, your doctor will know whether ovulation occurs and whether sperm can survive in your reproductive tract. If no problems are uncovered by the initial tests, additional information may be needed.

Hysterosalpingography is a test used to evaluate the condition of the uterus and the fallopian tubes. Fluid is injected into the uterus, and an X-ray image shows whether the fluid progresses out of the uterus and up the fallopian tubes. This test can detect blockages or problems that might be correctable with medications or surgery.

Another test is laparoscopy, a brief procedure performed with local or general anesthesia. A laparoscope is a thin, illuminated telescope. Through the laparoscope, the doctor can view blockages or irregularities of the fallopian tubes and uterus. Often a dye is injected into the cervix and through the uterus and fallopian tubes to determine whether they are open. This test can be done either in the hospital or on an outpatient basis.

Not everyone needs to undergo all or even many of these tests before the cause of infertility is found. However, a comprehensive infertility evaluation is recommended because up to 40 percent of couples have more than one cause of infertility. Successful treatment depends on identifying and correcting all significant abnormalities.

Treatment of Infertility

A starting point for many couples is recommendations on when and how often to have intercourse to improve the chances of conception. General sexual problems such as impotence or premature ejaculation can also be treated to improve fertility.

When the male has a decreased sperm count or activity, restoring or initiating fertility is sometimes possible. For example, treatment of infections such as sexually transmitted disease will sometimes restore fertility. In the woman, treatment also depends on the results of physical examination and tests.

If the fertility problem is related to anovulation (failure to release an egg), your doctor can attempt to bring about ovulation with medications.

Blockages or other problems in the fallopian tubes sometimes can be repaired surgically. However, most tubal problems are more successfully treated with in vitro fertilization (see page 10) than surgery.

Endometriosis occurs when bits of the endometrium (lining of the uterus) embed in other pelvic areas, such as the ovaries and fallopian tubes. Sometimes surgical removal of the endometrial tissues is necessary to improve fertility.

Artificial fertilization. For some couples, complex ethical issues are raised when fertilization is not possible through sexual intercourse but only through other methods such as artificial insemination. A significant distinction for many couples is using sperm from someone other than the partner. You and your partner should discuss these issues carefully. The best time to consider your ethical positions on fertility therapy is before pregnancy occurs as a result of such therapy.

Infertility support

Couples who need to come to terms with their infertility may benefit from RESOLVE, Inc., a national organization providing infertile couples with support and information. There are local chapters throughout the country.

Contact: RESOLVE, Inc.
1310 Broadway
Somerville, MA 02144-1731
Telephone: (617) 623-0744

In vitro fertilization. When a couple remains infertile despite treatment, when the cause is determined but can't be treated or even when the cause cannot be determined, pregnancy is still possible. Techniques include fertilizing a woman's egg with sperm from her partner or from a sperm donor. Fertilization can take place inside the woman's body or in a laboratory, in which case the fertilized egg is then transferred to her uterus.

The term "test-tube baby" actually is inaccurate because the baby develops within the mother. Only fertilization, the very earliest development of the fertilized egg (embryo), takes place in the laboratory. The correct term is "in vitro fertilization" (IVF). In vitro fertilization requires a surgical procedure. It's costly and complex. In IVF, eggs are removed from the woman's ovary by withdrawing them with a special needle. Semen is obtained from her partner or from a donor. Attempts are then made to fertilize an egg with the sperm in a laboratory. If fertilization occurs, the embryo is transferred to the uterus of the woman (embryo transfer). This technique achieves pregnancy in 20 to 40 percent of the attempts.

Artificial insemination. The partner's semen can be used for artificial insemination if it contains healthy sperm. The semen is collected, and the doctor places it directly into the woman's uterus at the time of ovulation. The probability of fertilization occurring is increased by placing sperm directly into the uterus, where fertilization is most likely to occur.

If the partner does not produce sperm or does not produce enough for successful fertilization, donor sperm can be used. Sometimes sperm from both the partner and the donor are mixed before being transferred to the uterus. Artificial insemination has a higher success rate with donor sperm than with the partner's sperm.

With a slightly different technique, called gamete interfallopian transfer (GIFT), a mixture containing sperm taken from the partner or donor and eggs from the woman is placed directly in the fallopian tube. This procedure is done with laparoscopy. The intent is to encourage fertilization to occur naturally. As with in vitro fertilization, the success of this procedure is by no means assured.

Overview of Pregnancy

The next two chapters provide an overview of pregnancy. Chapter 2 discusses the changes occurring in the mother; Chapter 3 describes how your baby develops before birth. Beginning with the earliest developments after conception, the chapter continues chronologically through the entire pregnancy. Some of the topics discussed in Chapters 2 and 3 are covered again in Chapters 10, 11 and 12, which provide details on the three trimesters of pregnancy.

CHAPTER TWO

Your Body During Pregnancy

At this very moment, a miracle is taking place inside your body. A sperm and an egg have joined to form a single cell—the starting point for an extraordinary chain of events. That microscopic cell will divide and redivide, again and again, until, in about nine months, it will have changed into about 2 trillion cells of different varieties, all intricately packaged as a new person—your one-of-a-kind baby.

While that tiny cell is becoming a full-sized infant, your body is being prepared to provide the nourishment and hormones that govern your baby's growth and development and to deliver him or her. A preset genetic timetable determines what happens and when as your body undergoes enormous changes during the course of your pregnancy.

Most pregnancies proceed smoothly, relatively free of complications, and most babies in the United States are born healthy. But you can take measures—as simple as eating a healthful diet, avoiding cigarette smoke and getting plenty of rest and exercise—to increase your chance of a successful pregnancy, birth and a healthy baby.

Receiving health care early and throughout your pregnancy is a crucial factor in a happy and successful outcome. When you have questions during your pregnancy, be sure to raise them with your caregiver.

About 4 million women will give birth this year in the United States, so you're not alone. But for each of these women, yourself included, it will be a unique experience. If this is your first baby, nothing that you have read or heard will quite prepare you for the experience of pregnancy. It will be exciting and boring, anxiety-producing and deeply satisfying. You will probably experience new, unexpected sensations, some comforting, others unsettling. This chapter provides an overview of changes and feelings you can anticipate during the coming months. Chapters 10, 11 and 12 provide more details and recommendations for coping with some of the common discomforts of pregnancy.

From Egg to Baby

In the first three months of pregnancy (the first trimester), your baby's major organs will begin forming. Your body will begin showing the first signs of pregnancy. Some changes, like breast changes, appear in the first month. By the end of the third month, a swelling abdomen may tell the world that you are, indeed, pregnant—though not all women show it this early. You will also likely feel most of the major discomforts of pregnancy, such as nausea, heartburn, frequent urination and fatigue, during the earliest months.

During the next three months (second trimester), your baby will grow from about 4 inches to almost a foot in length. Your uterus will expand and begin to push against the organs in your abdomen. Your baby will probably make itself known with beginning movements called "quickening" and, by the sixth month, possibly a few kicks. These months probably will be the easiest of your pregnancy.

During the final three months (third trimester), your baby will grow rapidly, gaining about one-half pound a week and reaching about 20 inches in length. You may feel some kicks and even be able to get a sense of how the baby is positioned. Your baby's growth may cause discomfort, such as increased frequency of urination and shortness of breath, as your uterus expands beneath your diaphragm (the muscle layer just below your lungs). As your body further prepares for birth, you may feel early contractions, your baby will move lower in your uterus, and your cervix, the opening at the neck of your uterus, will soften.

How Your Body Changes

About two weeks after the developing egg embeds itself in the lining of your uterus, your body begins to change, even before tests and a doctor's examination confirm the fact that you are pregnant. At this time, often before a missed menstrual period arouses your suspicions, your body starts preparing itself for your baby's arrival.

Some of the first changes, induced by hormones from the fetus and your own body, are described below.

Menstrual Flow

Contrary to popular belief, you may not entirely miss your first menstrual period. Spotting, or a scanty menstrual flow, and possibly a yellowish vaginal discharge may be a first sign of pregnancy. This spotting does not resemble a normal menstrual period; it comes from a small amount of bleeding that can occur when the developing egg implants into the lining of your uterus.

Breasts

Often the first hint of pregnancy is a change in the way your breasts feel. They may be more sensitive and tender. They may feel fuller and heavier. As early as two weeks after conception your breasts and nipples may start to enlarge. The areolas (rings of brown or reddish skin around the nipples) will begin to enlarge and darken.

Pregnancy may also announce itself by changes in the way your body functions and feels. You may experience fatigue, nausea ("morning sickness"), increased urination and bloating (abdominal fullness). These are all common and normal developments, signs that your body has begun the changes of early pregnancy.

Other Physical Changes

Within two weeks after conception, your uterus will begin to change. Its lining will thicken. Blood vessels in the lining will enlarge to nourish the growing fetus. If you've never been pregnant, your uterus is approximately the size of a small pear. During pregnancy, its capacity will expand about 1,000 times to accommodate your baby's growth before delivery.

Uterus

Your cervix, the opening of your uterus through which your baby will emerge, begins to soften. Your doctor will look for this change during your first examination to confirm your pregnancy.

Cervix

Major Hormone Changes During Pregnancy

Hormones are chemical messengers that regulate many aspects of your pregnancy. They prepare your uterus to accept the fertilized egg and tell it when to begin the process of birth. They ready your breasts for nursing, stimulate milk production and govern the growth of the fetus. Several important hormones work together before and throughout pregnancy.

Immediately after a menstrual period, follicle-stimulating hormone (FSH) fosters the development of an egg in your ovary. Every month several "follicles," each containing a single immature egg, develop in one of your ovaries (see the color photograph on page A1) and move into the fallopian tube, where, if an egg is fertilized by a sperm, pregnancy begins. Occasionally, more than one follicle matures, which can result in multiple births if fertilization has occurred. A hormone called luteinizing hormone (Lh) causes the follicle to swell, rupture and release the egg. The hormones involved in this process, called ovulation, also cause a slight increase in your body temperature and a change in secretions from your cervical glands.

When fertilization occurs, the corpus luteum that surrounds the developing egg starts to grow and produce minute amounts of the hormone progesterone. This helps support your pregnancy. Later, the placenta produces huge amounts of progesterone, 10 times as much as a nonpregnant woman produces. Progesterone keeps your uterus from contracting and promotes growth of blood vessels in the walls of your uterus, essential for your baby's nourishment.

As the fertilized egg travels and burrows into the lining of your uterus, it develops finger-like projections that will eventually become the placenta and begins to produce enormous amounts of the hormone estrogen. Some estrogen is produced by your ovaries, but a much larger amount comes from your placenta.

In fact, as researchers learn more about the placenta's role in hormone production, a new perspective on pregnancy itself is emerging. Instead of thinking of the mother's body as a protective haven, providing sustenance to the growing baby, doctors now view the events of pregnancy as being guided by hormones released by the fetus and the placenta. The mother's body changes in response to chemical messages from her developing baby.

Estrogen might be called the key hormone of pregnancy. Besides helping to promote fertilization, it causes growth and changes in your uterus and its lining (endometrium), your cervix, vagina and breasts. Estrogen also influences the control of some key body processes, such as the amount of insulin you produce.

Besides progesterone and estrogen, the placenta produces two other important hormones: human chorionic gonadotropin (hCG) and human placental lactogen (hPL). hCG is one of the very first hormones made by the placenta and is, so to speak, the announcer of pregnancy. Pregnancy tests can detect hCG in a urine sample. hCG is also thought to prevent the mother's body from rejecting the fetus as foreign tissue.

hPL is the hormone most involved in your baby's growth; it alters your metabolism to make sugars and proteins more available to your fetus. hPL also stimulates your breasts to develop and prepare to produce milk.

Different hormones will be produced at varying rates throughout your pregnancy to meet the demands of your growing fetus. These varying hormone levels help explain why your body and your moods change during the course of your pregnancy.

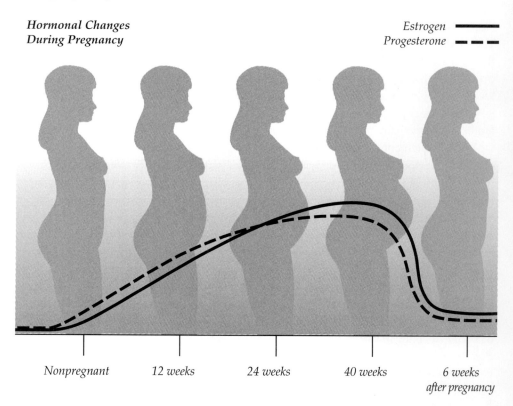

Hormonal Changes During Pregnancy

Estrogen ▬▬▬
Progesterone ▬ ▬ ▬

Nonpregnant   12 weeks   24 weeks   40 weeks   6 weeks
after pregnancy

Two of the major female hormones, estrogen and progesterone, increase during pregnancy to amounts 10 times more than in a nonpregnant woman. After approximately the first 12 weeks, the placenta and fetus produce more of the hormones than the mother's body.

Changes You May Notice During Pregnancy

Your body will undergo many changes during the next 40 weeks. Some will be readily apparent; others will be more subtle, or not apparent at all. Here is an overview of what you can expect.

Breasts

Stimulated by estrogen and progesterone, your breasts will enlarge as the milk-producing glands inside them increase in size. Breast enlargement will account for about a pound of the weight you will gain during your pregnancy. Some, but not much, of the increased breast size is due to fat. Responding to greater blood circulation, your areolas, the brown or reddish circles around your nipples, grow larger and darker—and may stay that way after pregnancy. The tiny bumps that circle the areolas, skin glands called Montgomery's tubercles, start enlarging. These glands contain oils that moisturize and soften the skin of your nipples and areolas.

Some women have inverted nipples that dimple back into their breasts. If you have inverted nipples, don't worry. They don't hinder nursing. But talk to your doctor about special techniques to prepare your inverted nipples for breastfeeding.

Blood vessels in the skin over your breasts will become engorged and more visible, showing through your skin as blue or pink lines. When delivery time approaches, your nipples may start to leak colostrum, the yellow-colored earliest milk. (For more on breastfeeding and techniques for successful nursing, see page 474.)

Abdomen

As your uterus expands to accommodate your growing baby, so does your abdomen—week by week. Up to the 12th week, your uterus will fit neatly inside your pelvis. By the 20th week, your uterus will reach your navel. Ultimately it will extend from your pubic area to the bottom of your rib cage.

Your expanding uterus presses on other organs—bladder, kidneys, stomach, intestines, diaphragm and blood vessels in your abdomen—affecting every organ's function. Toward the end of pregnancy, your protruding abdomen may sag lower; you may feel your baby settling down in your pelvis in preparation for birth.

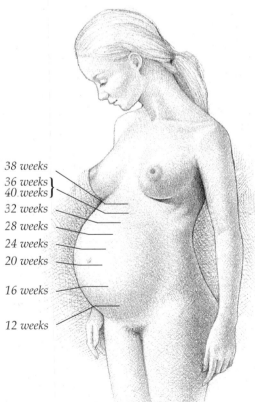

38 weeks
36 weeks
40 weeks
32 weeks
28 weeks
24 weeks
20 weeks
16 weeks
12 weeks

To accommodate your growing baby, your uterus expands from an area within your pelvis to just below your rib cage. During some office visits, your doctor will measure the distance from the top of your uterus to your pubic bone as a way of estimating the age and growth of the fetus. By the middle of pregnancy, for women of normal weight, the measurement, in centimeters, often equals the number of weeks of pregnancy.

Skin

You've probably heard about the "glow of pregnancy." Blood circulation increases during pregnancy, including the tiny vessels just beneath the surface of your skin. The result may be a healthy glow. You may notice some of the following less desirable skin changes too.

Stretch marks. Some women are prone to develop stretch marks—pink, reddish or purplish indented streaks on the abdomen, breasts, upper arms, buttocks and thighs. They appear in up to 50 percent of pregnant women, especially during the last half of pregnancy.

Stretch marks are not a sign of excessive weight gain. They seem to be caused, literally, by a stretching of the skin coupled with a normal increase in cortisone, a hormone produced by the adrenal glands. The increase may weaken elastic fibers of the skin. Fortunately, stretch marks often fade to light pink to grayish stripes, but they don't disappear.

Acne. If you commonly experience skin breakouts during your menstrual period, you may develop acne early in your pregnancy, or your acne may improve during pregnancy. The normal increase in progesterone, which stimulates oil secretion from skin glands, may explain why some women are prone to acne during pregnancy.

Skin pigmentation. It's common to notice changes in the color or pigmentation of the skin on your cheeks, chin, nose and forehead. These areas may grow darker as a result of increased amounts of estrogen and progesterone.

You are likely to notice that areas of skin that are already pigmented get even darker, most noticeably the areolas surrounding your nipples and the labia, the double folds of tissue on both sides of your vagina. Although some of this increased pigmentation fades after you have given birth, these areas are likely to remain darker than before you were pregnant.

You may experience other changes in skin pigmentation, as listed below.

Melasma. Sometimes referred to as chloasma, this brownish darkening of the facial skin has been called the "mask of pregnancy." It affects approximately 50 percent of women, mostly those who are dark-haired and fair-skinned. Melasma usually appears on the forehead, temples and the central part of the face. It may not be as intense as other increases in pigmentation and generally fades completely after delivery. Melasma may be caused or aggravated by exposure to sunlight.

Linea nigra. The barely noticeable white line (linea alba) running from your navel to your pubic hair often darkens and is termed the linea nigra.

Moles and freckles. Existing moles, freckles and skin blemishes may become darker. However, if a particular mole changes appreciably in size or appearance, see your doctor.

Vascular "spiders." Minute reddish spots with tiny blood vessels protruding outward (like spider legs) occur in about two-thirds of pregnant white women and about 10 percent of black women. Caused by increased blood circulation, vascular spiders may appear on your face, neck, upper chest or arms. They usually disappear within a few weeks after birth.

Puffiness of the face. During the last three months of pregnancy, about half of all pregnant women notice their eyelids and face becoming puffy, mostly in the morning. Normal puffiness is due simply to increased blood circulation. But if puffy eyelids occur along with a sudden weight increase (5 pounds or more within a week), see your doctor. Sudden weight gain and puffiness could indicate excessive fluid retention, which is often coupled with high blood pressure (preeclampsia; see page 192).

Red and itchy palms and soles. Your palms and the soles of your feet are likely to become red. Two-thirds of all pregnant women experience this skin change. It's probably caused by the normal increase in estrogen. Like most skin changes, the redness fades after delivery.

Generalized itching. Roughly one-fifth of pregnant women experience an itchiness on their abdomens, or all over their bodies. Such generalized itchiness typically vanishes spontaneously. Moisturizing your skin usually helps. Also, if you have itchiness, avoid getting overheated. Anything that itches will usually itch more if you're warm. If these measures don't provide relief, your doctor may prescribe a medication or ultraviolet light therapy.

Several itch-producing skin problems appear only during pregnancy, usually in the later months. Fortunately, they are uncommon. Pruritic urticarial papules and plaques (PUPP) of pregnancy occur in about one out of 150 pregnancies, most commonly in women pregnant for the first time or carrying twins. With PUPP, you break out with itchy bumps called papules or plaques on your abdomen or possibly on your thighs, buttocks or arms. PUPP can be relieved with prescription medications.

Another common problem that causes itching, one that occurs in the third trimester in up to one in 50 pregnancies, is called cholestasis of pregnancy. It may indicate altered liver function related to pregnancy and can cause severe itching and sometimes nausea, vomiting, loss of appetite, fatigue and possibly jaundice (a yellowing of the skin). If severe itching develops late in your pregnancy, your doctor may order blood tests to check your liver function. Prescription medications may help relieve the symptoms, but usually this problem will disappear after you give birth.

Bluish and blotchy legs. Especially in cold weather, a temporary skin discoloration caused by increased estrogen production develops in some women. Don't worry about it. This will disappear after your baby is born.

Varicose veins. In one in five pregnant women, protruding, bluish veins develop, particularly in their legs. Veins throughout your body become larger during pregnancy to accommodate increased blood flow to your baby. This change is especially noticeable in veins near the skin surface, as in your legs. Varicose veins are usually not serious, but they can be uncomfortable and may cause sore, aching legs. (See page 178 for tips on easing the discomfort.)

Perspiration and heat rashes. Pregnant women often perspire more as a result of the action of hormones on sweat glands distributed over the entire body. This makes heat rashes more common. Oddly, perspiration from glands under the arms, breasts and genital area is less frequent during pregnancy. You may notice more heat rash but less body odor while you are pregnant.

Other Skin-Deep Changes

Hair　Late in pregnancy, you may find yourself developing a more luxuriant head of hair than you ever had before. After pregnancy, you may temporarily lose more hair.

Normally, each of the 100,000 hairs on your head grows about half an inch a month for periods of six to eight years. Then they go into a resting phase, stop growing, and gradually fall out at a rate of about 100 hairs a day, mostly during brushing or washing, until the growth cycle starts again. During pregnancy, hair growth tends to remain in the resting phase longer. Because fewer hairs fall out each day, you may have a fuller head of hair.

After delivery, the picture changes. The resting phase shortens. More hairs fall out, and your hair follicles start to grow new hairs. Around six to 12 weeks after birth, you may notice a dramatic increase in hair shedding. For a few months your hair may feel thinner. But within six to 15 months you should enjoy the same head of hair you had before.

In some women, especially those who already have a fair amount of body hair, more hair may develop during pregnancy. Hormones produced by the placenta and increased cortisone levels stimulate blood circulation to your hair follicles. Hair growth may be especially noticeable on your face and extremities. This excess hair growth should subside in about six months, though it may recur in subsequent pregnancies.

Nails　Your fingernails and toenails, like hair, may start growing faster than normal. They may become brittle or soft and grooved, partly under the influence of pregnancy hormones and occasionally because of anemia.

Eyes　Your body retains extra fluid throughout pregnancy. This causes the cornea (the outer layer of your eye) to get about 3 percent thicker, a change that may become apparent by the 10th week of pregnancy and persist until about six weeks after delivery. Intraocular pressure (pressure of fluid within your eyeball) decreases about 10 percent during pregnancy. These two events, in combination, may cause slightly blurred vision.

If you wear contact lenses, particularly hard lenses, you may find them uncomfortable because of these changes. Still, there's no need to change your contact lenses during pregnancy. Your vision will return to its normal state after you give birth.

Mouth　Pregnancy does not cause cavities, as is commonly believed. However, increased blood circulation may make your gums softer. About 80 percent of pregnant women experience this softening, which may cause minor bleeding when brushing the teeth. If the problem persists, see your doctor or dentist.

New thoughts about weight gain

Other than the health of her baby, probably nothing concerns a pregnant woman more than her weight. Her biggest worry: gaining too much. This worry is understandable. For generations, women were taught that gaining too much weight could be hazardous. The fear was that excessive weight gain might cause the baby to grow too large and thus make birthing more difficult, painful and even dangerous for both mother and baby. This is not the case.

A major report issued by the National Academy of Sciences in 1990 concluded that pregnant women should gain a fair amount of weight to avoid having babies of low birth weight. Such babies may have more difficulties at birth, stay in the hospital much longer than bigger babies and not grow as quickly as infants of normal birth weight.

As recently as the 1950s, normal-weight women were cautioned to gain no more than 15 to 20 pounds. At that time, doctors generally believed that excessive weight gain could lead to the development of high blood pressure during pregnancy. Doctors now know that gaining weight does not cause high blood pressure in most pregnant women. However, some women do develop high blood pressure and gain striking amounts of weight in a short span of time. These changes occur not because they are adding fat but because their bodies are retaining fluid.

Keep in mind that most of the weight you will gain during pregnancy is not fat. It is mostly the weight of your baby, the placenta, amniotic fluid and the fluid that accumulates in your own body tissues.

How much weight gain is best for a healthy pregnancy and a healthy baby? **Doctors now advise a normal-weight woman to gain 25 to 35 pounds during pregnancy.** Most women gain about 10 pounds by their 20th week. However, the greatest weight gain occurs in the second half of pregnancy, and after the 33rd or 34th week, you are likely to put on a pound a week. If you are underweight to start with, an even greater weight gain may be recommended; if you're considerably overweight, you should gain less.

It is true that excess weight may be difficult to lose after you have had your baby and that being overweight is linked with medical problems later in life. But if you eat sensibly, exercise and keep yourself fit during pregnancy, you're not likely to need to trim pounds off afterward. In any case, you should never diet to lose weight during pregnancy. It could be harmful to you and your growing baby. (For more on weight, nutrition and pregnancy, see page 86.)

The Changes Taking Place Inside Your Body

Hormones released throughout your pregnancy by the placenta, the ovaries, adrenals and pituitary do two things simultaneously and automatically. First, they influence the growth of your baby. Second, they send signals that alter the way your organs function. In addition, the growing baby puts pressure on your abdominal organs. This sets off a series of changes that also influence the way your body functions. Here is what happens:

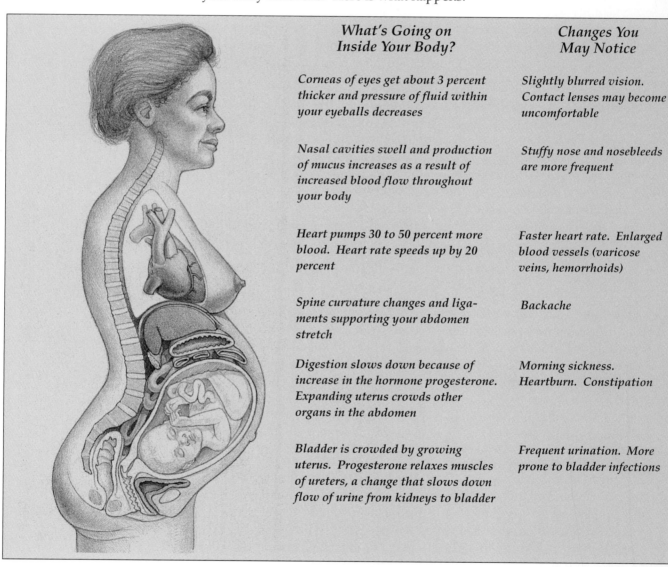

What's Going on Inside Your Body?	Changes You May Notice
Corneas of eyes get about 3 percent thicker and pressure of fluid within your eyeballs decreases	Slightly blurred vision. Contact lenses may become uncomfortable
Nasal cavities swell and production of mucus increases as a result of increased blood flow throughout your body	Stuffy nose and nosebleeds are more frequent
Heart pumps 30 to 50 percent more blood. Heart rate speeds up by 20 percent	Faster heart rate. Enlarged blood vessels (varicose veins, hemorrhoids)
Spine curvature changes and ligaments supporting your abdomen stretch	Backache
Digestion slows down because of increase in the hormone progesterone. Expanding uterus crowds other organs in the abdomen	Morning sickness. Heartburn. Constipation
Bladder is crowded by growing uterus. Progesterone relaxes muscles of ureters, a change that slows down flow of urine from kidneys to bladder	Frequent urination. More prone to bladder infections

Your Heart and Blood Circulation

Your blood is an indirect source of nourishment for your growing baby. It must constantly pass oxygen and nutrients through the placenta to the developing fetus. To meet these demands, your heart pumps more blood, faster, throughout pregnancy than it does normally.

The amount of blood your heart pumps increases by 30 to 50 percent. The increase is greatest during the first trimester, when pregnancy makes enormous demands on your circulation. Your heart beats progressively faster throughout pregnancy; by the third trimester your heart rate may be 20 percent faster than before you were pregnant.

To supply your oxygen needs and the needs of your growing fetus, your body will produce more blood. This additional blood also provides a reserve if you bleed excessively during or following birth.

Because of increases in blood volume and a speedier heart rate, heart murmurs develop in many women. Generally, doctors regard them as normal because blood is flowing faster. But occasionally the murmur may sound distinctly different enough to prompt the doctor to look into the cause. Heart murmurs can result from changes in the valves of the heart, as in the case of mitral valve prolapse, a problem that affects up to 7 percent of young women. Mitral valve prolapse rarely interferes with pregnancy.

Blood pressure. Your doctor will monitor your blood pressure regularly throughout your pregnancy. The first measurement is used as a baseline (point of comparison) for changes in blood pressure later in your pregnancy. High blood pressure may be a symptom of a condition called preeclampsia, or pregnancy-induced hypertension (PIH). PIH may affect the outcome of pregnancy in about one of every 14 women, usually in the second half of the pregnancy. (For more on preeclampsia, see page 192.)

Two numbers are recorded for a blood pressure measurement. The top number, typically 110 to 130 millimeters of mercury (mm Hg), is the systolic pressure, when the heart contracts. The bottom number, typically 70 to 85 mm Hg, is the diastolic pressure, when the heart relaxes between beats. Your systolic blood pressure will probably decrease during the first 24 weeks of pregnancy by 5 to 10 mm Hg and your diastolic pressure by 10 to 15 mm Hg. Then they will return to pre-pregnancy levels. It is normal for your blood pressure to swing back and forth during the day, up when you are excited or exercising and down when you are resting.

Only when your blood pressure stays high (more than 140/90 mm Hg) will it require medical attention. If you have symptoms that may warn of high blood pressure—severe and constant headaches, swelling or edema of your face, dizziness, blurred vision or sudden weight gain—see your doctor. If your doctor detects high blood pressure, he or she will probably take several readings to determine if it is persistently abnormal.

About one in 10 pregnant women has low blood pressure when lying down. The weight of the baby presses against the major vein (the inferior vena cava) that returns blood from the lower body to the heart. This pressure decreases the amount of blood returning to the heart and might cause light-headedness, dizziness, nausea or even fainting spells.

Dizziness or faintness may also occur during hot weather or when you're taking a hot bath or shower. This occurs because the tiny blood vessels in your skin dilate and temporarily reduce the amount of blood returning to your heart. If these symptoms develop during your pregnancy, mention it to your doctor.

Enlarged veins. Blood vessels often become larger to accommodate the increased blood flow during pregnancy. You may notice, for example, that the jugular vein on the side of your neck becomes more apparent.

Varicose veins may also develop on your legs and sometimes around your vaginal area. In some women hemorrhoids also develop, which are varicose veins in the rectum. These are caused by increased blood volume and the pressure from the uterus on the veins that return blood from the legs and pelvis. Generally, varicose veins and hemorrhoids recede or disappear after birth. If they are painful and troublesome during pregnancy, your doctor can suggest measures to relieve them.

Your Digestive System

Nausea, vomiting, heartburn and constipation are often the most common and exasperating discomforts you, and most other pregnant women, are likely to experience. There are usually ways to minimize them, and some discomforts, especially nausea, will probably taper off after the first trimester.

"Morning sickness" is the blanket term for the queasiness, nausea or vomiting that more than two-thirds of pregnant women experience during the first 14 to 16 weeks. It tends to be worse in the morning, but some women feel nauseated throughout the day, especially when the stomach is empty. The reason you feel nauseated is that progesterone slows the speed with which food passes through your digestive tract (intestinal motility). Fortunately, morning sickness seldom leads to significant weight loss or dehydration. It may, in fact, be a reassuring sign, because morning sickness is associated with fewer miscarriages. (For tips on coping with morning sickness, see page 131.)

About half of all pregnant women experience heartburn during pregnancy. For some women, it becomes a persistent problem. Heartburn results when digestive acid backs up into your esophagus, the tube that leads from your throat to your stomach. The backup is caused by a sluggishly functioning sphincter, the muscular ring that joins the esophagus to the stomach. Heartburn is more common during pregnancy because increased amounts of progesterone and estrogen tend to relax smooth muscle everywhere in your body, including your digestive tract. (For more information on heartburn and how to avoid it, see page 157.)

Pregnant women are less likely to have ulcers than nonpregnant women. Gastric acid secretion, which aids in food digestion and causes ulcers in some people, is lower than normal during most of pregnancy. The slower emptying of the stomach and increased mucus secretion also seem to help lessen the development and symptoms of ulcers.

At least half of all women become constipated sometime during their pregnancies. It is usually more troublesome in women who were prone to constipation before pregnancy. Constipation can be caused or encouraged by a slowing of intestinal motility and pressure from the ever-expanding uterus, which crowds your intestinal tract in later pregnancy. Your colon also absorbs more water during pregnancy. This tends to make stools harder and bowel movements more difficult. (For suggestions on dealing with constipation, see page 158.)

Your Respiratory System

Your blood needs to carry large quantities of oxygen to the placenta to sustain your growing fetus. Your blood also needs to remove more carbon dioxide, the waste product of respiration, than it does normally. To accomplish these crucial tasks, your respiratory system must make some adaptations.

Stimulated by progesterone, your lung capacity will increase. Your lungs will inhale and exhale 30 to 40 percent more air with each breath than before. You probably won't be aware of this change, but you may notice that you are breathing slightly faster. To accommodate this increased lung capacity, your rib cage will enlarge appreciably, by 2 or 3 inches in circumference.

Two-thirds of all pregnant women have shortness of breath, usually late in the first or early in the second trimester. There are two reasons for this. One, the carbon dioxide level in your blood decreases, making it easier to transfer more carbon dioxide from the baby to the mother. Two, you are breathing faster. Late in your pregnancy, when your baby begins to move down into your pelvis in preparation for birth, breathing probably will be easier.

Nasal stuffiness and frequent colds are common problems in pregnancy. Some women have nosebleeds, when they rarely did before. Often these symptoms are caused by swelling of the lining of your nose and airways, as well as an increase in nasal production of mucus. Like many of the other changes in your body, these problems are the result of increased blood flow throughout your body, including your nasal passages.

Your Urinary Tract

Particularly during the first trimester, you will probably feel like urinating more frequently. This urge, which you may feel even though you have just emptied your bladder, will probably ease during the next four or five months as your baby rests higher in your abdomen. But the need to urinate more frequently may return in the last month, when your baby moves deeper into your pelvis and presses on your bladder. In late pregnancy, you may find yourself waking up several times a night to urinate.

Your changing body may make you more prone to bladder and kidney infections for several reasons. For one thing, progesterone will relax the muscles of your ureters (the tubes that carry urine from your kidneys to your bladder), slowing the flow of urine. The increasing size of your uterus further slows the flow of urine through your kidneys and bladder. This slowing, plus a tendency to excrete more glucose in your urine, may lead to an increase in kidney and bladder infections.

Recognizing and treating urinary tract infections are especially important during pregnancy. These infections are a common cause of premature labor. Urinary frequency, burning on urination or fever are often the first symptoms, but abdominal pain and backache may also signal a urinary tract infection.

Kidney stones, which arise from an accumulation of minerals in the urine, are also more common during pregnancy. To avoid urinary problems and ensure the health of your baby, report any urinary symptoms to your doctor. (For more on urinary tract problems, see page 244.)

Skeletal Changes

About 50 percent of pregnant women experience backaches as their bones and muscles adapt to the stresses of carrying babies. For some women, backaches are merely an annoyance. But a third of pregnant women with back pain report that it significantly interferes with their daily activities.

Back pain is especially likely if it was a problem for you before your pregnancy. It may start any time during pregnancy, but most commonly begins at the fifth to seventh month. It is usually not related to excessive weight gain.

Backache is most likely to occur when you are tired or have been bending, lifting or exercising. Heavy work requiring lifting, twisting or bending forward can make back pain worse, as can prolonged sitting. You may feel back pain in the upper or middle portions of your back, but you are more apt to feel it in your lower back.

During pregnancy, the ligaments supporting your abdomen become more elastic. This will make it easier for your pelvis to expand during birth. Unfortunately, lack of the usual support from these ligaments increases the likelihood of strain and injury to your back.

Changes in your posture also may cause back pain. The lower portion of your spine will curve backward to compensate for a shift in your center of gravity as your abdomen protrudes under the weight of your growing baby. Without this change, you would tend to fall forward. But the change does put a strain on your back muscles and ligaments and may lead to back pain. (For more information on back pain, see page 155.)

Metabolic Changes

The process your body uses to convert food into energy undergoes many changes during pregnancy. Among the most important is altered regulation of glucose (a form of sugar), one of your body's main fuel sources.

Your body makes glucose from virtually all plant foods and milk. Normally, your body carefully regulates glucose levels, keeping them from becoming too low or too high.

This process is complicated. At night, or between meals, when you are not replenishing your body's fuel supply, your blood glucose (sugar) level drops. To keep your blood sugar within normal range, your liver converts glycogen, a stored energy supply, into glucose. Shortly after a meal, your glucose level will rise; your body will produce more of the hormone insulin to help it regulate glucose.

In some women, pregnancy leads to an inability to use insulin for proper glucose regulation. This can cause a form of diabetes (gestational diabetes). About 10 percent of all pregnant women have significant variations in glucose regulation. About 3 percent may require insulin for the treatment of gestational diabetes. Your doctor will probably take a blood sample to check your glucose levels and, between the 24th and 28th week, check specifically for the possibility of gestational diabetes. It can have adverse effects, not only on the mother but also on the fetus.

Diabetes mellitus is a common medical condition. If you have diabetes, you'll need to have optimal control of your diabetes before conception and throughout your pregnancy to protect your health and the health of your baby. Discuss your condition with your doctor. Your pregnancy will require special precautions and management. (For more on gestational diabetes, see page 189, and for more on pregnancy and preexisting diabetes mellitus, see page 232.)

Emotional Changes

If this is your first baby, nothing you have read or heard will quite prepare you for the mood swings you will undergo during the next nine months. Your emotions may range from exhilaration to exhaustion, delight to depression.

Some of these reactions may be linked to physical stresses your developing baby places on your body. Some may be from fatigue. Mood changes may also be caused by the release of certain hormones and changes in your metabolism.

The relation of hormones to the way your body functions and feels is extraordinarily complex, not only during pregnancy but also at other times. Altered hormone levels have, for example, been linked to the "blues" that some women experience during their menstrual periods and menopause. Though the mechanisms are unclear, doctors believe that similar hormonal changes are contributors to, or at least indicators of, mood swings during and after pregnancy.

The sudden fluctuations in progesterone, estrogen and other hormones after birth may play a role in the "baby blues" some women experience after giving birth. Conversely, the hormones that stimulate lactation also contribute to the elation women feel both before and after giving birth. The interrelationship of thyroid, adrenal and other hormones to a pregnant woman's emotions is receiving considerable scientific attention.

Adjusting to lifestyle changes and preparing for new responsibilities may leave you feeling up one day and down another. Your moods may change considerably during the course of a single day and are apt to be strongly affected by the nurturing and support you receive from your partner and family. Pregnancy often gives rise to conflicting emotions, not only in the prospective mother but also in the father. (For more on the complex issues that pregnancy raises for couples and families, see Chapters 37, 38, 39 and 40.)

The physical changes you experience throughout pregnancy may influence your moods and emotions. Preoccupation with body image, especially during your first pregnancy, can affect the way you feel. You may not like the way you look; you may feel less attractive in general and to your partner in particular. Perfectly normal changes in energy levels and bladder and bowel habits may give rise to fears that you have an underlying illness or other problems. Fatigue, changing sleep patterns and new bodily sensations may all influence your emotions throughout your pregnancy.

As necessary and remarkable as some of the changes may be, they still can be unsettling. But knowing more about why the changes are occurring and what you can do about them will make you more comfortable. You'll also be more confident that your body is prepared to nurture the development of your baby.

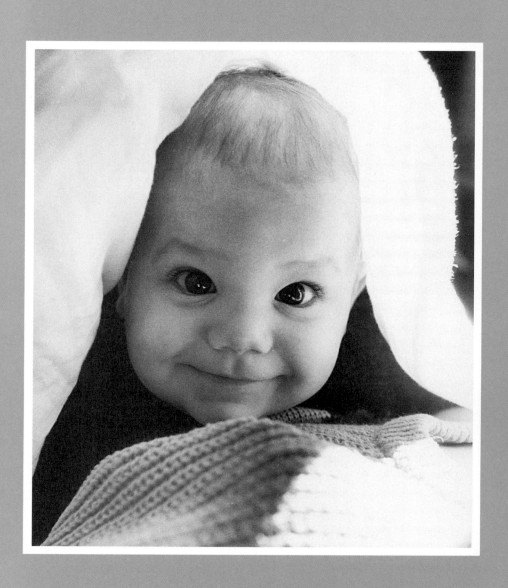

CHAPTER THREE

How Your Baby Develops

The inside story

During your pregnancy, you'll be concerned about your baby's development as well as the changes taking place in your own body. If you're like most expectant mothers, your mind will be full of questions:

- What does my baby look like right now?
- How big is she or he?
- Will I have a boy or a girl, and what determines the baby's sex?

Understanding how your baby develops can help you accept some of the changes taking place in your body. You may also feel a sense of elation at this miracle, the creation of a unique new person.

Boy or Girl?

Whether you will have a boy or girl is determined at the moment your baby is conceived. One pair of the baby's chromosomes, called sex chromosomes, determines its sex. Females have two chromosomes called X chromosomes. In males, the sex chromosomes are different; one is an X and the other is a Y chromosome. It is the presence of this Y chromosome that determines whether the embryo will develop as a male. Eggs contain only X sex chromosomes. Sperm, however, may contain either X or Y sex chromosomes.

Each month, during your menstrual cycle, a single egg leaves your ovary. This is called ovulation. At the instant of fertilization, sperm and egg join and pool their chromosomes, creating an embryo with a full complement of 23 pairs, or a total of 46 chromosomes. If a sperm containing an X chromosome meets the egg, a female embryo (with two X chromosomes) will result. If a sperm containing a Y chromosome joins the X chromosome in the egg, the embryo will be male. In this way, it is always the father's contribution that determines the sex of the fetus.

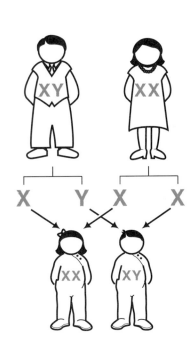

How old is your baby?

Health care providers generally calculate the age of the fetus from the start of the last menstrual period rather than from the actual date of conception, which usually occurs about two weeks later. That's why the "due date" is considered to be about 40 weeks (nine months) after the last period, when in fact only 38 weeks will have passed since conception occurred.

Very early in pregnancy it is most clear to refer to the age of the embryo by the interval since conception (post-conception age). Later in pregnancy it is customary to use dates based on counting from the first day of the last menstrual period (gestational age).

Even if the dating of a pregnancy is adjusted by the results of an ultrasound exam, your physician will almost invariably refer to the dates of your pregnancy using gestational age.

To minimize uncertainty, we've listed both dates in this chapter. Also, for variety, we occasionally used the familiar word "baby" as well as the more technically correct terms "embryo" and "fetus."

Earliest Changes After Conception

Within a day after the egg is fertilized, it begins to develop rapidly. In just three days, a cluster of 13 to 32 cells, called a morula, leaves the fallopian tube to enter the uterus. As the morula grows, a fluid-filled cavity begins to form. Now the developing morula is called a blastocyst. By day eight after fertilization, rapid cell division has increased the size of the blastocyst to several hundred cells.

After arriving in the uterus, the blastocyst embeds itself in the uterine lining, where it continues to grow at an amazing rate. During the first month, as the fertilized egg (zygote) grows and becomes an embryo, it increases in size by 40 times.

Three Weeks Since Conception
Gestational Age Five Weeks

How big is your baby? At conception, the single cell was microscopic in size. Now an embryo, your baby is about ¹⁄₁₇ of an inch long.

How is your baby developing? The embryo has divided into three layers from which tissues and organs will develop.

A groove, called the neural tube, has begun to take shape in the top layer, along the midline of the body. The brain, spinal cord, spinal nerves and backbone will develop from this region.

The middle layer of cells forms the beginnings of the heart and a primitive circulatory system—blood vessels, blood cells and lymph vessels. The foundations for bones, muscles, kidneys and ovaries or testicles also develop from the middle layer of cells. The first heartbeats occur at 21 to 22 days.

By the end of this week, the earliest blood elements and vessels have formed in the embryo and developing placenta. Circulation now begins, and the heart will develop rapidly. The circulatory system thus becomes the first functioning organ system.

The inner layer of cells will give rise to a simple tube, lined with mucous membranes, from which lungs, intestines and urinary bladder will develop. This week, however, not much is happening in the inner layer. Most of the growth is for the nervous and circulatory systems.

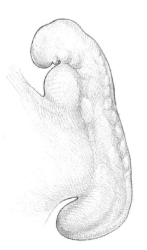

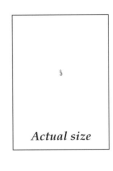

Actual size

Hazards to your baby's health

Infections or exposure to environmental factors such as drugs, cigarettes, alcohol, medications or chemicals in the first week to 10 days after conception can interfere with the embryo implanting in the uterus. This can result in a miscarriage, but generally does not cause birth defects. Don't take drugs or medications without first asking your doctor. This is particularly important during development of the embryo, when body organs are forming.

The developing embryo is most vulnerable during the period from three to eight weeks after conception. All major organs are forming at this time, and injury to the embryo can result in a major birth defect, such as spina bifida. Because the brain continues to develop throughout gestation, it can be harmed by drugs or alcohol at any point in the pregnancy.

For some women, the excitement of learning they are pregnant is soon dampened by anxiety that something might harm the fetus. Events as common as taking an aspirin for a headache, having an alcoholic drink or a minor illness may now become a source of worry. Be sure to share any of these concerns with your doctor.

How big is your baby? The embryo is no longer microscopic in size but is still less than ¼ of an inch in length. Growth is rapid during the fourth week. The embryo triples in size.

How is your baby developing? The embryo is starting to show rudimentary but recognizable physical features. The brain is growing and developing distinct regions. The eyes and ears are beginning to form. An opening for the mouth is formed by the ingrowth of tissue from above and from the sides of the face. Below the mouth, where the neck will develop, are small folds that ultimately will become the neck and lower jaw.

In front of the chest, the heart is already starting to pump blood. Forty small blocks of tissue developing along the embryo's midline will form the backbone, ribs and muscles of the back and sides.

*Four Weeks
Since Conception*
*Gestational Age
Six Weeks*

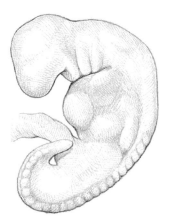

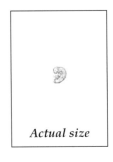

Actual size

Five Weeks Since Conception

*Gestational Age
Seven Weeks*

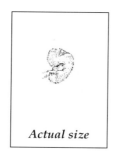

Actual size

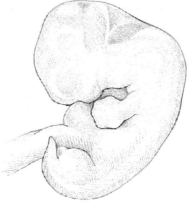

How big is your baby? The embryo is ⅓ of an inch in length.

How is your baby developing? The brain continues to develop in complexity. Cavities and passages necessary for circulation of spinal fluid have formed. The growing skull is still transparent; therefore, if you viewed an embryo under a magnifying glass at this stage, you might see the smooth surface of a tiny, developing brain.

The lenses of the eyes are forming, and the middle portion of the ears continues to develop.

Arms, legs, hands and feet are taking shape, though fingers and toes have yet to form. At this stage, your baby's hands and feet still are little more than stubs growing on the torso.

Six Weeks Since Conception

*Gestational Age
Eight Weeks*

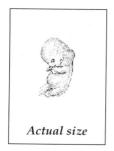

Actual size

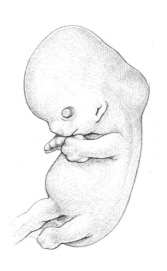

How big is your baby? It is just over ½ of an inch long. An ultrasound examination now can detect the developing embryo.

How is your baby developing? The eyelids are beginning to form; until their growth is complete the eyes look open. The pituitary gland is forming. Arms are growing, and wrists and elbows are evident. Hands and feet are shaped like paddles, and fingers are beginning to form. Ears are beginning to take shape, and the heart is pumping about 150 beats a minute, about twice the adult rate.

Seven Weeks Since Conception

*Gestational Age
Nine Weeks*

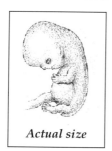

Actual size

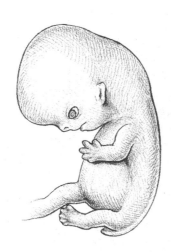

How big is your baby? The embryo is about 1 inch in length.

How is your baby developing? The embryo is becoming distinctly human in shape. The embryonic tail is disappearing, and the face is more rounded. Hands and feet that looked like paddles are forming fingers and toes. The pancreas, bile ducts and gallbladder have formed. The reproductive organs are starting to develop as male or female, but external genitals have no noticeable male or female characteristics.

How big is your baby? Because the embryo is curled into a snug position in the uterus, it is difficult to measure a total length including the legs. It is easier and more common to measure a "crown-rump" length, the distance from the top of the head to the buttocks. At this stage, your baby is about 1¼ inches long from head to rump. It weighs less than ½ ounce.

How is your baby developing? The beginnings of all the major body organs are formed. Bones of the skeleton are forming. Fingers have formed. The eyelids have grown, but the eyes look closed. The outer ears are forming.

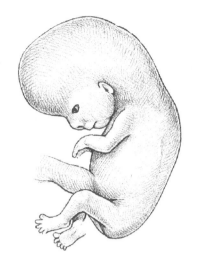

Eight Weeks Since Conception
Gestational Age Ten Weeks

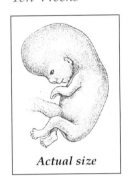

Actual size

How big is your baby? From the start of the ninth week after conception to the time she or he is full term, your unborn baby is called a fetus. By the end of 12 weeks, the fetus will be almost 3 inches long and will weigh about 1½ ounces.

How is your baby developing? All organ systems are in place. Equally significant, the brain, nerves and muscles are starting to function. The palate has completely formed by the end of this period. The genitals are beginning to have male or female characteristics. The baby moves his or her body in jerks, flexes the arms and kicks the legs, but you won't feel these movements until your baby grows a bit more.

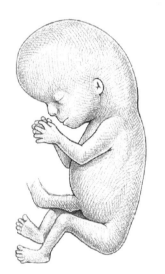

Eighty percent of actual size

Nine to 12 Weeks Since Conception
Gestational Age 11 to 14 Weeks

How big is your baby? She or he is about 5½ inches long, crown to rump, and weighs an impressive 7 ounces.

How is your baby developing? The eyes and ears will have a baby-like appearance. Eyebrows and scalp hair start to appear.

Although you may be unaware of it, your baby will be having frequent episodes of hiccups. Hiccups develop before fetal breathing movements become common. Because the trachea is filled with fluid rather than air, the hiccups don't generate sound.

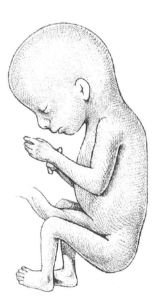

Fifty percent of actual size

13 to 16 Weeks Since Conception
Gestational Age 15 to 18 Weeks

Congratulations! It's a...

How and when can you tell whether you're going to have a boy or a girl? Until two decades ago, you waited for the doctor to hold up the newborn and announce "It's a boy!" or "It's a girl!"—or let you see for yourself. Today, parents-to-be can sometimes learn their unborn child's sex, if examination of the fetus is otherwise needed, by a test called a fetal ultrasound exam.

The images displayed by this technique reveal details such as the size and approximate age of the fetus, the shape and size of various organs, the position of the placenta and, although not foolproof, your baby's probable sex. Parents can have the extraordinary experience of seeing their baby—even the beating heart—on a television-like screen.

Other diagnostic tests, such as amniocentesis or chorionic villus sampling, can predict the sex of the fetus even earlier than the ultrasound exam. Because such tests carry a small risk of fetal injury, doctors don't use them merely to learn the baby's sex. (For more information on ultrasound exams, amniocentesis and chorionic villus sampling, see pages 72, 75 and 77.)

Although it is possible to learn the sex of your baby before birth, many parents ask their doctors and nurses to keep this information confidential. They prefer to find out at birth.

17 to 20 Weeks Since Conception

Gestational Age 19 to 22 Weeks

How big is your baby? The head-to-rump length is about 7½ inches, and the fetus weighs approximately 1 pound.

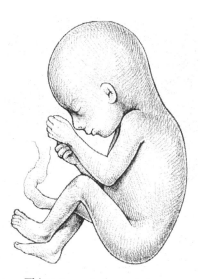

Thirty percent of actual size

How is your baby developing? Her or his skin is covered with a white, cheesy, protective coating called vernix. Fine, down-like hair called lanugo covers the skin. Your baby's kidneys are beginning to make urine. In females, the vagina, uterus and fallopian tubes have formed.

The uterus is a rather noisy environment. The fetus senses the sounds of the mother's heart, rumblings from her stomach and the pulsing of blood vessels. Sounds from a conversation are loud enough to be heard within the uterus. When parents sing and talk to their unborn babies, it is reasonable to expect that the fetus can notice them. Although it appears that the fetus can hear and react to sounds, it is less certain whether the fetus recognizes or remembers sounds.

21 to 25 Weeks Since Conception

Gestational Age 23 to 27 Weeks

How big is your baby? Babies born at this age typically weigh between 1 pound 5 ounces and 2 pounds 3 ounces; length with legs extended is 11 to 15 inches.

How is your baby developing? The body is well proportioned but still slender and with little body fat. The skin is thin and immature. The lungs are beginning to develop surfactant, a substance that covers the inner lining of the air sacs in the lungs, allowing them to expand easily. Blood vessels in the lungs are developing to prepare for breathing. The fetus makes breathing movements, but there is no air in the lungs yet. The fetus now swallows, but usually won't pass stool until after birth.

Because the retina of the eyes still hasn't finished forming, an eye problem called retinopathy of prematurity can occur in babies born at this time.

The blood vessels in the brain are still very immature, especially in rapidly growing regions deep in the middle of the brain, called the germinal matrix. The immaturity of these blood vessels in babies born prematurely increases the risk of spontaneous bleeding, called intracranial hemorrhage (ICH) or intraventricular hemorrhage (IVH).

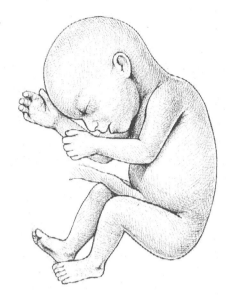

Twenty percent of actual size

Premature birth

Babies born after about 23 weeks gestational age, assisted with neonatal intensive care, can sometimes survive. By 24 weeks, survival rates are more than 50 percent, but complications are common. After 24 weeks, the survival rate steadily improves, complications become less likely and the intensity of care for the baby decreases.

Consequently, if labor starts prematurely (less than 36 weeks), your doctor will usually try to prevent the birth until later in pregnancy whenever possible. Still, a baby born even as early as 23 weeks, with optimal care and if fortunate enough not to develop complications, can grow up to be a healthy, normal child. (For more information on preterm labor, see page 169. For more on premature birth, see page 353.)

How big is your baby? Your baby probably weighs 2 to 3½ pounds. He or she is 12 to 16 inches in length.

How is your baby developing? The eyelids can open. The lungs are more developed. Still, babies born at this age are very immature, usually needing the help of a ventilator to breathe and a stay of six weeks or more in a newborn intensive care unit. The brain is more mature, and the risk of bleeding in the brain is reduced.

In a male fetus, the testicles are moving from their location near the kidneys through the groin on their way into the scrotum. In a female, the clitoris is relatively prominent. The labia are still small and don't yet cover the clitoris.

Babies born prematurely are short-changed on the supply of iron and antibodies they would get from their mother if they were delivered full term. As a result, they are more likely to develop anemia and are at increased risk for infection.

26 to 29 Weeks Since Conception

Gestational Age
28 to 31 Weeks

30 to 34 Weeks Since Conception
Gestational Age 32 to 36 Weeks

How big is your baby? There is incredible growth during this period. Babies generally range in weight from about 3 pounds to 6½ pounds. Length is approximately 16 to 19 inches.

How is your baby developing? Babies born during this period vary greatly in the amount of assistance they might require. This can range from needing help only with staying warm, and assistance with eating, to being as critically ill as a younger premature baby might be. (For information on premature babies, see page 353.)

In most males, the testicles have moved into the scrotum. Sometimes, however, one or even both testicles don't move into position until after birth, generally before the first birthday.

35 to 38 Weeks Since Conception
Gestational Age 37 to 40 Weeks

How big is your baby? Your baby is now considered to be full term. The birth weight of a typical full-term baby ranges from about 6 to 9 pounds. Length is perhaps 18 to 21 inches.

How is your baby developing? Your baby is fully developed and ready for birth. When labor begins, many changes take place to prepare your baby's body for birth. Fluid present in the lungs begins to be absorbed, "drying out" the lungs in preparation for breathing. There is also a surge in fetal hormones that may aid in maintenance of blood pressure and blood sugar levels after birth. When labor begins, fetal breathing movements are inhibited to save energy during birth.

The Fetal Support System

To assist the growth and safety of the embryo and later the fetus, an elaborate support system provides protection and nourishment for the fetus. It also functions as "lungs" for the fetus and helps support the kidneys and liver. The system is made up of the uterus and placenta. Major elements of the system include the following:

- Amniotic fluid—which cushions and protects the fetus and provides room for growth and movement
- The placenta—which provides nutrients and oxygen and removes wastes such as carbon dioxide
- The umbilical cord—which carries nutrients and oxygen from the placenta to the fetus and carries wastes away

Amniotic Fluid

The uterus contains the amniotic sac, sometimes called the bag of waters, which in turn contains the fetus and the amniotic fluid. Amniotic fluid is made from fetal urine, fetal lung fluid and fluid from the placenta. At full term, your baby is surrounded by 1 to 3 pints of amniotic fluid. It is usually sterile but can sometimes allow the growth of bacteria if, for example, the bag of waters has ruptured.

W ithin 12 days after conception, the placenta, a pancake-shaped, spongy mass of tissue, begins to form. Throughout pregnancy, until the final few weeks, the lining of the uterus thickens where the placenta is attached. Its blood vessels enlarge to nourish the developing fetus.

Initially, tiny projections sprout from the wall of the fertilized egg. From these sprouts, wavy masses of capillary-filled tissue, called chorionic villi, develop and then grow amidst the tiny blood capillaries of the mother's uterus. The chorionic villi ultimately cover most of the placenta.

The mother's blood and the baby's blood do not actually mix. Oxygen and carbon dioxide pass between mother and fetus through the placenta by a process called diffusion. The amount of oxygen in the mother's blood is always higher than that in the fetus. The fetus receives the oxygen it needs by the movement of oxygen molecules from the mother's blood into the capillary vessels containing the fetal blood. Correspondingly, fetal blood has a higher concentration of carbon dioxide than the mother's, and this waste product is eliminated by diffusion back into the mother's blood supply. Nutrition, in the form of amino acids, glucose and other carbohydrates, is transported across the placenta in more complex ways.

About two or three weeks before birth, the placenta begins to become less efficient in transferring nutrition. It becomes more fibrous instead of spongy. Blood clots and calcified patches appear, indicating that the placental blood vessels are aging.

The Placenta

T he vital link between placenta and fetus is the umbilical cord, which, at birth, may be up to 4 feet long. The umbilical cord contains two arteries and one large vein. Nutrients and oxygen-rich blood pass from the placenta to the fetus via the single vein and then back to the placenta through the two arteries. It takes about 30 seconds for a blood cell to make the round trip.

The Umbilical Cord

How Is Genetic Information Passed On?

One of the joys of parenthood is recognizing aspects of ourselves through our children. There is excitement in looking closely at your newborn baby to see if you can identify family characteristics, especially facial features. Perhaps the nose resembles yours or the chin your partner's. How is it that these characteristics are passed from one generation to the next?

The information that determines the growth and activities of cells is contained in your genes.

G enes are located in the central part of our cells, the nucleus. In the nucleus, the genes are located in large groups called chromosomes. Chromosomes are visible only under a microscope when cells divide.

The amount of information contained in our genes is immense; our entire collection of genes, called the human genome, consists of 50,000 to 100,000 individual genes. The genes themselves are made of more than three billion

Genes and Chromosomes

individual building blocks, the base pairs. Molecular genetics specialists around the world are hard at work analyzing the complete structure of our genes. This huge undertaking is called the Human Genome Project. A detailed understanding of the information in our genes will be extremely important to improve our understanding of how family characteristics are passed on. It also holds promise for improving the diagnosis and treatment of a wide variety of diseases.

Each of our cells contains 46 chromosomes. The chromosomes are grouped in pairs. There are two sets of 23 individual chromosomes. One member of each pair originally came from your mother, the other from your father.

When a sperm from your father combined with the egg (ovum) from your mother, you became the unique result of that combination. No matter how many brothers or sisters you have, unless you are an identical twin, no one else has your exact combination of genes.

The Egg

Development of the egg begins before a woman is born, when she is developing as a fetus. By the time she is born, her body has formed about 2 million undeveloped egg cells, called primary oocytes. The undeveloped eggs each contain 23 pairs of chromosomes (46 total).

Decades later, at a time of potential fertilization, this number will have been reduced so that only one of each pair (23 total chromosomes) is contributed by the mother. By the time a woman is born, each of the undeveloped eggs will have begun this reduction process. The undeveloped eggs do not complete this important reduction of chromosome number until many years later, just before ovulation. This "resting phase" may be useful for protection of the egg. Chromosomes appear to be most vulnerable to change (mutation) during cell division. The long rest may lessen the likelihood that the genes of the egg could become altered, which could lead to birth defects.

During childhood, most of the undeveloped eggs disappear, leaving only about 40,000 by puberty. During the remainder of a woman's reproductive life, a total of only 400 will develop fully.

Just before ovulation, the reduction in chromosome number is completed by a process of cell division. A single cell, with 23 pairs of chromosomes, separates into two new cells, each containing one chromosome from each previous pair. One of the new cells will become a mature egg. This separation helps decide which characteristics are passed on from mother to child.

After ovulation the egg begins to divide a second time. Again it proceeds only partly through the division process, then stops. Cell division will progress to completion only if the egg is fertilized. When the egg is released at ovulation, it is surrounded by a layer of cells called the corona radiata. To fertilize the egg, a single sperm must penetrate this covering. At this point, the egg is about $\frac{1}{200}$ of an inch in diameter—much too small to see without a microscope.

The Sperm

During male adolescence, testosterone stimulates development of cells that form sperm within the testicles. Like the egg, the chromosome pairs must divide to reduce the chromosome number from 46 to 23. Also like the egg, this process results in a vast number of possible combinations of chromosomes. However, unlike the development of the single egg, 350 million sperm cells are produced for each ejaculation. The maturation of sperm cells requires about two months.

Cell Growth

Starting from the genetic information contained in the fertilized egg, how is it that cells know how to divide and develop so perfectly? How do the basic early cells develop into the final tissues that are so varied: muscle, nerve, bone and skin? How do the variations we call "birth defects" arise? The science of molecular biology is beginning to provide answers to these questions.

Understanding how cells influence each other's growth holds tremendous promise for developments in medicine. It may explain why certain birth defects occur. It may explain why some wounds heal without a scar, whereas others leave large scars. It may also hold potential for new methods in the detection and treatment of cancer.

It is important to recognize the current limits of our knowledge. We do not understand the causes of many birth defects. Science has provided a glimpse of some of the possible answers. The next decade promises to hold many new insights to critical questions concerning such issues as cell growth, birth defects, repair of injury and the development and control of various forms of cancer.

Cell Growth

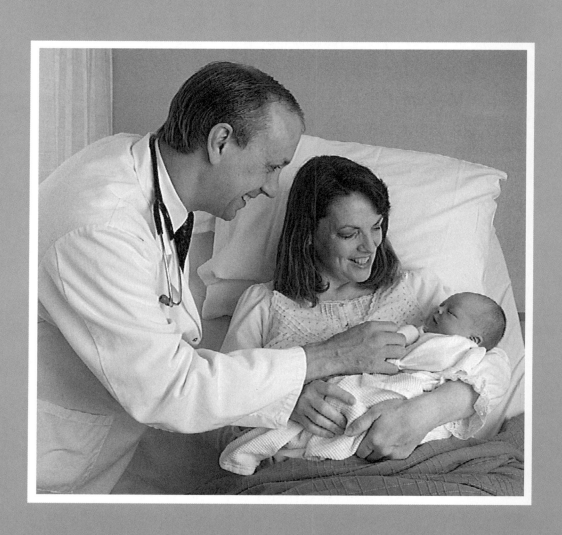

CHAPTER FOUR

Selecting an Obstetrical Caregiver

The person you choose for your obstetrical care can have a major influence on how satisfied you feel with your pregnancy experience. You may have a doctor or midwife in mind before you become pregnant, and your friends undoubtedly will pass along recommendations. But your needs and expectations will probably not be the same as those of your friends. Your needs may change during the pregnancy. And your choices may be limited by the insurance coverage you have.

This chapter will help you think about and understand your needs and preferences in a caregiver. It also explains four different options for an obstetrical caregiver: family physician, obstetrician, maternal-fetal medicine specialist and midwife. Individual physicians and midwives have unique personalities, practice styles and philosophies. Your chances of having a satisfying, productive relationship are increased by having realistic expectations of your caregiver and finding a caregiver who shares your perspective.

What Are Your Options?

After medical school, during a three-year program of specialized training called residency, a family physician gains experience in the various fields of medicine (for example, obstetrics, pediatrics, internal medicine and surgery). This experience enables a family practitioner to manage most pregnancies and to perform minor surgical procedures. A family physician's involvement with every member of your family, from newborns to grandparents, provides an opportunity for the doctor to know your whole family and to provide continuity from prenatal care throughout childhood and beyond.

Family Physician

Obstetrician/ Gynecologist

This physician specializes in the care of women during pregnancy and in diseases that affect a woman's reproductive organs. During the four-year residency, these doctors receive training in obstetrics, infertility and surgery. In addition to the residency, an obstetrician/gynecologist may complete additional training in an area such as the diagnosis and treatment of infertility. In some communities, only obstetricians perform cesarean deliveries and are consulted if a high-risk situation develops during a pregnancy.

Maternal-Fetal Medicine Specialist

A maternal-fetal medicine specialist, or perinatologist, is an obstetrician who has received special training and certification in the care of high-risk pregnancies. A perinatologist's training extends somewhat into the field of pediatrics because he or she often needs to manage problems that can occur in an unborn baby. Women who have had a prior complicated pregnancy, those who are carrying twins, triplets or more, or those who have preexisting medical conditions might see a maternal-fetal medicine specialist for part of or all their prenatal care. Commonly, a family physician or obstetrician may refer a woman to a maternal-fetal medicine specialist if complications develop during a pregnancy.

Midwife

In many parts of the world—England, France, Scandinavia and the Netherlands, for example—pregnancy care by midwives has been and remains traditional. It is growing in popularity in the United States. In 1990, the latest year for which figures are available, certified nurse-midwives delivered nearly 150,000 babies in the United States.

There are various types of midwives; one key distinction among the types is whether a midwife has nurse's training. If so, she is probably a certified nurse-midwife. If she is not a nurse, a midwife can be certified, licensed, registered, or none of these, depending on the state in which he or she lives. Certification or licensing usually requires some type of training and passing an exam. Each state determines which types of midwives are allowed to practice. Currently, state laws vary widely.

Nurse-midwife. A certified nurse-midwife has, at a minimum, a degree in nursing, specializing in obstetrics and gynecology, and has passed several examinations to receive certification. Nurse-midwives provide complete obstetrical care for normal, healthy pregnancies and are trained to screen mothers for potential problems. Generally, they are known for specializing in "low-tech" care that emphasizes support for the expectant mother. They are permitted to prescribe medications and vitamins in most states, but they do not perform cesarean births or administer anesthetics.

Some nurse-midwives have private, solo practices and will assist you if you decide to have your baby at home. Most, however, attend births in hospitals or birthing centers. All nurse-midwives are legally required to be associated with a backup physician or group of physicians they can call on to deal with pregnancy or birthing problems.

Choosing the Caregiver Who Meets Your Needs

If you begin pregnancy in good health and have no history of pregnancy problems, you may opt for care from a family physician, an obstetrician or a nurse-midwife. Not all risk factors can be identified in advance, however, and complications can develop during your pregnancy that might prompt your family physician or nurse-midwife to refer you to a specialist.

Different women may expect different approaches to their pregnancy care. For instance, you might be most comfortable with a collegial relationship with your caregiver, in which he or she acts as a consultant or resource person who is guiding, rather than directing, your pregnancy. ("I'm in charge of my own body, but I need expert advice for this particular problem."..."I've tried this—what do I do next?"..."We're partners in health care.") Or you might be more comfortable with someone who tends to give more clear-cut, specific recommendations. Your satisfaction, or lack of satisfaction, with a particular caregiver might be related to how closely his or her style meshes with your expectations. If, after discussing your expectations with your caregiver, you're still not satisfied, you might want to consider choosing a different one.

> ## *A Mayo physician's philosophy*
>
> The non-interventionist approach is very much a part of the way obstetrics is practiced with low-risk pregnancies at Mayo Clinic. As one Mayo Clinic physician puts it, "I see my job as helping a woman take charge of her own pregnancy. My greatest joy is standing by and watching things go normally, to not be needed. My other role is to provide 'insurance,' to be able to set matters right when they go wrong."

Whatever the particular practice style of your obstetrical caregiver, you deserve someone who listens to your concerns and provides helpful answers to your questions. Your caregiver should help you become as informed as you can be and allow you to participate in medical decisions affecting you and your baby.

Often, particularly if your caregiver is a member of a group practice, you will find yourself working with several physicians, nurses or certified nurse-midwives with different personalities and practice styles. These various individuals can complement one another, and if your primary caregiver is unavailable because of an emergency, illness or vacation, someone else will be available to cover.

Many sources of information are available to help you choose a caregiver. Most women start by seeking advice from family, friends, neighbors and co-workers. Doctors, nurses and other health professionals can also be a valuable source of information.

Your local county medical society will have a listing of all of the physicians in your area. The society can provide information about a physician's professional background, including his or her medical school, residency training, type of practice and hospital affiliation.

If you are interested, the following references can provide information about a physician's professional background. Look for them at your public library, medical society or libraries at a hospital or university medical school:

Where to Find an Obstetrical Care Provider

- *Directory of Physicians in the United States.* This book lists physicians who are located in the United States, Puerto Rico, Virgin Islands and certain Pacific Islands and U.S. physicians temporarily located in foreign countries. This is published by the American Medical Association (AMA). It lists members and non-members of the AMA. It provides such information as the doctor's address, type of practice, where he or she went to medical school and whether he or she is board-certified.

- *The Official ABMS Directory of Board Certified Medical Specialists.* This is published by Marquis Who's Who in cooperation with the American Board of Medical Specialties (ABMS). It lists physicians who are certified by the examining boards of recognized specialty organizations. It also provides information such as a doctor's medical school and internship training, hospital affiliation, address and telephone number.

  The Yellow Pages in many telephone directories throughout the country now lists local physicians who are recognized as specialists by the American Board of Medical Specialties (ABMS), noting their specialty or subspecialty. In addition, you now can call the ABMS toll-free at 800-776-CERT (800-776-2378) to verify a doctor's certification.

- American College of Nurse-Midwives. This is the professional organization that represents more than 5,000 certified nurse-midwives. It will give you the names and addresses of nurse-midwives in your community. Contact the American College of Nurse-Midwives, 818 Connecticut Avenue N.W., Suite 900, Washington, D.C. 20006. The telephone number is (202) 728-9860.

Your Relationship With Your Caregiver

A successful caregiver-patient relationship, like any partnership, is built, over time, on trust. You trust that your caregiver will give proper advice, make the correct diagnoses and prescribe the appropriate treatments. Similarly, the caregiver must trust that you will talk about your concerns, take responsibility for following recommended treatments and contact your caregiver if you are having problems.

Often, particularly in obstetrical care, your caregiver provides reassurance—reassurance that your concerns have been heard and appreciated, reassurance that nothing serious or life-threatening has been missed and reassurance that most problems are self-limited and will resolve on their own. However, you must trust your caregiver when reassurance, not extensive tests or medications, is required. You must also be able to trust that your caregiver will be available for follow-up or questions if your pregnancy does not proceed as expected. A strong relationship built on trust fosters teamwork between you and your caregiver.

Relationships With a Doctor's Group or Team

The solo practitioner of previous generations is becoming increasingly rare. You probably will work with a doctor who is a member of a group or team of doctors and nurses. This arrangement is particularly common in managed care settings.

Ask your doctor what his or her routine is regarding attendance at births. Some doctors try to deliver the babies of all of their own patients; others share "on-call" responsibilities with their partners or other doctors, particularly after hours or on weekends. If possible, arrange to meet the other professionals who might be helping you with your delivery.

If complications develop during your pregnancy or during your labor, you might be referred or, in some situations, even transferred to a different doctor or hospital. Discuss with your doctor, before any problems develop, what your options might be. For instance, would you be referred to another member of your doctor's group, or to someone outside the group? What role would your primary caregiver continue to play in these situations? What, if any, circumstances would necessitate transfer to a different medical center, and where would that be?

Particularly after hours or on weekends, you may not be able to see your regular doctor. Try to determine if you are comfortable with your doctor's on-call partners or backup, at least making certain that your doctor receives word of your after-hours care or has access to the results in your chart or medical record.

Other Important Considerations

In addition to the type of caregiver you choose and the development of a good working relationship, there are other practical considerations to keep in mind:

- Convenience. Is the location of the caregiver close to your work or home?

- Hospital privileges. Some women have a preference for a particular hospital in which to give birth. If this factor is important for you, ask the hospital to provide the names of caregivers who deliver there.

- Cost. Most providers charge one flat fee for prenatal care for low-risk pregnancies. Charges for specialized tests and treatment, should the need develop, are additional. Check your insurance coverage before choosing a caregiver to find out what, if any, limitations apply.

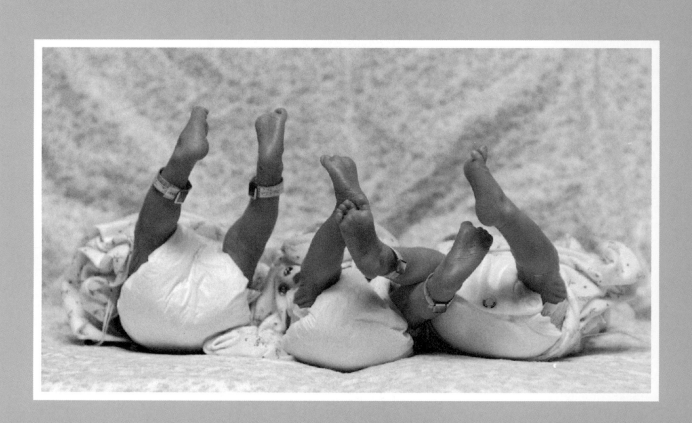

CHAPTER FIVE

Prenatal Care

Your first visit

Whether you only suspect you are pregnant or are already pretty sure, your first prenatal visit can make a big difference for your peace of mind. The first visit not only confirms your pregnancy but also gives you a chance to ask the many questions you may have. Determining your much-anticipated due date is just the beginning.

Your health and lifestyle at conception and in the following several weeks will affect your baby's welfare more significantly than at any other time in your pregnancy. Therefore, it's important to see your doctor, midwife or nurse-practitioner as soon as possible if you suspect you're pregnant. In fact, many health care providers advocate preconception (before you conceive) care for ideal preparation for pregnancy. Detecting conditions such as high blood pressure or diabetes before you become pregnant, or modifying the treatment of existing medical conditions, can decrease risks for you and your baby. (For more on preconception care, see page 5.)

Most likely your health care provider will reassure you that your pregnancy is proceeding normally and, if needed, will advise you about changes to make to minimize risks to you and to your baby. Engaging in activities such as smoking cigarettes, drinking alcoholic beverages or using some medications or drugs like marijuana

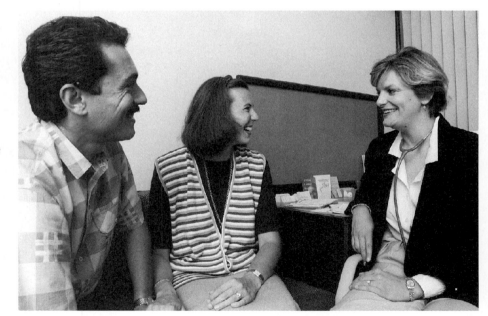

Taking time to get acquainted and discuss questions that you and your partner have is an important part of prenatal visits.

or cocaine may put your baby at increased risk for birth defects or miscarriage. (For more on these and other lifestyle factors that affect pregnancy, see page 103.)

Whether this is your first pregnancy or not, your prenatal visits provide an opportunity not only to review your health and lifestyle but also to express your hopes and fears about being pregnant and giving birth. Health care providers enjoy the celebration inherent in pregnancy and birth and want to enhance your celebration of it too.

Teaming Up for Good Care

You may envision selecting a health care provider you trust and have confidence in, and then seeing this person throughout your pregnancy and the baby's birth. However, depending on how a particular medical practice is set up, or the timing of vacations or emergencies, it's likely that sometime during the course of your pregnancy or delivery, someone other than your regular health care provider will be working with you. This substitution occasionally can be an awkward adjustment, especially during an experience as personal and important as pregnancy. But remember, everyone who works in obstetrical care wants what's best for you and your baby, and they'll do whatever is possible to ensure that you feel comfortable and safe.

Here are some recommendations to set the groundwork for a good partnership:

- Prepare questions in advance. Jot on paper the key questions you'd like answered. It's easier to collect your thoughts before your appointment than during a short visit.

- Assert yourself. More than likely, the question you're most reluctant to ask may be the one your doctor hears most often. If your doctor doesn't answer your questions to your satisfaction, or answers them in technical language you don't understand, persist until you understand. In addition, nurses and nurse-practitioners in many obstetrical practices are a great source of recommendations and answers to questions you may have. Your health care provider may also refer you to a registered dietitian or social worker for more assistance.

- Talk honestly and accurately. Because the quality of your health care hinges to some degree on the quality of the information you provide, it's important to be honest and accurate.

What to Expect During the First Visit

Allow plenty of time, up to two to three hours, so you won't feel rushed during the first visit. You'll be meeting several different people, including nurses and office staff, who work with your health care provider. Come prepared to answer questions about your health in general, your pregnancy and your insurance coverage.

At your first prenatal visit, one of the initial questions you may be asked is, "Were you surprised to learn that you're pregnant?" Another will be, "When was the first day of your last period?" And from there on, it may seem like the questions just don't stop. Gathering as much information as possible about your past and present health is one of your health care provider's biggest goals at your first visit. The answers you give have an impact on the care you receive.

The first visit usually begins with a review of your past and current health, sometimes called your medical history. Some health care providers make this a one-on-one conversation with just you, the mom-to-be; they'll invite your partner to join the appointment later. It gives you an opportunity to discuss, privately and confidentially, any concerns you may have that you might not want to share with your partner. Your health care provider may ask how you feel about being pregnant and how your partner feels about the pregnancy. If abuse is occurring, whether physical, verbal or emotional, it is important to talk about this with your doctor or a member of his or her professional staff.

As part of your medical history, you can expect questions about the following topics:

- Typical length of time between your periods

- Use of contraceptives

- Details of any previous pregnancies

- Medications (both prescription and non-prescription) you're taking

- Allergies you have

- Medical conditions or diseases you've had or now have

- Past surgeries, if any

- Your work environment

- Lifestyle behaviors such as exercise, diet, smoking, use of alcoholic beverages or recreational drugs

- Risk factors for sexually transmitted diseases (such as more than one sexual partner for you and your partner)

- Past or present medical problems in your partner's or your immediate family (father, mother, sisters, brothers)

Your Medical History

A word to expectant dads

She's right. You should offer to come along for her first prenatal visit.

The doctor may talk to you, too, in addition to talking with and examining your partner. Your medical history and your family's health history, not just your partner's, are important. Knowing about your lifestyle and habits such as smoking is also significant because they can affect the outcome of your partner's pregnancy and the baby. For example, even exposure to tobacco smoke can increase the risks of spontaneous abortion, fetal death, preterm labor and low birth weight.

Learning why certain recommendations are made can help prevent misunderstandings. For example, if she asks you to clean the cat's litter box, there's a good reason. (For information about toxoplasmosis, see page 113.)

If you're concerned about feeling out of place in the waiting area before the appointment, you'll probably be surprised to learn that there are a lot more dads-to-be there with their partners than you expected. Today, more and more men are playing an active role throughout their partner's pregnancy and not just in the delivery room.

Your presence is more important than even your role in providing health information. Your presence tells your partner that you care about her, that you care about the family you're planning together and that you want to share this special time with her.

Your Due Date

If you know when your baby was conceived, you may have already made a prediction of your baby's birthdate. Your health care provider is just as interested in estimating your due date as precisely as possible for several reasons. To monitor your baby's growth most accurately, it's best to establish the due date early in pregnancy. Also, because certain laboratory test results change during the course of pregnancy, a test result might appear abnormal if the estimate of the age of the baby is off. And knowing the due date significantly affects how doctors manage any preterm labor if it occurs. (See the chart on page 7.)

To estimate your due date, your doctor will probably take the date when your last period began, add seven days and then subtract three months. For example, if your last period began on September 10, adding seven days (September 17) and subtracting three months gives you a due date of next June 17.

Remember, though, your due date is only an estimate of when your baby will be ready for birth. Most babies arrive within two weeks before or after the due date.

Physical Examination

In addition to checking your weight, height and blood pressure, your doctor will assess your heart, lungs, breasts and abdomen. The pelvic exam will likely be more comprehensive than a typical physical exam.

Many women are apprehensive about the physical examination, especially the pelvic exam. During the exam, focus on relaxing. Breathe slowly and deeply. This can help prevent or relieve tension and anxiety, which can tighten your muscles and make the exam more uncomfortable. Remember, the pelvic exam usually takes only a couple of minutes.

Your doctor will look in your vagina with the help of a device called a speculum. This enables him or her to see your cervix, the opening to your uterus. Changes in your cervix and in the size of your uterus help your doctor determine how long you've been pregnant. Even within the first six to eight weeks of pregnancy, your cervix becomes bluish-tinged and softens.

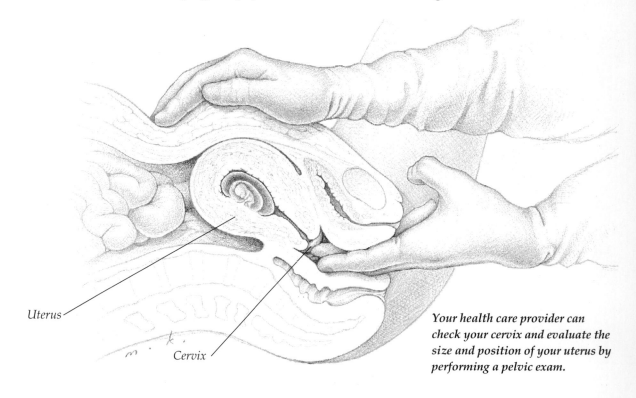

Uterus

Cervix

Your health care provider can check your cervix and evaluate the size and position of your uterus by performing a pelvic exam.

While the speculum is still in place, your doctor may obtain a small amount of material from your cervix for a Pap smear and to screen for infections. The Pap smear is designed to screen for abnormalities that indicate pre-cancer or cancer of the cervix. In young women, an abnormal Pap smear usually doesn't indicate cancer, but a follow-up Pap smear may be needed. Infections of the cervix may have significance for the progress of your pregnancy and the health of your child.

After removing the speculum, your doctor will insert two gloved fingers into your vagina to check your cervix and, with the other hand on top of your abdomen, check the size of your uterus and ovaries. (See the illustration on page 48.) By feeling bony landmarks, your doctor can determine the size and shape of your pelvis. These measurements can help predict whether problems might develop during labor. For example, if the exam shows that your pelvis seems too narrow for your baby's head to easily pass through the birth canal, your doctor will note this on your medical record. As your delivery date approaches, your doctor will monitor the size of your baby in comparison with the size of your pelvis. Often, late in pregnancy, ligaments in the pelvis relax and allow the birth canal to widen.

Laboratory Tests

During or after your first prenatal visit, you can expect to have several lab tests. Various tests can be conducted from a blood sample, a urine sample and a sample collected during the pelvic exam. The first prenatal visit typically includes the following tests:

- **Blood tests.** Although various blood tests are conducted, usually one needle stick is all that's necessary to collect the blood samples. It is important for your doctor to know your blood type (A, B or O) and Rh factor (negative or positive) and to check for antibodies. Antibodies can indicate differences in your blood type and your baby's, which may increase the risk of anemia and jaundice in your baby after birth. (For information on Rh incompatibility, see pages 167 and 223.)

  From the blood sample, your health care provider can also check for anemia and for infections such as hepatitis or syphilis.

  A blood test can also determine whether you are immune to rubella (German measles). Most Americans were vaccinated as children and still have antibodies that protect them against rubella. If the blood test shows that you aren't immune, you must avoid anyone who has rubella. Fortunately, rubella is not common in the United States. Rubella can have serious consequences on a developing fetus.

- **Urinalysis.** An analysis of your urine can determine if you have a bladder or kidney infection, which would require treatment. The urine sample may also be tested for increased amounts of sugar (indicating diabetes) and protein (indicating possible infection or kidney disease).

- **Cervical sample.** A sample of the cells and mucus from the cervix is checked for evidence of cervical cancer or for the sexually transmitted diseases gonorrhea and chlamydia.

If there is any uncertainty about your due date, or if you're having any bleeding or cramping, your doctor may do an ultrasound examination. (For details, see page 72.) Through the use of sound waves, this test gives a clear view of your developing baby. It's helpful for determining the size of your baby and for comparing his or her size to what is expected at different weeks of development. Health care providers vary in the use of ultrasound testing—some use it in only certain high-risk pregnancies, and others use it more often. Generally, though, if your doctor thinks you would benefit from one routine ultrasound exam, it's usually done at 16 to 20 weeks of gestational age.

During the course of your pregnancy, you will likely have some of the blood and urine tests again. See the Office Visits sections of Chapters 10 (page 139), 11 (page 164), and 12 (page 187) for descriptions of tests that are commonly performed after your first prenatal visit. You and your health care provider may also discuss other, less common tests, depending on your health and on your family's medical history. (For more on other prenatal tests, see pages 53 to 83.)

How to handle unsolicited advice

You're likely to receive unsolicited recommendations from family, friends and even strangers. "I heard on TV that you should…" "My mother read that you should…" "From my experience you should…" How do you sort good advice from well-meaning but bad advice? And what about the recommendations that seem plausible but are anxiety-provoking? Here are some suggestions:

- Make your own informed decisions—don't let others decide for you.

- Act only on information provided by the most reliable source— your health care provider. On medical subjects, your doctor is the most qualified. He or she not only has extensive obstetrical training and experience but also has the advantage of knowing you and your medical history.

- Don't feel guilty or feel that you should apologize if you don't necessarily follow advice from relatives and friends. Remember, this is your baby.

Some of the recommendations you receive from family and friends may in fact be appropriate; others may be out of date, or even dangerous. But whether the advice is about what to eat, how long you should work or how to prepare for breastfeeding, use your best judgment and discuss questions with your doctor.

Part of becoming a parent involves taking responsibility for making decisions. So while you may politely thank your well-meaning relatives and friends for their advice, or even cherish their sweet intent, what you should and shouldn't do is largely between you and your doctor.

Follow-Up Visits

Your health needs will determine the timing and number of follow-up visits your health care provider will recommend. Typically, your doctor will recommend monthly visits for the first seven months of your pregnancy. Then the visits become more frequent: every couple of weeks during your eighth month and then weekly until your baby arrives.

If you have a chronic health condition, such as diabetes or high blood pressure, your health care provider will recommend more frequent visits. If you're in good health and have previously been pregnant and gone through labor, your doctor may schedule fewer visits.

If any problems or concerns arise between visits, don't hesitate to contact your doctor or a member of his or her staff. See page 135 for a list of common concerns and recommendations on how quickly you should notify your doctor.

You and your partner may also want to attend childbirth education classes. Generally, these cover a wide range of topics, including fetal development, pain management skills for labor, breastfeeding and baby care. The classes provide helpful information, a chance to ask questions and an opportunity to meet other moms and dads. (See page 264 for more details on childbirth education classes.)

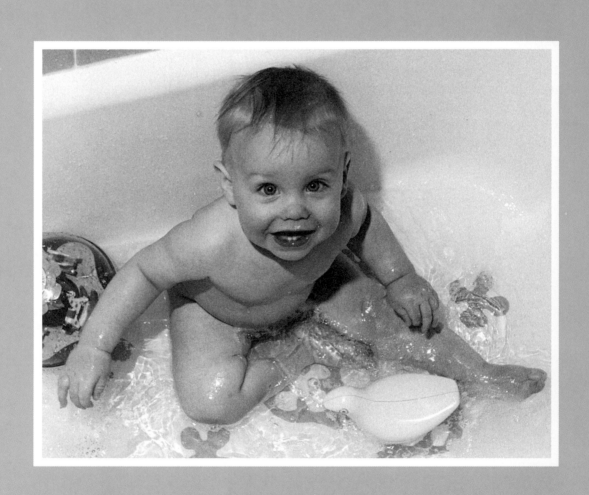

CHAPTER SIX

Prenatal Tests

Why they are used and how they are done

"Will my baby be healthy?" The question forms almost as soon as you find out you are pregnant. Like many women, you may seek medical reassurance about the health of the fetus you are carrying.

Although the development from embryo to baby is a very complex process, the odds of giving birth to a healthy child exceed 95 percent. At your first prenatal visit, your doctor may be able to tell you, "Things look good" or outline areas of concern, based on an evaluation of your medical and family history, physical examination and initial laboratory tests.

Even when "things look good," no doctor can promise that your child will be healthy. Everyone has a small background risk for having a child with a birth defect. Many, though not all, of these conditions can be detected during pregnancy. However, the most common result of a prenatal test is a normal finding.

Since the 1980s, prenatal testing has become available to any woman who needs information about the health of her fetus. This information can be helpful in determining any special care your fetus may require during pregnancy and at birth.

For some people, anxiety about the unknown makes prenatal testing of utmost importance. If the test results are normal, they feel they can relax and enjoy the rest of the pregnancy.

If the results indicate a problem, they want to know as much as possible so they can begin to make plans and can assist their physicians in managing the care of the fetus. Sometimes optimal prenatal care may significantly improve the outcome for the baby. For example, a woman who learns that her fetus has spina bifida may be encouraged to have a cesarean birth in order to minimize the chances of damaging the exposed nerves on the baby's back.

For some disorders, having the appropriate specialists ready to treat the baby immediately after delivery can make a big difference in the baby's chance of survival and the degree of health complications. For instance, a woman who learns her fetus has a congenital heart defect may want to give birth at a major

53

Prenatal tests at a glance

These tests and procedures are discussed in detail later in this chapter. The appropriate page number follows each definition.

- Maternal serum alpha-fetoprotein (MSAFP) test—a blood test designed to indicate an increased risk for fetal open neural tube defects, such as spina bifida. It may also indicate an increased risk for Down syndrome. (See page 68.)

- Triple test—a blood test that measures MSAFP, human chorionic gonadotropin and estriol. The test indicates which fetuses are at increased risk for open neural tube defects and improves the screen for Down syndrome. It is sometimes referred to as the MSAFP+ test. (See page 69.)

- Ultrasound exam—uses sound waves to obtain a "picture" of the fetus. (See page 72.)

- Amniocentesis—removal of a sample of amniotic fluid, from the sac surrounding the baby, for analysis. (See page 75.)

- Chorionic villus sampling (CVS)—removal of a small amount of the developing placenta for analysis. (See page 77.)

- Percutaneous umbilical blood sampling (PUBS)—also called fetal blood sampling, it involves direct sampling of the baby's blood for diagnosis of fetal infections (such as toxoplasmosis) or for enzyme studies, hematology studies or genetic analysis. (See page 79.)

Amniocentesis, CVS and PUBS provide samples of fetal cells, which are sent to the laboratory for genetic or biochemical studies. Because the blueprint to a person's genetic makeup is carried in every cell, only a tiny sample is needed to test for a specific gene or chromosome disorder.

Although laboratory tests have been developed to detect hundreds of disorders, not all of them will be performed on your sample. The specific tests performed are determined by the conditions for which your fetus is considered to be at increased risk.

medical center that does neonatal heart surgery, instead of at her local hospital. Some rare conditions can even be treated in the uterus, such as Rh incompatibility, which can be managed with in utero blood transfusions.

Knowing about birth defects before the baby is born can also help you and your partner prepare yourselves, your family and friends for any challenges ahead.

For parents who want the option of ending a pregnancy if their fetus has a serious health problem, early prenatal diagnosis allows for a less complicated termination, with fewer risks for the mother.

Other couples choose not to have prenatal tests for personal or religious reasons. Because they have decided the test results would not affect how they approach prenatal care and delivery, or their decision to continue the pregnancy, they feel they will have less anxiety during the pregnancy if they do not undergo tests.

As you consider which prenatal tests are appropriate for you, think about the risks and benefits of each, how the information obtained can help your doctor better care for your fetus and how it will help you make decisions.

You may choose to have prenatal testing if you discover there is effective technology that can provide the information you need. Or you may decide you don't want to have any tests. Many parents change their minds at several points during the testing process, and doctors expect this.

It is reassuring to know that serious birth defects are rare. However, some couples have a higher-than-average risk of bearing children with a specific birth defect or inherited disorder. If your doctor finds out that you have any special risks at your first prenatal visit, you may be offered specific prenatal tests.

Prenatal Testing Is Not a Crystal Ball

Your doctor may propose tests to determine whether your fetus has certain conditions, but these tests still can't guarantee that your baby won't have other problems.

As you talk with your doctor, you may want to replace the question, "Will my baby be healthy?" with questions such as, "How much information do I want about the future health of my baby?" "What can be done with this information to improve the health of my fetus?" "What factors might change my mind about continuing a pregnancy?"

These questions are not easy. How you as a couple choose to answer them will depend on your personal and religious principles, your relationship with each other, your own health and the amount of emotional and financial support you can count on. With this information, you will be better prepared to discuss your concerns with your partner and your doctor and to make sound decisions.

Birth Defects

Birth defects are congenital disorders, meaning the condition is present at birth. Birth defects vary from minor cosmetic irregularities to life-threatening biochemical disorders. Some children are born with multiple problems.

The March of Dimes Birth Defects Foundation recognizes more than 3,000 known conditions, including chromosome alterations, single gene defects, metabolic (body chemistry) defects, blood disorders, physical malformations present at birth and perinatal injuries (occurring just before or during the birth process).

Most birth defects are apparent at birth, but a few disorders can't be detected for months, or even years. Hundreds of conditions can be identified during pregnancy by prenatal diagnostic tests, if there is a reason in your family history or pregnancy history to suspect that they exist.

What Causes Birth Defects?

The majority (65 to 75 percent) of congenital conditions have no known cause, or may be considered multifactorial—due to a combination of genetic and environmental or other nongenetic factors. Of the remaining birth defects:

- Genetic (hereditary) factors (either chromosomal or single gene defects) are involved in most known causes, about 20 to 25 percent.
- Maternal diseases (such as diabetes, heart disease or alcohol abuse) are implicated in about 4 percent. (See pages 105, 231, and 239.)
- Infections passed from the mother to her baby (such as rubella or toxoplasmosis) are responsible for 3 to 5 percent. (See pages 216 and 219.)
- Drugs and medications taken by the mother cause less than 1 percent. (See page 106.)

To assess your risk for any of these known causes, your doctor will probably ask you to fill out an extensive questionnaire at your first prenatal visit. It will require information about medications you have taken and your use of alcohol, tobacco and recreational drugs. Answer honestly about your use of these substances so your doctor can assess whether your fetus is at risk.

The form may ask about your exposure to agents known to cause birth defects (such as methyl mercury, lead and radiation). It will also require a detailed medical history, including your immunization status.

In addition, most questionnaires ask about your family history, as well as your partner's, to determine your risk of passing on a hereditary disorder to your child. It may be helpful to ask relatives for this information before your first prenatal visit.

It is important that you answer the questions as accurately and completely as possible. Some questionnaires do not require much family medical information. If your doctor doesn't bring up the subject, make a point of asking whether any concerns you may have about your family history (or your partner's) are relevant to your pregnancy.

What are my chances of having a child with a birth defect?

Of every 100 babies born in the United States, 95 to 97 are born healthy (no major medical or surgical intervention is necessary). According to the March of Dimes Birth Defects Foundation:

- One of every 175 is born with a congenital heart defect.
- One of every 400 is born with clubfoot.
- One of every 700 is born with cleft lip and palate.
- One of every 800 is born with Down syndrome.
- One of every 2,000 is born with spina bifida.

To put this list into perspective, consider the following:

- The odds of having twins are about one in 100.
- The odds of having triplets are about one in 8,000.

Medical Geneticists and Genetic Counselors

If your doctor finds anything that may increase your risk of having a child with a birth defect, a medical geneticist or a genetic counselor could help you in better understanding diagnoses and clarifying risks. A medical geneticist is a physician who specializes in genetic disorders. A genetic counselor has completed master's-level training in medical genetics and is certified in genetic counseling. Genetic counseling is designed to provide information in a supportive and non-judgmental manner and to assist in decision making. A medical geneticist or genetic counselor can help parents understand the consequences of a particular diagnosis, the options regarding treatment and the possibilities of the condition recurring in future pregnancies.

A medical geneticist may also assist your doctor in determining which genetic studies may be needed and what information may be necessary to make informed decisions about the pregnancy.

To understand how birth defects occur and whether your fetus has any special risk for them, consider the genetic and environmental causes and a combination of both.

Genetic Causes

Just as a baby's eye color and hair color are inherited, some birth defects are the result of genes or chromosomes inherited from the parents. An estimated 50,000 to 100,000 genes, which determine traits for appearance, function and development, are located on the chromosomes.

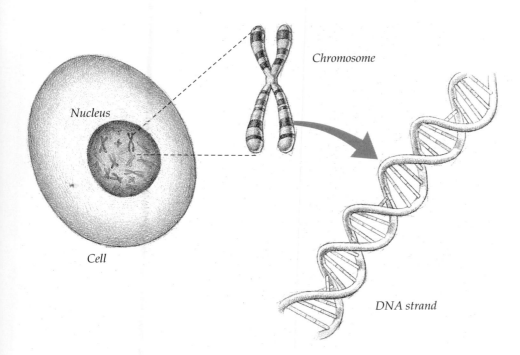

Nucleus

Chromosome

Cell

DNA strand

Each of the 60 trillion cells in your body has a center (nucleus) that contains 46 chromosomes (23 pairs), half coming from each of your parents. Each chromosome consists of spiral strands of deoxyribonucleic acid (DNA), divided into units called genes. Your genes, (shown on the chromosomes as bands that represent hundreds of genes) control the physical traits you inherit and pass on to your children. Each gene has a unique task. One gene, for example, might govern the color of your eyes or hair and another could determine whether you'll be, or your children will be, at risk for a genetic disorder such as cystic fibrosis, a serious health condition affecting the lungs.

Under normal circumstances, every cell in a person's body has 23 pairs of chromosomes except egg and sperm cells (which have 23 single chromosomes). At conception, the egg and sperm join, forming an embryo with 23 pairs of chromosomes, for a normal total of 46. The sex chromosomes are called X and Y, and the non-sex (autosomal) chromosome pairs are numbered 1 to 22.

Normal eggs always carry an X; a normal sperm may carry an X or Y. When the egg is fertilized by the sperm, the XX combination will produce a girl and the XY combination will be a boy. (See page 27 for more details.)

Genetic disorders may occur when there are abnormalities in the number or structure of chromosomes (chromosome abnormalities) or defects in a single gene (dominant, recessive or X-linked disorders).

Some genetic disorders are not inherited from either parent. Instead, a spontaneous alteration (mutation) may take place in the egg or sperm or, after conception, in the embryo. Not all causes for this are known. Some may be due to errors in cell division causing an extra or missing chromosome, or piece of a chromosome. Some result from single gene changes caused by exposure to certain chemicals, radiation or other agents that damage genetic material (DNA). Sometimes it is simply an error in DNA copying that the cell does not detect and repair.

Sometimes an abnormal chromosome pattern is inherited from one or the other parent. Approximately one in 500 people are carriers of chromosome abnormalities. They themselves have no symptoms, but they have a much higher chance of having multiple miscarriages, unexplained infertility or children with birth defects.

Sometimes something goes wrong in the development of the egg or the sperm, and there is either extra or missing chromosome material in the embryo. This can cause the fetus to develop physical defects or a loss of mental capacity. It might also result in early miscarriage. Approximately half of all miscarriages that occur during the first trimester are due to chromosome abnormalities.

Chromosome Abnormalities

Down syndrome (trisomy 21). This is the most common chromosome disorder. People with Down syndrome have extra genetic material from the number 21 chromosome. Most commonly, they have three of the number 21 chromosomes instead of the normal two. This extra chromosome (trisomy) disrupts normal development. Children with Down syndrome have a distinct facial appearance (a small head, flat face and upslanting eyes) and various degrees of physical problems and mental retardation. About half of these children have congenital heart defects and may require surgery at an early age. They are also at risk for the development of gastrointestinal complications, thyroid problems, hearing loss and vision impairment.

Many children with Down syndrome are happy, loving and easygoing. In some, behavior problems may develop later in life. Past the age of 35, one in three people with Down syndrome will have increasing senility similar to Alzheimer's disease. The average life expectancy is about 50 years, but this varies greatly depending on the severity of health problems. Down syndrome support groups can be very helpful for the families of these children.

Early intervention with specialists from many professions (doctors, nurses, physical and speech therapists) can optimize development. Many children with Down syndrome can attend community schools, learn to read and write and perform various levels of jobs as adults.

What causes Down syndrome? Ninety percent of the time, Down syndrome is caused when an egg or sperm cell divides unequally, resulting in one cell having an extra number 21 chromosome. The risk of this condition increases with the mother's age.

In the United States, one of every 800 babies is born with Down syndrome. Among 25-year-old mothers, the incidence of Down syndrome is only one in 1,250 births. Among 35-year-old mothers, the incidence increases to one in every 378 births, and by age 45 it is one of every 30. (See the chart on page 59.)

Down syndrome can also result when one parent who is completely normal has a genetic structure rearrangement (translocation) involving chromosome 21 in many or all body cells, including the egg or the sperm. A person with this chromosome 21 rearrangement has a greater risk of having a child with Down syndrome. A couple that has previously had an infant with Down syndrome is also at greater risk.

How is Down syndrome diagnosed prenatally? Down syndrome is identified by looking at a sample of fetal cells in the laboratory to determine whether they have a number 21 chromosome abnormality. Chromosome analysis can be performed on cells obtained through amniocentesis, CVS or PUBS. Chromosome analysis cannot predict the severity of mental retardation.

Women at age 35 have about the same risk of having a chromosome abnormality (including Down syndrome) detected in their fetus (one in 192) as they do of having a miscarriage caused by amniocentesis (about one in 200, although in some medical centers this risk may be as low as one in 400). Consequently, amniocentesis is usually offered to women older than 35 years to test for Down syndrome.

Amniocentesis is also offered to women whose MSAFP test or triple test indicates a very low level of alpha-fetoprotein. For reasons that are not yet understood, a low level of this protein is sometimes associated with certain chromosome abnormalities, including Down syndrome. However, there are many other reasons for low levels of AFP, which you will read about later in this chapter.

Parents who are known to have a chromosome rearrangement will also be offered prenatal testing.

Chromosome abnormalities: What are your risks?

Age	Risk for Down syndrome	Total risk for clinically significant chromosome abnormalities
20	1/1,667	1/526
21	1/1,667	1/526
22	1/1,429	1/500
23	1/1,429	1/500
24	1/1,250	1/476
25	**1/1,250**	**1/476**
26	1/1,176	1/476
27	1/1,111	1/455
28	1/1,053	1/435
29	1/1,000	1/417
30	1/952	1/385
31	1/909	1/385
32	1/769	1/322
33	1/602	1/286
34	1/485	1/238
35	**1/378**	**1/192**
36	1/289	1/156
37	1/224	1/127
38	1/173	1/102
39	1/136	1/83
40	1/106	1/66
41	1/82	1/53
42	1/63	1/42
43	1/49	1/33
44	1/38	1/26
45	**1/30**	**1/21**

Trisomy 18. This is the next most common non-sex chromosome trisomy. Children with this disorder have three number 18 chromosomes. A less common condition is having three number 13 chromosomes, **trisomy 13**. Both disorders severely affect physical and mental development, and affected infants rarely live more than two years. There are several other less common chromosome disorders, all of which can be diagnosed prenatally through chromosome analysis of cells obtained from amniocentesis, CVS or PUBS. Unfortunately, it may be difficult to know which pregnancies are at risk for these rarer chromosome abnormalities.

Sex chromosome disorders. These occur when there is an alteration in a sex chromosome, or an extra or missing X or Y. Most are caused by a mistake in cell division. Some of these conditions may cause varying degrees of disabilities in learning and behavior. They may be associated with infertility, but usually they do not affect life expectancy. If a fetal chromosome analysis is performed for any reason during your pregnancy, these conditions can be discovered prenatally. They include Turner syndrome (45, X), trisomy X (47, XXX), Klinefelter syndrome (47,XXY) and 47,XYY syndrome.

Single Gene Disorders

Sometimes birth defects are the result of abnormalities in (or loss of) a single gene. Genes are the DNA molecules that determine the characteristics you inherit from your parents. They occur in pairs. For instance, a gene located on the chromosome number 7 you inherited from your mother is paired with a gene located at the same "address" on the chromosome you inherited from your father. Single gene disorders can be

- Recessive (both genes in the pair are altered)
- Dominant (only one gene in the pair is altered, but it overrides the normal one)
- X-linked (there is an abnormal gene on an X chromosome); X-linked disorders may be recessive or dominant

Certain disorders are passed on from one generation to the next through affected genes. Your risk as a couple for some of these conditions may be determined with complete family histories. If your risk is high, there may be a blood test available to determine whether you or your partner is a carrier.

What is a carrier? Carriers are people who have only one copy of a recessive gene for a particular disorder and have no symptoms themselves. Scientists estimate that we are all carriers of four to eight altered genes, but they are usually not expressed when the normal gene of the pair performs the necessary functions.

These abnormal genes are expressed only if the same gene is altered or missing in your partner and your child inherits both faulty genes. The likelihood that you and your partner have the same altered genes increases if you are blood relatives.

Recessive disorders. Recessive disorders occur only when both parents contribute an altered gene to the pair. When both parents are carriers for the same autosomal recessive disorder, each of their children has a one in four chance of being affected with the disorder, and a one in two chance of being a carrier.

If there is a family history of one of these conditions on both the mother's side and the father's side, you may want to ask whether a test is available to determine if both of you are carriers. Carrier status can be established with a blood test for certain conditions, but such testing is still not available for most autosomal recessive disorders (recessive disorders involving chromosomes that are not sex chromosomes).

If both you and your partner are found to be carriers, you may be offered amniocentesis, CVS or PUBS. Complicated genetic analysis can be performed on fetal cells obtained from these procedures to determine whether your fetus is affected.

Phenylketonuria (PKU) is an autosomal recessive disorder resulting in a deficiency of a specific enzyme. This disrupts normal metabolism and can result in mental retardation if diet is not carefully regulated beginning in early infancy.

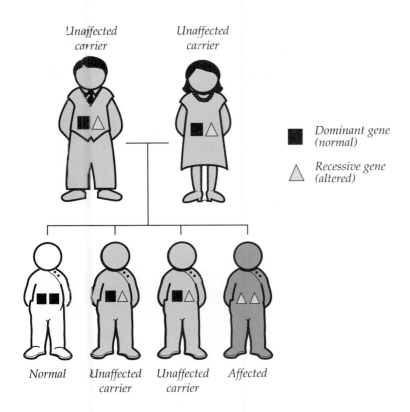

Unaffected carrier — Unaffected carrier

■ Dominant gene (normal)

△ Recessive gene (altered)

Normal — Unaffected carrier — Unaffected carrier — Affected

Recessive disorders, such as cystic fibrosis, can be passed along to children even if neither parent has the disorder. Both parents in this example are healthy, but they are carriers of an altered recessive gene. The chance is 25 percent that their baby will be born with cystic fibrosis, 50 percent that the baby will be an unaffected, healthy carrier (just like his or her parents) and 25 percent that the baby will neither carry nor have the disease. The sex of the baby has no bearing on the outcome.

(In the United States, approximately one of every 10,000 babies is born with PKU, so all infants born in this country are tested for PKU at birth.)

Specific geographic and ethnic groups are at significantly greater risk of having certain recessive disorders, as follows:

- **Whites of Northern European descent—Cystic fibrosis (CF)** is much more common among whites of northern European descent; about 4 percent of the white population carries the CF gene. It is rare among blacks, Jews and Asians. CF is an inherited metabolic disorder affecting cells lining certain glands in the body. Symptoms include chronic lung disease, digestive problems and related complications, resulting in a shortened life expectancy. Physical and respiratory therapy improve breathing; a controlled diet and supplements aid digestion. Complications may require various medical interventions.

  Although scientists have located the gene that causes CF, they have found that it can have as many as 200 different alterations instead of just one. This large number has made development of a screening test difficult, but currently it is possible to detect 85 to 90 percent of carriers.

- **Blacks—Sickle cell disease** is much more common in American blacks and people with mixed African heritage. In the United States, 7 to 8 percent of blacks carry a gene for sickle cell disease, an inherited blood disorder that causes abnormal oxygen-carrying capacity in red blood cells. Symptoms include anemia, fatigue, delayed growth and development and also other complications. Clogging of blood vessels by abnormally shaped red blood cells causes severe attacks of pain.

  Treatment includes medication for pain and infections, vitamin supplements, occasional oxygen therapy and blood transfusions. Blood tests can determine carrier status.

- **Ashkenazi Jews—Tay-Sachs disease**, an inherited metabolic disorder in which the enzyme necessary for breaking down certain fat and protein complexes is missing, has a carrier rate as high as one in 30 among Ashkenazi Jews. Children with this condition die in early childhood.

- **People from Southeast Asia and Mediterranean countries—Alpha thalassemias** are more common among people of Southeast Asian descent; **beta thalassemias** are predominantly found in people descended from Mediterranean countries such as Greece, Italy or Middle East countries. Thalassemias are anemias resulting from inherited defects in the production of hemoglobin.

Is my child at risk for a recessive disorder? If you answer "yes" to the following questions, ask your doctor if your pregnancy could be affected:

- Are both you and your partner members of the same ethnic group that has a high carrier rate for one of the disorders listed above?

- Do you or your partner have any family members who had stillbirths or children who were severely ill or who died at an early age? If so, there may have been an abnormality caused by a recessive disorder.

- Are you and your partner related by blood (for example, first cousins) or members of a small, closed community?

Dominant disorders. Dominant disorders are usually transmitted from parent to child through a single altered gene that overcomes the normally functioning gene in the pair. The child of a parent who carries this gene has a 50 percent chance of inheriting it.

Sometimes, even though neither parent is a carrier, there can be a mutation in the child's genes, or in the single egg or sperm from which the child was

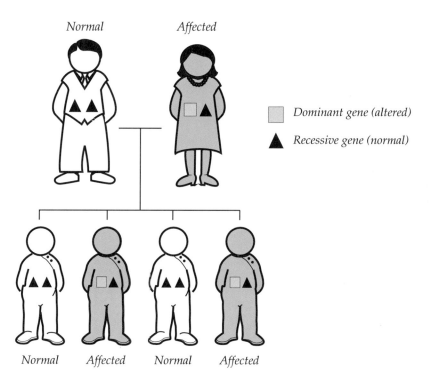

Dominant disorders: If one parent-to-be carries an altered dominant gene, such as the gene for Huntington's disease, the chance is 50 percent that the couple's baby, regardless of sex, will be born with the disease.

formed, that causes a dominant genetic disorder. Advanced paternal age is one factor that is associated with new mutations, such as **achondroplasia**—a rare skeletal condition resulting in short arms and legs.

Many dominant disorders that run in families are characterized by illnesses occurring after childhood, such as **Huntington's chorea (Huntington's disease)**—a degenerative condition that causes movement problems and increasing senility beginning in adulthood. This is the condition that affected the famous folksinger and songwriter Woody Guthrie.

Is my child at risk for a dominant disorder? To screen for dominant disorders that may run in the family, ask yourself, "Are there people in my family or my partner's family who had an unusual illness?" Some inherited conditions may include serious cholesterol problems, early colon cancer or early breast cancer. Although no prenatal tests exist for these conditions (and some aren't screened for even in late childhood), it is important to discuss them with your doctor if you discover any such illnesses in your family history.

Dominant disorders tend to be variable in severity, even among members of the same family. If an autosomal dominant condition is found in your family, ask your doctor about the range of symptoms and age at onset you might expect. Even if you and your partner seem healthy, mild evidence of the disorder may be detectable by a doctor familiar with the condition.

X-linked (sex-linked) disorders. X-linked disorders involve an altered gene on the X chromosome. Normal males have one X and one Y chromosome, and normal females have two X chromosomes. A woman can be normal but carry the altered gene on one of her X chromosomes. X-linked disorders can be recessive or dominant.

X-linked recessive conditions. In X-linked recessive conditions, the altered gene is usually expressed only in males because they have only one X chromosome. Females who inherit one X chromosome with an abnormal gene usually have no symptoms because the normal gene on their second X chromosome will dominate.

These disorders are generally passed from normal women carriers to their affected male children. Female children can be carriers, but will usually not have any symptoms of the disorder. If you are a carrier of an X-linked disorder, each of your sons will have a one in two chance of being affected, and each of your daughters will have a one in two chance of being a carrier. In certain conditions, however, females sometimes have mild symptoms of the disorder.

- **Duchenne muscular dystrophy**—The most common form of muscular dystrophy, this is an X-linked recessive condition affecting males, usually before age 5. However, one-third of cases are caused by new mutations, in which there is no family history of the condition. Prenatal diagnosis is often possible with amniocentesis, CVS or PUBS.

- **Fragile X**—This is an X-linked recessive condition that causes mental retardation and characteristic features, affecting between one in 1,000 and one in 2,000 children (mostly boys). Prenatal diagnosis of this condition is complex .

- **Hemophilia**—This includes several X-linked recessive blood conditions in which males are born deficient in specific factors that are necessary for blood clotting Family history can identify those at risk, and a blood test

X-linked recessive disorders: Some genetic conditions affect only males; females can be carriers of the disorder. When a couple has a son who has hemophilia, for example, the mother is a carrier and the father is normal. The chance is 50 percent that a daughter would be normal and 50 percent that she would be a carrier, like her mother. For a son of this couple, the chance is 50 percent that he would be normal and 50 percent that he would have the condition.

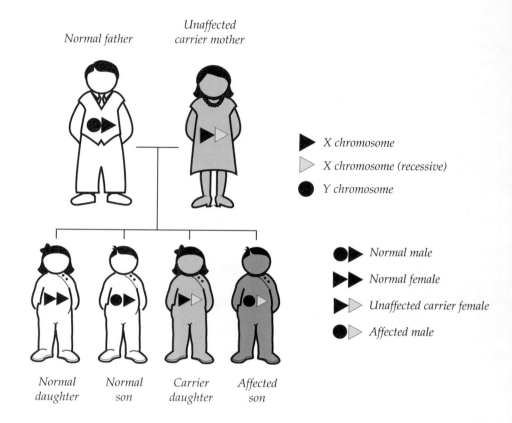

Normal father

Unaffected carrier mother

▶ X chromosome
▷ X chromosome (recessive)
● Y chromosome

Normal daughter   Normal son   Carrier daughter   Affected son

●▶ Normal male
▶▶ Normal female
▶▷ Unaffected carrier female
●▷ Affected male

may be helpful to identify some carriers. Prenatal diagnosis can be made with amniocentesis, CVS or PUBS.

X-linked dominant conditions. X-linked dominant conditions are less common conditions in which a single copy of an altered gene is sufficient to cause symptoms (even when the gene on the other X chromosome is normal). In this type of inheritance, a woman can pass the condition to her sons or daughters, and a man can pass it only to his daughters.

Genetic Centers

Thousands of genetically caused conditions have been identified, and hundreds of these can be diagnosed prenatally. More than 200 genetic centers across the country are linked by computer to keep abreast of new advances. Still, it may take years to develop laboratory tests for prenatal diagnosis once the specific gene that causes a condition has been identified for the first time.

Keep in mind that prenatal diagnostic tests are not mandatory for your care, nor are most of them routine. They will be offered only if your medical or family history warrants them. If they are not medically indicated, the costs of the tests may not be covered by your insurance.

If a genetic condition has been detected in your family, and you are concerned about what this means for you and your children, a medical geneticist can help you to understand the implications. You may want to ask your doctor for a referral to a medical geneticist or genetic counselor, or you can make the call yourself. Your local chapter of the March of Dimes can provide information on genetic services in your area.

Environmentally Caused Birth Defects

A fetus develops in an environment designed for its safety: an amniotic sac filled with fluid to protect it within your uterus. Certain factors can change that environment to cause birth defects in the developing child: radiation, some chemical pollutants, a few maternal diseases, certain prescription drugs, recreational drugs and alcohol. Problems can also occur with the amniotic sac itself, or complications can arise during labor and delivery, either of which can result in disabilities.

There is nothing you can do to prevent some of these birth defects, but you do have control over others:

- Try to lead a healthful lifestyle while pregnant. (See Chapters 7, 8 and 9.)

- Avoid X-rays, recreational drugs, smoking and alcohol while you are pregnant.

- Find out whether your job exposes you to any known environmental causes of disabilities (for example, lead, radiation or industrial chemicals such as PCBs), so you may request a transfer or can take necessary precautions.

- Ask your doctor before you become pregnant whether any medications you take might affect pregnancy.

If you are concerned that you may have been exposed to any substance that could harm your fetus, discuss it with your doctor or genetic counselor.

The specific effects of many drugs or other environmental factors on the fetus have been well documented. When your doctor knows what to look for, there may be a prenatal test available. For instance, isotretinoin (Accutane), an acne medication taken orally, is known to cause birth defects such as hydrocephalus or cardiac abnormalities that may be detected on an ultrasound exam. However, some abnormalities associated with this medication, such as ear defects, might or might not be detectable prenatally. Women who take Accutane **must** wait at least three months after stopping use of the medication before becoming pregnant.

If a serious infection develops while you are pregnant, fetal blood sampling or other prenatal testing may be suggested to determine whether your fetus has been affected.

Prenatal Tests for Environmentally Caused Birth Defects

Birth Defects Caused by Environment and Heredity

Most congenital conditions are probably due to some combination of genetic and environmental factors. Often, it is not known how such factors affect each other, so an exact cause for these "multifactorial" or "sporadic" birth defects is impossible to pinpoint. Examples of multifactorial conditions include many congenital heart defects, clubfoot, cleft lip and cleft palate.

Neural tube defects are one of the most common and most serious multifactorial conditions. Some families are more susceptible than others to environmental factors that cause neural tube defects, such as folic acid deficiency (see page 69). Because they occur in about one or two of every 1,000 pregnancies in the United States, your doctor will probably talk to you about screening tests to determine whether your fetus is at risk for neural tube defects.

Neural Tube Defects

Neural tube defects are birth defects resulting from incorrect development of the brain or spinal cord. The most common types are anencephaly and spina bifida.

The neural tube is the embryonic structure that eventually develops into the baby's brain, spinal cord and the tissues that enclose them. The formation of the neural tube is usually complete by day 28 after conception. When the tube does not grow closed, delicate neural tissue is exposed and does not develop normally.

At age 21 days (left drawing), folds of tissue on the back of a developing embryo are rapidly growing together (see arrows). Just a day later (center drawing), the growth is almost complete. If the tissue fails to close completely (right drawing), development of the spine, muscle and skin in this region is affected and the baby will be born with a serious health problem called spina bifida.

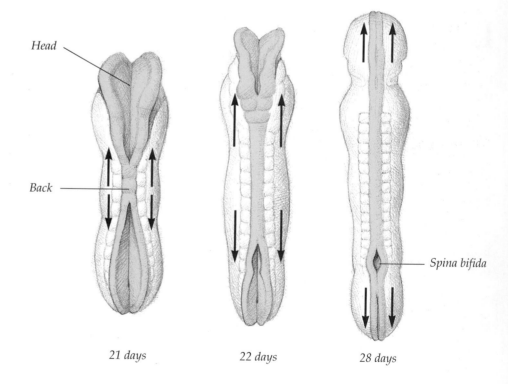

Head

Back

Spina bifida

21 days   22 days   28 days

- **Anencephaly**—This condition results when the head end of the neural tube does not close as it should and the brain and skull do not develop properly. Babies with this condition usually die shortly after birth.

- **Spina bifida**—In this disorder, a section of the developing spinal cord, usually the lower back, does not grow closed properly and the vertebrae do not form as they should.

  Open spina bifida—This disorder is also called myelomeningocele. The spinal cord and nerves are not covered by skin, muscle and bone. Instead, they are covered by only a thin membrane. Newborns who have this condition can die from meningitis, an infection in the fluid surrounding the brain. The majority survive, but they experience problems, including paralysis of the legs, various degrees of hydrocephalus (increased size of the fluid-filled cavities of the brain) and lack of normal bowel and bladder control. These children are also at a higher risk of having other birth defects. (See page 383 for more information.)

  Closed spina bifida—In babies with this condition, the backbone and spinal cord have not formed properly, but the overlying skin looks almost normal. Although this type of spina bifida tends to be less severe, the range of problems depends a great deal on how much of the spinal cord and which vertebrae are involved.

What causes neural tube defects? No one knows for sure why most neural tube defects occur, but a few risk factors have been identified:

- A previous pregnancy in which the baby had a neural tube defect.

- The mother was born with a neural tube defect, or has a close relative with one.

- An increased requirement for folic acid in some genetically susceptible individuals. Folic acid is a part of the vitamin B complex. Although folic acid is found in many foods, green, leafy vegetables are a particularly good source. There is increasing evidence that vitamin supplements of folic acid help reduce the recurrence of neural tube defects. Many doctors recommend that women begin taking folic acid supplements while they are trying to conceive, because the neural tube begins developing before most women even realize they are pregnant.

- Certain drugs prescribed for seizures, such as valproic acid or carbamazepine (perhaps because they interfere with the body's ability to use folic acid). If you are taking any seizure medication, ask your doctor for precautions to observe if you are trying to conceive or are already pregnant.

- Elevated body temperatures in the mother during the first trimester. Studies have shown an association between neural tube defects and hot tubs, saunas and illnesses that cause an increase in body temperature. (For more details, see page 110.)

Because 90 percent of pregnancies with neural tube defects occur in women who have none of the known risk factors listed above, the MSAFP and triple tests are useful for identifying affected fetuses. Most neural tube defects are detectable on a detailed ultrasound exam.

Prenatal Screening Tests

Knowing the causes of many birth defects helps determine whether your fetus may be at risk for certain conditions. But because most birth defects are due to unknown causes, the only way to determine your risk (or to make a diagnosis before your baby is born) is to test prenatally. The rest of this chapter discusses prenatal screening tests and prenatal diagnostic tests.

Screening tests try to identify those who are more likely to be at risk for certain conditions. They cannot diagnose disorders. Diagnostic tests are more complicated tests that can diagnose certain conditions quite accurately.

Screening tests are safe, relatively inexpensive tests that are offered to large groups of people. Their purpose is to indicate who might benefit from further, more complex diagnostic tests.

Prenatal screening tests to determine whether your fetus is more likely to have chromosome abnormalities or neural tube defects are commonly recommended. These screening tests are not mandatory (except in California, where all pregnant women must be offered the MSAFP test discussed below). Your doctor will usually ask whether you want to be tested.

Negative vs. Positive Results

Usually, the result you want to hear is that the screening test is "negative," meaning that your fetus is at low risk for having a certain condition. Screening tests are not perfect. If the result of a screening test is "negative," there is still a small chance that further tests or time will reveal that the condition is actually present (the initial results are then "false negative"). If a screening test has a "positive" result, there is a higher likelihood that your fetus has the condition. It is still possible that no disease exists (the results are then "false positive"). The proportion of false negative and false positive results varies from test to test.

Maternal Serum Alpha-Fetoprotein Test

What is it? A small sample of your blood can reveal useful information about the health of your fetus. The maternal serum alpha-fetoprotein (MSAFP) test is a common test that measures the level of alpha-fetoprotein (AFP) in the mother's blood. Its main purpose is to screen for neural tube defects; it's also used to help in screening for chromosome abnormalities in the fetus.

AFP is a protein produced naturally by the fetus and passed into the mother's bloodstream. The function of AFP is uncertain, but it may help transport materials in the blood. Health professionals often shorten the name of this test, referring to it as an AFP test.

What is the triple test? The triple test is another method of screening maternal blood to detect fetal spinal defects and chromosome abnormalities, especially Down syndrome. It consists of lab tests performed on one blood sample between the 15th and 20th week of pregnancy to analyze three substances normally present in pregnant women:

1. MSAFP
2. Human chorionic gonadotropin (HCG), a hormone produced in the placenta
3. Estriol, an estrogen produced by both the fetus and the placenta

Sometimes the triple test is referred to as an MSAFP+ test.

The values obtained from these three tests are interpreted on the basis of your age, weight and race, the age of the fetus and a few other factors relating to your current health. This information is compared with data that show the range of the three levels for thousands of women who had normal pregnancies.

One study showed that in addition to detecting open neural tube defects, these three test results, examined together, increase the detection of Down syndrome to 60 percent (compared with 20 percent for the AFP test by itself).

When is AFP testing done? Levels of AFP vary with different stages of pregnancy, so it is essential that your pregnancy is correctly dated for accurate assessment of the results. Although the AFP test can be done between 15 and 20 weeks of gestational age, it is most accurate when performed between the 16th and 18th week after the first day of your last menstrual period.

Why is it done? High levels of AFP are often linked to neural tube defects and a few other rare conditions; low levels are sometimes associated with Down syndrome and other chromosome abnormalities.

The triple test is used to indicate whether your fetus is at a higher risk for having one of these conditions. In other words, an abnormal test result does not necessarily mean your child will have a birth defect. Conversely, a normal result does not guarantee a healthy child.

Although some cases of neural tube defects and chromosome abnormalities will not be detected with maternal serum testing, the tests do serve as useful indicators of which fetuses are at higher risk for these conditions. The results of these tests are sometimes better predictors of these conditions than using maternal age or prior medical history alone to define risk.

Why do open neural tube defects increase the level of AFP? Open neural tube defects leave an exposed opening on the body of the fetus. Without a protective cover of skin, it is much easier for the alpha-fetoprotein to leak from the open surface into the amniotic fluid. With more AFP in the amniotic fluid, increased amounts can diffuse into the mother's bloodstream.

What else can cause elevated levels of AFP? Of 1,000 women who undergo AFP screening, between 25 and 50 will have results that are higher than normal. Only about two of the 1,000 will have a fetus with a neural tube defect.

If your test shows elevated levels of AFP, other causes include the following:

- Your pregnancy is not dated correctly. AFP levels normally increase during the first 20 weeks of pregnancy. If the gestational age of your fetus is

> *"I didn't want to have an amnio because I did not want to be faced with the decision of whether or not to continue the pregnancy, but I didn't mind having the ultrasound and the AFP blood test. The results of my AFP came back negative, which I found very reassuring."*
>
> —A mother's experience

> *"I think you assume your child is healthy, so even though my triple test came back negative for my first pregnancy, it didn't provide any extra reassurance for me. During my second pregnancy, the triple test showed a higher risk of Down syndrome, and I felt we were being hurried into making a decision about whether to continue testing and even whether to continue the pregnancy. Looking back, I wish we had made a decision, before the test, about how we would handle a positive result. We decided not to have further tests, but it did make me question what was going on for the rest of the pregnancy, until our little girl was born healthy."*
>
> —A mother's experience

actually older than was estimated, then AFP levels will be higher than expected.

- You are carrying twins. Your AFP levels will be elevated because there are two babies producing the AFP instead of one.

- Your fetus has a less common "open" birth defect that can also cause an increase in AFP. For example, if the baby's abdominal wall does not close completely, there will be an opening through which more AFP will leak out. Some rare skin conditions or intestinal blockages also increase AFP levels.

- A fetal blood vessel in the placenta has bled, allowing fetal cells containing high amounts of AFP to cross over to the mother.

- There is a defect in the placental wall. This also enables more AFP to cross over to the mother. Placental wall defects sometimes occur in pregnant women who have high blood pressure or who contract other illnesses that damage the placenta.

- The initial interpretation of your test results did not consider your weight, race or the presence of diabetes, all of which also affect AFP levels.

What if my AFP levels are high? Although abnormally high levels of AFP are sure to cause anxiety, the great majority of pregnant women with high AFP levels will be found to have nothing wrong.

Some doctors will recommend repeating the AFP or triple test to compare the results with those of your first test; most doctors will suggest an ultrasound exam to view the fetus. This procedure establishes whether there is more than one fetus and confirms the gestational age. Many neural tube defects and other structural problems can actually be seen on the scan.

When an ultrasound exam can't explain the high levels of AFP, the next step is often amniocentesis to check the amniotic fluid level of AFP. Of every 50 pregnancies investigated with amniocentesis after a high result on the AFP or triple test, 48 will have normal levels of amniotic fluid AFP, which indicate that the risk of a neural tube defect is low. For the remaining two pregnancies, the chance of having a fetus with a neural tube defect is high.

What can cause low levels of AFP? The most common reason is an incorrect estimation of the age of the fetus. Some fetuses with Down syndrome, trisomy 13 or trisomy 18 may have a low level of AFP. Maternal diabetes can cause a low level of AFP.

Sometimes there is an undetected miscarriage or a molar pregnancy, which will result in miscarriage. (See page 144 for a discussion of molar pregnancy.)

What if my AFP levels are low? The next step is usually to offer an ultrasound exam to assess the age and development of the fetus or to determine whether it has died. If the ultrasound exam does not provide an explanation, amniocentesis may be offered to obtain fetal cells for chromosome analysis, especially for Down syndrome.

What are the risks of AFP testing? There are no direct risks to you or your fetus, because maternal testing requires only a small blood sample from the mother, but increased anxiety is common. For women who are told there is a problem with their test results, there may be a great deal of emotional stress, and further testing such as an ultrasound exam or amniocentesis may be recommended. Although most of these women will not have an affected baby, they may experience anxiety waiting to find out.

How long does it take to get the results? The results are usually ready in a few days, depending on the lab performing the tests. Ask your doctor when you can expect to hear.

Is the AFP test accurate? The AFP test was developed to screen for the possibility of a fetal neural tube defect, and it has proved to be a very useful test for this purpose. About 90 percent of neural tube defects are detected accurately.

Although the AFP test is not the primary test for Down syndrome, it can detect some cases of Down syndrome and other trisomies.

The triple test is just as accurate at screening for neural tube defects and has the advantage of improving the screen for Down syndrome. The potential for false positive and false negative results inherent in screening tests makes the AFP and triple tests somewhat controversial. However, their safety to mother and fetus, relatively low cost and usefulness for detecting most neural tube defects are the reasons many doctors offer these maternal screening tests to all pregnant women.

Do you want a prenatal screening test?

Before you say "yes":

- Ask yourself how you will feel if the results are abnormal.
- If the results are abnormal, will you want to continue with more prenatal testing to find out whether your fetus has a congenital condition?
- Do you need to ask the cost first, and whether insurance will cover it?

Before you say "no":

- Would you want to know during your pregnancy whether there is a problem affecting your fetus's health?
- Will you worry more not knowing?
- If a problem was identified prenatally, could anything be done to improve the health of your fetus?

Prenatal Diagnostic Tests

Prenatal diagnostic tests are designed to identify certain birth defects in the fetus. Although prenatal diagnostic tests can diagnose some conditions very accurately, a normal test result does not guarantee a healthy infant. There are still many birth defects for which no prenatal tests exist, such as vision loss, hearing impairment or learning disabilities. But the number of disorders that can be detected prenatally is increasing rapidly, and some diagnoses can be made as early as the first trimester.

There are many reasons why prenatal diagnostic tests may be recommended, based on your medical and family history, physical examination and results of lab tests:

- Mother is 35 or older (the risk for some birth defects increases with advanced maternal age)
- Previous child with a chromosome abnormality
- Previous child with a neural tube defect
- Abnormal results from screening tests or MSAFP test
- Parents are at risk for (or are known carriers of) a genetic or metabolic condition that can be diagnosed prenatally
- Exposure to a known cell-destroying agent during pregnancy (such as radiation, chemotherapy or certain other medications)

- Previous child with malformations or mental retardation
- Previous unexplained stillbirth or more than two miscarriages
- Pregnancy at risk for conditions diagnosable by ultrasound examination, such as skeletal abnormalities
- Father is 45 or older (the risk for new autosomal dominant conditions, such as skeletal abnormalities, increases with paternal age)
- Pregnancy is at risk for conditions that can be treated with prenatal therapy, or for which special interventions may be required at birth (Rh incompatibility or certain congenital heart defects)
- Parental anxiety

Ultrasound Exam

What is an ultrasound exam? An ultrasound exam is a non-invasive (non-surgical) method of getting a picture of what is going on inside your body without radiation. An ultrasound exam uses high-frequency sound waves that cannot be heard by humans. When used in obstetrics, the sound waves are directed into your uterus with a small plastic device called a transducer. The sound waves reflect off bones and tissue and are converted into black and white images on a small screen, where you will be able to "see" the fetus.

When is it done? An ultrasound exam can be done at any time during pregnancy. It may be repeated at different stages to monitor the baby's growth and development if there is cause for concern. An advanced-level ultrasound exam is offered only when a problem is suspected.

Some medical centers offer ultrasound examinations between the 16th and 20th weeks of pregnancy. By that time, major structural abnormalities can be diagnosed and all four chambers of the heart can be seen, and thus some congenital heart defects can be detected. Fathers are usually welcome to stay for the ultrasound examination, and most enjoy watching the baby move. It is helpful to have your partner or a close friend with you for support in case a problem is detected on the scan.

Why is it done? Ultrasound examination is usually performed for the following reasons:

- Confirm pregnancy (or detect miscarriage)
- Date the pregnancy (an ultrasound exam is extremely accurate for judging the fetal age before 20 weeks of pregnancy)
- Learn the number of fetuses
- Evaluate risks to pregnancy (such as implantation of the embryo in an abnormal location)
- Examine the fetus for structural variations (one large study reported that

---

"The ultrasound was scary at first. It was the only prenatal test we did, so it was the only clue we had as to the baby's health. It was somewhat comforting to hear that everything they could see on the ultrasound looked normal, but I knew there were some things it couldn't tell.

"In the beginning, pregnancy is focused on how you feel. But when I saw the baby on ultrasound, it was the first time I realized there was a person inside. I thought, 'Wow, I've got to take care of this child,' as opposed to focusing on 'Gee, I'm getting fat.'

"I was very teary-eyed as I watched. Until I felt the baby kick, which may not have been for another month or two, I needed more than a heartbeat to bond with the baby."

—A mother's experience

"Watching the ultrasound exam, it was eerie to be able to see inside (my wife's abdomen), but I felt joyous seeing the fetus move around and knowing it was my child-to-be.

"All along, my wife had been the one experiencing the pregnancy—I wasn't the one feeling nauseated or tired. The ultrasound exam served as a reality check: I was able to experience seeing the baby move.

"My biggest fear was that we'd see something abnormal. It was a tremendous relief to see that everything looked good."

—A father's experience

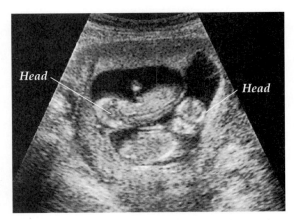

Most ultrasound scans show a healthy, normal fetus, like the 16-week-old at left. But there can be a surprise, such as the healthy, normal twins at right.

more than 50 percent of malformations were detectable with advanced-level ultrasound testing)
- Determine the location and development of the placenta
- Evaluate the growth rate and development of the fetus
- Assess the health of the fetus by monitoring the movements (especially in later pregnancy)

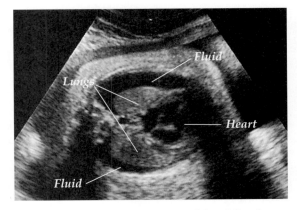

Sometimes an ultrasound exam can reveal the sex of the fetus, if the baby's genitals can be seen clearly. (Inform the technician if you would prefer not to be told.) This information is not always accurate, however, because a loop of umbilical cord between the legs can easily be mistaken for male genitals on an ultrasound scan.

Most of the time, babies are completely healthy, and an ultrasound exam is an exciting and rewarding experience for the parents. They can actually see the shape and form of their unborn baby and the heart beating in the tiny chest. Sometimes the fetus will kick or suck a thumb, and the parents begin the bonding process, perhaps perceiving the fetus as an individual for the first time.

This advanced-level (level two) ultrasound scan zooms in on the baby's chest and shows fluid beside the lungs (pleural effusion). Physicians use advanced-level ultrasound testing, which takes more time and equipment, only when they suspect a serious health problem.

What types of ultrasound examinations are there? You may undergo different types of ultrasound exams during your pregnancy.

Standard ultrasound exam. This test creates a two-dimensional picture, called a sonogram, of your uterus and the fetus within. This is useful for taking measurements and assessing development of your fetus and placenta. This type of exam, sometimes called a level one ultrasound exam, lasts about 20 minutes and may be available in your doctor's office.

Advanced-level ultrasound exam. This exam is sometimes called level two ultrasound. It is a more thorough examination that requires more expertise and sophisticated equipment. The exam may last more than an hour. It takes a rapid series of sonograms to document fetal movement, which may be important in diagnosing certain conditions. Advanced-level ultrasound exams are often used in high-risk pregnancies, or those that have had irregularities found on a routine ultrasound exam. State-of-the-art machines may have color flow imaging to show blood flow patterns.

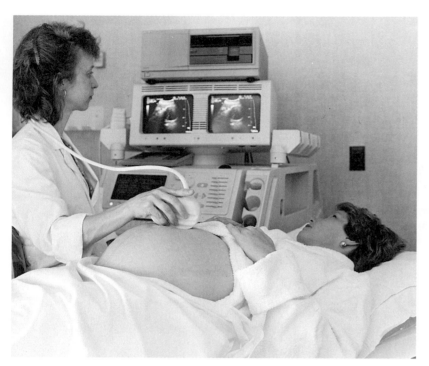

In an ultrasound exam, high-frequency sound waves penetrate your uterus to reveal on a nearby monitor screen an image of your developing baby. The test is painless, safe and often exciting, offering the first actual glimpse of your developing baby.

Transvaginal ultrasound exam. For this test, a small transducer is inserted in the vagina up to the entrance of the uterus to create images of the fetus on a monitor. This method is sometimes preferred for investigating pregnancy complications during the first trimester.

Fetal echocardiography. In this procedure, sound waves are observed reflecting from the baby's heart. It is used when fetal cardiac defects are suspected.

What are the risks of ultrasound examination?
Ultrasound has been used in obstetrics for more than 20 years, and there is no evidence that the sound waves harm the mother or the fetus. It does not involve the use of radiation or X-rays. The exam is painless, except for the discomfort of pressure on a very full bladder.

How is an ultrasound exam done?
You will be asked to drink several glasses of water before your exam. A full bladder serves as a useful landmark on the monitor, and the uterus is put into a position that allows it to be examined more easily.

You will lie flat on a table, and some oil or gel (which may feel cold) will be put on your exposed abdomen. This gel acts as a conductor for the sound waves.

The doctor or ultrasound technician uses a transducer to direct sound waves into your uterus. Although the images on the monitor are difficult to sort out at first, the ultrasound operator will explain what you are seeing. As the transducer is moved back and forth, you can watch a "tour" of your uterus on the screen. Occasionally, the operator will stop to measure the head, abdomen or length of the thigh bone (femur) to document growth or to take a picture (sonogram) to document important structures.

After the examination, your doctor or technician will explain the findings.

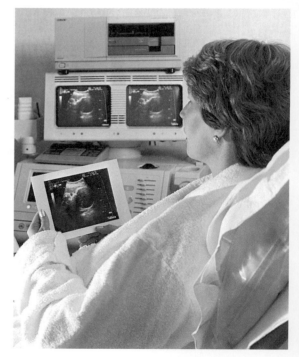

Some medical centers offer copies of ultrasound scans, which make good keepsakes for your baby's photo album.

Amniocentesis

What is amniocentesis? Amniocentesis ("amnio" or "tap") is a procedure in which a needle is used to remove a sample of fluid from the amniotic sac surrounding the fetus. Ultrasound is used to help your doctor guide the needle to a safe area away from your fetus. The amniotic fluid, which contains cells shed by the fetus, is then studied in a laboratory for genetic analysis and biochemical tests.

When is it done? If done for chromosome analysis or molecular DNA analysis, amniocentesis is usually performed after the 16th week of pregnancy, but it can be performed up to a month earlier at some medical centers.

If a woman needs to give birth early for some medical reason, amniocentesis might be performed shortly before delivery to assess fetal lung maturity.

Why is it done? In the first half of your pregnancy, your doctor may offer amniocentesis if your fetus is suspected to be at increased risk for chromosome abnormalities, inherited disorders or neural tube defects.

Chromosome abnormalities. Conditions such as Down syndrome may be detected by examining the fetal chromosomes under a microscope. A chromosome analysis will also establish the sex of your fetus, so let your doctor know if you don't want to be told. (Amniocentesis is not offered for sex determination alone.)

Genetic disorders. Disorders known to run in your family (such as cystic fibrosis) often can be tested for by studying the DNA in fetal genes. Complex techniques involving genetic probes and markers are used to identify malfunctioning genes.

Neural tube defects. Conditions such as anencephaly and spina bifida may be found by analyzing the amniotic fluid. Although amniocentesis cannot indicate the severity of these birth defects, very high levels of alpha-fetoprotein (AFP) may indicate the presence of a neural tube defect or other "open wall" birth defect (one not closed over by skin and other tissue). The AFP level can be falsely elevated if any fetal blood gets into the sample, but advanced-level ultrasound can detect the physical changes caused by most neural tube defects. The AFP level will be in the normal range in 10 to 30 percent of fetuses with closed spina bifida, but in some of these cases the disorder can be detected with advanced-level ultrasound at 18 to 20 weeks.

Fetal lung assessment. This is important if you need to deliver early. By testing the amniotic fluid, doctors can tell whether the baby's lungs are developed enough to breathe on his or her own. This is done during the last half of pregnancy.

> "My husband and I decided to have amniocentesis because my age (35) put our fetus at an increased risk for Down syndrome.
>
> "For me, the anesthetic was like a little prick, but the amnio needle felt like a puncture wound for a split second as it entered my uterus. After that, it was not uncomfortable as the needle probed around.
>
> "Two weeks later, we celebrated the normal results by going out to dinner and opening the envelope that told us the baby's sex."
>
> —A mother's experience

> "There was a problem with my AFP results, so my doctor offered amnio. I had a severely retarded uncle, and my husband and I felt it would be too scary to go through pregnancy not knowing if the baby had Down syndrome. We had decided we would have the baby anyway, but we had to know.
>
> "I thought the needle would be a little poke, but it was painful. I was surprised when the doctor told me I should take it easy for the rest of the day.
>
> "We had to wait a long time for the results. My doctor called and told me the chromosomes looked normal. I said, 'So my baby will be fine?' He said, 'I can't promise that, but the chromosomes are normal.'"
>
> —A mother's experience

Rh disease. This causes antibodies in the mother's blood to attack fetal blood cells. Amniocentesis is useful for evaluating the condition of the fetus to reduce complications. This testing is also done during the last half of pregnancy.

What are the risks of amniocentesis?

Amniocentesis is performed about 200,000 times a year in the United States and is considered to be a relatively safe procedure. The risk of a miscarriage caused by amniocentesis ranges from one in 200 to one in 400. At centers where doctors do the procedure frequently and use continuous ultrasound to monitor placement of the needle, the risk is closer to one in 400. (After the third month of pregnancy, three to four of every 100 pregnancies will end in miscarriage even when no prenatal tests are used.)

In the rare instances that amniocentesis causes a miscarriage, it is usually because an infection develops in the uterus, the water breaks or labor is induced prematurely. The fetus is rarely poked by the needle when continuous ultrasound is used.

It is not uncommon for women to experience mild complications such as cramping or leakage or discomfort around the needle site. Be sure to call your doctor if these symptoms continue or become severe.

Women's descriptions of the procedure range from "uncomfortable" to "like a bee sting" to "fleetingly painful" (when the local anesthetic or the brief needle puncture is experienced). Because the uterine wall cannot be numbed, you will feel the puncture sensation of the amniocentesis needle. One woman said it was so fascinating to watch the baby on the monitor that she was unaware of any discomfort at all.

Women who feel tense at the very mention of a needle may find it helpful to practice relaxation or breathing exercises.

How is amniocentesis done?

The procedure may be performed in your doctor's office, or it may be done in a hospital on an outpatient basis. It usually takes about 45 minutes, with only five minutes needed for the needle insertion and withdrawal of fluid.

Because you will be having an ultrasound exam, you will need to drink several glasses of water before the test. The preliminary ultrasound exam is done to determine whether you are carrying more than one baby, determine the gestational age, measure the baby and evaluate the shape and position of your uterus and placenta.

Your abdomen is cleansed with an antiseptic. Then a sterile ultrasound transducer is placed on your abdomen to determine a safe site for the needle to enter. Some doctors offer a local anesthetic, which can be injected near the site to numb your abdomen if you choose.

A long, hollow needle is inserted through your abdominal wall and into your uterus, where it passes through the amniotic sac and enters the amniotic fluid. A small sample of fluid is withdrawn (approximately one to two tablespoons). If the doctor can't obtain enough fluid from this site, the needle is taken out and inserted in another spot. Because the amniotic fluid is partly composed of fetal urine, it should be clear and slightly straw-colored.

Your doctor will watch the fetus on the ultrasound monitor to make sure all is well. A small bandage will be placed on your abdomen to cover the puncture site. The samples are labeled and sent to the laboratory.

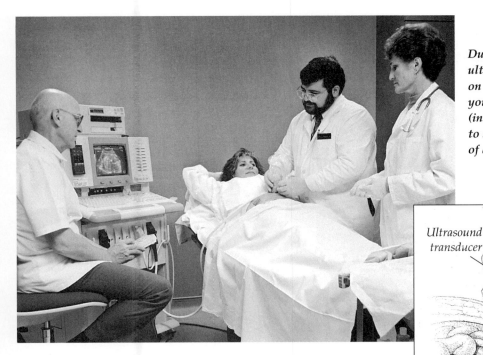

During amniocentesis, an ultrasound transducer shows on a screen the positions of your fetus and the needle (inset), enabling your doctor to safely withdraw a sample of amniotic fluid for testing.

Ultrasound transducer

How long do I have to wait for my test results? Many of the biochemical test results are back in a few hours or a few days. Some chromosome results can be available in seven days, but it sometimes requires two weeks to obtain the results. Extremely rare tests may need to be sent to labs across the country, and it may take longer to get the results. Chromosome studies are highly accurate and usually serve to reassure women, so they can enjoy their pregnancies and minimize anxiety.

***W**hat is chorionic villus sampling (CVS)?* The chorionic villi are microscopic finger-like projections that line the chorion, a part of the placenta. Introduced in 1984, CVS is a procedure to remove a small sample of chorionic villi cells from the placenta at the point where it attaches to the uterine wall.

There are two ways to obtain the cell sample. In the more common transcervical method, ultrasound is used to guide a thin tube called a catheter through your cervix to the placenta. A small amount of chorionic villi cells are then gently suctioned into the catheter.

The transabdominal method is similar to amniocentesis, and also depends on ultrasound guidance. A long, thin needle is inserted through your abdomen to the placenta, where a small tissue sample is withdrawn.

These cells are useful for genetic testing because the placenta is made of the same genetic material as the fetus.

When is CVS done? CVS is usually performed between nine and 12 weeks from your last menstrual period.

How long does it take to get the results? Because CVS provides a larger sample of cells than amniocentesis, results take a little less time to obtain. Preliminary results may be possible within a day or two, but laboratory studies may take up to seven days (or longer for tests on extremely rare disorders).

Chorionic Villus Sampling (CVS)

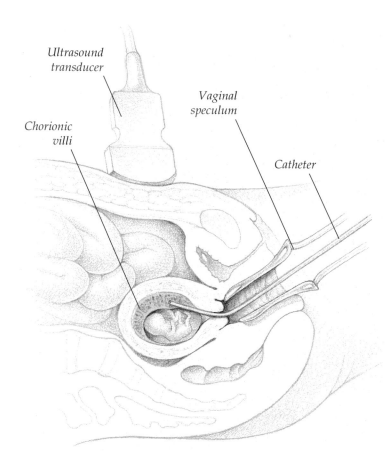

Ultrasound transducer

Vaginal speculum

Chorionic villi

Catheter

A vaginal speculum opens the vagina, and a catheter is inserted through the cervix into the chorionic villi during a transcervical chorionic villus sampling (CVS) test. A sample is gently removed by suction, for testing in a laboratory. As with amniocentesis, the doctor uses an ultrasound image to check the position of the fetus and to guide the catheter into position.

Why is CVS done? The primary reason for CVS is for early detection of chromosome abnormalities, such as Down syndrome, and other genetic disorders. CVS cannot diagnose neural tube defects because it does not sample any amniotic fluid for testing levels of alpha-fetoprotein (AFP).

Although CVS does not provide as much information as amniocentesis, it has the advantage of being available earlier in pregnancy. (Early detection, once considered the main benefit of CVS, is now possible with early amniocentesis at some medical centers.) There are also certain extremely rare autosomal recessive disorders for which CVS is preferred over amniocentesis.

What are the risks and accuracy of CVS? The risks of a pregnancy ending in miscarriage are higher with CVS (one in 100) than with amniocentesis (about one in 200, and one in 400 at some centers). Both methods of CVS require more expertise than amniocentesis, so it is important to have an experienced obstetrician. If your doctor does not do CVS, he or she may be able to recommend an experienced obstetrician who does.

Recent studies suggesting an association between CVS and limb malformations have made some doctors hesitant to offer this procedure.

With CVS, there is a 1 percent or less risk of getting false positive results (indicating that your fetus has a chromosome abnormality when it does not). Such results occur in rare cases, because the placenta can have chromosome abnormalities that the fetus does not have. If your CVS test results are positive for chromosome abnormalities, most doctors will offer to confirm the diagnosis with amniocentesis. A negative test result is considered accurate in establishing that there are no chromosome abnormalities in the fetus.

Other complications of CVS are similar to those of amniocentesis: infection, spotting (vaginal bleeding), cramping and pain at the needle site. If you experience any persistent or severe spotting or leaking of amniotic fluid, fever, chills or cramping, call your doctor.

Most women find the transcervical procedure painless, although perhaps as uncomfortable as any vaginal procedure. Women who have the transabdominal method describe much the same experience as women who have amniocentesis.

How is CVS done? CVS is usually done at a medical center on an outpatient basis by an obstetrician with specialized training in CVS.

An ultrasound exam will be done to determine the position of the placenta and whether

"Trying to decide whether the risk of CVS was worth the benefit was the most morally difficult decision of my life.

"CVS was very easy to tolerate, but I had some bleeding afterward, which was scary. I felt a sense of relief when I learned that my son's chromosomes were normal."

—A mother's experience

the sample should be obtained through the cervix or the abdomen.

If the transabdominal method is chosen, ultrasound is used to guide a thin needle through the lower abdomen into the chorionic villi, where a small sample is aspirated into the needle.

For the transcervical method, you lie on your back with your feet in stirrups, as you do for routine pelvic exams. A speculum is inserted into your vagina, and your cervix is cleansed. With ultrasound guidance, a catheter is inserted through your cervix into the chorionic villi, where a small amount of the tissue is gently suctioned into the tube.

The tissue sample is removed and put into special containers. If there is not enough tissue, the procedure may be repeated. Your doctor will observe your fetus on ultrasound after the procedure to watch for signs of trouble. The entire procedure takes about 45 minutes, including the ultrasound exam.

CVS is not recommended for women who:
- Have experienced vaginal bleeding during pregnancy
- Have an active infection (such as genital herpes)
- Are carrying twins

Transcervical CVS is not recommended for women who:
- Have uterine fibroids
- Have their uterus at an angle that would make passage of the catheter difficult

---

Percutaneous Umbilical Blood Sampling (PUBS)

What is percutaneous umbilical blood sampling (PUBS)? PUBS was developed in 1983 as an improved method of obtaining fetal blood samples. The procedure is performed with ultrasound guidance to insert a needle through the mother's abdominal and uterine walls into a vessel in the umbilical cord, where a sample of fetal blood is withdrawn for laboratory analysis. This procedure, which requires highly skilled personnel, is available only at some large medical centers in the United States. Its safety and success are largely dependent on the experience of the person performing the test. It is performed in an outpatient setting and takes 45 minutes to an hour.

Why is it done? PUBS is done when you can't get the information you need from amniocentesis, ultrasound or CVS. The most common reason for performing PUBS is for rapid chromosome analysis or for evaluating fetuses at risk for certain blood disorders (such as fetal hemolytic disease or fetal anemia). PUBS can also determine drug levels in the fetus or detect whether the fetus has contracted a serious infection from the mother who has been exposed during pregnancy (such as toxoplasmosis or cytomegalovirus). Some genetic conditions or other metabolic disorders may also be diagnosed with PUBS.

When is it done? PUBS is usually performed between the 18th and 36th week of pregnancy. Although it is a very delicate test, and blood vessels may be very fragile before the 18th week, some medical centers perform the test as early as the 16th week and right up until the end of pregnancy.

What are the risks of PUBS? The risk of miscarriage attributed to PUBS is generally thought to be higher than that with amniocentesis, or about 2 percent at centers where PUBS is done often. Other complications are similar to those of amniocentesis (including infection, cramping, and bleeding and leakage and discomfort around the needle site). There is a small risk of a blood clot in the umbilical cord or a tearing of the umbilical vein, which may cause fetal death.

How is PUBS done? As with amniocentesis, you lie on a table, and oil or gel is spread on your abdomen. Advanced-level ultrasound is used to find the site of the umbilical cord insertion on the placenta. Then your abdomen is cleansed and covered with an antiseptic solution. The transducer is covered in sterile plastic. In some circumstances, a medication may be given to keep the fetus from moving during the procedure.

Using ultrasound guidance, the doctor inserts a needle through your abdominal and uterine walls to the umbilical cord, and a small amount of fetus blood is withdrawn and sent to the laboratory.

Other Procedures

While research continues for safer, more accurate prenatal tests that can be offered in the first trimester, many other procedures are being developed to examine fetuses that have specific risks.

One experimental procedure is fetoscopy, in which a viewing instrument is inserted through a small incision in the mother's anesthetized abdomen, under ultrasound guidance, to actually view parts of the fetus and placenta. This may be used to confirm a limb abnormality or other suspected visible defect. The major risk with fetoscopy is miscarriage or preterm labor, which may occur in 5 percent of pregnancies when fetoscopy is done by experienced physicians.

Another test is fetal skin sampling, done during fetoscopy, in which tiny snips of skin are taken from the baby's scalp, trunk or buttocks. These tissue fragments can be analyzed for congenital skin conditions.

Common Anxieties About Prenatal Testing

How Do I Decide Whether to Have a Prenatal Test?

Your doctor will recommend tests that will provide the information you need based on your family history, screening test results, medical evaluation and other risk factors. In addition, you will want to consider the following:

Usefulness. What can you do with this information? Will the results affect your decision to continue with the pregnancy? Will they enable you and your doctor to provide better care for the fetus during pregnancy or at delivery? If you would not do anything with the information, why test?

Timing. Find out when the test is given and how long it takes to get results. This information is important for couples who choose to keep news of their pregnancy private until they know their test results. If you want to have the option of terminating your pregnancy, early abortion has fewer maternal risks.

Risks of the procedure. If you have had problems with infertility, even a slight difference in risks of miscarriage may be significant to you. In addition to pregnancy loss, ask your doctor what side effects you can expect with the procedure (bleeding, cramping or possible harm to the fetus).

Cost. Ask your doctor what the total costs are for the procedure (prices may vary a great deal among medical centers), including laboratory fees. Find out whether your insurance will cover all the expenses. If you have no coverage, a social worker or genetic counselor may be able to help you get information about possible financial assistance.

I t is your life and your baby, and you have every right to ask your doctor about his or her experience regarding a certain procedure, especially the less common procedures such as PUBS or early amniocentesis. There is no minimal number of tests performed that makes someone an expert, but you should ask the following questions:

- How often do you perform this procedure? (Is it something you usually do? Do you feel comfortable doing it?)
- What kind of pregnancy loss rate have you had with this procedure? (Most doctors are willing to discuss their experience with you.)
- What kind of follow-up has been done to determine potential late effects of this procedure (such as limb deficiencies that may be associated with CVS)?

There is more to choosing doctors than simply knowing their expertise. You want a doctor you have confidence in, but also one with whom you can communicate and feel comfortable.

If your doctor does not perform the procedure you need, or you decide to seek a second opinion, a genetic counselor can assist you in finding someone with the necessary expertise. Counselors can make suggestions and can contact colleagues in their field to obtain names of providers in your area.

How Do I Choose the Best Doctor to Do My Test?

D iscussing your feelings and options with your partner before testing can help a great deal to prepare you for this possibility. If you have already talked about it at a calmer time, communicating with each other will be much easier. Couples often change their minds several times about how they want to proceed.

The most likely result of all prenatal tests is a normal finding. But this information is of little comfort if you are the one who has just been told that your fetus has a life-threatening condition or a disability that will require medical intervention. After the initial shock, you may find yourselves feeling sad, angry, guilty, afraid or disbelieving.

The first thing to do is to schedule a meeting with your doctor to discuss the findings and learn as much as you can about the diagnosis. If the diagnosis may have a genetic component, you might want to ask for an immediate referral to a geneticist or a genetic counselor. Genetic disorders are often complicated, and you will need current information. A public health nurse can be of assistance in finding local specialists to help after the baby is born, and a social worker may be able to recommend financial assistance programs.

Make a list of all of your concerns so you don't forget any at this emotional time. Some questions you may want to ask include these:

- How accurate are the test results? Could there be a mistake?
- Can the baby survive with the condition? If so, what is the life expectancy?
- How will the baby be affected physically?
- Will he or she feel pain? If surgery is needed, what degree of pain will the baby experience and for how long? How will the pain be recognized and treated?
- Will my child have to undergo one or more operations or other therapies to manage the condition?
- How might the baby's mental functioning be affected?

What If the Test Results Show an Abnormal Finding?

- Are there special learning programs that can assist my child's mental development?
- What is involved in caring for a child with this condition?
- Can we talk to parents whose children have a similar condition?
- Is there a support group in our community for the families of children with this condition?
- Are there other health care professionals who can provide us with additional information to assist us in making this decision?
- What resources are available to us should we choose to terminate the pregnancy? What counseling resources are available? Is there a support group for people who have terminated pregnancies?
- What are the chances that this condition will affect our next pregnancy?

Your doctor or genetic counselor will help you acquire the information you need to make your own choices in light of your personal circumstances. In addition to the medical questions, you will want to consider your emotional and physical strength, financial resources and the family, community and state support available to you. Here are options to consider:

- Continue the pregnancy, making plans for parenting—If you choose this option, you will want to learn how the diagnosis will affect the management of your pregnancy and delivery. You may learn about therapeutic interventions for treating your baby during pregnancy or immediately after birth to improve his or her health.

  Your counselor or a social worker can help your whole family to prepare emotionally for the changes you will be making in your lifestyle, and provide you with information about resources within and beyond your community to meet your child's special needs.

- Continue the pregnancy, making plans for adoption—Your counselor can put you in touch with a social worker in the adoption office of your state's Department of Human Services, or other adoption agencies.

- End the pregnancy—The decision to have an abortion is never an easy one, even if your fetus has been diagnosed with a condition that is "incompatible with life." Even though many parents in these circumstances feel they are releasing their baby from the prospect of a limited life and do not want to prolong a dying process, they are still devastated to lose the child they have been dreaming about and planning for. Counseling, both before and after such a decision, can be invaluable in helping you to sort out your feelings.

  If you want to consider this option, get all the information you need as quickly as possible. The earlier a pregnancy is terminated, the less risk there is of having complications. Although the federal limit for performing abortions is 24 weeks, regulations vary from state to state, and finding a doctor who will terminate a pregnancy beyond 20 weeks is difficult in some communities. Your doctor or genetic counselor can help you explore your options.

  Some communities or medical centers have support groups specifically designed for couples who have chosen to terminate pregnancies after diagnosis of a genetic condition. If you feel you would benefit from such a group, don't hesitate to ask whether one is available in your area.

Know Your Options

Prenatal tests do not prevent birth defects, but they can often let you know whether an abnormality exists before your baby is born. Testing can be reassuring when the results are normal, but normal results are still no guarantee that your baby won't have a birth defect. Also, women sometimes have "false alarm" screening test results and may find themselves going through expensive and anxiety-producing procedures to prove their child is healthy.

In a malpractice climate that requires doctors to offer all medical options and document that all options were discussed, some women might feel pressured to have tests simply because the tests are available and offered. Now that you understand a little more about the types and causes of birth defects and the prenatal tests available, you will be better prepared to seek the information and guidance you need to make your own decisions.

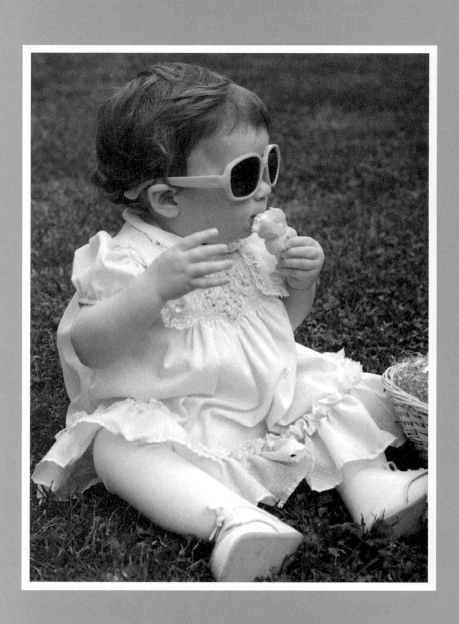

CHAPTER SEVEN

Nutrition During Pregnancy

Eating for two doesn't mean eating twice as much.
It means eating twice as well.

The best time to start thinking about good nutrition is before you plan to become pregnant. Then you can be sure that your baby will have all the essential nutrients from the moment of conception. In fact, the improvements you make in your own diet now can spark a healthful change for the whole family.

If you have a history of good eating habits, you begin your pregnancy with optimal amounts of all nutrients needed for your baby's tremendous growth and development. However, a background that includes chronic dieting, skipping meals or eating a limited variety of foods can put you both at nutritional risk.

Just how much do you know about eating right during pregnancy? Nutrition is one of those medical topics that seem to be changing constantly. Less than a fourth of Americans get information about diet and nutrition from their doctors or registered dietitians. We rely more on the mass media or our family and friends than on the experts for advice about what to eat. Although friends and relatives may mean well, it's essential that you know the facts about eating right for both you and your baby.

Extremely poor eating habits before or during pregnancy can harm both you and your baby. If you eat too few calories or nutrients, cell development can be less than ideal and your baby may be underweight at birth. Low-birth-weight babies have a greater chance for short- and long-term health problems.

In the first weeks of your pregnancy, perhaps even before you know you're going to have a baby, most of your fetus's major organs will be forming. That is why it is so critical to make nutritious eating habits part of your decision to begin a new life.

Nutrition risk factors

You may be at increased risk for poor nutrition if you:

- Have a history of chronic dieting, skipping meals or fasting
- Do not ordinarily consume a wide variety of nutritious foods
- Use cigarettes, alcohol or recreational drugs
- Are significantly underweight or overweight at the time of conception
- Are carrying more than one baby

After the first couple of months of pregnancy, your rate of metabolism and circulation increase to provide more nutrients for your developing baby. Your intestines and other organs are working harder to absorb the nutrients that will increase your ability to nourish your baby. The development of your baby's bones, tissues and organs requires different nutrients at different times throughout pregnancy. Maintaining a nutrient-rich diet will ensure that those nutrients are ready and available when your baby needs them.

Weight Gain

Pregnancy is the one time in your life when you're encouraged to gain weight. But weight gain in pregnancy doesn't mean getting fat. Your size increases for various physical reasons, including the weight of the baby you will deliver.

Over the years, the recommended amount of weight to gain during pregnancy has varied dramatically. Your mother was probably told to gain no more than 15 pounds. Twenty or 30 years ago, a minimal weight gain was thought to be best for mother and baby. Now, research has proved that women who are normal weight at the time of conception have the healthiest pregnancies and babies if they gain 25 to 35 pounds.

Your caregiver will estimate the right amount of weight for you to gain during your pregnancy. Individual recommendations will vary based on various factors, including your pre-pregnancy weight, your medical history, your health and the health of your developing baby.

Your baby's weight is partly determined by how much weight you gain during your pregnancy. And a normal birth weight is important for good health. A desirable weight for a full-term newborn is between 6½ and 9 pounds. Babies born at these healthy weights have:

- A lower rate of infant death
- Fewer mental and physical handicaps
- Fewer serious childhood illnesses
- A head start, both physically and mentally, over smaller babies

Strive for a slow and steady increase in your weight, but keep in mind that individual women gain weight at different rates. Here are some general guides to weight gain:

- First trimester   1 to 1½ pounds a month
- Second trimester   ½ to ¾ pound a week
- Third trimester   ¾ to 1 pound a week

Calorie Needs

To gain extra weight, you will need to consume more than 100,000 extra calories during your pregnancy. That may seem like a lot of extra calories, but over the course of the nine months you'll be pregnant, it's not.

Early in pregnancy, your developing fetus is almost exclusively dependent on the calories you provide through eating and drinking. This need by the fetus does not mean that you have to eat excessively, but you may need to eat more often. In fact, some of the discomforts of early pregnancy—feelings of hunger, nausea or vomiting—are often relieved by intermittent snacking. If you feel more comfortable snacking, eat smaller meals to avoid excessive weight gain.

As the placenta develops into the second trimester, hormones are produced that begin to ensure a more steady supply of nourishment for the fetus, and frequent snacking becomes less necessary. By this time, you'll probably be feeling better and eating regular meals.

During your first trimester, an extra 200 calories a day over your normal intake will provide for the recommended 1 to 1½ pounds of weight you should gain each month. It's important that these calories are from foods that offer the most nutrition for you and your unborn baby. For example, a slice of whole-grain bread, a glass of skim milk and 1 ounce of lean meat will add about 200 calories.

In your second and third trimesters, you'll need a total of 300 to 500 extra calories a day beyond your normal diet. The more active you are, the more calories you will need.

Your health care provider will monitor your weight gain at each prenatal visit.

Where you'll gain the weight

Your baby	6½ to 9 pounds
Placenta	1½ pounds
Amniotic fluid	2 pounds
Breast enlargement	1 to 3 pounds
Uterus enlargement	2 pounds
Fat stores and muscle development	4 to 8 pounds
Increased blood volume	3 to 4 pounds
Increased fluid volume	2 to 3 pounds
Total	22 to 32½ pounds

Nutrition Basics

There are lots of ways to keep track of your food intake. The key is finding a system that works for you. No, you don't have to keep a food diary or analyze your meals and snacks—but you do need to pay attention to some basic guidelines.

Food Guide Pyramid

The Food Guide Pyramid, developed by the U.S. Department of Agriculture and endorsed by the Department of Health and Human Services, is a good model for healthful daily eating. This graphic pyramid, shown on page 88, replaces the old basic four food groups and is designed to help you plan a nutritious diet.

The steps of the pyramid show how to make the best food choices for you and your baby. Each of the food groups provides some, but not all, of the nutrients required for a healthful diet. Because foods in one group can't replace those in another, you can't skip or eliminate any category of food if you want to eat right. No one food group is more important than another—for good health and a healthy baby you need them all.

The pyramid conveys three essential elements of a healthful diet:

1. Proportion. The shape of the pyramid tells you at a glance that grains, vegetables and fruits should make up the bulk of your diet.

2. Moderation. Foods from the meat and milk groups, in moderate amounts, contribute to a healthful diet. The tip of the pyramid shows the fats and sweets group, which is not omitted from healthful eating but is proportionately the smallest food group in the pyramid.

3. Variety. Choose different foods from each major food group every day. The pyramid doesn't make any food off-limits, but guides you to choose appropriate amounts of different foods.

Eating at least three meals daily is important. When you eat three meals a day, you're more likely to consume a greater variety of foods and to keep your appetite in check. Healthful snacks can also help ensure that you remain on target.

We have modified the Food Guide Pyramid to reflect a pregnant woman's special nutritional needs. The recommended servings provide between 1,800 and 2,800 calories daily. You might find it helpful to keep a tally of the foods you eat. This way you can become aware of your food selections and work toward meeting the recommendations. If you find you're low in one or more categories and higher in others, try to balance your selections. If you're too full at meals, try to include healthful snacks. If you're routinely unable to meet the recommendations for any of the food groups, discuss this with your health care provider.

Remember that a "serving" of food as described in the pyramid is not necessarily the amount that you should eat at one time. A serving is simply a way to measure foods so that you can keep track of your intake. A plate of spaghetti may have three half-cup servings of pasta, but that doesn't mean you've had too much. You don't need to measure servings, just use the amounts listed as a general guide. For combination foods like pizza, do the best you can to estimate the food group servings of the main ingredients. For example, a slice of cheese pizza would count toward servings in the bread (crust), vegetable (tomato sauce) and milk (cheese) groups.

The Food Guide Pyramid is your guide to healthful eating throughout your pregnancy. The servings shown are the minimal numbers you should eat daily.

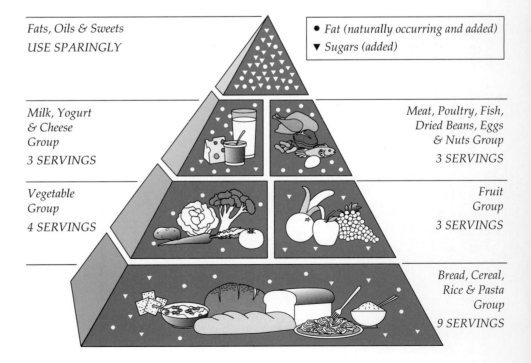

Fats, Oils & Sweets
USE SPARINGLY

• *Fat (naturally occurring and added)*
▼ *Sugars (added)*

Milk, Yogurt & Cheese Group
3 SERVINGS

Meat, Poultry, Fish, Dried Beans, Eggs & Nuts Group
3 SERVINGS

Vegetable Group
4 SERVINGS

Fruit Group
3 SERVINGS

Bread, Cereal, Rice & Pasta Group
9 SERVINGS

Eat at least the minimal recommended servings from each level of the pyramid. If you need to gain more weight or if you have special nutritional concerns, seek help from a registered dietitian or your doctor.

The base of the pyramid includes breads, cereals, rice, pasta and other grain foods. You need plenty of servings from these foods daily to maintain an adequate supply of vitamins, minerals and fiber. Most grains are naturally low in fat and high in nutrition. If you are gaining weight too rapidly, cut back on the toppings you add to bread and other grain foods, but don't cut back on these staples of a good diet. However, if you're having trouble gaining enough weight, this is one of the food groups from which to add extra servings.

Breads and Cereals

Best-bet grains
Bagels and muffins (low-fat)
Brown and white rice
Enriched breads and cereals
Fruit and nut breads (low-fat)
Pancakes
Tortillas and pita bread
Whole-grain breads, cereals, rolls and crackers
Whole-wheat pasta and noodles

What's a serving?
1 slice bread
½ bagel or bun
1 ounce cold cereal (½ to ¾ cup)
½ cup cooked cereal, rice or pasta

The second level of the pyramid also includes foods that come from plant sources. Fruits and vegetables are essential sources of many vitamins and minerals, including folic acid, vitamin A and vitamin C. Fresh and frozen fruits and vegetables are also good sources of fiber. Aim for at least one food high in vitamin A and one high in vitamin C each day.

Fruits and Vegetables

Best-bet fruits and vegetables

Apples	Papaya
Apricots	Pears
Bananas	Peas
Broccoli	Pineapple
Cantaloupe	Raspberries
Carrots	Red and green peppers
Citrus fruits and juices	Spinach
Corn	Strawberries
Dried fruit	Sweet potatoes
Grapes	Tomatoes
Greens	Vegetable juice
Leaf lettuce (romaine, endive)	Winter squash
Mango	

What's a serving?
1 cup raw salad greens
½ cup vegetables, cooked or chopped raw
¾ cup vegetable or fruit juice
1 medium piece of fruit
½ cup cooked or canned fruit

Protein Foods

The third level of the pyramid includes two groups of foods that come mostly from animal sources. Milk and dairy foods provide an important source of calcium and protein. Meat, poultry, seafood, dried beans, eggs and nuts are important for the protein, iron and zinc they contain. Although it is possible to have a nutritious diet that does not include animal foods, it is more difficult if you eliminate whole categories of foods.

Best-bet dairy products and meat or meat alternatives

Buttermilk
Eggs
Ice milk and frozen yogurt
Low-fat cheese
Low-fat cottage cheese
Low-fat fruit yogurt
Low-fat yogurt
Milk shake
Puddings and custard
Skim or 1 percent milk

Canadian bacon
Dried peas and beans
Fish and shellfish
Lean beef (round, sirloin)
Lean pork
Nuts and seeds
Peanut butter
Poultry (chicken and turkey)

What's a serving?
1 cup milk or yogurt
1½ ounces natural cheese
2 ounces processed cheese
2 to 3 ounces cooked lean meat, poultry or fish
½ cup cooked dried beans or peas
1 egg
2 tablespoons peanut butter
¼ cup nuts

Fats and Sugars

Limit cake, pie, chips, soft drinks, sugar, candy and other foods high in fat and sugar. These foods make up the small tip of the pyramid and tend to replace more nutritious foods. They can compromise the quality of your diet.

How much fat you need depends on your calorie requirements. Remember that small amounts of fat are essential for a well-balanced diet. When possible, choose lean meats and skim or low-fat dairy products. If you're gaining weight too fast, cut back on salad dressings, butter, margarine and oils.

Sugar supplies calories but little else nutritionally. So limit your consumption of table sugar and sweets. White sugar, brown sugar, honey and corn syrup are common ingredients in many processed foods. Develop the habit of reading the ingredient list and nutrition facts panel on food labels.

In the past, it was common to encourage pregnant women to limit their sodium intake. New research suggests that it is much better not to overly restrict sodium in normal pregnant women. In the last few weeks of pregnancy, almost all women have some swelling in their ankles, legs, fingers or face. This is a normal response to the high levels of estrogen circulating in your body. Attempting to cut back on salt drastically to reduce this swelling will cause your body to conserve sodium and water. This can actually make the swelling worse.

Of course, we're not suggesting that you dive into a bag of salty chips and other snack foods. Just don't make drastic changes in your sodium intake unless directed by your physician. If you have high blood pressure or develop complications later in your pregnancy, your physician may suggest you limit your intake of foods high in sodium and table salt.

Salt Sense

Vitamin and Mineral Supplements

Pregnant women often wonder about taking vitamin supplements. On the one hand, guidelines from the National Research Council advise that pregnant women who eat a well-balanced diet don't need supplements. On the other hand, research shows that multivitamins taken early in pregnancy may help prevent birth defects. Still, taking individual vitamins in excessive amounts, especially vitamin A, can actually harm your baby. What's the solution?

Pregnant women need more of almost every vitamin and mineral than do women who are not pregnant. Most of these increased nutrient requirements can be met through a carefully planned, nutritious diet. But it is highly unlikely that most women can eat enough foods high in iron and folic acid to meet current recommendations. And some women can't or won't eat enough high-calcium foods to meet the increased need for this mineral during pregnancy.

Many doctors prescribe a prenatal vitamin specially formulated to provide various essential nutrients. Keep in mind that even if you are taking a daily prenatal vitamin, eating a balanced diet is still the best nutrition for a healthy baby. Most registered dietitians agree that a bad diet supplemented with vitamins is still a bad diet. And taking supplements will not "make up" for poor eating habits.

Doctors and scientists agree that use of folic acid supplements can reduce the recurrence of a birth defect called a neural tube defect. Neural tube defects include spina bifida (incomplete closure of the spine), anencephaly (a partially or completely missing brain) and encephalocele (a hernia of the brain). In the United States, neural tube defects occur in approximately one or two of every 1,000 births. The usefulness of folic acid (a B vitamin) as a means of preventing first-time occurrences of these defects is still under investigation. Preliminary studies suggest folic acid supplementation may reduce the risk of first-time neural tube defects, but these early findings have not been confirmed.

The U.S. Public Health Service recommends 0.4 milligram of folic acid daily for all women of childbearing years, whether or not they intend to become pregnant. This can be attained by eating foods high in folate, or taking over-the-counter vitamins containing folic acid. Because side effects of large amounts of folic acid

Folic Acid

Key nutrients in pregnancy

There are more than 50 nutrients that are essential for good health when you're pregnant. Here's a summary of nutrients most critical for you and your baby.

Nutrient	Why you and your baby need it	Best sources
Protein	It's the main building block for your baby's cells; provides reserves you'll need for labor and delivery	Eggs, lean meats, poultry, fish, cheese, milk, dried peas, beans
Carbohydrate	Provides energy for you and your baby; allows protein to be used for tissue growth	Whole-grain and fortified breads and cereals, fruits, vegetables, rice, pasta, potatoes
Fat	Provides long-term energy for growth; is critical for the development of your baby's brain	Lean meat, fish, poultry, eggs, nuts, seeds, peanut butter, oils, margarine, butter
Fluids	Help increase fluid volume; prevent constipation and dry skin; are needed for amniotic fluid	Tap and bottled water, juice, soup
Vitamin A	Promotes healthy skin, eyesight and bone growth	Sweet potatoes, carrots, dark leafy greens, cantaloupe, apricots
Vitamin C	Forms healthy gums, teeth and bones for your baby; keeps your tissues in top shape; improves iron absorption	Citrus fruits, broccoli, tomatoes, peppers, berries, melons, potatoes with skin
Folic acid	Helps blood cell and hemoglobin formation; early in pregnancy, it may prevent neural tube defects	Dark leafy greens, dried peas and beans, whole-grain breads and cereals, citrus fruits, bananas, cantaloupe, tomatoes
Calcium	Helps form strong bones and teeth	Milk, cheese, yogurt, collard greens, kale, sardines and canned salmon (with bones), broccoli, dried beans
Iron	Develops red blood cells needed to deliver oxygen to your baby; prevents fatigue	Lean red meat, spinach, tofu, dried fruits, whole-grain and fortified breads and cereals

remain unclear, the Public Health Service cautions that women should not exceed an intake of 1 milligram of folic acid daily. Physicians agree that excessive amounts of folic acid can complicate the diagnosis of a vitamin B_{12} deficiency.

The American College of Obstetricians and Gynecologists (ACOG) recommends higher amounts of folic acid daily for women who have had a fetus with a neural tube defect in a previous pregnancy. Supplementation of 4 milligrams daily (which requires a doctor's prescription) should begin one month before the time the woman plans to become pregnant and continue through the first three months of pregnancy. By four weeks after conception, the neural tube is closed; consequently, there may be no benefit in beginning supplementation after that time. ACOG does not currently recommend routinely prescribing folic acid supplements for women who are not at risk for a neural tube defect. Certain other conditions may put you at risk for neural tube defects.

Before becoming pregnant, talk to your caregiver about your potential need for a folic acid supplement. You may already have unusually low levels of folic acid in your blood if you regularly have poor eating habits, are prone to strict dieting, abuse alcohol or smoke cigarettes. Taking oral contraceptives is also associated with low levels of folic acid.

If you take a folic acid supplement, keep in mind that more is not always better. Too much of any supplement can harm your health.

Good dietary sources of folic acid include fortified breakfast cereals, leafy green vegetables, liver, lentils, black-eyed peas, kidney beans and other cooked dried beans, oranges and grapefruits.

Iron

Iron is a critical nutrient during pregnancy. In fact, the amount of iron you need is double the amount recommended for non-pregnant women. It is practically impossible to eat enough foods to provide the recommended 30 milligrams of iron you'll need daily. The typical American diet provides about 6 milligrams of iron per 1,000 calories. Because eating 5,000 or more calories a day is not practical or prudent, iron supplements are necessary.

You'll need extra iron because your blood volume expands greatly to accommodate the changes in your body during pregnancy. Iron is also required for the formation of tissue for both your baby and the placenta. At birth, your newborn needs enough stored iron to last for the first six months of life.

If you don't get enough iron, you may develop a condition commonly referred to as iron-deficiency anemia. Some side effects of this anemia include lowered resistance to infection, fatigue and reduced physical performance. In addition to the iron you receive in your prenatal supplement, you'll need to obtain iron by eating as many foods rich in iron as possible.

Good sources of iron

Food source	Serving	Milligrams of iron
Bran cereal, fortified	1 cup	12
Molasses, blackstrap	1 tablespoon	3
Baked potato, with skin	1 large	3
Red meat (beef, lamb)	3 ounces	2*
Kidney beans	½ cup	2
Spinach, cooked	½ cup	2
Split-pea soup	1 cup	2
Perch, broiled	3 ounces	2*
Chicken or pork	3 ounces	1*
Raisins	1 ounce	1

*The iron you consume in animal products is more easily absorbed by your body.

Here are additional ways to add iron or to foster absorption of iron:

- Take your prenatal or iron supplement with beverages high in vitamin C (such as orange, tomato or vegetable juice)

- Eat foods high in vitamin C at the same time you eat iron-containing foods as a means to enhance iron absorption (for example, eat strawberries with iron-fortified breakfast cereal)

- Cook foods in a cast-iron skillet.

Calcium

Calcium is another crucial mineral during pregnancy. If you enjoy milk and dairy products, it's easy to meet your need for this nutrient. The recommended number of servings increases from two a day for non-pregnant women to three servings. If you can't or won't drink milk, you still need to get at least 1,200 milligrams of calcium every day. Your baby is building a whole new skeleton, and calcium is an essential part of healthy bone tissue. Keep in mind that alcohol and caffeine can interfere with your body's handling of calcium, so that's another reason to avoid them during your pregnancy.

The amount of calcium in most prenatal supplements is not sufficient if you don't regularly eat dairy products such as milk, cheese and yogurt. If your doctor recommends a calcium supplement, make sure you buy one that is made from calcium carbonate or calcium citrate because they are the most absorbable forms available. Never take oyster shell or bone meal calcium. They not only are in a form that is difficult for your body to use but also may be contaminated with lead and other harmful chemicals.

Check the aisles in the grocery store for calcium-fortified foods such as orange juice, selected breakfast cereals and applesauce. Read the labels to determine the level of fortification. A serving of calcium-fortified orange juice that contains 300 milligrams of calcium is equivalent to a glass of milk.

Large doses of vitamin or mineral supplements, exceeding, for example, the amount contained in a prenatal supplement, are not recommended. Be sure to tell your caregiver if you have been taking any individual supplements before pregnancy. Big doses of vitamins may actually harm your baby. For example, large amounts of vitamin A (more than 25,000 international units) taken daily can cause defects in the bones, heart, nervous system, head and face of your baby.

The best advice is to eat a healthful diet and take only the supplements recommended by your caregiver.

Calcium comparison chart

Food source	Serving size	Milligrams of calcium
Lasagna	2½-inch square	460
Yogurt, plain non-fat	1 cup	450
Tofu (made with calcium sulfate)	½ cup	430
Macaroni and cheese	1 cup	360
Milk	1 cup	300
Swiss cheese	1 ounce	270
Cheeseburger (with 1 ounce of cheese)	3 ounces	180
American cheese	1 ounce	175
Pizza	¼ of 12-inch	165
Spinach	½ cup, cooked	140
Turnip greens	½ cup, cooked	125
Almonds	¼ cup	95
Ice cream or ice milk	½ cup	90
Taco (with ½ ounce of cheese)	1 small	80
Tempeh (soybean product)	½ cup	75
Orange	1 medium	50
Broccoli	½ cup, cooked	35
Molasses, blackstrap	1 tablespoon	30

Meal Planning

Now that you've reviewed the facts and figures on nutrient needs, just how do you translate all that information into a plan of daily meals and snacks? After all, you eat foods and not individual vitamins and minerals.

The first step in planning a nutritious diet is to figure out what you are already doing well. Choose a typical day and write down all the foods you eat. Look at the portion sizes and estimate how many servings from each group you consumed. Then tally the totals for all your meals and snacks that day. Chances are you'll come up short for one or more of the recommended servings outlined in the Food Guide Pyramid. Work with your menu and add the foods you need. It may take a little practice, but soon you will develop a good sense of how to choose foods that ensure a balanced diet.

Use the following sample menus, for two typical days, as guides to help you tailor your own daily menu plans.

Day One

Number of servings of:

	Bread	Vegetable	Fruit	Milk	Meat	Other fats and sweets
BREAKFAST						
1 scrambled egg					1	
Toasted bagel	2					
Jam or preserves						1
½ grapefruit			1			
1 cup skim milk				1		
LUNCH						
Chef salad made with						
2 cups salad greens		2				
½ cup raw sliced						
vegetables		1				
1 oz. turkey breast					½	
1 oz. extra-lean ham					½	
1½ oz. Swiss cheese				1		
2 tbsp. salad dressing						1
1 whole-grain roll	1					
1 tsp. margarine						1
1 cup skim milk				1		
1 small banana			1			
DINNER						
2 oz. baked fish					1	
1 baked sweet potato		1				
1 tsp. margarine						
or brown sugar						1
1 cup seasoned noodles	2					
1 large breadstick	1½					
1 cup skim milk				1		
SNACKS						
¾ cup fruit juice			1			
1 large blueberry muffin	1½					
Day One total servings	**8**	**4**	**3**	**4**	**3**	**4**

Day Two

	Bread	Vegetable	Fruit	Milk	Meat	Other fats and sweets
			Number of servings of:			
BREAKFAST						
1 cup oatmeal	2					
1 cup skim milk				1		
½ cup strawberries			1			
1 slice whole-grain toast	1					
1 tsp. margarine or jam						1
LUNCH						
Sandwich made with						
2 oz. lean roast beef					1	
2 slices whole-grain bread	2					
Lettuce and tomato slices		1				
Mustard or mayonnaise						1
½ cup cole slaw		1				
½ cup sliced melon			1			
1 cup skim milk				1		
2 small oatmeal raisin						
cookies	1					
DINNER						
4 oz. broiled						
chicken breast					2	
½ cup brown rice pilaf	1					
½ cup steamed broccoli		1				
1 cup mixed salad greens		1				
1 tbsp. salad dressing						1
1 cup skim milk				1		
SNACKS						
½-inch slice banana						
nut bread	1					
1 cup frozen yogurt				1		
1 piece fresh fruit			1			
Day Two total servings	8	4	3	4	3	3

Smart Snacking

Snacks can be an important addition to your daily food intake. Snacking is the perfect opportunity to add the extra calories and nutrients essential during pregnancy. Registered dietitians agree that cereals, whole grains, fruits and vegetables lead the list of smart-snack choices. If you have trouble drinking enough milk, include calcium-rich snack foods too, such as low-fat cheese and yogurt.

Well-planned snacks are also helpful for the times during your pregnancy when you can't eat a full meal. In the early part of your pregnancy, frequent smaller meals and snacks can help control nausea. In the last weeks you may notice that the pressure of your baby limits the amount of food you can comfortably eat at one time. Sensible snacking, in addition to nutritious meals, assures a steady stream of nutrition for your baby to grow on.

Sample snacks

Crunchy
Raw vegetables with dip
Whole-grain crackers

Sweet
Fresh fruit
Dried fruit
Low-fat yogurt
Low-fat muffin

Thirst quenchers
Ice water or sparkling bottled water
Fruit juice fizz (½ juice and ½ sparkling water)
Fruit shake made with skim milk
Vegetable juice

Hearty
Fruit muffins or breads
Cereal with low-fat yogurt
Vegetable soup
Tuna sandwich

Vegetarian Diets

If you are a vegetarian, you can continue your vegetarian diet throughout your pregnancy and still have a healthy baby, but you will need to pay additional attention to meal planning to ensure the right food choices. Be careful to make time to plan and review your food intake on a regular basis. If you include fish, milk and eggs in your diet, it is easier to balance, from a nutritional standpoint. Simply follow the eating recommendations outlined in this chapter and include one to two extra servings of plant foods high in iron. It is no longer necessary to combine complementary proteins at each meal. The best advice for a healthful vegetarian diet is to eat a wide variety of foods and balance your intake each day according to the Food Guide Pyramid.

Vegans. If you eat no animal products at all, you'll need to plan your daily food intake in even greater detail to meet your need for protein and calories during your pregnancy. Vegans often do not get enough zinc, vitamin B_{12}, iron, calcium and folic acid. A prenatal vitamin/mineral supplement will be essential for you.

Vegan diets are usually high in plant fiber. This may make you feel full before you eat enough calories to gain the recommended amount of weight for your pregnancy. Try including more energy-rich foods such as nuts, nut butters, seeds and dried fruits if your weight gain is not following a smooth curve. Because of the complexity in designing a high-quality vegan diet for pregnancy, seek the help of a registered dietitian.

Food Safety

Now that you're pregnant, you'll need to be particularly careful in handling food. Changes in your metabolism and circulation during pregnancy may increase your risk of food poisoning. A small amount of bacteria in your food can cause big problems.

If you do get sick, your symptoms will probably be more severe than if you were not pregnant. And because bacterial toxins pass from mother to baby, if you have food poisoning your developing baby can become sick too.

The most common food-borne bacteria are *Salmonella* and *Listeria*. *Salmonella* bacteria are often found in raw poultry, eggs, milk, fish and products that contain these ingredients. Symptoms of *Salmonella* poisoning occur 24 hours after eating contaminated food and include fever, headache, diarrhea and abdominal pain. Most people recover in two to four days, but if you are pregnant it may take longer.

Listeria bacteria are common, and one particular species, *Listeria monocytogenes*, can be harmful. The main sources of the bacteria are soft cheeses, undercooked poultry and hot dogs. The symptoms of listeriosis are similar to those of the flu and include fever, fatigue, nausea, vomiting and diarrhea. A third of all documented cases of listeriosis occur during pregnancy, and severe cases may lead to miscarriage or newborn infections in the fluid surrounding the brain (meningitis) or in the bloodstream.

During the past several years, new recommendations have been made by the Food and Drug Administration concerning food safety for individuals at high risk. There is no way to tell by sight or smell if a food has been contaminated with bacteria. The best way to prevent all types of food infection is to wash your hands frequently during food preparation and to store and heat foods properly.

Handling Food

To make sure that the food you eat is safe, start at the supermarket. Purchase highly perishable items such as meat, poultry, fish and eggs last to reduce the amount of time they are not under proper refrigeration. Unpack and store foods immediately when you get home.

Keep your refrigerator set between 34 and 40 degrees Fahrenheit, and your freezer at or below zero. You can purchase an inexpensive refrigerator thermometer to monitor the temperature. Now is a good time to clean out the refrigerator. Toss any food that is past its expiration date.

Hand washing is perhaps the most effective tool to prevent food-borne disease. Always wash your hands, and under your fingernails, before any food preparation. Keep raw and cooked foods separate to prevent cross-contamination. Use separate cutting boards for meats and produce, and wash cutting boards with hot, soapy water after each use.

And don't forget the old adage, "Keep hot foods hot, cold foods cold and keep everything clean," because it's as true today as it was 100 years ago.

Raw eggs carry the risk of being contaminated with *Salmonella* bacteria. Do not eat any home-prepared foods that contain raw eggs such as Caesar salad dressing, eggnog or ice cream. The commercial forms of these products sold at grocery stores are safe because they are made with pasteurized egg products.

Cook all eggs thoroughly until both the yolk and the white are firm and not runny. This preparation will kill bacteria that might be present. Don't forget that sampling uncooked batters when you prepare foods can be a source of raw eggs. Lightly cooked foods such as soft custards, French toast, meringue and soft scrambled and sunny-side-up eggs do carry some risk and are best avoided. Pasteurized liquid egg products and powdered dried eggs are good substitutes if you have favorite recipes that call for raw or undercooked eggs.

Ground meat products, including hamburger, ground chicken and sausage, require special handling. *Escherichia coli* and other bacteria that are commonly found on the surface of meat are distributed throughout the whole product as part of the grinding process. If you cook a steak or pork chop, the surface bacteria are almost instantly killed. However, a hamburger that is cooked to medium doneness will not have reached an internal temperature high enough to kill bacteria that might be present. Eat only well-done burgers and sausage, and cook all ground meat until it is light gray and the juices run clear.

Fish and shellfish are nutritious foods you should include in your diet. Seafood is a good source of high-quality protein that is low in fat and high in nutrients, including iron and zinc. Proper cooking eliminates viral or bacterial contamination in fresh or frozen fish. Use the "10-minute rule"—measure fish at its thickest part and cook for 10 minutes per inch at 450 degrees Fahrenheit. Boil or steam clams, oysters and shrimp for four to six minutes.

Environmental toxins may be a problem with some freshwater fish and ocean seafood. Despite being banned in 1979, polychlorinated biphenyls (PCBs) remain in our waterways and can accumulate to potentially dangerous levels in fish. Just as hazardous is methyl mercury, a byproduct of industrial waste and fuel burning. To limit your exposure to environmental contaminants that may be present in some seafood:

- Eat various seafoods. Small fish have had less exposure to environmental contaminants than large fish of the same species.

- Avoid all raw and undercooked seafood, especially clams, mussels and oysters.

- Limit your consumption of shark, swordfish and fresh tuna to once a month. These species tend to have the most chemical contaminants.

- Buy fresh fish and seafood the same day you plan to eat it, and always buy from a reputable store.

- Pay attention to local advisories that warn pregnant women, nursing mothers and young children not to eat fish from certain recreational lakes, rivers and streams. Warnings may be posted at the water's edge or included with information on your local fishing license.

Artificial Sweeteners

More than 1,500 artificially sweetened foods line the shelves of your local grocery store. They include chewing gum, soft drinks, pudding, gelatin, drink mixes, yogurt and candy. The National Academy of Sciences landmark report titled "Diet and Health" suggests that although there is no recommendation either for or against the use of artificial sweeteners, pregnant women might want to consider limiting the amount in their diet. We suggest you keep your use down to no more than two or three products a day.

Caffeine

Caffeine is a drug that has been part of the human diet for thousands of years. It occurs naturally in coffee, tea, chocolate and cocoa. Caffeine is frequently added to soft drinks and over-the-counter drugs, including headache and cold tablets, stay-awake medications and allergy remedies. An abundance of research indicates that moderate consumption of caffeine (200 milligrams daily) has no negative effects during pregnancy. Consumed in high amounts (500 milligrams or more daily), caffeine increases the amount of time a fetus spends in an active, awake state and may cause a decrease in your baby's birth weight and head circumference.

Coffee is the most common source of caffeine. Drinking more than two or three cups of coffee a day is not recommended. Other foods that contain caffeine include tea, carbonated beverages and chocolate. To reduce the amount of caffeine in hot beverages you drink, consider changing how you brew them. The shorter the brewing time, the lower the caffeine concentration. You can also lower your caffeine consumption considerably by switching from perked to instant coffee.

If you love a soothing hot cup of tea, brewing a tea bag for just one minute, instead of five, can reduce caffeine content by as much as half. Because little is known about herbs and their effects on pregnancy, avoid herbal teas. Don't take anything that contains comfrey; this herb can cause serious liver disease.

The best advice is to avoid caffeine-containing foods and drugs whenever possible. If you can't give up caffeine during pregnancy, keep your intake below 200 milligrams daily.

Caffeine content of common foods

	Milligrams of caffeine	
	Average	Range
Coffee, 5 ounces		
Brewed, percolator	115	60-180
Brewed, drip method	80	40-170
Instant	65	30-120
Tea, 5 ounces		
Brewed, imported	60	25-110
Brewed, U.S. brands	40	20-90
Instant	30	25-50
Iced (12 ounces)	70	67-76
Soft drinks, 12 ounces	36	30-50
Cocoa, 5 ounces	4	2-20
Chocolate milk, 8 ounces	5	2-7
Semisweet chocolate, 1 ounce	20	5-35
Milk chocolate, 1 ounce	6	1-15
Chocolate syrup, 1 ounce	4	4-5

A Final Word

Start now to improve your diet, so that you can feel good and give your baby a healthful head start. Good nutrition can be easy if you take the time to plan. It won't mean giving up your favorite snack foods or treats.

Don't forget to share your healthful eating habits with your partner. Remember that after your baby is born, the foods you both eat will help to guide your child's eating habits. Now is a good time to make the small changes that can offer a significant improvement in the diet of your whole family.

Pregnancy nutrition myths and facts

Take this simple quiz to test your knowledge of nutrition during pregnancy.

True or False

T F 1. Everyone should gain 25 pounds to have a healthy baby.
T F 2. It's okay to fast when you're pregnant.
T F 3. Pregnant women must drink milk to get enough calcium.
T F 4. I need to double my intake of iron during pregnancy.
T F 5. I have to give up chips and candy to have a healthy baby.
T F 6. I should try to eliminate fat from my diet.
T F 7. Vegetarians can have healthy babies.
T F 8. Snacks are a good way to get important nutrients.
T F 9. I should restrict my intake of salt and sodium while pregnant.
T F 10. Raw eggs are a safe source of protein.

Answers:

1. False. Weight gain for a healthy baby depends on many factors. For example, an underweight woman may need to gain up to 40 pounds, whereas an overweight woman can have a healthy pregnancy and baby with as little as a 15-pound weight gain.

2. False. If you fast, your body won't be able to provide the steady stream of nutrients your baby needs for optimal growth and development.

3. False. Milk is one of the richest sources of calcium, but other dairy products such as cheese and yogurt also can supply this essential nutrient.

4. True. In fact, it is almost impossible to get the recommended amount of iron from foods you eat. Almost all pregnant women need iron supplements.

5. False. All foods can be included in a healthful diet if they are eaten in moderation. Your first priority is to eat the recommended amounts of nutritious foods, but an occasional treat won't harm you or your baby.

6. False. Fat is an essential component of all diets. It's best to decrease but not eliminate fat by choosing low-fat meats and dairy products, but you do need to have some fat for your baby's normal growth and development.

7. True. Vegetarians must work much harder to ensure an adequate diet during pregnancy, and they may need the assistance of a registered dietitian.

8. True. Eating nutritious snacks can help meet the increased calorie and nutrient needs of pregnancy.

9. False. Healthy women should not limit their intake of salt. Newer research shows an ordinary intake of sodium is important during pregnancy. If you have high blood pressure, or develop complications during pregnancy, your doctor may change this advice.

10. False. Raw eggs are a possible source of food poisoning. Don't eat them.

How did you rate?
Nine or 10 correct answers: Great! You really know your nutrition.
Seven or eight right answers: Good, but you need a little fine tuning.
Five or six correct: Poor. It's time to learn the facts.
Less than five correct: Oops! Better re-read this chapter.

CHAPTER EIGHT

Lifestyle During Pregnancy

As an expectant mother, the sheer volume of health information reported in the news may be overwhelming. And, to make matters worse, some of the information is conflicting. You might find yourself questioning virtually every aspect of your day-to-day life for fear of harming your baby. Is an occasional glass of wine at dinner harmful? Is it safe to continue my exercise routine? Is soaking in a hot tub risky? Will sexual intercourse cause me to miscarry?

Being pregnant obviously involves major changes in your body, but rest assured, you probably won't need a complete overhaul of your lifestyle. Remember, most women give birth to healthy babies. Certainly many things that you took for granted before you were pregnant take on a new importance now that you are pregnant. You probably won't need to change your life dramatically, other than set a few limits, as highlighted in this chapter. Some activities, however, you should avoid altogether: smoking, drinking alcohol and using recreational drugs.

The key is to be cautious about applying information unless you've checked it with your doctor first. You're an individual, not a statistic. The life you led before becoming pregnant doesn't need to come to a sudden halt—pregnancy is a special opportunity for you to focus on being good to yourself and to your unborn child.

Isn't an Occasional Smoke Okay?

No question about it, smoking tobacco when you're pregnant is unwise: Women who smoke during pregnancy are more likely to have a stillbirth or to deliver babies whose birth weight is lower than average. Sudden infant death syndrome (SIDS), a condition in which an apparently healthy baby dies unexpectedly during sleep, occurs more often in children born to mothers who smoked during pregnancy. And women who smoke during pregnancy have a greater risk of a miscarriage. Even breathing the tobacco smoke of others (secondhand smoke) while you are pregnant may be harmful to your health and to your baby's.

Cigarette smoke contains thousands of chemicals. Little is known about many of them. Others, such as carbon monoxide and nicotine, are toxins that can move through your bloodstream and harm your developing baby. Both carbon monoxide and nicotine can reduce the flow of oxygen to your baby. And nicotine, which causes your heartbeat and blood pressure to increase and your blood vessels to constrict, can also decrease your baby's supply of nutrients.

Take action to stop smoking

Stopping the chemical addiction requires a solid game plan for dealing with withdrawal symptoms: craving cigarettes, irritability or restlessness, difficulty concentrating, headaches, sleeplessness, depression and stomach or digestive problems. Breaking the habits associated with smoking also requires specific strategies. Here are guidelines to help you:

- Set a stop date.
- Get support from your partner, family, friends and coworkers.
- Identify specific circumstances that prompt you to light up, whether they're instances of stress or relaxation. Then develop a strategy to eliminate each one—try distracting yourself by changing your routine, engaging in new activities and doing deep-breathing exercises to promote relaxation.
- Persevere—although the time varies with individuals, if you can cope for two weeks, you'll probably gain relief from many, if not all, withdrawal symptoms.

Because success may hinge on more than your personal reserves, consider getting professional assistance from your health care provider. Your doctor may prescribe nicotine replacement in the form of chewing gum or a medicated skin patch. These products can help decrease withdrawal symptoms, allowing you to be more comfortable while your body adjusts to the loss of nicotine. Keep in mind, however, that there are risks associated with use of these products by pregnant women. Many of the medications are not approved by the Food and Drug Administration for use during pregnancy. Your doctor will decide whether the risks of continued smoking outweigh the risks associated with use of these medications.

Several major medical centers offer comprehensive smoking cessation programs. The programs include hospitalization and are patterned after more widely available programs for alcohol and drug addiction. Your local hospital may also offer smoking cessation classes. For more information on how to stop smoking, contact the American Lung Association (800-LUNG-USA), the American Cancer Society (800-ACS-2345) or the American Heart Association (800-AHA-USA1).

But what if you're hooked on smoking? Smoking is an addiction—a chemical need for the nicotine. Smoking is also a habit—an established behavior pattern. It may be tough to stop smoking, but it's not impossible, no matter how many times you've tried. Thousands of people are former smokers. You can be too. Even cutting down on how much you smoke may yield benefits to you and your baby. A fresh attempt to quit, despite past setbacks, is well worth your effort.

One Alcoholic Drink Can't Hurt, Can It?

We don't know the answer for sure—there is no known safe level of alcohol consumption during pregnancy. What we do know is that excessive use of alcohol during pregnancy can harm an unborn baby. The hazards of minimal to moderate use are less apparent. So why take a chance? Alcohol is a drug. If you drink alcohol, so does your baby—and your baby's ability to metabolize alcohol is much less than your capability.

Although a single drink may not pose a hazard, sustained drinking during pregnancy does: You have a higher risk of having a miscarriage, and your baby has a higher risk of death. Alcohol can damage brain cells and limit oxygen flow to developing tissues.

Every year, approximately 5,000 babies are born (one out of every 750 births) in the United States with fetal alcohol syndrome (FAS). "FAS" is a term used to describe a group of birth defects caused by excessive use of alcohol during pregnancy. These defects include facial malformations, such as a smaller-than-normal sized head, exceptionally thin lips, small eyes and a deep nasal bridge; retarded physical growth before and after birth; mental retardation; short attention span; and behavioral problems.

Women who drink even moderately (as well as those who drink heavily) during pregnancy may also cause their children to be born with a condition called fetal alcohol effect (FAE). Children born with FAE have some but not all of the characteristics of those with FAS.

Sadly, the effects of alcohol on babies are 100 percent permanent. They are also 100 percent preventable. As soon as you know you're pregnant, don't drink alcohol. Or if you're planning to get pregnant, it's also probably best to refrain from consumption of alcohol.

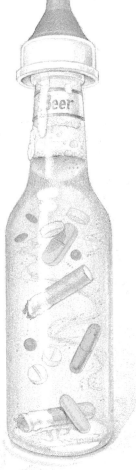

You wouldn't think of giving your baby alcohol, a cigarette or recreational drugs. But unfortunately, if you drink, smoke or take drugs while you're pregnant, your unborn baby is exposed to dangerous substances that can have permanent effects.

What's So Bad About Recreational Drugs?

In the United States and throughout large regions of the world, the use of recreational or street drugs for enjoyment or coping purposes has reached epidemic proportions. Women who use cocaine during pregnancy risk miscarriage, placental abruption (see page 194) and preterm labor and delivery. The risks for the unborn child are apparent as well: growth retardation and birth defects. Cocaine can even pass into breast milk.

The risks of using illegal drugs are especially high, not only because the drugs themselves may be harmful but also because of other dangerous aspects of their use. Drugs that are used intravenously may cause infections, including HIV (the AIDS virus). Illegal drugs have no guarantee of purity and can be mixed with additional harmful substances. Money wasted on drugs may lead to hardships for the family, including inadequate housing and poor nutrition.

If you are pregnant, don't risk using cocaine, marijuana, heroin, methadone, lysergic acid diethylamide (LSD), phencyclidine (PCP) or any other kind of recreational or street drug. And don't believe anyone who claims these drugs are harmless.

Should I Avoid All Medicines?

Medicines should not be used unless needed. Even seemingly mild over-the-counter agents such as aspirin or cough syrup may cause side effects for you or your baby. Before you take any nonprescription or prescription medicine, check with your doctor for specific advice based on the nature of your pregnancy and health history. Your pharmacist can also provide general advice.

If you have a health condition that requires regular medication, your doctor will evaluate whether it's safest for you to continue taking the medication, discontinue its use or switch to a different medication that poses less risk or eliminates risk to you or your baby. Keep in mind that your health care provider can't give you any guarantees. Determining whether a particular drug is entirely safe for a pregnant woman is not always easy or possible. Because of the risk of legal action, pharmaceutical manufacturing companies have little incentive to test their drugs on pregnant women.

The following pages contain a partial list of commonly used nonprescription drugs and a description of the risks they may pose to you and your baby if they are taken during pregnancy.

Pain Relievers   **A**cetaminophen. This widely used non-aspirin substitute is available under various brand names, including Aspirin Free Excedrin, Panadol and Tylenol. In addition to relieving pain, acetaminophen can lower a fever. You can use acetaminophen when you're pregnant without worrying about it causing birth defects. But also consider a non-pharmaceutical alternative. For example, instead of taking acetaminophen for a headache, try resting or eating a snack. If you need relief from sore muscles or arthritic aches, try a warm bath or massage.

Aspirin. Avoid taking aspirin when you're pregnant, unless your doctor specifically recommends it. There is conflicting information about the safety of taking aspirin when you're pregnant. Some doctors point to a link between aspirin use and the incidence of fetal heart defects and infant and maternal bleeding, especially during and directly after birth. Other evidence indicates that low doses of aspirin may help prevent miscarriages in women at high risk for a miscarriage. And aspirin may sometimes help prevent complications of pregnancy such as pregnancy-induced hypertension (high blood pressure).

Ibuprofen. This is another medication that's best left in the bottle when you're pregnant. Ibuprofen (common brand names include Advil, Ibuprin, Motrin IB and Nuprin) could pose risks similar to those of aspirin.

Antacids

Antacids are generally safe when taken as directed, but you might not appreciate their side effects. Sodium, a common ingredient in antacids, can cause swelling and water retention. Antacids containing aluminum can cause constipation. Those containing magnesium can lead to diarrhea. Antacids that contain magnesium or calcium may reduce your absorption of some prescription medications. The Food and Drug Administration now requires this label: "Antacids may interact with certain prescription drugs; do not take this product without checking with your physician or other health professional." If you experience trouble with indigestion or gas, before you reach for an antacid, try eating small meals frequently and avoid lying down immediately after eating.

Cold Medications

The aisles of your local pharmacy and grocery store are stacked with cold remedies. Options include wide varieties of decongestants, cough syrups, antihistamines and nasal sprays, but you're best off avoiding them unless your doctor recommends one. Although these medicines are intended to relieve your cold symptoms, they don't actually affect the severity or duration of your cold. The symptoms of a common cold can be unpleasant, but they pose no hazards to you or your baby. If you're pregnant, the best treatment for a common cold includes rest, fluids, increased humidity and time. (For specific tips on how to avoid catching a cold in the first place, or how to treat the symptoms without medications, see page 136.)

Weight-Loss Aids

Do not use any weight-loss medications while you're pregnant. Pregnancy is not the time to suppress your appetite or to trim down. Phenylpropanolamine, an appetite suppressant, is a common ingredient in over-the-counter weight-loss medications. This medicine may increase your blood pressure. Pregnancy is the time for an especially well-balanced, nutritious diet. (For more information on nutrition during pregnancy, see page 85.)

Laxatives

Constipation is one of the most common aggravations of pregnancy. Non-prescription laxatives are generally safe to use, but check with your health care provider for a recommendation. Overuse of laxatives can cause diarrhea. Prevention is the best treatment. To avoid constipation, eat high-fiber foods and drink plenty of liquids. Regular, moderate aerobic exercise throughout your pregnancy should also help.

Is It Safe to Exercise During Pregnancy?

If you have no known complications, moderate aerobic exercise while you're pregnant can help you feel healthy and boost your spirits. Even if you've been a "couch potato" up until now, pregnancy is a good incentive for getting started. Throughout pregnancy, the conditioning that results from exercise can help prevent back pain, muscle cramps, swelling and constipation. It can also reduce fatigue and encourage a good night's sleep.

Exercise during pregnancy can help prepare you for labor and birth. Increased stamina and muscle strength can decrease stress on ligaments and joints when that exciting time arrives. If you're in reasonably good physical condition, your labor and recovery times may be shortened.

But whether or not you've been exercising regularly before you became pregnant, remember that pregnancy is physically demanding. You can expect to gain 25 to 35 pounds. Your heart will pump about 50 percent more blood. Your body will consume up to 20 percent more oxygen while you rest—and even more when you exercise. As your abdomen increases in size, your posture will shift forward, putting new strain on your back muscles and changing your balance. Toward the end of your pregnancy the joints and ligaments in your pelvis will loosen in preparation for labor. All of these changes will affect the way your body responds to exercise. For example, muscle and joint injuries are more likely to occur if you're not careful.

Sports to Avoid

It's best to avoid certain sports altogether while you're pregnant. These include activities at high altitudes and those that are associated with a risk of falling or colliding with another participant, such as horseback riding, climbing and snow and water skiing. Also, avoid scuba diving. Snorkeling is a safer alternative. And after the first trimester, avoid floor exercises that require you to be on your back for a prolonged time.

How Do I Get Started?

If you're not now exercising regularly, it's best to begin modestly and gradually increase the frequency and length of each session. Your goal should be three or four 20-minute sessions weekly. Allow three or four weeks to work up to this goal.

Walking is an outstanding exercise to start with. It provides moderate aerobic conditioning and minimal wear on your joints. You don't need membership in a club or special equipment, other than a good pair of walking shoes. Other non-weight-bearing activities, such as swimming and cycling, are also good ways to get a safe aerobic workout.

Before you begin any activity, be sure you get your doctor's approval. And to reduce the chances of muscle cramps after exercise, be sure to stretch your muscles before and after you exercise.

The type of exercise you do should be enjoyable in addition to being safe. Pick times and places that are convenient. Avoid exercise programs that feature massive doses of discipline. You may find you'll get discouraged and give up exercising entirely. Many hospitals or birthing centers offer prenatal fitness classes. Exercising with other pregnant women can help motivate you to be more active. Your goal is to make exercise a healthful habit, and enjoyment and convenience are important to long-term success.

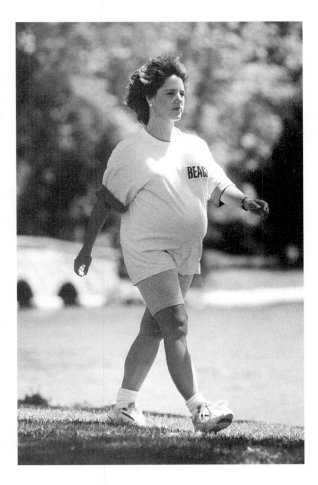

An invigorating walk is one of the safest, easiest forms of exercise during pregnancy. If you weren't physically active before pregnancy, walking is a good way to get started.

So What Should "Moderate" Mean for Me?

Listen to your body, and it will tell you if you're overdoing it. That's the key to exercising safely, whether you're a novice exerciser or a competitive athlete. If you are already in good condition, you probably can safely work out at about the same level as you did before you became pregnant, as long as you are comfortable and your doctor approves.

If your body's telling you to slow down, heed that advice. Dizziness, nausea, blurred vision, fatigue or shortness of breath can signal heat stroke, which can threaten your life and your baby's. Chest pain, abdominal pain and vaginal bleeding are other danger signs. Don't take a chance. Slow down or stop and get help if you need it—even if you're competing. Talk to your doctor as soon as possible if you're having any problems.

Practice some preventive measures also to keep your exercise routine safe. Drink fluids during exercise whether you are thirsty or not. And don't push yourself to the point of being short of breath or let your heart rate exceed 140 beats per minute. The runner who's passing you probably isn't pregnant. In 10 years the glow of a victory is a memory; your child will be an important part of your life.

Some pregnant women have medical conditions that may warrant a particularly cautious approach to exercise. These include anemia, thyroid disease, diabetes, a seizure disorder such as epilepsy, an irregular heartbeat and a history of premature labor. Other pregnant women have health conditions that require special monitoring during exercise or that prohibit any exercise. Examples include heart disease, an infectious disease such as hepatitis, severe high blood pressure, lung disease, a history of miscarriages, uterine bleeding or placenta previa (when the placenta blocks the cervix). Other circumstances can also affect your exercise program; for example, you may be expecting twins or have other conditions that place you at risk for premature labor; or your fetus may have poor weight gain. If you have any of these conditions, carefully review with your doctor what exercise may be permissible. If you're not restricted to bed rest, even minimal walking may help you feel better.

Is It Safe to Use a Hot Tub, Whirlpool or Sauna?

Nobody knows the answer to this question for sure. But prolonged immersion in hot water or the heat of a sauna could increase your internal body temperature high enough to harm your baby. The condition of a dangerously high internal body temperature is called hyperthermia. Hyperthermia can also result from a high fever or extreme exertion.

Evidence indicates that if a pregnant woman's internal temperature exceeds 104 degrees Fahrenheit (40 degrees Centigrade) during the early weeks of pregnancy, the risk that her baby will have a neural tube defect (a type of birth defect) increases. Your baby's neural tube, which forms during the first month of pregnancy, may be sensitive to an increase in your internal temperature. Spina bifida and anencephaly are both neural tube defects. (For more information on these birth defects, see page 67.)

An occasional warm bath to encourage relaxation or to relieve sore muscles poses no significant health hazards. But play it safe. Avoid prolonged exposure to high temperatures when you're pregnant, particularly during the first trimester. If you do decide to use a hot tub, whirlpool or sauna, especially after exercising, limit the temperature and the length of your exposure. You're more likely to develop hyperthermia in a hot tub than in a sauna. Limit your immersion in a hot tub to 10 minutes—this time may pass before you even feel hot. Ten minutes in a sauna is unlikely to raise your temperature to a worrisome degree, but it is possible that a longer stay could.

Is It Safe to Travel?

Whether travel is for business or pleasure, determining if it's safe for you and your unborn baby to travel depends on several considerations: your destination, how you plan to travel, how long you expect to be away, how many weeks pregnant you are and your general health.

Roads and Highways

Regardless of whether your trip is to the neighborhood grocery store or a campground hundreds of miles away, if you travel in a car, use your seat belt every time. Among pregnant women, auto accidents are the most common cause of death. If you're in an accident and you don't survive, your baby probably won't either.

Many states have laws requiring drivers and passengers to wear safety restraints. Restraints reduce the death toll to mothers and babies alike. But it's important to use them properly. Position the lap portion of the belt snugly under your abdomen and across your upper thighs. The safety restraint should not cross your abdomen. If the lap belt is positioned properly, the shoulder-strap portion will lie between your breasts. It will neither chafe your neck nor cross your abdomen.

Many pregnant women avoid using seat belts because they are uncertain about risks to their unborn babies. Don't make this mistake. When you buckle up, you and your baby are safer. For your own sake and the sake of your baby, make buckling your seat belt a habit.

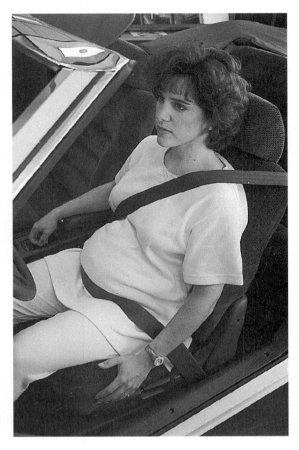

Protect yourself and your unborn baby every time you're in a vehicle by wearing your seat belt. Place the lap portion of the belt below your abdomen and across your upper thighs, and position the shoulder strap between your breasts.

Air Travel

If you're an expectant mother in good health and you're more than five to six weeks away from your due date, traveling by air should be fine. But ask your doctor first, and take along a note from your doctor verifying the date that your baby is due. Many domestic and international airlines don't allow pregnant women on board if they are more than 35 to 36 weeks pregnant.

Don't worry about the safety of metal detectors through which all passengers must pass before boarding a plane. These devices won't harm you or your developing baby.

Similarly, changes in air pressure on a high-altitude flight should present no unusual problems for you or your developing baby. During flight, the air pressure in the cabin of a jet is adjusted to approximate the pressure you'd experience around 5,000 to 8,000 feet above sea level, about what you'd feel driving around Denver, Colorado. At this height, you and your baby will each have less oxygen in your blood than you would at sea level. But your bodies will adjust, and you should get along fine.

If possible, select a seat directly behind a bulkhead or an aisle seat so you'll have more leg room. While seated, fasten your seat belt snugly beneath your abdomen, across the tops of your thighs. If possible, also periodically get up and move about, especially on a lengthy flight. Blood can pool in your legs if you sit idle for extended periods, leading to blood clots.

Drink plenty of non-alcoholic liquids before you board and during your flight. The humidity aboard the aircraft is generally low, and extra fluids can help prevent dehydration, which can lead to nausea.

Don't bother with special diets that supposedly prevent jet lag. You'll have better results if you change your sleeping patterns gradually for several days before traveling to a new time zone.

If you are experiencing health problems during your pregnancy, air travel can be unwise. For example, if you have anemia or sickle cell anemia, decreased air pressure during the air travel could cause complications that risk your health and your baby's. Other medical conditions that may necessitate postponing air travel include heart or lung disease, a blood clot in an inflamed vein (thrombophlebitis), preterm labor or vaginal bleeding; also, if you're expecting twins, triplets or more, air travel may not be advisable.

Besides checking with your doctor before leaving on any trip, you may want to check with your health insurance agent about coverage in another city or state or especially overseas. Travel can alter insurance benefits. You may want to consider additional coverage.

Immunizations for International Travel

Regardless of travel plans, it's best to receive vaccinations before you become pregnant. But sometimes, of course, the need is unforeseen. Consult your doctor before receiving any vaccine.

Your need for immunizations before departure on a trip outside the United States depends on the region into which you plan to travel. Most countries don't require immunizations before entry. However, if you're traveling to a developing country or one in which there's a known outbreak of disease, your doctor may recommend one or more vaccines, or advise you not to go at all. Your doctor or travel agent can help determine whether a particular geographic region poses unusual health hazards.

Your doctor will also recommend whether you should receive the vaccine on the basis of how far along you are in your pregnancy and the safety of the vaccine. Some vaccines are made from killed viruses. Others are made from live, inactivated viruses (weakened but not dead microorganisms). If at all possible, avoid any vaccine within the first trimester of your pregnancy. But throughout your pregnancy, avoid live vaccines. If you're proposing a trip to a country in which diseases such as typhoid, cholera or yellow fever are prevalent, your doctor may advise against travel.

Avoiding Traveler's Diarrhea

If you're traveling to a country outside the United States, you may be more likely to experience diarrhea. So before you leave, take steps to minimize your risk of picking up a diarrheal illness. Also, have a backup plan in case prevention fails. Some suggestions are listed below.

Recognize your risks. Largely due to inadequate sanitation standards, traveler's diarrhea is common in developing nations. High-risk areas include Latin America, Africa, the Middle East and Southeast Asia. In the Caribbean islands, the risk varies based on local sanitation standards. Risk is minimal within the United States, Canada, northern Europe, Australia and New Zealand.

Be careful. Don't use tap water in high-risk areas—don't drink it, brush your teeth with it or use ice cubes made from it. Don't drink water purified with iodine. Stick to bottled drinks. Pay attention to what you eat too. Be sure meat, shellfish and vegetables are cooked thoroughly. Don't eat fruits that you haven't peeled, or dairy products and food offered by street vendors.

Be prepared. Many medications, prescription or over-the-counter, are unavailable in other countries. For symptomatic relief of diarrhea, several over-the-counter medications are safe to use: products that contain attapulgite (such as Kaopectate, Diasorb) or kaolin and pectin (such as Kapectolin, Kao-Spen). Avoid products that contain salicylate, such as Pepto-Bismol. Before you travel to an area where poor sanitation poses a risk for traveler's diarrhea, talk to your doctor about prescribing an antibiotic for you to take along in case you need it.

Do I Need to Take Precautions Around the House?

There are a few precautions to observe, especially if you have a cat or if you're planning to decorate a room for your baby or elsewhere in your home. Whether you just learned you're pregnant or you are nearing the final weeks of your pregnancy, you may experience a compelling urge to rearrange rooms or tidy up for visitors who may be planning to come soon after your baby arrives. As long as you feel comfortable and enjoy the "nesting," go ahead—but remember to follow these precautions.

Painting

If you're determined to do stripping, painting, wallpapering or furniture refinishing yourself, avoid exposure, especially during the first trimester, to oil-based paints, lead, mercury (contained in some latex paints) or other substances that have solvents (chemicals used to dissolve other materials). Most of the studies investigating the risks to pregnant women exposed to these substances involved women who were exposed for long periods because of their occupations. Even if you're expecting only minimal exposure, it's best to be cautious. Make sure to work in a large, well-ventilated area to minimize breathing fumes. Wear protective clothing and gloves. Don't eat or drink in the work area.

Housecleaning

Disinfecting your toilet or polishing your furniture is not likely to harm your baby in any way. No evidence indicates a link between the normal use of household cleaners and birth defects. It's a good idea, however, to avoid oven cleaners and dry-cleaning agents while pregnant. Also, never mix ammonia with chlorine-based products. The combination produces toxic fumes. Be sure to wear gloves when you are cleaning, and don't directly inhale any strong, caustic fumes.

Cleaning the Litter Box

The solid wastes (feces) of cats may contain a parasite that can cause toxoplasmosis, a rare but serious blood infection. If you pass this infection on to your baby, birth defects such as blindness, deafness and mental retardation may occur. The chances of these are slim, but be cautious. Wear rubber gloves when cleaning the litter box or, better yet, delegate the task to someone else. Also avoid yard work or gardening in areas that your pet may have contaminated. (For more information about toxoplasmosis, see page 219.)

Exposure to Electrical Fields

Since the late 1970s, experts have speculated on whether exposure to weak electrical fields produced by computer display screens, electric blankets, heated waterbeds or other electric household devices is a health hazard while you're pregnant. Some studies have looked for risks of miscarriages or birth defects from prolonged use of computers by pregnant women. Studies also have assessed the potential risks of using electric blankets and heated waterbeds. Most scientists agree on the need for additional study. To date, however, no convincing evidence indicates significant risks associated with using these devices while pregnant.

Will Lovemaking Harm My Baby?

If your pregnancy is proceeding normally and your physician has not told you that you're at risk for premature labor, your lovemaking can proceed well into the third trimester of your pregnancy. Granted, you might find your bulging abdomen an obstacle, but with a willingness to try new positions and a spirit of adventure, you and your partner may find the effort well worthwhile.

Many expectant mothers are especially concerned that intercourse will cause a miscarriage, particularly in the first trimester. Most miscarriages during this time, however, would occur regardless of sexual activity. They commonly result from genetic defects unrelated to any influences after conception.

Orgasms can cause uterine contractions. But the vast majority of studies indicate that if you have a normal pregnancy, orgasms with or without intercourse do not lead to premature labor, premature rupture of your membranes or premature birth.

As you approach your due date, you do not need to worry about intercourse itself physically harming your baby. Intercourse more than once a week in late pregnancy, however, might increase the risk of intrauterine infection. So your physician may recommend abstinence during the last weeks as a precaution.

If vaginal bleeding, an incompetent cervix (premature softening and widening of the cervix) or placenta previa develops at any point in your pregnancy, your doctor may recommend no intercourse. Other conditions of pregnancy, such as expecting twins, may also rule out intercourse late in pregnancy.

Decreased interest in sex early in your pregnancy also may play a significant role in your sexual activity. Changing hormones, added weight and a decrease in your energy level may take their toll on your desire. The lackluster interest may continue through the first trimester, when exhaustion and nausea are most likely to occur. During the second three months, however, you may find your interest changing. Increased blood flow to your sexual organs and breasts may rekindle your desire, or even increase your normal interest in intercourse. You may even experience a moderate feeling of sustained readiness due to the effects of increased blood flow to your sexual organs and breasts. As you enter the final trimester you may find your desire waning again. Besides a large abdomen that makes intercourse physically challenging, increased fatigue or back pain can dampen your enthusiasm for lovemaking. Experiment with positions that make intercourse comfortable for you and your partner.

Throughout your pregnancy, try to sustain the romance in your relationship. Cuddling, caressing and massage can be just as pleasurable as intercourse. Focus on the "love" part of lovemaking.

Take Care of Yourself

Physical and emotional changes are a normal part of pregnancy. But as long as you have no known complications, you don't need to change your daily life dramatically. Following the various precautions recommended here will help reassure you that you're doing what you can to create a safe environment for your unborn baby. Pregnancy is a time to take especially good care of yourself and your unborn child. It can even motivate you to establish healthful habits such as exercising or quitting smoking.

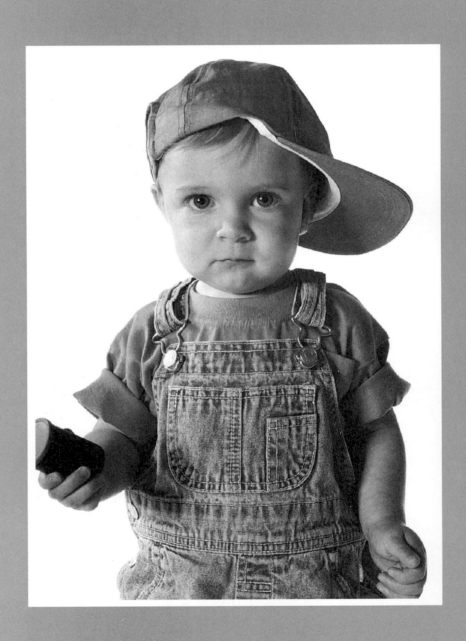

CHAPTER NINE

Pregnancy and Work

During pregnancy, you work hard 24 hours a day, seven days a week. (This is true even if you are resting at home.) Your heart pumps faster. You breathe faster. You need more food and rest. Your metabolism and hormones are altered. In addition, your body undergoes outward physical changes, some of which may make you uncomfortable.

You may be working overtime mentally, too, worrying about the baby and about whether you will be a good parent. Some days you may feel as if you are on an emotional roller coaster. Coping with these highs and lows can be stressful.

This chapter is about working wisely during your pregnancy, while your body undertakes the most demanding job of all: nurturing a developing baby.

The Myth of Superwoman

Superwoman has a highly paid, demanding job and keeps a beautiful home without help. She gives generously to her partner, family, friends and co-workers, but needs nothing from them in return. Pregnancy does not slow her down. It does not seem to have much effect on her at all. During labor, she cracks jokes. When she returns to work, her life is flawlessly organized and running smoothly. Superwoman never has to puzzle out an insurance form, never is tired at the end of the day and never worries about the responsibilities of motherhood.

Everyone knows Superwoman from books, movies and television. But no one has met her. She is a myth. She does not have these traits because she is superior to you; it is because she does not exist.

Reality

Unlike this mythical Superwoman, you live in the real world. Therefore, working during your pregnancy means making choices and getting information.

Some or all of the following questions might be important:

- Is it safe to work while pregnant?
- How can you make your work environment as physically comfortable as possible?
- What steps can you take to reduce stress and fatigue?
- Can you count on support from your employer and co-workers?
- What health insurance and maternity leave benefits are you entitled to?
- How much maternity leave will you take? Will your partner take paternity leave?
- What plans can you make that will allow you to breastfeed after you return to work, if that is your choice?
- What if you don't want to work full-time after the baby is born?

In considering these questions, you are not alone. Discuss your concerns about working during pregnancy with your doctor at the first prenatal visit. Your company personnel office can provide information on health insurance, disability benefits and family/maternity leave policies.

Your employer and co-workers are important people in your life. A positive attitude and a frank discussion of your needs while pregnant will go a long way toward enlisting their support.

The Good News

"You're working at a job and at the same time making a baby. It's even more satisfying."
—Susan, architect

For almost all women, it is safe to work while pregnant. This is true even if you have a physically strenuous job. If you have an uncomplicated pregnancy, you likely will be able to work right up until the onset of labor, if you choose.

In fact, working can be good for you. Employment provides money (which may be especially important right now). It may also provide other important benefits, such as access to health and disability insurance, social support and increased self-esteem. Work is also a distraction. You may worry less and feel better with a job to occupy your mind. According to some studies, pregnant working women reported having fewer physical and psychological symptoms than pregnant homemakers.

Jean, an office worker in a duplicating shop, worked full-time during her first pregnancy but not during her second and third pregnancies. She said that she felt "physically and mentally healthier" while working. She credited her increased sense of well-being to close relationships with her co-workers. "I got a lot of support and advice from them," she said. "It really helped—especially because this was my first baby."

Each pregnancy is unique. Some women work fewer hours, stop working altogether or perform different tasks during pregnancy. Others continue all their job duties for the entire nine months. You and your doctor will decide what is best based on your health, how your pregnancy is progressing, how you feel and how you spend your working day.

Your Working Day

Balancing Activity and Rest

The great trick of working is balancing the demands of your job with your equally important needs for play, rest and relationships with other people. Finding that balance can take time and experimentation, whether or not you are pregnant. However, when you are pregnant, it may be especially important to reflect on how you spend your time.

When you are pregnant, you need more rest. In the first and third trimesters, especially, you may feel tired much of the time. This fatigue is your body's way of telling you to slow down. In most cases, slowing down does not mean quitting your job. It means working smarter.

Working smarter. Regular rest periods throughout the day improve your productivity rather than decrease it. Schedule frequent, short breaks. As one pregnant woman remarked, "Even 10 minutes of rest could make me feel really rejuvenated." Taking regular breaks may let you pace yourself. As a result, you might be able to work longer each day and perhaps for a greater length of time during your pregnancy.

Working smarter can also mean reorganizing your day. Schedule easier tasks during the periods of the day when you feel most tired. If mornings are particularly difficult, you might investigate the possibility of starting work later and staying that much longer at the end of the day. You may also need to consider reducing or eliminating some of your other activities outside of work to ensure that you get enough rest. Even small changes could make a big difference in your comfort and productivity.

If your job is physically strenuous, it makes sense to take it easy in the evenings and on weekends. The more strenuous your job, the more rest you need. However, if you sit at a desk all day, a walk, a prenatal exercise class or a night out might be just what you want and need. Balance is the key. Because so much of your energy is going toward nurturing your unborn baby, it makes sense to avoid overdoing it in other areas of your life.

Buying time

Contrary to popular belief, you can buy time. Any of the following services can give you and your partner some precious additional hours of rest and relaxation.

- Home maintenance services—for all the little jobs around the house that never seem to get done: fixing faucets, washing windows, caulking, doing yard work.

- Housecleaning services—coming home to a clean house will free up some time and lift your spirits too.

- Mail-order shopping—those slick catalogs make shopping easy and fast.

- Grocery shopping by phone—groceries delivered to your door.

- Errand services—whatever you need picked up or dropped off.

Making Yourself Comfortable

Try to be as comfortable as possible when you're at work. Doing stretching exercises when you get up and periodically throughout the day will help reduce muscle aches and tension. Also, be sure to empty your bladder every few hours. Here are some other suggestions that you might find helpful, depending on the type of work you do.

Sitting. You'll be more comfortable if your office chair:

- Is adjustable for height and tilt
- Has a firm seat and back cushions
- Has adjustable armrests
- Provides good support for your lower back

If you need more support than your chair provides, bring a small pillow from home or invest in a cushion specifically designed to support the lower back. (Such a cushion may help for driving, too, if you have a long commute.)

It is better to sit with your feet elevated on a footrest or box than to cross your legs. This position will help take some of the strain off your back and reduce the chances of developing varicose veins or clots in the veins of your legs. Using a footrest may also help reduce the swelling in the feet and legs that so many pregnant women experience. Also, be sure to get up occasionally and walk around because this is good for your circulation and helps stretch your muscles. Some footrests are round-bottomed, enabling them to be rocked. This gentle motion is good for your circulation and may be soothing if you feel restless.

Standing. If you have to stand for prolonged periods, put one foot on a box or low stool to take pressure off your back. It may also help to wear support hose and to take frequent breaks throughout the day. Some doctors recommend shoes with low, wide heels rather than high heels or flats. If your job requires you to stand four or more hours each day, be sure to tell your doctor.

Bending and lifting. For recommendations on proper lifting technique, see page 155.

Reducing Stress

"It's imperative for people to continue exercising. They'll feel 100 percent better."
—Danielle, advertising sales representative

Stress can inspire you to try harder, dig deeper and do better work than you ever believed possible. Stress can also burn you out, make you feel depressed and exhausted and tempt you to do things that won't help you or your baby (for example, neglecting to eat right and exercise).

During pregnancy, you have heavy responsibilities but only limited control. Such a role is stressful, so it is important for pregnant women to reduce stress in other areas of their lives.

People who respond negatively to stress believe that there are no solutions to their problems. They suffer silently rather than trying to change their circumstances or their attitudes. As a result, the pressure builds.

Positive responses to stress include talking out problems with supportive people, finding harmless ways to blow off steam (crying, taking a brisk walk, writing an angry letter and then tearing it up) and making changes to avoid or minimize a problem. Your health care provider may have insights and suggestions that can be helpful in dealing with stressful situations. Prenatal educators, social workers or nurses may also serve as good sources of information and support.

A sense of humor helps, and so does the company of positive, optimistic people. It is wise to keep the big picture in mind as you decide what is and is not important. It is also wise to ask yourself whether it is worth getting angry about events you cannot change. As the saying goes, "You can be right, or you can be happy." Given the choice, choose being happy.

Relaxation tips. Reducing your stress level will make you a better, more productive employee. It is far better to spend five or 10 minutes doing a relaxation exercise than to spend an hour worrying or fuming (while neglecting your work).

The following three exercises are simple stress relievers. You may even be able to use some of these techniques during labor and birth. The breathing exercise can be done anywhere, anytime. The others can be done during breaks or other "down" periods.

- *Breathing.* Inhale slowly through your nose. Hold your breath for the count of five. Exhale slowly and deeply. Repeat three or four times.

- *Drift away.* Look at a picture or object that has a pleasant meaning for you. Lose yourself in the positive thoughts that it inspires. Listening to favorite music might help you relax. If that's not possible at your workplace, turn up your inner stereo and indulge yourself silently.

- *Write down your feelings.* Buy an inexpensive notebook and write for five or 10 minutes when you feel restless or frustrated. Write without stopping, and pay no attention to grammar or spelling. Expressing your feelings—if only on paper—is better than pretending that they don't exist. And don't be surprised if insights and solutions to problems suddenly present themselves as you write.

Workplace Cautions

Physical Stress

Several studies indicate that certain physical activities and working conditions can increase the risk of preterm labor and low birth weight:

- Heavy, repetitive lifting
- Prolonged standing
- Heavy vibration (such as that from large machines)
- Long, stressful commutes to and from work

The risk from prolonged standing may not seem obvious at first. However, during pregnancy there is increased dilation of blood vessels and pooling of blood in the legs with standing. These effects may cause dizziness and even fainting, which could lead to accidents and injuries in some circumstances.

Other job conditions might also require modification during pregnancy. For example, frequent shift changes may make it difficult for a pregnant woman to get all the rest she needs. A hot working environment may decrease her stamina and ability to perform strenuous physical tasks. Activities that require agility and good balance may become more difficult and risky later in pregnancy.

You may need to review these issues with your health care provider and, possibly, your employer. If your work involves one or more of the conditions listed above, you may need to stop working earlier in your pregnancy or modify your job duties. Your doctor will make specific recommendations as your pregnancy progresses.

Safety of VDTs

A VDT (video display terminal) is a monitor connected to a computer or word processor. Like color televisions, VDTs emit a small amount of non-ionizing radiation.

In the 1980s there was much controversy about whether the non-ionizing radiation emitted by VDTs posed a threat to the fetus. However, studies to date indicate that this low level of radiation is not dangerous.

If you continue to be worried, or just want to be cautious, it's simple to be safe. Sit 22 to 28 inches (about one arm's length) from the front of your terminal and 3 to 4 feet from the backs and sides of other people's terminals. At these distances, the amount of non-ionizing radiation drops off dramatically.

Newer VDTs manufactured to the "Swedish standard" emit less non-ionizing radiation than older ones.

Certain substances in the workplace are known to be harmful to the developing fetus. These include lead and mercury, ionizing radiation (X-rays) and drugs used to treat cancer. Anesthetic gases and organic solvents such as benzene are suspected to be harmful, although results of studies are inconclusive. Women who work in health care or any type of manufacturing, especially, should be aware of the substances to which they are exposed at work.

The good news is that few birth defects are caused by environmental agents. Of the 4 to 6 percent of birth defects that can be traced to an environmental cause, most involve alcohol, tobacco or drugs used during pregnancy—not substances in the workplace. Nevertheless, exposure to known or suspected harmful substances should be avoided.

Tell your doctor about exposure you have to chemicals, drugs or radiation on the job. Also tell your doctor about any equipment in the workplace designed to minimize exposure, such as gowns, gloves, masks and ventilation systems. He or she will use that information to determine whether a risk exists and, if so, what can be done to eliminate or reduce it. You might be asked to keep a diary of your workplace activities for a week or so.

Industries in the United States are required by federal law to have Material Safety Data Sheets on file that report hazardous substances in the workplace. It is also required that this information be made available to employees. Your doctor may have access to the latest data on hazardous substances through computerized databases and specialized resource centers.

Exposure to Harmful Substances

Health care and child care workers, schoolteachers, veterinary workers and meat handlers may be exposed to infections in the course of their jobs. Infections of greatest concern for pregnant women are rubella (German measles), chickenpox, fifth disease (parvovirus), cytomegalovirus, toxoplasmosis, herpes simplex, hepatitis B and AIDS. (See page 212 for more information about infections during pregnancy.)

You may already be immune to some of these diseases, either because you've had them or been vaccinated against them. If not, you should avoid situations in which you are exposed to the infection, such as close contact with a person who has the illness.

Doctors, nurses and other health care workers practice infection-control procedures such as wearing gloves, washing hands and avoiding eating on the job. Good hygiene is also important at child care centers. If you work at a child care center, wash your hands after changing diapers or helping children use the bathroom, and before eating. Avoid contact with saliva, which means not kissing your young charges or sharing food with them.

If you are concerned about getting an infection at work, speak with your doctor. Depending on your health, immune status and job duties, he or she may want you to take special precautions to avoid exposure.

Infections

Support From Your Employer and Co-Workers

Most women of childbearing age have jobs outside the home. Also, more than half of the mothers of children younger than 6 work outside the home. Because women, including pregnant women and working mothers, are such a big part of the American workforce, it is important that policies continue to be developed that promote ongoing productivity while protecting the health and well-being of the individual woman and her unborn child.

Family-Friendly Policies

"Working during my pregnancy was a really good experience. And I think that was because of the people around me."—Barbara, nursing assistant

"Family-friendly" policies include flexible time, health insurance, paid sick leave, job-protected maternity leave and direct child care benefits. There is some evidence that these policies are good for both employees and employers. A recent study sponsored by the U.S. Department of Labor indicated that pregnant women who worked for employers with family-friendly policies were more productive, had more job satisfaction, worked longer into their pregnancies and planned to return to work earlier than pregnant women whose employers did not provide these benefits.

However, if you were recently hired, work part-time or work for a very small company, you might not have these benefits. (The possible exception is flexible time, which is relatively inexpensive for employers to offer.) In some cases, employers offer unpaid leave or flexible time on an individual basis.

Your Legal Rights

The Family and Medical Leave Act. The Family and Medical Leave Act of 1993 might make it easier for both women and men to balance their need to work with their family responsibilities. The basic provision of the Act is simple: Employers with 50 or more employees must provide workers with up to 12 weeks of unpaid leave a year for the birth or adoption of a child, for the foster care of a child, to care for a child, spouse or parent with a serious health condition or because of an employee's own serious health condition.

Here are the main requirements:

- To be eligible for benefits under the Family and Medical Leave Act, employees must have worked for their employer for at least 12 months and have worked at least 1,250 hours during the previous 12-month period.

- Employers may require employees to substitute sick leave, vacation days, personal leave or other available family leave for any part of the 12 weeks of leave provided by federal law. Employees may also elect this option.

- With the exception of a few highly paid "key" employees, persons taking family leave are entitled to return to the jobs they left or to equivalent positions.

- When leave is foreseeable, employees must give at least 30 days' notice.

- Employees taking leave are entitled to the same health insurance benefits they had while they were working.

Your state may also have a maternity/family leave policy. If the state provisions for leave are more generous than those in the Family and Medical Leave Act, employers must comply with the state law. State provisions for maternity/family leave vary dramatically—from none at all to benefits that exceed the new federal requirements. Your state department of labor or human rights commission can tell you what maternity/family leave benefits are available.

Note that the Family and Medical Leave Act makes it possible for fathers, as well as mothers, to take time off to care for a newborn child.

The Pregnancy Discrimination Act of 1978.

The Pregnancy Discrimination Act of 1978 makes it illegal for employers to discriminate against pregnant employees. A pregnant woman cannot be fired or forced to take leave from her job just because she is expecting a baby. Furthermore, if a woman has a disability related to pregnancy or childbirth, she is entitled to the same benefits offered to other disabled employees. These benefits might include paid disability leave, job protection or, in some cases, reassignment to different duties.

The Pregnancy Discrimination Act does not apply to federal employees or to businesses that employ 14 or fewer workers. Nor does the Act force employers to provide benefits where none existed in the first place. In other words, if an employer does not provide medical, disability or leave benefits for any employees, the employer does not have to provide these benefits for pregnant employees either.

As of 1993, five states (California, Hawaii, New Jersey, New York and Rhode Island) and Puerto Rico had temporary disability insurance laws that provide partial salary replacement for non-work-related conditions. Those conditions include childbirth and pregnancy-related disabilities. Information on this insurance can be obtained from the states' departments of labor.

The right to work.

In 1991 the U. S. Supreme Court ruled that fertile women cannot be banned from jobs to protect their unconceived fetuses. Some jobs (for example, battery manufacturing) might expose workers to toxic substances that could damage their ability to become parents or have harmful effects on a fetus. However, a policy that bans fertile women (but not fertile men) from certain jobs amounts to sex discrimination. In addition, the Pregnancy Discrimination Act indicates that the responsibility for making decisions related to work and pregnancy rests with the individual woman, not with her employer.

Chances are that you will be able to work throughout your pregnancy. But what if you can't? Nicole, a systems analyst with a government agency, had to quit working full-time during her second trimester because of medical complications. Although she was able to arrange to work part-time at home for her employer, weeks went by before she received approval for doing so. If she had it to do over again, she said, she would have a contingency plan in place from the time she knew she was pregnant. "Women should find out as soon as possible what their options are, before they are pregnant, if possible," she said.

"What If?" Planning

Attitudes of Your Supervisor and Co-Workers

Women who are conscientious workers may think that they have to over-compensate for being pregnant. At work, they may resist asking for help, ignore their need for extra rest and even feel guilty about being pregnant. Such an attitude does no one any good. It increases fatigue and stress in the expectant mother. Furthermore, it may leave her co-workers feeling bewildered and hurt. They may not understand why their help is being rejected.

"I was close to my co-workers," one woman said. "People were concerned about my pregnancy and eager to give advice."

Chances are that your co-workers want to support you. However, they may not know how. That is why it is important to talk openly with them about your needs.

One pregnant woman got extra rest by closing her office door, turning out the lights and putting her head down for a few minutes each day. Her co-workers supported her by taking her phone calls and not interrupting her during these breaks. Another woman was very sensitive to odors during the first trimester of her pregnancy—so sensitive that the scent of a co-worker's aftershave made her sick. Rather than be a martyr, she asked him to stop wearing the aftershave temporarily. "He took it fine," she said.

Apart from practical help, co-workers can provide emotional support. Christine, an accounts-payable supervisor at a real estate investment firm, said that her co-workers' support was extremely important. "It's hard to work and be pregnant," she said, "but the people here at work were really supportive—interested and excited. It helped a lot."

Support from your supervisor means a lot too. That support could take several forms. Supervisors could enable a change of duties if certain activities (for example, standing for long periods) become difficult or uncomfortable. One woman mentioned that her supervisor helped her arrange her job duties so that all major projects were finished about a month before the baby was due. For the last month, she worked on short-term projects that other people could easily take over.

Don't feel guilty about accepting help when it's offered. A positive, cooperative attitude on your part will inspire positive, cooperative responses in the people around you.

Planning for Maternity Leave

Don't wait until the last minute to find out about maternity leave. Get information from your company's personnel department on the type of leave available for new mothers and fathers. Ask whether you can use paid sick leave, vacation days or personal days to substitute for part of your maternity leave or to extend it. Make sure you understand what benefits will continue during your leave and what benefits will cease. If the baby's father plans to take family leave, all these questions are important for him to ask too.

If you feel that you are not receiving all the benefits you should, either under the law or under your employer's benefit plan, contact an attorney familiar with employment law.

Preparing for Life
After the Baby Is Born

Start planning for child care as soon as possible. Some providers have long waiting lists, especially for infants. Start investigating your options and thinking about what you and your child are going to need in a child care situation. Talk to family, friends and co-workers who have faced the same issue. Just knowing what they decided—and how they felt about their decisions—may help you. Chapter 35 has specific advice on choosing a child care center or in-home caregiver for your baby.

Planning for Child Care

You won't know how you feel about combining work and motherhood until you become a mother. Perhaps you will decide that you would rather stay home with your baby. Perhaps you will decide that returning to work is more important than ever. This is a personal decision that no one can make for you.

Because you won't know for sure how you will feel, play the "what if" game. What if you decide not to return to your job? What will be the cost in lost income, benefits, social support and professional advancement? What will you gain? Thinking about the consequences of either choice in advance may help you make a decision when the time comes.

Ambivalence About Returning to Work

The era in which everyone worked for a rigid amount of time in one location is giving way to an era of more choices. Flexible hours, for example, can be a great boon for working parents. Job sharing or part-time work may be other possibilities.

Some people with information-based jobs (a fast-growing segment of the labor force) find that they can "telecommute." Home computers, modems, fax machines and electronic mail (e-mail) can enable telecommuters to do part or all of their work at home. The technological advances that enable telecommuting have also promoted a boom in freelancing and home-based businesses. This option may be possible for you. Look for information on home-based businesses in libraries and bookstores.

Before exploring any of these possibilities with your supervisor, try to imagine the company's point of view. You should present a win-win scenario. Show how both you and your employer will benefit from the changes you propose.

Get in touch with someone who has worked out an alternative approach to her job. Ask how she presented this alternative to her employer and what she might have done differently. Her advice may make a difference in the way you develop your strategy.

Creative Approaches for Returning to Work Later

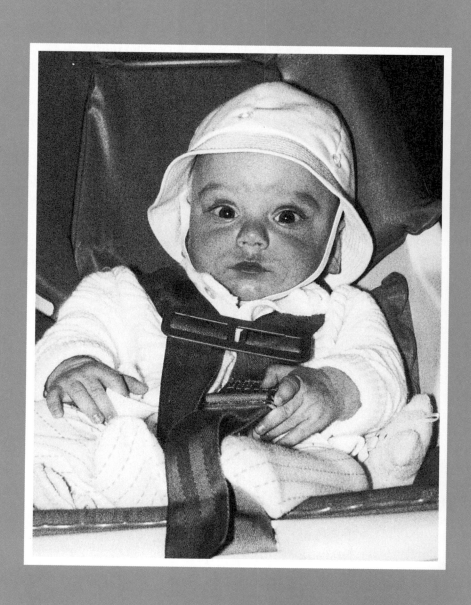

CHAPTER TEN

The First Trimester

First 12 weeks

Pregnancy typically lasts 40 weeks, counting from the first day of a woman's last menstrual period, and is often referred to in three parts, called trimesters. The first trimester lasts 12 weeks, the second from 13 to the end of 27 weeks, and the third from 28 to 40 weeks. These divisions, however, are somewhat arbitrary, and you may encounter slightly different versions of these time periods. Actually, your doctor will probably refer to your pregnancy by the age of the fetus in weeks.

Certain important milestones in pregnancy occur during each trimester. For example, specific tests are done during the first trimester, and certain problems, if they develop, almost always arise during the third trimester. Although there is nothing crucial about these trimester divisions, they do help both you and your doctor in planning the management of your pregnancy.

The first trimester is a time of profound changes inside your body, and you'll experience these changes in your own individual way. For example, some women know right away that they have conceived, whereas others may not be convinced that they're pregnant even after a positive pregnancy test and confirmation by their physician. The first trimester may bring increased energy and a sense of well-being, yet other women feel increasingly tired and emotional; still others don't notice many changes until much later in pregnancy.

Physical Changes and Symptoms

Although the physical changes of early pregnancy may make you uncomfortable, they don't endanger your health or the health of your baby. Each pregnancy, of course, is unique, and you may experience many, some or none of the changes and symptoms described here. Knowing what the symptoms mean, in terms of what is happening inside your body, and knowing what you can do to make yourself more comfortable will help you cope with the adjustments in early pregnancy.

Fatigue

What causes it? Most, if not all, women are more tired than usual in early pregnancy. This feeling is understandable: your body has a lot of work to do. During the first weeks of pregnancy, your body begins to produce more blood to carry nutrients to the fetus. Your heart multiplies its efforts to accommodate this increased blood flow, and your pulse quickens by as much as 10 to 15 beats per minute. Your body changes the way it uses water, protein, carbohydrate and fat. The combination of these profound changes translates into the fatigue you feel.

In addition to the physical changes that make you feel tired, you are also adjusting to new feelings and concerns. Whether your pregnancy was planned or unplanned, you may have conflicting feelings about it. Even if you are overjoyed at being pregnant, there are probably added emotional stresses in your life at this time. You may have fears about whether the baby will be healthy, anxiety about how you will adjust to motherhood and concerns about increased expenses. In addition, if your work is demanding, you may worry about being able to sustain your productivity throughout pregnancy.

Anxieties can occur whether this baby will be your first or your fourth. These concerns are natural and normal. It's important to recognize that they, too, play a part in how you feel physically.

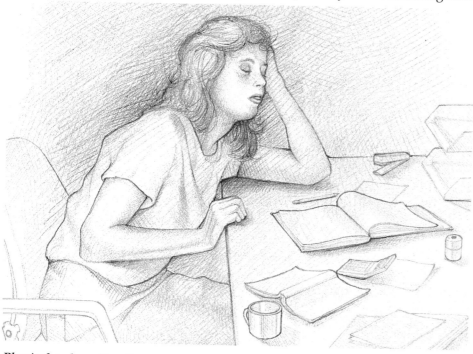

Physical and emotional changes are a normal part of early pregnancy, but they may sap your energy.

What can I do? Rest. Try to get the rest you need. After the birth of your baby, your lifestyle is sure to change, and there are adjustments you can make even now. In addition to eating well and avoiding the harmful effects of smoking and alcohol, you need to find ways to feel as rested as possible.

Take naps when you can during the day. At work, finding time to rest comfortably with your feet up can renew your energy.

If you can't nap during the day, maybe you can do so right after work, before dinner or evening activities. If you have a partner or other children, get them to help as much as possible. Also, cut down on social events if they're wearing you out. Those who care about you will understand and will be more than happy to make allowances for you. Ask for the support and understanding that you need during this time, keeping in mind that you will almost certainly have more stamina in later pregnancy.

If you need to go to bed at 6:30 or 7:00 to feel rested, do it. It may also help if you avoid drinking fluids for a few hours before bedtime so you won't have to get up as frequently during the night to empty your bladder.

Exercise. One of the best ways to increase your energy level is to exercise. The more you exercise, the more energy you seem to have to continue exercising, as well as to perform your daily tasks. Even moderate exercise, such as walking for 30 minutes each day, can really help you feel energized. (See page 108 for more about exercising during pregnancy.)

Eat right. Eating a balanced diet is even more important when you're pregnant than it was before. The fatigue that is natural in early pregnancy can be aggravated if you're not getting enough iron or protein. Check with your doctor to make sure your diet is nutritious and balanced. (See page 85 for more about eating a healthful diet during pregnancy.)

Nausea and Vomiting

W*hat causes it?* One theory is that nausea and vomiting in early pregnancy may be due to hormone changes produced by the placenta and the fetus. Changes in your gastrointestinal system may also play a role—the stomach empties somewhat more slowly under the influence of the hormones of pregnancy. Nausea and vomiting may also be aggravated by emotional stress and fatigue.

Even though it is commonly called "morning sickness," the nausea and vomiting in early pregnancy can occur at any time of day. This symptom is common, affecting up to 70 percent of pregnant women. It can be more severe in a first pregnancy, in young women and in women carrying multiple fetuses. Usually, it begins at four to eight weeks of gestation and subsides by 14 to 16 weeks. But some women have nausea and vomiting beyond the first trimester, and a few even throughout their entire pregnancy. In rare instances, nausea and vomiting may be so severe that a pregnant woman cannot maintain proper nutrition and fluids or gain enough weight. (See "Hyperemesis gravidarum," page 141.)

What can I do? Modify your eating habits. Eating smaller meals more frequently throughout the day often helps alleviate nausea. Drinking less fluid with meals may also provide relief. The idea behind these measures is to avoid having your stomach completely empty or completely full, either of which can make nausea worse.

Eat morning snacks. If nausea is worse when you first wake up, try nibbling on soda crackers or sipping weak tea before you get out of bed. Rise slowly, allowing a little time to digest before you get up.

Rest. The fatigue that is so common in early pregnancy can also contribute to nausea. Additional sleep each night may help.

Avoid displeasing smells and foods. Many women find certain smells or foods unpleasant when they are pregnant, even if they had no such reactions before. Whenever possible, try to avoid foods or smells that seem to aggravate your nausea.

Other possible remedies. It may be possible to alleviate nausea with an over-the-counter antacid. Don't take one, though, before getting your doctor's advice. Some types of antacids can cause fluid buildup. Vitamin B$_6$ has also been proposed as a remedy, but talk to your doctor before taking a vitamin supplement during pregnancy. Some women have successfully used acupressure or motion-sickness bands to combat nausea. These bracelets exert a steady pressure on the inside of the wrist.

Urinary Frequency

What causes it? The increasing size of the uterus in the first trimester, along with more efficient functioning of the kidneys, may cause you to feel the need to urinate more often. You may also have leaking of urine when sneezing, coughing or laughing. This is due to the growing uterus pressing against your bladder, which lies directly in front of and slightly under the uterus during the first few months of pregnancy. By the fourth month, the uterus will have expanded up out of the pelvic cavity, so that the pressure on your bladder is not as great.

What can I do? You may find that if you avoid drinking anything for a few hours before bedtime you will get up less often—and sleep better—throughout the night. It's not a good idea, though, to otherwise restrict your fluid intake during pregnancy.

Urinate as often as you feel the need to. Holding in your urine can result in incomplete emptying of the bladder, which may in turn lead to a urinary tract infection. Leaning forward while you urinate will help to empty your bladder more fully. Completely emptying the bladder may also have the added benefit of cutting down on how often you need to urinate. If you leak urine throughout the day, wearing panty liners will make you more comfortable.

Breast Tenderness

What causes it? The increased production of the hormones estrogen and progesterone is the primary reason for the changes in a pregnant woman's breasts. By a few weeks of gestation, you may notice tingling sensations in your breasts, and they may feel heavy, tender and sore.

What can I do? A good support bra can help alleviate breast soreness. Try a maternity bra or a larger-sized athletic bra; they tend to be breathable and comfortable. If you have large breasts that make you uncomfortable at night, you might want to try wearing a bra while you're sleeping too.

Headaches and Dizziness

What causes them? Occasional headaches trouble many women in early pregnancy. The cause is uncertain, but like so many other discomforts of the first trimester, changes in your hormone levels and blood circulation may be factors. Other possible causes are the stress and fatigue that often accompany the emotional and physical adjustments to pregnancy. If you suddenly eliminated or cut down on caffeine once you learned you were pregnant, this change may also cause headaches for a few days.

Dizziness is common in pregnant women and can result from circulatory changes during pregnancy. Stress, fatigue and hunger can also be causes of dizziness or faintness. A more serious cause may be an ectopic pregnancy, especially if dizziness is severe and occurs with abdominal pain or vaginal bleeding (see ectopic pregnancy, page 141). For this reason, it's always a good idea to tell your doctor about this symptom.

Although headaches and dizziness at this point in your pregnancy may be nothing to be concerned about, call your doctor right away if these symptoms are persistent or severe. Migraine-like, throbbing headaches or fainting spells should also prompt you to call your doctor immediately.

What can I do? Sinus headaches can be soothed by applying warm compresses to the front and sides of your face, around your nose, eyes and temples. A tension headache may be relieved by applying a cold compress to the back of your neck.

Relaxation exercises can help alleviate headaches as well as give you a greater overall sense of well-being. These exercises may consist of simply closing your eyes and imagining a calm, peaceful scene. Eating well and getting enough rest and exercise are important too.

It's easier said than done, but minimizing the stresses in your life will help you get through the first trimester, as well as the rest of pregnancy. Some sources of stress, of course, can't be avoided; the key, then, is to improve your coping skills. If you are under more stress than you feel you can handle, talking with a therapist or counselor, even if only on a one-time basis, to get advice and ideas can be very helpful.

Talk to your doctor before using pain relievers, even over-the-counter medications such as aspirin or ibuprofen (Advil, Ibuprin, Motrin IB, Nuprin). Acetaminophen (Aspirin Free Excedrin, Panadol, Tylenol) is a better choice during pregnancy, but it's best to avoid taking any medication during pregnancy unless absolutely necessary, and only when prescribed or advised by your doctor.

To prevent mild, occasional dizziness, move slowly as you get up from lying or sitting down. Try to keep your blood sugar level on an even keel by munching occasionally on snacks such as dried or fresh fruit, whole-wheat bread, crackers or low-fat yogurt.

Weight Gain

Although you'll probably gain about 25 to 30 pounds during the course of your pregnancy, you'll put on only a small percentage of this amount during the first trimester. A normal weight gain during the first trimester is only about 2 pounds. (See page 19 for more on recommended weight gain in pregnancy.)

The "warming up" effect: second and subsequent pregnancies

If you've already been pregnant once, you may notice that some of the changes you experienced the first time seem to be happening earlier in this pregnancy. You may notice that you're bigger than you were at the same time during your last pregnancy. You may also notice that some of the side effects you had last time—such as nausea, heartburn or abdominal twinges—seem to be happening earlier this time.

There is a likely explanation: It's known that a pregnant woman's abdomen often expands more and earlier in a second or subsequent pregnancy than it did the first time. The bigger size and earlier growth of your uterus, in turn, can give rise to the earlier appearance of side effects that are related to the expansion of the uterus.

For instance, nausea and heartburn may be aggravated by the uterus pushing up against the stomach. Twinges in the lower abdomen can be due to the stretching of ligaments and muscles. Because the uterus is getting bigger earlier, these symptoms may appear sooner in this pregnancy than they did in the first.

This result can be thought of as a "warming up" effect. Like a balloon that's easier to blow up the second or third time, your uterus expands more easily in subsequent pregnancies, because the muscles and ligaments have already been stretched. Because some of the tone of the abdominal muscles is lost after a first pregnancy, they stretch more as the uterus expands. In extreme instances, the abdominal muscles are so weakened that the abdomen sags forward and down.

The degree to which your uterus expands might depend on how big you became the first time, how much muscle tone you were able to gain back after delivery and also how much natural muscle tone you have. But even if you are in top shape, have good natural muscle tone and were rigorous in your approach to postpartum exercises after your first pregnancy, don't be surprised if you get at least somewhat bigger during this one.

What's Happening With the Baby?

All of your baby's essential structures and organ systems are formed during the first trimester. During the rest of the fetus's time in the uterus, those features are continuing to grow and develop and the baby is gaining weight.

By the end of the first trimester, the average fetus is about 2½ to 3 inches long and weighs about an ounce. Several organs and organ systems have formed and are beginning to function:

- The heart has been beating since about day 26.
- Reproductive organs have formed, although they cannot be seen well enough to determine the fetus's sex.
- The first bone cells are forming.
- Fingers and toes are present, along with the beginnings of nails.
- The circulatory and respiratory systems are working.
- The liver is making bile, and the kidneys are secreting urine into the bladder.

The fetus also begins to move during the first trimester, although it's unlikely that you will feel movement until later in pregnancy (see page 159).

Common Concerns in the First Trimester

Along with the common side effects of early pregnancy, many women experience other signs that may be more troubling. These are not necessarily cause for worry, but you should be aware of what symptoms should prompt you to contact your doctor.

Spotting or Bleeding

Vaginal bleeding in the first trimester is not uncommon, occurring in one out of every four to five women. Depending on several factors, such as whether it is heavy or light, how long it lasts and whether it is continuous or sporadic, bleeding can indicate many things. Bleeding in early pregnancy may be a warning sign, but it can also be due to normal events of pregnancy.

You may notice a small amount of bleeding or spotting very early in pregnancy, about a week to 10 days after fertilization. This is known as implantation bleeding, and it commonly happens when the fertilized egg first attaches to the inside of the uterus. This type of light bleeding usually lasts only briefly.

Because bleeding may signal a problem, however, call your doctor if you have spotting that persists for more than a day or two. Call immediately if:

- Bleeding is heavy
- Pain, cramping or fever is present with the bleeding
- You seem to have passed some tissue

These symptoms may be a cause for concern (see "Ectopic pregnancy," page 141, "Molar pregnancy," page 144, and "Miscarriage," page 145). Your doctor will want to examine you if you have bleeding in the first trimester.

Pelvic Pain

You may notice many new aches and pains when you are first pregnant. Many women tend to feel tired, achy or crampy during the first trimester. Pain in the lower abdomen can be explained by some of the normal processes taking place during this time. If it is severe and unrelenting, however, it may be a sign of a problem.

As the uterus expands, the elastic tissues (ligaments) that support it stretch to accommodate its growth. This process can cause twinges, cramps or pulling sensations on one or both sides of your lower abdomen. Although uncomfortable, it's usually nothing to worry about. You may get relief by soaking in a warm bath or doing relaxation exercises.

If pain is severe, persistent or accompanied by fever, call your doctor right away. These symptoms could signal a more serious problem.

Some Common Questions

Q: *I always get a bad cold in winter, and this year is no exception. But this time I'm pregnant. Is there any safe way I can treat the symptoms? Can my illness harm the baby?*

A: The symptoms of even a bad cold or flu, though they can make you miserable, are usually not harmful to your baby. Being run down, however, is a strain on your body. And unfortunately, colds tend to last longer during pregnancy, because of changes in your immune system.

Eating well, getting plenty of rest, exercising and avoiding close contact with anyone who has the sniffles or a sore throat are the best ways to keep from catching a cold or flu. If you're around family or co-workers with colds, wash your hands often. Cold germs are easily passed hand to hand, especially if you touch your eyes, nose or mouth after contact with the sick person.

The best way to deal with colds and flu during pregnancy is to take care of yourself without taking medications. Treat the symptoms first with plenty of rest and extra fluids. In addition to helping your body fight the cold, drinking plenty of fluids may help keep your stuffy nose clearer. Nasal congestion can also be helped by using a humidifier in your bedroom at night, sleeping propped up with your head elevated or breathing the steam from a pan of simmering water with a towel over your head. A sore throat may be soothed by sucking on ice chips, drinking warm liquids or gargling with very warm salt water. Cool baths can help lower a fever.

Although your appetite may be affected by a cold, take care to continue eating well. Eat smaller amounts more frequently throughout the day if you can't tolerate large meals.

Call your doctor if:

- Your fever reaches 102 degrees Fahrenheit
- You are coughing up greenish or yellow mucus
- Your symptoms are bad enough to keep you from eating or sleeping
- The symptoms persist for more than a few days with no signs of improvement

It may be possible to treat your symptoms with a cold remedy—or a secondary infection (such as bronchitis or sinus infection) with an antibiotic—but this decision must be made by your doctor.

Q: *Are X-rays harmful during pregnancy? Should I avoid getting them during a dental checkup? What about other types of X-rays?*

A: Although exposure to high doses of X-rays, such as radiation treatments for cancer, can harm the fetus, the low doses used for diagnostic purposes are unlikely to cause damage. If you had a diagnostic X-ray before you knew you were pregnant, don't become alarmed; talk with your doctor.

At doses of less than 10 roentgens (a unit of radiation exposure), there is no significant increase in the risk of birth defects. Dental X-rays and other common diagnostic procedures deliver far less than this amount. Even a direct X-ray of a pregnant woman's abdomen delivers a very tiny exposure (only about 0.05 roentgen). A chest X-ray of the mother exposes the uterus to an even smaller fraction (0.001 roentgen).

As with any medical procedure or medication during pregnancy, however, it's best not to have an X-ray unless it becomes necessary. Routine dental X-rays are usually put off until after delivery, or at least until the third trimester. But if a complication or injury makes an X-ray necessary, let your care provider know that you are pregnant before undergoing the procedure. Usually, the abdomen can be shielded with a lead apron.

Q: *My 2-year-old child wants to be carried all the time. Is it true that lifting her, or any heavy weight, can cause a miscarriage?*

A: Picking up your toddler or lifting heavy objects is more likely to harm your back than your fetus. It is not true that this can cause a miscarriage. As long as you don't exhaust yourself or strain your back, you should have no fears about lifting.

This will become more of a concern in later pregnancy, as your center of gravity changes and your enlarging abdomen starts to affect the way you normally move, lift, stand and carry. It's a good idea to get in the habit now of lifting by bending at the knees, not the waist, and pushing up with your legs, keeping your back as straight as possible. This is the best way to lift anything heavy, even if you're not pregnant. (See page 155 for photographs of the correct way to lift.)

Certain conditions in pregnancy require a woman to avoid heavy lifting after the first trimester. These include cervical incompetence (see page 172) and the risk of preterm labor (see page 169).

Q: *I'm pregnant with my second baby. Do I need to be concerned about diseases such as chickenpox that my small son may be exposed to?*

A: Although it's possible for childhood diseases to affect pregnant women, fortunately, they're rare in adults. The most common, such as chickenpox, rubella and mumps, are viral diseases that usually infect children younger than 15 years. And once you've had these diseases, you're immune to them for life. Even if you haven't had them, you were probably vaccinated against rubella and mumps as a child.

If you are unsure whether you had these diseases or the vaccines for them, there is still little reason to worry. It is true that these viruses can potentially harm a fetus in early pregnancy, but they cannot be transmitted directly to the fetus from infected people. The only way your fetus can be affected by them is if you yourself become ill. So unless you know you're immune, avoid contact with anyone who has chickenpox, measles, mumps or rubella, especially during the first trimester.

Of course, your own child should be vaccinated at 15 months of age for measles, mumps and rubella if he or she hasn't been already. The same goes for you, too, but not during pregnancy because the vaccines for rubella and mumps can potentially harm the fetus. There is as yet no widely used vaccine for chickenpox. If you have never had chickenpox but become exposed during pregnancy, contact your doctor to find out whether tests or medications would be helpful.

Q: *Should I be concerned about having sex while I'm pregnant? Can vigorous sex or orgasm trigger a miscarriage?*

A: There is usually no need to refrain from making love or having an orgasm at any stage of pregnancy. However, doctors sometimes advise women to refrain from lovemaking in the last few weeks before delivery. But it is not true that intercourse or orgasm will cause a miscarriage in early pregnancy.

Your doctor may advise you against having intercourse if you have had a previous miscarriage or preterm labor. Infection, bleeding and pain are also reasons to refrain from having sex (and to call your doctor).

The way that women feel about sex during the first trimester varies. You and your partner may enjoy the freedom from birth control. Or fatigue and nausea may dampen your interest. The important thing is for you and your partner to follow your feelings. There's no need to restrict lovemaking in early pregnancy unless you want to, or your doctor advises it.

Q: *My sleep patterns are totally different now that I'm pregnant; I often have insomnia, and my dreams are very vivid. Is this difference normal?*

A: Yes. Considering all the changes you're going through, both physically and emotionally, it's not surprising that your sleep is affected.

Although many women sleep more during the first trimester than before they were pregnant, some have trouble sleeping through the night. Insomnia won't harm your baby, and it won't hurt you, either, unless you become exhausted from it. Here are a few suggestions if you can't sleep through the night:

- Don't lie awake worrying about not sleeping; get up and read, write a letter, listen to a book on tape, do needlework or knitting or involve yourself in some other activity.
- If you get sleepy during the day but can't sleep at night, try taking short naps in the afternoon or early evening.
- If anxiety is keeping you awake, ask your doctor about relaxation exercises that may help.

Vivid dreaming or nightmares are also common during pregnancy. Dreams may be the mind's way of processing unconscious information, such as emotional or physical changes. You may find that you are dreaming more now than before or that you are remembering your dreams more clearly once you awaken. If disturbing dreams or nightmares are a cause of great concern or distress, it may be helpful to talk with a therapist or counselor to help sort out what's troubling you.

Q: *I've been nauseated quite a bit during these first months of my pregnancy. On top of that, I seem to have an unusual problem: I'm salivating a lot. It gets to be almost embarrassing at times. Am I imagining this?*

A: No, you're not. Excessive salivation, called ptyalism (TIE-a-lism), is a somewhat unusual side effect of pregnancy, but it is nonetheless real and can be an annoyance. It is not an indication that anything is wrong. Ptyalism seems to occur with nausea in some women. In fact, it may be that women are not producing any more saliva than usual, but rather, because of their nausea, they are not swallowing as much as they normally would.

Excessive salivation in pregnancy may be linked to eating starchy foods, so cutting down on these may help. When your nausea begins to decrease in the next trimester, this problem is likely to ease off as well.

Office Visits

Your first visit to the doctor after you've learned you're pregnant will focus mainly on assessing your overall health, identifying any risk factors for this pregnancy and determining the age of the fetus. Your doctor will take a detailed history, including information about any chronic medical conditions you have and problems you had during past pregnancies. The baby's due date will be estimated according to when you had your last period. A physical exam will include a look at the cervix through a speculum (a device inserted into the vagina, allowing the cervix to be seen) and feeling the shape of the uterus and ovaries (see page 48). For the first 28 weeks of your pregnancy, you'll probably see the doctor once a month unless a reason arises for more frequent visits.

Routine lab tests during the first trimester include blood tests to determine your blood type and Rh type (see page 167) and to find out whether you have been exposed to syphilis, rubella or hepatitis B. You may also be offered a test for HIV (the virus that causes AIDS). These will probably be done on the first visit, along with a blood count, urinalysis and a Pap smear.

It is not unusual for women to have some vaginal bleeding after a Pap smear. This may occur within 24 hours after your visit to the doctor. The bleeding may consist of a small amount of spotting or may be a little heavier, and it usually goes away within a day. If you are concerned, call your doctor's office. Be sure to do so if you are still spotting or bleeding bright-red blood after a day.

After the exam and tests, your doctor may want to spend some time talking with you about your general lifestyle, including nutrition, exercise, smoking, alcohol use and your workplace.

The first visit is a good time to raise any concerns or fears you may have about your pregnancy. Developing a strong relationship with your caregiver starts now, at the very beginning of your pregnancy.

Whom to call with questions—and when

It's normal to have fears and worries about the physical changes you're experiencing. So many of these sensations can seem ambiguous: Is a little spotting normal for early pregnancy, or is it a sign of an early miscarriage? How do you know when nausea and vomiting becomes severe enough to worry about? Is a nagging headache just from stress, or is it something more serious? How can you tell the difference between what is normal and when you should take action?

In making these judgments, your doctor is your primary resource. At your very first visit, ask for a list of the symptoms that she or he wants to hear about right away. Then you'll have an idea of what your doctor considers an emergency.

If you're still unsure about other symptoms, you can rely on the other care providers in your doctor's office. At your office visits, learn the names of the nurses, nurse-practitioners, physician assistants (PAs) and other staff you see most often. Then, if something comes up that has you worried, you can ask for someone by name or by title. The staff will know from your symptoms whether to consult your doctor. The bottom line, though, is this: When in doubt, call. It's better to have a needless worry eased than to have a real source of concern ignored out of embarrassment or fear.

Symptom	When to notify your doctor
Vaginal bleeding or spotting	
Slight spotting that goes away within a day	Next visit
Any spotting or bleeding that lasts more than a day	Same day
Moderate to heavy bleeding	Immediately
Any amount of bleeding accompanied by pain, fever or chills	Immediately
Pain	
Occasional pulling, twinging or pinching sensation on one or both sides of the abdomen	Next visit
Occasional mild headaches	Next visit
Moderate, bothersome headache that won't go away	Same day
Severe or persistent headache, especially with dizziness, faintness or visual disturbances	Immediately
Moderate or severe pelvic pain	Immediately
Any degree of pelvic pain that doesn't subside	Immediately
Pain with fever or bleeding	Immediately
Vomiting	
Occasional	Next visit
Once every day	Next visit
More than two or three times a day	Immediately
With pain or fever	Immediately
Other symptoms	
Chills or fever (temperature of 102 degrees Fahrenheit or higher)	Immediately
Painful urination	Immediately
Steady or heavy discharge of watery fluid from the vagina	Immediately
Sudden swelling of face, hands or feet	Immediately
Visual disturbances (dimness, blurring)	Immediately

Complications

Most pregnancies are healthy and untroubled by complications, but problems sometimes do arise. In most cases, risks to the mother and the baby are decreased if warning signs are recognized and dealt with early. So it's important to know about some of the more common complications of early pregnancy, how to recognize warning signs and when to call your doctor.

Hyperemesis Gravidarum

What causes it and who's at risk? Hyperemesis gravidarum, the medical name for excessive vomiting in pregnancy (*hyper* means "over"; *emesis* means "vomiting"; *gravidarum* means "pregnant state"), affects about one in every 300 pregnant women. This condition is defined as vomiting that is frequent, persistent and severe. If not treated, hyperemesis can keep the mother from getting the nutrition and fluids she needs. If it persists long enough, it can also threaten the fetus.

The causes of hyperemesis are not known with certainty, but it appears to be linked to higher-than-usual levels of the hormones hCG and estrogen. It is more common in first pregnancies, young women and women carrying multiple fetuses.

What's the treatment? Before treating you for hyperemesis, your doctor will first want to rule out other possible causes of the vomiting, such as gastrointestinal disorders, thyroid problems or a molar pregnancy (see page 144). Mild cases are treated with dietary measures, rest and antacids. More severe cases often require a stay in the hospital so that the mother can receive fluid and nutrition through an intravenous line.

If you have nausea and vomiting so severe that you cannot keep any food down, or if it persists well into the second trimester, contact your doctor. Do so right away if vomiting is accompanied by pain or fever.

Ectopic Pregnancy

An ectopic pregnancy is one in which the fertilized egg attaches itself in a place other than inside the uterus. Almost all (more than 95 percent) ectopic pregnancies occur in a fallopian tube; hence the term "tubal" pregnancy. Rarely, the egg may implant elsewhere, such as in the abdomen, ovary or cervix.

Because the narrow fallopian tubes are not designed to hold a growing embryo, the fertilized egg in a tubal pregnancy cannot develop normally. Eventually, the thin walls of the tube stretch to the point of bursting. If this happens, a woman is in danger of life-threatening blood loss (hemorrhage).

During the 1980s, the rate of ectopic pregnancy increased. Ectopic pregnancy now occurs in about seven of every 1,000 reported pregnancies in the United States. Even so, death from ectopic pregnancy is rare, occurring in fewer than one of every 2,500 cases. This low rate is largely a result of new techniques to detect ectopic pregnancy at an early stage, when the risk to the pregnant woman is much lower.

What causes it and who's at risk? Most cases of ectopic pregnancy are caused by an inability of the fertilized egg to make its way through a fallopian tube into the uterus. This is often caused by an infection or inflammation of the tube which has caused it to become partly or entirely blocked. Scar tissue left behind from a previous infection or an operation on the tube may also impede the egg's movement. Previous surgery in the pelvic area or on the tubes can also cause adhesions (bands of tissue that bind together surfaces inside the abdomen or the tubes). A condition called endometriosis, in which tissue like that normally lining the uterus is found outside the uterus, can also cause blockage of a fallopian tube. Another possible cause is an abnormality in the shape of the tube, which may be caused by abnormal growths or a birth defect.

Most ectopic pregnancies occur in women 35 to 44 years of age. The major risk factor for ectopic pregnancy is pelvic inflammatory disease (PID). This is an infection of the uterus, fallopian tubes or ovaries. The risk of ectopic pregnancy is also higher in women who have had any of the following:

- Previous ectopic pregnancy
- Surgery on a fallopian tube
- Several induced abortions
- Infertility problems or medication to stimulate ovulation

An ectopic pregnancy is one that occurs outside the uterus. The most common site of an ectopic pregnancy is inside one of the fallopian tubes; thus, ectopic pregnancies are sometimes called tubal pregnancies. The highlighted circles show other areas within the reproductive system, or even, rarely, the abdomen, where ectopic pregnancies can also occur.

What are the symptoms? In many cases, a pregnant woman and her doctor may not at first have any reason to suspect an ectopic pregnancy. The early signs of pregnancy, such as a missed period and other symptoms and signs, also occur in ectopic pregnancies.

Pain is usually the first sign of an ectopic pregnancy. The pain may be in the pelvis, abdomen or even the shoulder and neck (due to blood from a ruptured ectopic pregnancy building up under the diaphragm). Pain from an ectopic pregnancy is usually described as sharp and stabbing. It may come and go or vary in intensity.

Other warning signs of ectopic pregnancy include:

- Vaginal bleeding
- Gastrointestinal symptoms
- Dizziness or light-headedness

Although there may be other reasons for any of these symptoms, they should be reported to your doctor.

How is it diagnosed? If your doctor suspects an ectopic pregnancy, she or he will probably first perform a pelvic exam to locate pain, tenderness or a mass in the abdomen. Lab tests may then be ordered. The most useful of these is the measurement of hCG. In a normal pregnancy, the level of this hormone approximately doubles about every two days during the first 10 weeks. In an ectopic pregnancy, however, the rate of this increase is much slower. An hCG level that is lower than what would be expected for the stage of the pregnancy is one reason to suspect an ectopic pregnancy. The hCG level may be tested several times over a certain period to determine whether it is increasing at a normal rate.

Progesterone is another hormone that can be measured to help in the diagnosis of ectopic pregnancy. Low levels of this hormone may indicate that a pregnancy is abnormal. Further tests will be needed to confirm whether the pregnancy is ectopic and, if it is, where it is located.

Ultrasound exams may also be used to help determine whether a pregnancy is ectopic. With this technique, a device called a transducer, which emits high-frequency sound waves, is moved over the abdomen or inserted into the vagina. The sound waves bounce off internal organs and create an image that can be viewed on a TV-like screen. With this procedure, your doctor may be able to see whether the uterus contains a developing fetus. (See page 72 for more details about ultrasound exams.)

A procedure called culdocentesis is occasionally used to aid in diagnosing ectopic pregnancy. This technique involves inserting a needle into the space at the very top of the vagina, behind the uterus and in front of the rectum. The presence of blood in this area may indicate bleeding from a ruptured fallopian tube.

What's the treatment? Treatment of ectopic pregnancy usually consists of surgery to remove the abnormal pregnancy. Surgery is generally scheduled soon after an ectopic pregnancy is diagnosed.

At one time, a major operation was needed for ectopic pregnancy. General anesthesia was used, and the pelvic area was opened with a large incision. Now, however, it is often possible to remove an ectopic pregnancy with a less extensive technique called laparoscopy.

In this procedure, a small incision is made in the lower abdomen, near or in the navel. The surgeon then inserts a long, thin instrument, called a laparoscope, into the pelvic area. This instrument is a hollow tube with a light on one end. Through it, the internal organs can be viewed and other instruments can be inserted. Sometimes a second small incision is made in the lower abdomen, through which surgical instruments can be placed. The laparoscope allows the surgeon to remove the ectopic pregnancy and repair or remove the affected fallopian tube. Laparoscopy may be performed possibly with local anesthesia but more likely with regional or general anesthesia.

A fallopian tube that has ruptured from an ectopic pregnancy usually must be removed. Less extensive surgery can be done if the ectopic pregnancy has been found early, before the tube has been stretched too much or has burst. In these instances, it may be possible to remove the ectopic pregnancy and repair the tube, allowing it to continue to function.

Occasionally, a medication called methotrexate can be used to dissolve an ectopic pregnancy. This medication may be used either with or without laparoscopy, depending on how far the pregnancy has developed.

What about the future? After treatment for an ectopic pregnancy, your doctor will want to see you on a regular basis to recheck your hCG level until it reaches zero. An hCG level that remains high could indicate that the ectopic tissue was not entirely removed. If this is the case, you may need additional surgery or medical management with methotrexate.

The outlook for future pregnancies after an ectopic pregnancy depends mainly on the extent of the surgery that was done. Although the chances of having a successful pregnancy are lower if you've had an ectopic pregnancy, they are still good—perhaps as high as 60 percent—if the fallopian tube has been spared. Even if one fallopian tube has been removed, an egg can be fertilized in the other tube. The chances of having a successful pregnancy with one tube removed may be more than 40 percent.

If you've had one ectopic pregnancy, though, you're more likely to have another one. And the risk increases with the number of ectopic pregnancies. If you've had an ectopic pregnancy, talk to your doctor before becoming pregnant again so that together you can plan your care.

Molar Pregnancy

What causes it and who's at risk? Technically called hydatidiform mole (*hydatid* means "a drop of water"; *mole* means "a spot"), molar pregnancy is a relatively rare condition that occurs in only about one of every 1,500 to 2,000 pregnancies in the United States. In a molar pregnancy, an abnormal mass, instead of a normal embryo, forms inside the uterus after fertilization. A molar pregnancy does not consist of a growing baby, but rather something more like an abnormal placenta.

A molar pregnancy occurs when the cells that normally make up the chorionic villi (the tiny, finger-like projections that attach the placenta to the uterine lining) do not develop properly. Instead, they form bubble-like, watery clusters that cannot support a growing embryo. The risk of molar pregnancy is higher in women older than 40 years than in younger women.

Molar pregnancy is caused by chromosome problems in the sperm that fertilized the egg, the egg itself, or both. Molar pregnancies are of two types: complete and partial. In a complete molar pregnancy, the uterus contains a small cluster of clear, blister-like pouches instead of an embryo. In a partial molar pregnancy, the embryo is abnormally formed and usually does not survive.

Women who have had a molar pregnancy are at risk for development of a type of malignant tumor, or invasive disease, inside the uterus. Some of these tumors are highly metastatic (likely to spread to other parts of the body). Although it is rare and its cure rate is high, any woman who has had a molar pregnancy is at risk for invasive disease.

What are the symptoms? Molar pregnancy is nearly always signaled by bleeding by the 12th week of pregnancy. Another possible sign of molar pregnancy is a uterus that is much larger than would be expected for the age of the fetus.

How is it diagnosed? Most cases of molar pregnancy are diagnosed in the first trimester. Bleeding and an hCG level that is much higher than in a normal pregnancy are possible warning signs. They may prompt your doctor to listen for a fetal heartbeat. If none is detected, she or he may suspect a molar pregnancy. An ultrasound exam may then be performed, which allows the doctor to see whether the uterus contains a normal fetus or a molar pregnancy.

What's the treatment? When a molar pregnancy is diagnosed, the treatment consists of removing it. This is most often done by a technique called suction curettage. For this procedure, the woman is given an anesthetic, her cervix is dilated and the contents of her uterus are gently removed by suction. A medication called oxytocin may be given at the same time to stimulate the uterus to contract.

What about the future? Treatment of molar pregnancy is successful in most cases. Because of the risk of invasive disease after a molar pregnancy, however, your doctor will want to monitor you for a period of time afterward. Invasive disease after molar pregnancy is usually marked by an hCG level that remains high or increases after the pregnancy has been terminated. For this reason, your doctor will want to test your hCG level on a regular basis. Most women who have had a molar pregnancy are advised not to become pregnant again for at least a year.

The relatively rare forms of malignant disease that may follow a molar pregnancy are managed with chemotherapy. The success rate of treating these tumors is very good, approaching nearly 100 percent.

Miscarriage

What causes it and who's at risk? Miscarriage, technically called spontaneous abortion, is defined as the loss of a pregnancy before 20 weeks of gestation. It has been estimated to occur in 15 to 20 percent of all pregnancies. The actual number, however, is probably higher. Many miscarriages occur very early, going unnoticed before a woman is even aware that she is pregnant.

More than 80 percent of miscarriages occur in the first 12 weeks of pregnancy. Of these early miscarriages, at least half are thought to be caused by problems with the fetus's chromosomes. (See page 57 for details about chromosome abnormalities.)

Most of the time, the chromosome problems that cause a miscarriage are not inherited from the parents. In other words, the chromosome defect in the fetus is not caused by a similar defect in the chromosomes of the mother or father. Rather, these errors usually happen by chance as the fertilized egg begins to divide.

A miscarriage caused by a chromosome defect often happens when the fetus would not have been able to survive. Miscarriage early in pregnancy can occur as many as several weeks after the embryo or fetus has actually died. And sometimes there was no fetus at all inside the membranes that normally surround the baby.

Other causes of miscarriage may be factors related to the mother's health. Miscarriage from these causes usually occurs later in pregnancy. They include infection, chronic diseases such as diabetes or high blood pressure, and problems with the immune system. Abnormalities of the uterus or cervix can also cause miscarriage. Among these problems are cervical incompetence, in which the cervix begins to dilate too early in pregnancy. This nearly always occurs in the second trimester (see page 172).

Recurrent or repeated miscarriage is defined as three or more miscarriages in a row. (You may hear this referred to as habitual abortion.) The causes of this are much the same as those for a single miscarriage. Although tests can be done to find the reason for repeated miscarriage, the tests can be costly and the treatment options are somewhat limited. Even so, many couples go on to have a successful pregnancy later.

If you've had a miscarriage, or are worried about having one, it's also important for you to understand what *doesn't* cause it. You are not alone if you have fears about being somehow responsible for the loss of your pregnancy. Such fears are common among pregnant women, whether or not they have been through this experience.

Miscarriage is not caused by exercising, having sex, working or lifting heavy objects. Nausea and vomiting in early pregnancy, even if severe, will not cause a miscarriage. (In fact, there is some evidence that women who have these symptoms are less likely to miscarry.) Finally, it is unlikely that a fall, a blow or a sudden fright can cause miscarriage. The fetus is unlikely to be harmed by an injury unless the injury is serious enough to threaten your own life.

What are the symptoms? Nearly all miscarriages are preceded by the warning sign of vaginal bleeding. Up to 25 percent of all pregnant women have bleeding at some point in pregnancy, and of these women, about half will have a miscarriage. Bleeding that signals a miscarriage may be scant or heavy. It may be constant, or it may come and go. Bleeding may be followed by cramping abdominal pain and, in some women, lower backache. Although there may be other reasons for these symptoms (see "Spotting or bleeding" and "Pelvic pain," page 135), you should contact your doctor if you have any type of bleeding or severe pain in pregnancy.

How is it diagnosed? If you come to your doctor's office with bleeding, the first thing she or he will want to do is to perform a pelvic exam to check whether your cervix has begun to dilate. If it has, this situation is called threatened abortion—a miscarriage will not necessarily happen, but there is a chance that it might.

Your doctor will also check whether the membranes that surround the fetus have broken. If they have, and your cervix is dilated, then a miscarriage is certain. This is referred to as inevitable abortion because a miscarriage can't be stopped.

If you have passed tissue, your doctor may suspect that a miscarriage has already occurred. If the tissue is available, he or she may be able to examine it to see whether it contains any fetal tissue or is actually a clot or a piece of placenta.

An ultrasound exam is often used to try to determine whether there is a live fetus inside the uterus. With this test, your doctor will try to see the sac that surrounds the fetus or, using a special kind of ultrasonography, check the fetal heartbeat. If the fetus is not alive but has not been passed out of your body, this is called a missed abortion.

What's the treatment? In cases of threatened abortion, bed rest and pain medication may be prescribed until the bleeding or pain has passed. If bleeding or pain is severe, you may need to be hospitalized.

When the fetal membranes have broken, a miscarriage often occurs soon afterward. If it doesn't, however, and there is continued bleeding, pain or a fever, there is a risk of serious infection. In this case, the fetal tissue must be removed from the uterus. In this procedure, which is done under anesthesia, the cervix is gradually dilated and the tissue is gently scraped or suctioned out.

If you have had a miscarriage or a procedure to empty the uterus, call your doctor right away if you have heavy bleeding, fever, chills or severe pain. These could be a sign of an infection.

What about the future? Most women who have had a miscarriage go on to have successful pregnancies later. Even women with repeated miscarriages (three or more in a row) have a 70 to 85 percent chance of carrying another pregnancy to term. It is usually advised, however, to wait awhile before becoming pregnant again. Your doctor can advise you about when to attempt pregnancy after a miscarriage.

I f you've had a pregnancy loss, whether because of ectopic pregnancy, molar pregnancy or miscarriage, you may be having intense and sometimes confusing feelings. This reaction may occur no matter how early the pregnancy ended—even if it was only a few weeks along. Grief is a natural and normal response to an important loss. It is a way of learning to accept the loss, to heal from it and to always remember it.

You're not abnormal or unfeeling, however, if you don't feel sorrow or grief after a pregnancy loss. Each person responds in a unique way. You may feel only disappointed. You may even feel relieved that a difficult period of anxiety and uncertainty is now over. Or you may be overwhelmingly sad or confused.

Regardless of your reaction to a pregnancy loss, this section will help you understand your feelings and reactions. You can't wish away your feelings, but with insight you can try to understand them, eventually coming to terms with your loss.

A broken bond. When you were pregnant, you may have spent hours daydreaming about what your baby would look like, and what kind of person she or he would turn out to be. This is part of the normal process of bonding, the unique attachment between a mother and baby that often begins well before birth.

Grieving is the process of letting go of your emotional attachment to your baby. You are grieving that the bond you felt with her or him now has been broken. Thus, when it comes to grief, it doesn't matter how early in pregnancy you were struck by this loss. Your feelings are real, and they ought not be denied.

The stages of grief. There is a process of emotional healing common to many people who have suffered an important loss. It is often said to be characterized by certain recognizable steps or stages.

These so-called stages of grief are not a given timetable for your emotional healing, but they are a description of experiences common to many grieving people. As you mourn a loss, it is normal to move from one stage to another, and even back again.

Knowing a little about the grieving process may help you to gain perspective on what you're going through. It may also help you to recognize when you can't handle the burden alone and need to seek help. And if you know someone who is grieving, this insight can help you to be sensitive.

Shock and denial

> "My pregnancy turned out to be ectopic, which was completely unexpected. I know I should be upset, but I don't know what I'm feeling. I wanted this baby so much, and now I don't seem to feel anything at all."

> "I just don't believe that this has happened to me."

A natural first reaction to any upsetting event, a sense of numbness and disbelief is the mind's way of protecting itself from emotional trauma. Just as natural processes in the body are sometimes activated to block physical pain immediately after a severe injury, so too do similar mental mechanisms shield

Grieving the Loss of a Pregnancy

you when first confronted with emotional trauma. This reaction is normal and does not mean you are an unfeeling, uncaring person. It will usually pass as the reality of the event sinks in.

Guilt and anger

"There must have been something I did to cause my miscarriage. I feel like I'm being punished."

"After trying for almost a year to get pregnant, I had a molar pregnancy. I know it doesn't make sense, but I feel so resentful of my sister-in-law, who has three beautiful children."

You are not alone if you feel somehow responsible for what has happened. Above all, however, don't blame yourself for the loss of your pregnancy. It is highly unlikely that anything you did or could have done contributed to the problems that arose. Nor is the loss anyone's way—that of Nature, or God, or Fate—of punishing you for something you did. This knowledge may not erase feelings of guilt, but it may help you understand that these feelings are normal.

You may also feel anger toward others, even though this doesn't seem to make sense. Envy, jealousy and resentment toward women with healthy pregnancies and babies are normal reactions to your own loss. Anger toward doctors or nurses, toward your partner and toward family and friends is normal. There's no need to worry about feelings of anger unless they cause you to become hostile to, or to physically hurt, other people or yourself. Turning anger inward, on yourself, is no better; it's what causes depression.

Depression and despair

"I don't know what's happening to me. I'm constantly tired, even though I sleep more than I ever have. I just don't have the energy to do anything; nothing interests me anymore."

"Sometimes I'm afraid that I'll never be able to stop crying."

Depression is not always easy to recognize. Sometimes it comes out as a profound feeling of fatigue or a loss of interest in things you used to enjoy. It may alter your appetite or affect your sleeping patterns. It may also be expressed in the more obvious symptoms of tearfulness and crying.

Some women worry that they're literally going crazy. This too can be a normal and understandable reaction to a pregnancy loss.

Acceptance

"It's been a year and a half since my miscarriage, and now I'm thinking about becoming pregnant again. I know I can never replace the first baby, and I'll always wonder what she would have been like. But after all I've been through, I'm finally able to look forward to the future again."

At the moment, this attitude may be hard to believe: You will eventually come to terms with your loss. It can't be said that the pain will go away completely, but gradually it will become easier to function. One day you will begin to look forward instead of back.

Shadow grief. Sometimes termed "anniversary reaction," shadow grief is the recurrence of grief on the anniversary of an important date. This may be the date you miscarried or had surgery for an ectopic or molar pregnancy. It may also be your baby's due date, the date you first learned you were pregnant or the date you first heard the fetal heartbeat. During these times, you may feel shaky or vulnerable. It may even seem like the loss is happening all over again.

When you might need professional help. If you feel "stuck" emotionally and can't seem to move on, consider looking for outside help. There are many counselors, therapists, support groups and self-help groups that understand how to help you get through your grieving.

Don't be afraid to talk out your feelings with someone. Acknowledging your feelings and hearing yourself describe them out loud are very helpful. A common myth is that the way to heal is to forget. But in reality, it is remembering that allows us to grieve and to heal.

It is especially important to get professional help if your feelings:

- Are so overwhelming that you cannot function adequately at work or at home
- Interfere with your relationships with those close to you
- Cause you to become violent or hostile to others
- Keep you from getting up in the morning or taking care of yourself— your personal hygiene suffers, for instance, or you can't eat or sleep

Even if your feelings are not this overwhelming, it can be extremely helpful to talk to a counselor or therapist, especially if you are worried in any way about whether your feelings are "normal."

Effects on your family. **Your partner.** Your partner is probably grieving his loss, too, but it may be hard for you to recognize this. Men and women often have very different ways of dealing with painful emotions. Your partner may tend to keep his feelings to himself because of fears of increasing your burden. He may have difficulty listening to your concerns as you attempt to resolve your grief by talking. He may think he has to be "strong" for both of you, to keep things running smoothly in your relationship and around the house. He may seem distant from you at a time when you need him the most and may, in fact, try to "run away" from his grief by spending more time at work.

None of these reactions mean that your partner doesn't care about you, or about the loss of the pregnancy. Talk to each other. Try to listen and respond to his feelings, to accept them for what they are. Consider seeing a couples' counselor or therapist to provide a "neutral" place where you can both be heard— and can more easily listen to each other.

Your children. If you have other children, they may also be affected by the loss, especially if they have been eagerly looking forward to having a new brother or sister. Just as common, though, is for children to feel that they are somehow responsible for the loss. They may have secretly "wished away" the new baby and may now feel that their wishes have come true. Or they may think that the baby died because they behaved badly or were disobedient. Even very young children are aware of their parents' sadness, and they often feel it is somehow their fault. Be sure to talk with your children about what has happened and reassure them that they are blameless.

Future pregnancies. Most professionals who counsel people who have lost a pregnancy think it's best not to become pregnant again immediately. You will need time to absorb this loss, to let yourself heal and to allow your body to return to normal before becoming pregnant again.

The responses of others. Without meaning to, persons closest to you may say things that they think are helpful but that only make you feel worse (see page 151). Poorly thought-through comments can be hurtful during this time, when you're feeling particularly vulnerable.

It may help to understand that people often make these well-meaning remarks because they don't know what else to say. Those who care about you may believe that they have to say something to make you feel better.

However, your friends, family and co-workers may also avoid talking about your loss, or may avoid you altogether. Many people have problems confronting loss, especially death. Many people are uncomfortable around someone whom death has affected. What has happened to you may remind them of their own mortality, as well as that of their loved ones. It may even, perhaps on an unconscious level, seem like "bad luck" to be too close to you. People may want to avoid the topic, either because of their own attitudes or emotions or because they fear that it will cause more pain for you.

When confronted with hurtful remarks, it may help to say something like, "Thank you for caring, but I just need time to work through my grief." It usually doesn't help to be unpleasant in response to insensitivity. Letting others know what you do need, as specifically as possible, will be more helpful. Tell others whether you prefer to talk about your feelings or the plans you had, or not to talk at all.

Grieving is a process. Grieving is ongoing, unpredictable and painful. It may last a few weeks or as long as a few years. The loss will always be there, but eventually you will think of it without tears or overwhelming sadness.

Allowing others to grieve
Some do's and don'ts

If you know someone who's lost a pregnancy, a baby or another loved one, you may find it difficult and awkward to be around that person. This reaction is not unusual—many people are uncomfortable around matters of loss. But don't make the mistake of avoiding someone you love who has experienced such a tragedy. Gather up your courage and let the person know you care.

Anyone who has had someone close to them die—whether a parent, a friend or a baby not yet born—will tell you that it is a comfort to talk about, and to hear others talk about, the loved one. With a lost pregnancy, this may take the form of talking about the pregnancy itself and the parents' feelings. Don't be afraid to bring up what has happened, but be sensitive, and let the other person take the lead. If the person wants to talk about it, communicate that you want to listen. If the person seems withdrawn, respect this feeling and just make it known that you care.

Some of the more common things that may occur to you to say, however, can actually be hurtful, no matter how well-meaning. The common remarks made by others in an effort to "take care" of a grieving person often have the effect of making the pain seem trivial. Here are some guidelines for how to talk to someone who has lost a pregnancy.

What not to say:
- *"It's all for the best."* This statement can hardly seem true to someone who is trying to understand why her or his fondest hopes have been taken away.
- *"Next time, things will be better"* or *"You can always have another pregnancy."* These comments can make a person feel as though the lost pregnancy was somehow "replaceable" or "didn't count."
- *"I know just how you feel."* Even if this statement could be true, it doesn't help a person who is in pain, and who is probably feeling that no one understands what she or he is going through.

What to say instead:
If you don't feel comfortable talking directly about another's loss, or if it doesn't seem appropriate, here are some things you can say:

- *"I'm so sorry."*
- *"I care about you, and I want to help."*
- *"Please let me know if you want to talk about it."*

These statements may seem simple, but they may be all a grieving person needs to hear.

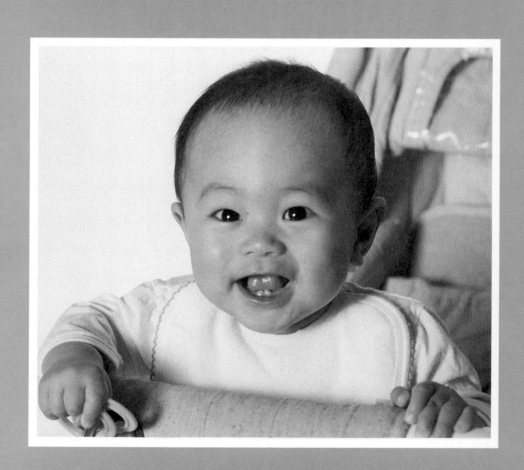

CHAPTER ELEVEN

The Second Trimester

13 to 27 weeks

The second trimester, typically said to last from the beginning of the 13th week of pregnancy until the end of the 27th, is sometimes called the "golden period" of pregnancy. This label is appropriate because many of the side effects of early pregnancy have diminished, whereas the discomforts of the third trimester, when the growing baby will put increased demands on your body, have not yet begun. During the second trimester, you are likely to find that your nausea is easing off, you are sleeping better and your energy is returning.

In addition, the baby will probably begin to seem more "real" to you during these weeks. Using a special listening device, your doctor will probably hear the baby's heartbeat for the first time at around 12 weeks. And somewhere between 16 and 20 weeks, you will feel the first fluttering movements.

The risk of miscarriage in the second trimester, although it still exists, is lower than that in the first trimester. For this reason, now is the time that many women—especially those who have had a miscarriage before—feel comfortable in spreading the news about being pregnant. Your enlarging abdomen will begin to be much more noticeable by four or five months. You'll need to begin to change your wardrobe during these months and to make plans to prepare your home for your new baby.

Now is the time you'll also want to think about childbirth classes for you and your partner (see page 264) and perhaps also sibling and grandparent classes for others in your family. You'll want to explore the options concerning maternity and paternity leave for you and for your partner after the baby is born and to look into child care options if both of you will be returning to work. There are plans to be made, and luckily, now is the time you are likely to feel a return of your energy.

The second trimester, however, is not always trouble-free. A whole new set of symptoms and sensations are common during this time, as well as potential problems and complications. Like the changes of the first trimester, those of the second, and the particular way in which you experience them, will be unique to you. It helps to know about what is normal and what may not be, as well as what routine tests and care may be advised by your doctor.

Physical Changes and Symptoms

The changes that began in the first weeks of pregnancy increase and accelerate during the second trimester. Of these, your growing uterus is probably the most obvious. But many other, unseen events are also taking place.

During the mid-trimester, more blood is produced to supply the placenta with oxygen and nutrients for your baby's growth. Your digestive system slows the rate at which food moves through your system. And every organ system in your body continues to adapt to pregnancy under the influence of increasing hormone levels. These and other changes may give rise to some of the signs and symptoms described in this chapter.

Aches and Pains

You'll notice a rapid increase in the size of your uterus during the second trimester. By the end of 27 weeks, the fetus will be about four times bigger than it was at 12 weeks. As the uterus becomes too big to fit within your pelvis, internal organs are pushed out of their usual places, and greater tension is placed on surrounding muscles and ligaments.

All of this growth is likely to result in some discomfort. The common aches and pains of the second trimester mostly stem from the increase in the size and weight of the uterus, as well as from the effects of pregnancy's hormones.

Normally, two bands of muscles, called the rectus abdominis muscles, meet in the middle of the abdomen, as shown in the left illustration. Some pregnant women experience a separation or relaxation of the two bands of muscles, as shown on the right. You might notice this separation (diastasis) because it can cause a bulge where the two muscles separate. The separation of these muscles can contribute to back pain. The condition may first appear during the second trimester, may become more pronounced in the third trimester and sometimes persists after delivery.

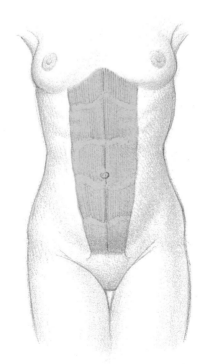
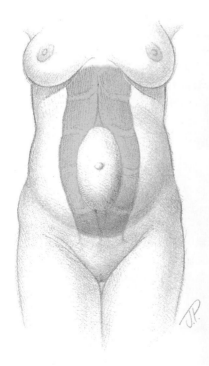

Back pain. **What causes it?** During pregnancy, the joints between your pelvic bones begin to soften and loosen in preparation for the baby to pass through your pelvis during birth. In the second trimester, your uterus becomes heavier, changing your center of gravity. Gradually—and perhaps without even noticing it—you begin to adjust your posture and the ways in which you move. Compensations you make for the change in your center of gravity can result in back pain, strain or other injury.

Another contributor to back pain may be separation (diastasis) of the muscles along the front of the abdomen (the rectus abdominis muscles). These two parallel sheets of muscles run from the rib cage to the pubic bone. As the uterus expands, these muscles sometimes separate along the center seam, and back pain can then become worse. Your doctor can evaluate whether the amount of separation is more than usual and may suggest ways to remedy the separation after your baby is born.

What can I do? To prevent or ease back pain, try to be aware of how you stand, sit and move:

- Practice correct posture. Stand with your pelvis tucked in and your shoulders back.
- When standing for long periods, rest one foot on a low step stool if possible.
- Sit with your feet slightly elevated, and don't cross your legs. If you must sit for long periods, take breaks at least every half hour.
- Lift correctly. Place your feet a shoulder's width apart; lower your body by bending at the knees, not the waist; and lift by pushing up with your thighs, not with your back.
- Don't make sudden reaching movements or stretch your arms high over your head.
- When sleeping or resting, lie on your side, with your knees and hips bent. Place a pillow between your knees and another one under your abdomen. This position will take the pressure off your lower back.

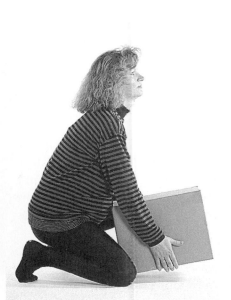 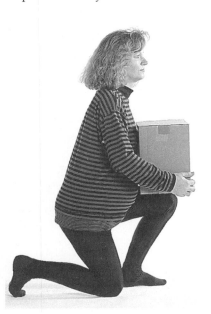 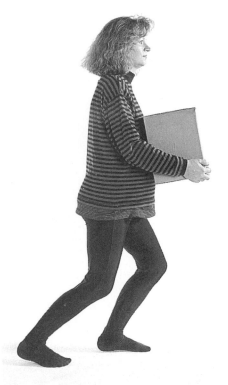

To lift correctly, squat and grasp the load, keeping your back as straight as possible. Keep the load close to your body while using your leg muscles to lift you and the load.

It's important to bend at your knees, rather than at your waist, to pick up something from the floor. Don't twist your body while lifting.

- Exercises to strengthen the muscles in your abdomen will help minimize back pain. (For specific exercises to strengthen the abdomen and back, see page 267.)

If none of these measures bring relief, your doctor may recommend a special elastic sling or back brace to support the weight of your abdomen and ease the tension on your back.

Abdominal pain. **What causes it?** Pain in the lower abdomen during the second trimester is often related to the stretching of ligaments and muscles around the expanding uterus. Although this cause of abdominal pain doesn't pose a threat to you or your baby, it's important to report it to your doctor because abdominal pain can be a symptom of ectopic pregnancy (see page 141), preterm labor (see page 169) or other problems.

A fairly common cause of abdominal or groin pain in mid-pregnancy is stretching of the round ligament. Actually made of muscle cells, the round ligament is a cord-like structure that supports the uterus. Before pregnancy, the round ligament is less than a quarter of an inch thick. By the end of pregnancy, it has become longer, thicker and more taut. A sudden movement or reach can stretch the round ligament, causing a pulling or stabbing pang in your lower pelvic area or groin or a sharp cramp down your side. The discomfort usually lasts several minutes and then goes away.

If you've had abdominal surgery, especially infertility surgery, you may have pain from the pulling or stretching of adhesions. These are bands of scar tissue that adhere to other structures, such as the walls of the abdomen. The increasing size of the uterus can cause these bands of tissue to stretch or even to pull apart, which can be painful.

Sometimes pain from an inflamed appendix or gallbladder can appear in unusual locations during pregnancy. This pain develops because the organs inside the abdominal area are crowded out of their usual positions by the growing uterus. A nonpregnant woman would probably feel pain from appendicitis in the lower right side of her pelvis, but a woman in the second trimester of pregnancy is more likely to feel this pain higher up in the abdomen.

What can I do? It may help to sit or lie down when abdominal pain becomes bothersome. Relaxation exercises may help, as may soaking in a warm bath. The relatively minor aches and twinges described here are probably nothing to worry about and will diminish as your pregnancy progresses, but if the pain is severe, call your doctor immediately.

Leg cramps. **What causes them?** Cramps in the lower leg muscles are fairly common in the second and third trimesters. They often occur at night and may disrupt your sleep. The exact cause of leg cramps is uncertain, but they may be due to an inadequate amount of calcium in your diet, fatigue or pressure of the uterus on nerves in your legs.

What can I do? If you're bothered by leg cramps, try doing exercises to stretch your calf muscles. Other measures to ease or prevent leg cramps include wearing support hose, especially if you stand a lot during the day. Take frequent breaks from sitting or standing for long periods. If you do get a cramp, you might be able to relieve it by straightening your knee and gently flexing your foot upward. Applying local heat may also help.

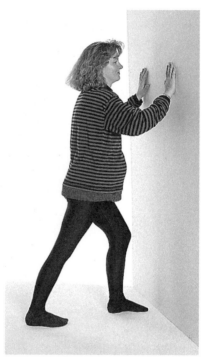

Calf Stretches: Stand about 18 inches from a wall and lean forward against it with your hands, keeping your back straight (don't bend at the waist). Placing your right foot behind you, bend your left knee and push with your right heel until it is flat on the floor, keeping your right leg straight. Don't let your bent knee extend forward beyond the tip of your toes. You should feel the stretch in your right calf muscle, but don't overdo it, and don't bounce. Stretch gently and then release. Repeat with the other leg.

If leg cramps persist and are severe, tell your doctor about the problem. Rarely, they can indicate that a blood clot has formed in a vein, which would require medical treatment.

Heartburn. What causes it? Heartburn actually has nothing to do with your heart. It's caused by the contents of the stomach backing up into the esophagus (the tube that carries food from the mouth to the stomach). When this happens, stomach acids irritate the lining of the esophagus. The resulting burning sensation at about the level of the heart gives this condition its misleading name.

There are many reasons why heartburn is more common during pregnancy. For one thing, your growing uterus is continually pushing on your stomach, moving it higher and higher up in your abdomen and compressing it. For another, your digestive system as a whole, under the influence of hormones, has been slowed down. The wavelike movements of the esophagus that push swallowed food down into your stomach tend to become slower during pregnancy. Your stomach also takes longer to empty, and food moves more slowly along your gastrointestinal tract. The purpose of this general slowdown is to allow nutrients more time to be absorbed into your bloodstream and to reach the fetus. Unfortunately, it can also cause bloating and indigestion.

What can I do? Some of the things you did to ease nausea and vomiting during the first trimester (see page 131) may also help your heartburn during the second trimester. For example, remember to eat frequent and small meals and not to overfill your stomach. Avoid movements and positions that seem to aggravate the problem. When picking things up, bend at your knees, not your waist. Avoid lying flat on your back—when resting or sleeping, prop yourself up on pillows.

If heartburn is bothersome enough to keep you from eating properly, your doctor may prescribe an antacid. But do not take any antacid without talking to your doctor first. Some antacids contain sodium, which can cause fluid buildup in body tissues during pregnancy.

Rarely, an inflammation of the esophagus may cause heartburn. When this is suspected, a procedure (endoscopy) can be done to view the inside of the esophagus. The condition can be treated with medication during pregnancy.

Skin darkening. What causes it? The hormones at work in your body during pregnancy can cause several changes in your skin. One of the most common, occurring in 90 percent of all pregnant women, is skin darkening. This symptom is more pronounced in dark-skinned women. Its exact cause is unknown, but it may be related to increased levels of estrogen.

Skin darkening during pregnancy is typically noticeable on or around the nipples, in the area between the vulva and the anus (the perineum) and around the navel. You may also notice it on your armpits and inner thighs. The pale line that runs from the navel to the pubic bone, called the linea alba ("white line"), also often darkens during pregnancy, when it is referred to as the linea nigra ("black line"). In some pregnant women, mild skin darkening on the face also develops. This is commonly called the "mask of pregnancy," or chloasma.

Skin Changes

What can I do? Skin darkening during pregnancy is made worse by exposure to sunlight or to other sources of ultraviolet (UV) light. If you have this problem, avoid getting too much sun. Always wear a sunblock with a skin protection factor (SPF) of at least 15 when outdoors, whether it's sunny or cloudy—the sun's UV rays also reach your skin on overcast days. A wide-brimmed hat that shades your face will also help.

Skin darkening almost always fades after delivery. If it is extreme, especially on your face, covering makeup can help. But avoid agents that bleach the skin. If yours is a severe case, it might be improved with a medicated ointment that can be prescribed by your doctor.

Other skin symptoms. Below are other common skin changes that usually disappear after delivery:

- Red and itchy palms and soles, which may be relieved by using moisturizing creams.

- Blotchy patches on your legs and feet may appear at times, particularly when you are chilly. They do not signal a problem or cause discomfort.

- Skin tags—very small, loose growths of skin—may appear under your arms or breasts. They usually disappear after birth but can be easily removed if they don't.

- Moles may become more numerous, but the ones that appear during pregnancy are usually not the type that are linked to skin cancer. (Just to be sure, though, it is still a good idea to show any new moles to your doctor.)

- Fingernails may become brittle and soft. Using nail polish may make them worse. Moisturize your nails as well as your hands with lotion, and wear rubber gloves when working with detergents or cleansers.

- Heat rash can be soothed by applying cornstarch after bathing, avoiding very hot baths or showers and keeping the skin cool and dry.

Constipation

What causes it? Unfortunately, constipation is one of the most common and uncomfortable side effects of pregnancy. It is due to the general slowdown in the digestive system and to the pressure of the uterus on the lower bowel. Constipation also tends to give rise to hemorrhoids later in pregnancy (see page 179).

What can I do? The first strategy in dealing with this problem is evaluation of your diet. Foods high in fiber will help prevent or ease constipation, as will drinking plenty of fluids. Fruits, vegetables and whole-grain foods may provide the fiber you need. Fruit juices, particularly the age-old remedy of prune juice, can also ease constipation.

Increasing the amount you exercise will help too. Just adding a little time to your daily walks or other exercise regimen can be effective.

If these measures fail, your doctor may recommend a mild laxative such as milk of magnesia, a bulking agent or a stool softener. But take these remedies only on the advice of your health care provider. Don't take cod liver oil during pregnancy because it can interfere with the absorption of certain vitamins and nutrients. Also avoid other harsh laxatives and enemas.

How much weight will you gain during the second trimester? The answer varies somewhat depending on your weight before pregnancy, but you'll probably gain about a pound a week after the first trimester. It is typical to fluctuate somewhat—gaining a pound and a half one week and only half a pound the next. But as long as your weight gain is steady, without any sudden increases or decreases, you're doing fine. (See page 86 for more about weight gain during pregnancy.)

Weight Gain

What's Happening With the Baby?

By 26 weeks gestational age, the baby has grown to about 9 inches long (crown to rump, see page 33) and weighs about 1½ pounds. Fat is being laid down under the red, wrinkled skin, which is covered with fine, downy hair called lanugo. Fingerprints and toe prints, as well as eyebrows and lashes, have formed. By 28 weeks, the baby's eyes open and close, and the baby sleeps and wakes at regular intervals. By that time, the baby will be about 10 inches long (crown to rump) and will weigh about 2 pounds.

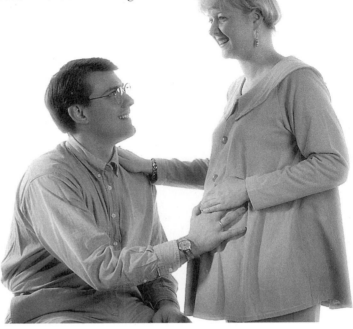

Feeling your baby move, and sharing that with your partner, is often a special milestone during the second trimester.

You will probably have begun to feel your baby's movements by 20 weeks gestational age. It is normal during this trimester for these movements to be somewhat erratic; later, they typically become more regular. The most active time is between 27 and 32 weeks.

Feeling the Baby Move

As your baby's activity increases, your pregnancy will begin to seem much more "real" to you. In the first trimester, you may have been constantly reminded of being pregnant because of nausea or other symptoms. But now the reminder begins to take the much more pleasant and exciting form of feeling your baby move. As time goes on, your partner will be able to feel movements through your abdomen, and you'll both begin to become more emotionally involved with your baby.

About the time you begin to feel the baby move, she or he in turn is beginning to be able to hear you. Hearing is well established by 24 weeks, when the baby begins to respond to outside sounds. The baby can now hear your voice and is likely to recognize it after birth. The environment inside the uterus is relatively quiet, but your baby can hear your heart thumping, your blood whooshing through your veins and arteries and the rumblings of your stomach.

The Baby's Senses

The rest of your baby's sense organs also continue to develop during the second trimester. Beginning at 16 weeks, your baby is sensitive to light, and by 29 weeks a baby can open his or her eyes and turn the head to find the source of a continuous, bright light.

"Superbabies": fact or fiction?

Studies have been done to find out whether stimulating the baby inside the uterus can accelerate the child's future intellectual development. Some have thought that, for instance, reading to a baby through a pregnant woman's abdomen will produce a literary child, or playing classical music will give rise to a music lover. But so far, there is no convincing evidence of such a result.

The newborn does seem to recognize voices that were heard in the uterus. And loud noises, such as common household sounds, that were familiar before birth do not seem to startle a newborn. Whether parents can influence their baby's learning and development before the baby is born is still unknown. Cuddling, singing to and playing with the baby after birth are far more important.

Common Concerns in the Second Trimester

Although many women find the second trimester to be easier than the first, mid-pregnancy often brings new physical side effects and other concerns. Knowing about potential problems and knowing when to contact your doctor are just as important now as they were during the first trimester. Some common concerns during mid-pregnancy are discussed on the following pages.

Vaginal Discharge and Infections

Many women have an increased vaginal discharge during pregnancy. It is caused by the effects of hormones on glands in the cervix, which stimulate the production of mucus. A normal vaginal discharge in a pregnant woman is thin and white and has a mild odor. Its high acidity is thought to play a role in suppressing growth of potentially harmful bacteria.

Normally, the vagina contains various organisms that tend to keep one another in check. When this balance is thrown off—by stress, illness, substances (such as douches) introduced into the vagina, medications (such as antibiotics) or the hormones of pregnancy—one type of organism may grow faster than the others, causing a vaginal infection.

If you have a vaginal discharge that is greenish or yellowish, strong-smelling or accompanied by redness, itching and irritation of the vulva, you may have a vaginal infection (vaginitis). This is common during pregnancy because of hormone changes.

The two most common types of vaginal infection during pregnancy are candidiasis and trichomoniasis. Neither presents a direct hazard to the baby, and both can be treated during pregnancy.

Candidiasis. Vaginal infections caused by the organism *Candida albicans* are commonly referred to as yeast infections, or candidiasis. The *Candida* organism can be found in about 25 percent of pregnant women near the time of delivery. This organism can be present without causing symptoms, in which case no treatment is needed. But it may result in a thick, curd-like discharge along with burning, which is a sign of infection.

Candidiasis is treated during pregnancy with a vaginal cream, ointment or suppository containing an antifungal drug. These medications are now available without a prescription, but do not use one without consulting your doctor first. Because other types of vaginal infections may produce similar symptoms, your doctor needs to confirm the diagnosis and type of vaginitis before you start treatment.

Once you've had a yeast infection during your pregnancy, it can be a recurring problem until after delivery, when it usually subsides. It may be necessary to treat yeast infections repeatedly throughout your pregnancy.

Trichomoniasis. The organism that causes trichomoniasis, *Trichomonas vaginalis*, is found in up to 20 percent of pregnant women and often causes no symptoms. When symptoms do occur, they may consist of a gray or green, foamy discharge, along with itching around the vulva. This infection may be linked to preterm labor, but this relationship is not known for certain.

Trichomoniasis can be treated during pregnancy with a medication called metronidazole, which is given in pill form. Although this drug does not appear to harm the baby, it's best to avoid taking it during the first trimester. Your doctor may also recommend treatment for your sexual partner to help prevent reinfection.

Preventing vaginitis. To ward off vaginal infections during pregnancy—especially if you were prone to them before you were pregnant—follow these guidelines:

- Keep the vulvar and vaginal area as clean and dry as possible.
- Wear comfortable, loose-fitting clothing, and avoid synthetic and other fabrics that don't "breathe."
- Wear underwear and pantyhose with a cotton crotch.
- Do not use feminine hygiene sprays or douches.
- If you do get a vaginal infection, ask your doctor whether your partner should also be treated.

Cravings

Many women have strong desires for certain types of food during their pregnancies. The old stereotype of pregnant women craving pickles and ice cream probably has its origins in this fact. Especially during the first trimester, you may have noticed changes in your appetite, which are probably due to the hormones of pregnancy. In the second trimester, you may still have cravings or distaste for some foods. As long as you continue to eat a healthful diet and get all the nutrients you need, such appetite changes are of no consequence.

Rarely, some women have a craving for a nonfood substance during pregnancy. Substances range from relatively harmless to potentially dangerous and include the following:

- Clay
- Laundry starch
- Dirt
- Baking powder or baking soda
- Ice chips or frost from the freezer

The name for this uncommon craving is pica. Why some women experience it isn't known, although it's more common in certain cultures. It is sometimes caused by an iron deficiency. Pica probably won't be harmful if it consists of an occasional desire for ice chips, but other substances may cause gastrointestinal problems. Dirt and clay may contain parasites, and laundry products are likely to contain harsh chemicals and perfumes. If you experience a craving for something that isn't food, report it to your doctor.

Some Common Questions

Q: *I feel so clumsy lately, and I'm worried about falling and hurting my baby. Is there something wrong with me?*

A: What you're feeling is perfectly normal. Because of the changes in your posture and balance as pregnancy progresses (see page 155), it's not abnormal at all for your usual ways of moving, standing and walking to change. When you are back to your usual size and shape after the baby is born, you'll feel like your old, graceful self again.

If you do fall, your baby probably won't be harmed. An injury would likely have to be severe enough to hurt you before it would harm your baby. But if you're worried about the welfare of your baby after a fall, see your doctor right away for reassurance or treatment.

Because of changes in your center of gravity, avoid wearing even moderate heels or pumps. Instead, wear stable, flat shoes with soles that provide good traction. Avoid situations that require careful balance, such as perching on ladders and stools. Take a little extra time during tasks that require numerous changes of position.

Q: *Why do my gums bleed so much when I brush my teeth? Is this something to be concerned about?*

A: Like the other mucous membranes in your body, your gums are receiving more blood flow during pregnancy. As a result, they can become swollen and inflamed and tend to bleed when you brush. There's no reason to be concerned unless the pain and redness of an infection develop.

Don't neglect your dental care during pregnancy. Although routine dental X-rays are usually postponed until after birth (see page 136), brushing, flossing and regular dental exams and cleaning are important. Professional cleaning prevents a buildup of plaque, which, left untreated, can make your bleeding gums worse. If the bleeding is profuse or accompanied by pain or inflammation, make an appointment with your dentist soon to check for infection.

Q: *I never had nosebleeds before I was pregnant, but now I have them a lot. Also, my nose seems to be stuffed up much of the time, although I don't have a cold or allergies. What can I do?*

A: Nosebleeds and nasal congestion are other possible results of the increased blood flow to the mucous membranes in your body. Your nasal tissue tends to become swollen, tender and more prone to bleeding, especially when you blow your nose. This change won't harm your health or the baby's, but it can be disconcerting and annoying.

Avoid over-the-counter remedies for your stuffed-up nose. Instead, increase your intake of fluids and use a humidifier in your home to loosen nasal secretions. Blow your nose gently, one nostril at a time, to avoid putting too much pressure on delicate nasal membranes. If the weather is cold and dry, apply a small amount of petroleum jelly inside each nostril to keep your nose from becoming dry. A saline nasal spray may also be helpful.

To stop a nosebleed, sit up or stand—don't lie down or tilt your head back. Gently pinch your nostrils shut for a few minutes and then release, repeating several times until the bleeding stops. If this method doesn't work, or if the bleeding becomes heavy, contact your doctor.

Q: *My moods are so unpredictable that I sometimes feel I'm going crazy. I'll be feeling fine and then get weepy for no apparent reason. What's going on?*

A: Even if your overall feelings about your pregnancy are feelings of joy, it can still be a stressful experience, for both your body and your state of mind— and the two are intertwined. Your fatigue and discomfort are reasons enough to feel stressed emotionally. In turn, feeling "down" affects how you feel physically. Sometimes you may find your stress relieved by an emotional outburst.

Because many pregnant women don't get enough rest and because rest is so important in helping to relieve stress, pay attention to how much sleep you get. A healthful diet and regular exercise are also important.

Moods that actually interfere with your ability to function may be more than a passing, mild case of fatigue, stress or the blues. If you're consistently down in the dumps, and you notice that your eating and sleeping are affected (either less or more), that your work is disrupted or that your pleasure in the things you normally enjoy is diminished, you may be having more than just mood swings. These symptoms are the hallmarks of depression. Women can be prone to depression, even when they're not pregnant. And even though severe depression does not occur often during pregnancy, mild depression is quite common.

Depression during pregnancy is most often treated through counseling and psychotherapy. Although many new medications are now available to combat depression, they are usually not recommended during pregnancy. These drugs have been studied very little in pregnant women, so their effects on the baby are not known with certainty. But if you have significant depression, a psychiatrist can advise your obstetrician on safe and effective medications that may be helpful to you.

If your mood swings seem to be more than you can handle alone, talk to your doctor about seeing a counselor or therapist. And if you are feeling overwhelmed, don't hesitate to seek the help you need—and deserve. Pregnancy can be hard enough without struggling with depression. (For more information on depression and psychiatric disorders during pregnancy, see page 242.)

Q: *I've noticed that my once-concave navel is being pushed out until it protrudes from my belly. My doctor says this is a type of hernia. Am I going to need surgery?*

A: No—this is an umbilical hernia, and unlike other types of hernias, it does not signal a problem or require surgery. It's simply due to the pressure of the growing uterus. After delivery, your "outie" will go back to being an "innie."

Q: *I'm nervous about the way my heart pounds sometimes, especially when I get up from sitting or lying down. Could there be something wrong with my heart?*

A: Probably not. Your circulatory system expands rapidly during the second trimester. This expansion tends at first to lower your blood pressure. As your blood pressure returns to normal, you may feel a fluttering or pounding sensation around your heart, as though it has skipped a beat. Although this feeling may be alarming, it is usually not a symptom of anything serious. Often it eases later in pregnancy. But tell your doctor about it—especially if you are also having shortness of breath and chest pain. These symptoms may signal a problem for which further evaluation may be needed.

Office Visits

Until you have reached 28 weeks of pregnancy, you will probably visit your doctor about once a month. Depending on factors such as problems you had in previous pregnancies and any medical conditions you may have now, you may need to be seen more often. Visits during the second trimester focus on tracking the growth of the fetus, fixing the due date more exactly and watching for any problems with your own health.

Routine Care

By 20 weeks, you will probably have felt the baby move for the first time. Make a note of this, and tell your doctor at your next visit. This date will help to determine the age of the baby more accurately.

The size of your uterus is another measurement used to determine the baby's age. It is determined by checking the fundal height—the distance from the top (fundus) of your uterus to your pubic bone. After you have emptied your bladder, the doctor finds the top of your uterus by gently tapping and pressing on your abdomen and measures from that point down along the front of your abdomen to your pubic bone. During the middle of pregnancy—from about 18 to 34 weeks—the fundal height, in centimeters, often equals the number of weeks of pregnancy.

In addition, your blood pressure and weight are checked at every visit, and you'll be asked about any symptoms you may be experiencing.

Special Tests

There are tests available which are aimed at detecting problems at an early stage of pregnancy. They allow specialized care to begin as early as possible. (For more details about these tests, see page 53.)

Alpha-fetoprotein. Between 15 and 18 weeks, you may be offered a test to determine the level of alpha-fetoprotein (AFP) in your blood. AFP is a substance normally produced by a growing fetus. Measuring the level of AFP in your blood can help determine the presence of a type of birth defect called a neural tube defect.

Neural tube defects are an abnormality in which the spinal cord or brain does not form properly. An increased level of AFP may be found in the blood of a woman whose fetus has a neural tube defect. An AFP level that is lower than normal may be linked to an increased risk of Down syndrome.

In AFP testing, a blood sample taken from a vein in your arm is analyzed. If the test shows that your AFP level is higher than normal, further tests will be done to confirm or rule out a diagnosis. (For more details on AFP testing and what the results mean, see page 68.)

Ultrasound exam. Ultrasound exams are being used more often during pregnancy. Although not necessarily done in every pregnancy, an ultrasound exam can be used to help date your pregnancy and to obtain information about the health of the fetus.

During an ultrasound test, high-frequency sound waves are used to create an image of the fetus which can be viewed on a monitor. Some of the things that may be looked for in an ultrasound exam during the second trimester include the following:

- Whether you are carrying twins or other multiples
- Fetal heart movements
- The location of the placenta
- The amount of amniotic fluid (whether there is too much or too little)
- Measurements of the fetal head, abdomen and thigh bone (femur), all of which help in dating the pregnancy and observing growth of the baby

An ultrasound exam may also be done during the second trimester as a follow-up procedure when the result of an AFP test is positive.

The information gained from an ultrasound exam may affect how you are cared for during the rest of your pregnancy. For instance, if you are carrying twins, you will need to take in more calories and to visit your doctor more often. You also have a greater risk for certain problems, such as preterm labor and high blood pressure, that require special care. (See page 201 for more information about expecting twins, triplets or more.) Or if your pregnancy is not as far along as previously thought, the timing of certain routine tests may be affected.

Ultrasound testing also provides information about the placenta. Through the placenta, nutrients are brought to the growing baby and waste products are carried away.

Sometimes an ultrasound exam done in the mid-trimester reveals the placenta to be lying low in the uterus. If it partly or completely covers the cervix at delivery, problems can result (see page 195). But at this point in your pregnancy, this positioning is probably not a reason for concern. As pregnancy progresses, the placenta tends to move upward as the uterus expands and, near term, the cervix begins to dilate. By the time the baby is ready to be born, the placenta has usually moved safely out of the way of the cervical opening.

An ultrasound exam is not invasive or painful. The only discomfort you are likely to feel is from a full bladder. This is frequently necessary for the procedure because it allows the fetus to be seen more easily.

While lying on your back on an examining table, you'll have a gel or oil placed on your abdomen. A transducer, a small device somewhat like a high-tech microphone, is then placed on your abdomen. The transducer sends out sound waves that bounce off inner organs and are relayed back to form an image on a screen. (A different type of transducer, which is placed in the vagina, is sometimes used for ultrasound examinations.)

It's a thrill for most parents to see these first views of their baby. Depending on the baby's position, you may be able to make out a face, tiny hands and fingers or arms and legs.

A word of caution: It is often difficult to determine the sex of the baby on an ultrasound view. You can't be certain until after the baby is born. (For more information about ultrasound testing, see page 72.)

Amniocentesis. The amniotic fluid that surrounds the growing fetus can yield important information about the health of your baby. Amniocentesis allows a small sample of this fluid to be collected for analysis.

Amniocentesis may be done in the second trimester for many reasons. One of the most common reasons is to identify genetic defects. Genes carry the "master plan" of a person's physical makeup. Because the amniotic fluid is formed from the same cells that gave rise to the developing fetus, it has the same genetic makeup as the fetus. The amniotic fluid can therefore be studied to see whether the fetus's chromosomes are normal.

Amniocentesis for this purpose is usually offered to women who are at an increased risk for having a baby with a birth defect. These women include those who will be age 35 or older on their due date and those who have a history of birth defects in their close family. Amniocentesis may also be done as a follow-up procedure if the result of an AFP test is positive (see page 164). Or if problems arise later in pregnancy, it may be performed to find out whether the fetal lungs are mature enough for an early birth.

Amniocentesis begins with an ultrasound exam to determine the position of the fetus and the location of the placenta. With the ultrasound images used for guidance, a long, thin needle is then passed into the uterus. A small amount of amniotic fluid is withdrawn through the needle. (For more details on the procedure, see page 75.)

Amniocentesis for genetic testing is usually done at 16 to 18 weeks, when there are enough cells in the amniotic fluid to be tested. Sometimes the procedure is done earlier—as early as 11 to 14 weeks. There is a slightly increased risk of miscarriage after amniocentesis, and some women experience mild cramping.

Glucose tolerance testing. Your doctor may perform a glucose tolerance test to determine whether you have gestational diabetes. Diabetes involves an abnormality in the hormone insulin, which regulates levels of blood sugar (glucose). In a person with diabetes, the body does not produce enough insulin, or it does not properly use the insulin it does produce. The result is an excess amount of glucose in the blood, which can give rise to numerous health problems.

Gestational diabetes is a form of diabetes that can develop in a pregnant woman who did not have diabetes before her pregnancy. It is caused by changes in a pregnant woman's metabolism and hormone production. Gestational diabetes poses many potential problems for the baby. The baby may put on excess weight before birth, a condition called macrosomia. There is no universal agreement as to what birth weight constitutes macrosomia, although most authorities define it as more than 9¾ pounds (4,500 grams). Overly big (macrosomic) babies can make delivery more difficult for both mother and child; as a result, birth injuries are more common in these babies.

The risk of gestational diabetes is higher in some women, particularly those who:

- Are older than 30 years
- Have a family history of diabetes
- Had a macrosomic, malformed or stillborn infant in a previous pregnancy
- Are obese

Women with any of these risk factors are usually given a glucose tolerance test. Some doctors believe that all pregnant women should be screened for gestational diabetes, because half of women with gestational diabetes have none of these risk factors. Your doctor will talk to you about her or his approach to this screening test.

A glucose screening test is usually done between 24 and 28 weeks of pregnancy. You will be asked to drink a glucose solution. After you have waited an hour, blood is drawn from a vein in your arm, and the glucose level is checked. About 15 percent of pregnant women who are given a glucose screening test will have abnormal levels of blood glucose. If this is the case, a second test, called an oral glucose tolerance test, is done.

For the follow-up test, you will first be asked to fast overnight. You are then given another solution to drink; this one contains a higher concentration of glucose. Blood tests are taken during a three-hour period, during which your blood glucose is measured several times. Of the women whose first test result was abnormal, gestational diabetes will be diagnosed in 15 percent with this follow-up test.

The main goal for a pregnant woman with diabetes is to avoid problems during delivery because of an oversized infant. To achieve this, careful control of blood glucose is important throughout pregnancy. If you are found to have gestational diabetes, your blood glucose level will need to be checked at regular intervals until delivery. (See page 189 for information about how diabetes is managed during pregnancy.) Because there can be other complications for you and your baby if gestational diabetes occurs, your doctor may do additional tests during the last weeks of your pregnancy. Tests may include ultrasound exams (see page 72) and non-stress tests (see page 188).

Hemoglobin testing. Hemoglobin is a protein found in red blood cells. By measuring your hemoglobin level during pregnancy, your doctor can determine whether you have anemia, a deficiency in hemoglobin (see page 170).

A certain decrease in hemoglobin is normal in the second trimester. The level decreases even in pregnant women who take iron supplements. If your hemoglobin level drops during the second trimester, there is no reason to be concerned unless it falls lower than expected. If you do become anemic, your doctor will advise you about changes you may need to make in your diet and in the amount of iron supplements you need to take.

Rh factor. Among the routine tests done early in pregnancy—often at the first visit—is one to determine whether the Rh factor is present in your blood. The Rh factor is a type of protein sometimes present on red blood cells. Whether or not you have the Rh factor is determined by genes passed on from your parents. A woman who carries this protein on her red blood cells is said to be Rh-positive, whereas someone without it is Rh-negative.

Your Rh status, whether positive or negative, does not affect your health before pregnancy. But during pregnancy, if you are Rh-negative and your fetus is Rh-positive, problems can arise.

If an Rh-negative woman is carrying an Rh-positive fetus, her immune system may begin to produce antibodies against the Rh factor in the fetus's blood, which it recognizes as a foreign substance. The result can be mild or severe damage or death in the fetus from Rh disease (also called hemolytic disease or erythroblastosis).

The risk of Rh disease in a first pregnancy is thought to be lower than in subsequent pregnancies. It is probably lower because, before delivery, you're exposed to very little of the fetus's blood—not enough to trigger an immune response. But by the time you become pregnant again, the levels of antibodies in your blood will have reached a point at which they can threaten the well-being of the fetus.

If you are Rh-negative and your fetus is Rh-positive, it is not necessary to carry a pregnancy to term to develop Rh antibodies. Antibodies can form during a pregnancy that ended in miscarriage or abortion, or during an ectopic or molar pregnancy—any pregnancy with an Rh-positive fetus. If you become pregnant again, an Rh-positive fetus is at risk.

Your immune system can be prevented from making Rh antibodies if you are given an injection of Rh immunoglobulin (RhIg). This substance causes the Rh-positive cells in your blood to be destroyed. With no Rh factor to fight, antibodies do not form, and the fetus is protected. Because of the development of RhIg, fetal Rh disease is now very rare.

Your Rh status is found by testing blood drawn from a vein in your arm. If you were found to be Rh-negative early in pregnancy, you will be tested for Rh antibodies later in pregnancy, usually at 28 or 29 weeks. If you are not producing antibodies, then RhIg will be given by injection into a muscle. This will prevent Rh antibodies from forming.

RhIg will not work, however, in rare cases in which the mother's body is already producing Rh antibodies. In these cases, the fetus needs to be monitored carefully throughout the pregnancy. The tests that may be done to monitor the fetus include the following:

- Amniocentesis, in which a sample of the amniotic fluid is withdrawn from the uterus and analyzed to determine whether and how much the fetus is affected. (For more information on amniocentesis, see page 75.)
- Sampling of the blood in the baby's umbilical cord to determine whether it is Rh positive or negative. (For more information on the procedure, called percutaneous umbilical blood sampling, see page 79.)

If you are one of the few women who do have Rh antibodies, you will be tested on a regular basis throughout the second trimester to determine the level of antibodies in your blood. If the levels become too high, measures can be taken to prevent harm to the fetus. These measures may include blood transfusions to the fetus while still in the uterus or, in some cases, early delivery.

Complications

For many women, the second trimester can be relatively problem-free—mostly a matter of keeping prenatal appointments, having routine exams and tests and maintaining a healthful lifestyle. But potential problems do exist during this stage of pregnancy.

Most complications in the second trimester are more successfully dealt with when they are identified early, so it will benefit both you and your baby if you are familiar with possible warning signs. Some of the problems that can arise during mid-pregnancy are described here.

Although miscarriage is less common in the second trimester than in the first, a risk still exists. As with first-trimester miscarriage, vaginal bleeding is the chief sign of miscarriage in mid-pregnancy. Report any bleeding in your second trimester to your doctor.

If bleeding is slight or spotty, there may be no cause for concern. But report moderate to heavy bleeding in mid-pregnancy as soon as possible, because it may be a sign of one of the following problems:

- Miscarriage (if it occurs before 20 weeks)
- Preterm labor (if it occurs between 20 and 37 weeks)
- Problems with the placenta—conditions in which it lies too low in the uterus (see page 195) or begins to separate from the inner wall of the uterus before birth (see page 194)

If you have any bleeding along with pain or cramping during pregnancy, immediately call your doctor or go to an emergency department. (See page 135 for more information about bleeding during pregnancy.)

A "term" pregnancy is defined as one in which birth occurs between 37 and 42 weeks. Labor and delivery before the end of the 37th week of pregnancy are considered "preterm." Babies who are born this early often have low birth weight—they weigh less than 5½ pounds (2,500 grams) at birth. Their low weight, along with various other problems related to early birth, puts these infants at risk for numerous health problems (see page 353).

What causes it and who's at risk? The exact causes of preterm labor are not known. Often it occurs in the absence of known risk factors. Still, factors that seem to increase a woman's risk of early labor have been identified. These factors include the following:

- Previous preterm birth
- Pregnancy with twins, triplets or more
- Several previous miscarriages or abortions
- Infection of the amniotic fluid or the fetal membranes
- Hydramnios (an excess of amniotic fluid)
- Abnormalities of the mother's uterus
- Problems with the placenta
- Serious illness or disease in the mother

What are the symptoms? The signs that labor is beginning too early in pregnancy may be subtle or severe. Preterm labor is usually, but not always, signaled by contractions of the uterus. If you notice more than five contractions during an hour, it is time to contact your doctor or your hospital. Contractions at first may consist of a tightening feeling in your abdomen, which you may be able to feel with your fingertips.

Other signs of labor. Uterine contractions may be accompanied by lower back pain and a feeling of heaviness in the lower pelvis and upper thighs. Changes in vaginal discharge are also typical. There may be light spotting or bleeding along with the contractions. Or you may notice a watery fluid leaking from your vagina. This may be amniotic fluid, a sign that the membranes surrounding the fetus have ruptured. If you pass the mucus plug—the mucus that accumulates in the cervix during pregnancy—you may notice this as a thick discharge tinged with blood.

For some women, the changes described above may occur without any sensation of uterine contractions. If you have doubts about what you're feeling—and especially if you have vaginal bleeding along with abdominal cramps or pain—call your doctor. Don't be embarrassed about mistaking "false labor" for the real thing.

How is it diagnosed? If your doctor suspects that you may be having early labor, you will need to be examined. Two of the first questions to be answered will be whether your cervix has begun to dilate and whether the fetal membranes have broken. A cervical examination will be necessary to answer these questions. A uterine monitor may be used to measure the duration and spacing of your contractions. With this information, your doctor will determine whether you are actually in labor.

What's the treatment? When preterm labor is diagnosed, a decision must be made as to whether to try stopping labor or allow it to continue. Many factors will enter into this decision. Both your baby's and your own well-being must be weighed against the benefits and risks of delivery versus stopping labor. (See page 247 for more about factors that enter into the decision of postponing birth.)

Anemia

The demands of your growing fetus during pregnancy create a need for increased stores of iron in your own body. Iron is a mineral that plays an important role in the production of red blood cells. Before you were pregnant, you needed about 15 milligrams (mg) of iron a day. Now you need twice this amount, or 30 mg.

If you're like most women, you won't have enough iron stores to provide this amount each day throughout your pregnancy. And it's difficult to get this much from your diet, even if you overeat, which is not good for you or your baby. Because up to 20 percent of all pregnant women are iron-deficient, iron supplements are often prescribed during the second half of pregnancy.

What causes it and who's at risk? Anemia is due to a decline in the concentration of hemoglobin in the blood. Hemoglobin is a type of protein located in red blood cells. It plays a crucial role in the transport of oxygen to body tissues. The reason hemoglobin concentrations tend to decrease during pregnancy has to do with an increase in blood volume.

The volume of blood in your body expands dramatically during pregnancy—by about 45 percent. Most of this increase is due to an increase in blood plasma, the fluid portion of blood (as distinct from the part made up of red and white blood cells). During the first half of pregnancy, the volume of plasma increases more rapidly than the volume of red blood cells. As a result, the concentration of red blood cells decreases during this time, until they have a chance to catch up with the increase in blood plasma.

Anemia can develop when there's not enough iron to fuel the increased production of red blood cells. The result is a decrease in hemoglobin concentrations in the blood.

Besides iron deficiency, other causes of anemia may include excessive blood loss (hemorrhage) from injury or surgery, chronic illness (such as serious infections or kidney disease) or a deficiency in folic acid (a vitamin needed for the production of red blood cells). In pregnant women, though, iron deficiency is the most common cause of anemia.

In the United States, many women of childbearing age don't get enough iron, even when they're not pregnant. Women lose iron along with the blood and tissue shed during their periods, which is one reason why they are more prone to anemia. Inadequate diet is another common reason. During pregnancy, the increased need for iron to fuel the fetus's growth compounds the problems many women already have in getting enough iron.

Women who receive prenatal care and take iron supplements during pregnancy generally avoid the problems associated with iron-deficiency anemia. Among women who don't receive prenatal care, especially women who have little or no access to health care, iron-deficiency anemia is much more common.

Anemia in a pregnant woman can cause excessive fatigue and stress and make her more susceptible to illness, but it is unlikely to harm the fetus. Even when a woman is iron-deficient, the required amount of iron continues to be provided to the placenta and fetus.

What are the symptoms? If anemia is mild, you may not notice symptoms. In moderate to severe anemia, you may experience some of the following:

- Excessive fatigue and weakness
- Pale complexion
- Shortness of breath
- Heart palpitations
- Dizziness, light-headedness or fainting spells

How is it diagnosed? Your blood will be checked early in pregnancy, probably at the first visit to your doctor, to make sure that your hemoglobin levels are normal. But even if you're not anemic at that point, your pregnancy may cause you to become at least mildly anemic later on, as your blood volume expands and more and more nutrients need to be delivered to the growing fetus. In fact, iron-deficiency anemia develops most often after 20 weeks of pregnancy. Many doctors prescribe an iron supplement to all their pregnant patients as a safeguard against the development of anemia.

What's the treatment? Treatment for anemia consists of taking in enough iron, which is prescribed in capsule or tablet form, to increase your hemoglobin concentrations to normal levels. Most likely you will already be taking extra iron by the second trimester, but if anemia develops despite this treatment, your dosage may need to be increased.

Taking iron supplements may sometimes make nausea and vomiting worse. You may want to take your iron supplements near bedtime if they tend to give you an upset stomach. You may find it helpful to keep them near your toothbrush as a reminder to take them every day. Like any medication, keep iron capsules or tablets away from children.

Very rarely, blood transfusions may be required in a pregnant woman who is severely anemic and has had significant blood loss. Transfusions may also be needed in a severely anemic woman who needs surgery.

Cervical Incompetence

A cause of miscarriage and preterm birth in the second and third trimesters, cervical incompetence is a condition in which the cervix begins to open (dilate) and thin (efface) before a pregnancy has reached term. In a woman with cervical incompetence, dilation and effacement of the cervix occur without pain or uterine contractions. Instead of happening in response to uterine contractions, as in a normal pregnancy, these events occur because of a weakness in the cervix, which opens under the growing pressure of the uterus as pregnancy progresses. If the changes are not halted, rupture of the membranes and birth of a premature baby can result.

If you have an incompetent cervix, the medical name for this condition may give you the impression that you are somehow faulty, inadequate or weak. This is not the case—"incompetent" in this sense simply means that the muscle of the cervix is not able to withstand the pressure of the uterus. Because you cannot voluntarily control this muscle, it cannot possibly be due to any failure on your part.

What causes it and who's at risk? Cervical incompetence is relatively rare, occurring in only 1 to 2 percent of all pregnancies. But it is thought to cause as many as 20 to 25 percent of miscarriages in the second trimester. It may have any of several possible causes, such as:

- A previous operation on the cervix (D&C or biopsy)
- Damage to the cervix during a prior difficult delivery
- A malformation in the cervix due to a birth defect (such as in DES-exposed women; see page 173)

These risk factors make it more likely for the problem to recur in another pregnancy.

Other women at risk for this problem include those who are pregnant with more than one fetus and those who have an excess of amniotic fluid (a condition called hydramnios) in the current pregnancy. For these women, cervical incompetence is less likely to recur in a subsequent pregnancy.

What are the symptoms? Cervical incompetence may cause some of the typical symptoms of miscarriage or preterm labor. When the following signs or symptoms occur in the absence of abdominal pain, cervical incompetence may be the cause:

- Spotting or bleeding
- A vaginal discharge that is bloody or thick and mucus-like (the latter may be the passing of the mucus plug from the cervix; see page 160)
- A sensation of pressure or heaviness in the lower abdomen

You need to be especially alert to these signs if you had a miscarriage or preterm labor in a previous pregnancy which was due to cervical incompetence.

How is it diagnosed? Some attempts have been made to diagnose cervical incompetence before it causes problems, but these efforts have not been very successful.

What's the treatment? If you were diagnosed with cervical incompetence in a previous pregnancy, your doctor might take steps to prevent the problem from recurring in this pregnancy. Treatment may include cerclage, a surgical technique to reinforce the cervical muscle.

Several procedures are used for cerclage, but they all involve placing sutures above the opening of the cervix to narrow the cervical canal.

Cerclage is most successful if it is performed relatively early in pregnancy—by about 18 or 20 weeks. Depending on what type of procedure was used, the sutures may either stay in place or be removed close to your due date. Placement of a cervical cerclage does not completely protect a woman from miscarriage or preterm delivery. Additional treatment, such as bed rest or tocolytic therapy (medication to stop uterine contractions), may also be needed. Even with a cerclage and additional therapy, the risk of preterm birth is high (about 25 percent in some studies) in women with cervical incompetence.

If your mother took DES

During the 1950s and 1960s, more than a million pregnant women took a medication called diethylstilbestrol (dye-ethel-still-BESS-trawl), or DES. It was thought that this drug helped prevent pregnancy complications such as hypertension, diabetes, preterm labor and miscarriage.

In the early 1970s, it was found that DES did not have these beneficial effects. As a result, pregnant women were no longer given this drug. Unfortunately, though, DES has been found to have lasting effects in some of the daughters born to women who took it.

The daughters of mothers who took DES while pregnant have an increased risk of abnormalities of the reproductive tract. Up to two-thirds of these women have an abnormally shaped uterus, defects in the fallopian tubes or structural abnormalities of the vagina and cervix. Changes in vaginal and cervical tissues, which have been linked to a rare type of cancer, have also been found in some women whose mothers took DES, although the risk is small. Other, noncancerous, changes in the vagina and cervix are also more common in DES-exposed women.

Ironically, DES, once given to pregnant women in the belief that it would prevent complications, is now thought to cause or contribute to some of those same problems in their daughters. DES-caused abnormalities in the cervix are believed to result in cervical incompetence, leading to preterm labor and miscarriage. In addition, abnormal fallopian tubes are the cause of infertility in some DES-exposed women. In others, the risk of ectopic pregnancy is increased.

If there is a chance that your mother took DES while she was carrying you, talk to your doctor before you become pregnant. During your pregnancy, your doctor may want to perform ultrasound exams and other tests more frequently. If it can be confirmed that you were exposed to DES while your mother was pregnant, you will need to be monitored carefully for early cervical dilation. Finally, it's important to have regular examinations to check for abnormal changes in the cells of your vagina and cervix. These changes, if identified early, can be successfully treated.

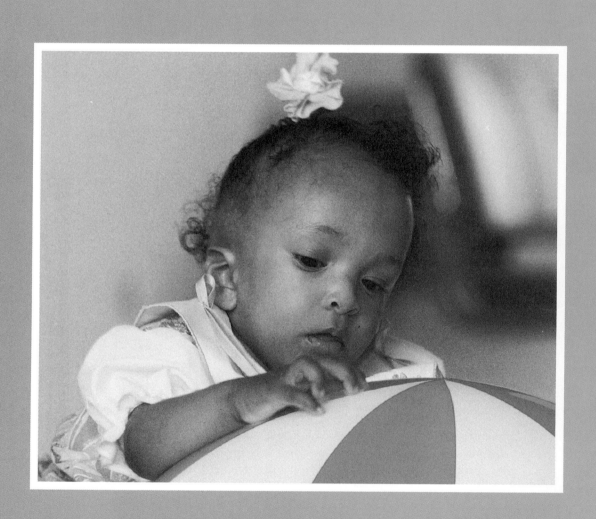

CHAPTER TWELVE

The Third Trimester

28 to 40 weeks and beyond

The third trimester begins at the 28th week of pregnancy and lasts until birth. This is usually a time of growing excitement and anticipation of the baby's arrival. After all, you're coming down the home stretch!

You're probably thinking a lot these days about when labor will start and how your delivery will go. A growing sense of tension during this time is understandable, as are worries and fears about whether your baby will be healthy. Like many women during late pregnancy, you may be tired of being pregnant. You may find yourself wishing for the time to pass quickly until the birth so that you can begin to enjoy your new baby.

It's natural for your thoughts to turn now to the plans that need to be made. Now is the time, for instance, to start thinking about whether you will breast-feed. You'll also need to choose a doctor or other health care provider for your child. You may want to meet with this caregiver before your baby's birth to get acquainted and discuss any questions.

Like the rest of your pregnancy, you'll experience the third trimester in your own way. Some of the common signs and symptoms experienced by many women are described in this chapter, along with potential problems and what to expect during office visits in late pregnancy.

Physical Changes and Symptoms

Before you were pregnant, your uterus, a small, almost-solid organ, weighed only about 2 ounces and could hold a volume of less than half an ounce. At term, it will weigh about 2½ pounds and will have stretched to hold your baby, the placenta and about a quart of amniotic fluid. Nearly all of the physical symptoms of late pregnancy arise from this increase in the size of the uterus.

Shortness of Breath

What causes it? If you're like many women in late pregnancy, you may be feeling as though you can't get enough air. This is because your diaphragm—the broad, flat muscle that lies under your lungs—is being pushed up out of its normal place by the expanding uterus. The diaphragm rises about 1½ inches from its usual position during pregnancy. That may seem like a small amount, but it's enough to decrease your lung capacity (the amount of air your lungs are able to take in).

At the same time, though, the hormone progesterone acts on the respiratory center in the brain, causing you to breathe more deeply. As a result, although your total lung capacity is decreased, the volume of air you are taking in with each breath is actually increased during pregnancy.

Despite your own discomfort, you don't need to worry about your baby. Your expanded respiratory and circulatory systems are seeing to it that the baby is getting plenty of oxygen. Your body is now carrying more blood and more oxygen-rich hemoglobin. These increases cause the oxygen level in your blood to increase, ensuring an adequate supply to your growing baby.

What can I do? Improving your posture will help you to breathe better, both during pregnancy and afterward. Practice sitting and standing with your back straight and your shoulders back, relaxed and down. Aerobic exercise is also beneficial throughout pregnancy. It will improve your breathing and lower your pulse rate. Take care, however, not to overexert yourself. Consult your doctor about a safe exercise program for late pregnancy. When sleeping, lying propped up on pillows or on your side may help lessen the pressure on your diaphragm.

If none of these measures seem to help enough, hang in there. Your breathlessness will subside during the last few weeks of pregnancy, when the baby drops farther down into your pelvis and takes the pressure off your diaphragm.

Although mild shortness of breath is common in pregnancy, more severe breathing problems may be a sign of a more serious problem, such as a blood clot in the lung. If you develop severe shortness of breath along with chest pain, discomfort while taking a deep breath, rapid pulse or rapid breathing, contact your doctor right away or go to an emergency room promptly.

Other Minor Discomforts

Hip pain. The increased hormones of pregnancy tend to cause the connective tissue in your body to soften and loosen up. One result is that the joints between the bones of your pelvis become more relaxed. The greater flexibility of these bones makes it easier for the baby to pass through them during birth. Unfortunately, it can also have the added effect of producing hip pain.

Hip pain in late pregnancy usually occurs on one side. The changes in your posture, along with lower back pain, that result from the heavier uterus can add to your discomfort.

Exercises to strengthen your lower back and abdominal muscles may ease hip pain. Warm baths and compresses may also be helpful.

Sciatica. Pain, tingling or numbness running down the buttock, hip and thigh is called sciatica. It can be caused by the pressure of the pregnant uterus on the sciatic nerve. Two sciatic nerves run from your lower back down your legs to your feet.

Sciatic nerve pain during pregnancy is usually not a cause for concern. You should still tell your doctor about it, though, because there are other, rarer causes of sciatica that could be more serious.

When your baby changes position closer to the time of delivery, sciatic pain is likely to ease. Warm baths, a heating pad and sleeping on the opposite side may help until then.

Vaginal pain. Some women occasionally feel a sharp, stabbing pain inside the vagina during late pregnancy. This is probably linked to the cervix starting to dilate, which can happen weeks, days or hours before labor begins. It is usually nothing to be concerned about, but tell your doctor if it causes a great deal of discomfort. Any severe pain in the lower abdomen should be reported to your doctor right away.

Sciatic nerve

Pressure on your sciatic nerve may cause pain, tingling or numbness in your buttock, hip or thigh late in your pregnancy. Called sciatica, it's unpleasant but temporary and generally not serious.

Sleeping Problems

W ***hat causes them?*** As you get closer to delivery, you may be finding it more and more difficult to sleep through the night. There could be several reasons for this. One is the size of your abdomen, which may make it seem impossible for you to find a comfortable position. Another is the natural anticipation, or even anxiety, you may be feeling about your baby's arrival. Insomnia can be troublesome for you, but there's no need to worry about it harming your baby.

What can I do? The best position for sleeping in late pregnancy is on your left or right side, with your legs and knees bent. Lying on your side is better than on your back because it takes pressure off the large vein that carries blood from your legs and feet back to your heart. The side position is also good for taking pressure off your lower back.

Try using a pillow to support your abdomen and another one to support your upper leg. Also try leaning against a bunched-up pillow or rolled-up blanket placed at the small of your back. This can help take some of the pressure off the hip you're lying on.

To deal with anxiety, the relaxation exercises you learned in childbirth classes can help you even now, well before labor begins. If you're feeling restless and anxious at night instead of getting the sleep you'd like, try some of these techniques to calm your mind and allow your body to rest. (See page 138 for more suggestions about coping with insomnia.)

Skin Changes

Itchy abdomen. The stretching and tightening of the skin across your abdomen during late pregnancy tend to leave it dry, making you want to scratch. But try not to, or at least do as little as possible. Keep your abdomen lubricated with a good moisturizing cream to help alleviate the discomfort. You may also want to try an anti-itch cream, such as one with 0.5 percent hydrocortisone in it.

Varicose veins. Varicose veins are more common in women than in men, and they often tend to run in families. Caused by a weakness in the small veins that carry blood back to the heart, they show up as fine bluish, reddish or purplish lines under the skin, most often on the legs and ankles.

The circulatory changes of pregnancy that are designed to support the growing fetus can produce this unfortunate but common side effect. Varicose veins may surface for the first time or may worsen during late pregnancy, when the uterus exerts greater pressure on the veins in the legs.

Varicose veins may cause no symptoms or may be accompanied by mild to severe pain. Measures to help prevent them, keep them from getting worse or ease their discomforts include the following:

- Avoid standing for long periods.
- Don't sit with your legs crossed. This position can aggravate circulatory problems.
- Elevate your legs whenever you can. When sitting, rest them on another chair or a stool. When lying down, raise your legs and feet on a pillow.
- Exercise regularly to improve your overall circulation.
- Use compression stockings to help improve the circulation in your legs. Ask your doctor to recommend a good brand.

Although varicose veins don't go away by themselves, they generally improve greatly after delivery. In severe cases, they can be removed surgically, but this procedure is not normally done during pregnancy.

Vascular spiders. Spider nevi, or vascular spiders, usually arise only during pregnancy. Their name comes from the way they look—tiny, red, raised lines that branch out from the center, like a spider. They appear most often on the upper body, face and neck and are due to the effects of hormones on the circulatory system. Unlike varicose veins, spider nevi don't cause pain or discomfort, and they usually go away after delivery.

Stretch marks. The reddish or whitish streaks you may notice on your breasts, abdomen and upper thighs are common to about half of pregnant women. These are stretch marks, and women who aren't pregnant also get them.

Stretch marks are not necessarily related to gaining weight. In some women they can be severe even when little weight has been gained during pregnancy. Heredity is thought to play the biggest role in their development.

There is no proven treatment for stretch marks. Because they develop from deep within the connective tissue underneath the skin, they cannot be prevented by anything applied externally. Contrary to some beliefs, there are no "miracle" creams or ointments that will make them magically vanish. They will, however, tend to fade slowly after delivery.

PUPP. The term "PUPP" refers to a condition called pruritic urticarial papules and plaques of pregnancy. Occurring in about one of every 150 pregnancies, PUPP is characterized by itchy, reddish, raised patches on the skin. These usually show up first on the abdomen and often spread to the arms and legs. In some women, the itching can be extreme. Although PUPP can be quite uncomfortable for the mother, it doesn't seem to cause a risk for the baby.

It's not known for certain what causes PUPP, but there appears to be a genetic factor involved because it tends to run in families. Unlike so many of the other symptoms of pregnancy, PUPP doesn't seem to be linked to increased hormone levels. When it occurs, it is nearly always in first pregnancies, and it rarely recurs in subsequent ones.

Treatment of PUPP consists of oral medications or anti-itching creams that are applied to the skin. Oatmeal baths or baking soda baths may also provide some relief. The rash-like symptoms will go away after you deliver.

Hemorrhoids

What causes them? Hemorrhoids are firm, swollen pouches formed underneath the mucous membranes inside or outside the rectum. A form of varicose veins, hemorrhoids are more common during pregnancy because of increased pressure on the rectal veins. They may occur for the first time or may become more frequent or severe during pregnancy.

Bleeding, itching and pain in and around the anus are among the uncomfortable symptoms of hemorrhoids. Although they sometimes require surgical treatment, they usually eventually shrink and go away on their own.

What can I do? As with so many other conditions, the best way to deal with hemorrhoids is prevention. If you have had this problem before pregnancy, taking preventive measures is especially important from early pregnancy onward.

Avoid becoming constipated by including high-fiber foods, fruit and vegetables and plenty of fluids in your diet. (See page 158 for more about avoiding constipation.) Straining during bowel movements puts pressure on the rectal veins and can cause or aggravate hemorrhoids.

To treat hemorrhoids and ease their symptoms, try the following:

- Keep the area around your anus clean. Gently wash the area after each bowel movement. This can be done with hygienic witch hazel pads (sold over the counter) or in a warm sitz bath (a shallow basin that fits over the toilet and in which the buttocks and hips are submerged). Use only soft, non-dyed, unscented toilet paper.
- Warm soaks—in a tub or a sitz bath—will help shrink hemorrhoids and provide soothing relief. Add an oatmeal bath formula or baking soda to the water to relieve itching.
- Apply compresses with an ice pack or hygienic pads.
- Avoid sitting for long periods, especially on hard chairs.
- Consult your doctor before using any over-the-counter remedy for hemorrhoids.

Occasionally, a hemorrhoid may become thrombosed (filled with blood clots). In this case, it is impossible for the swollen vein to shrink to its normal size, and minor surgery may be needed to remove the hemorrhoid.

Leaking Urine

What causes it? The increased pressure of your pregnant uterus on your bladder may cause you to leak urine from time to time. You may notice this annoying symptom when you laugh, cough or sneeze. It will most likely disappear after delivery.

What can I do? Empty your bladder whenever you have the urge to—don't hold urine in. Frequent emptying will keep your bladder from becoming over-full, which contributes to leakage. Wear panty liners to help keep you dry.

Kegel exercises can help strengthen the muscles that control urination. These exercises are done by contracting the muscles of the pelvic floor. You can feel these muscles contract during urination by stopping the flow of urine. The exercises themselves, however, should not be done regularly during urination, or when the bladder is full—this practice could actually weaken the muscles.

Tighten the muscles as if you are stopping a stream of urine. Try it at frequent intervals for five seconds at a time, four or five times in a row. These exercises may help cut down on urine leakage.

Weight Gain

By the end of pregnancy, the "average" woman has gained 25 to 35 pounds. How much you gain will depend greatly on your weight before pregnancy. The Institute of Medicine recommends that underweight women gain 28 to 40 pounds, normal-weight women gain 25 to 35 pounds and overweight women gain 15 to 25 pounds.

During the third trimester, most women gain an average of 11 pounds. Your own weight gain may vary somewhat from this amount, however, and still be normal. (See page 86 for more about weight gain in pregnancy.)

What's Happening With the Baby?

Size and Weight

The fetus continues to grow and put on weight throughout the last trimester of pregnancy. By the end of the 28th week, it weighs about 2½ to 3 pounds and measures about 14 to 16 inches long. Because little fat has yet been laid down, the skin appears thin, red and wrinkled. A slick, white, fatty substance called vernix caseosa covers the skin. The eyes open and close, and the fetus may suck his or her thumb.

The fetus continues to put on weight steadily—about half a pound each week—until about 37 weeks. As the pregnancy reaches term, the baby begins to gain weight more slowly. As fat is laid down, the body becomes rounder. By the ninth month, the baby usually settles into a position for delivery, with the head down and arms and legs pulled up tightly against the chest.

At 40 weeks, the average baby weighs about 7 to 7½ pounds and measures about 18 to 20½ inches long. Your own baby may have a weight and size of less or more, though, and still be normal and healthy.

Fetal Movements

As the baby's weight and size increase throughout later pregnancy, so too does the activity you feel inside your uterus. From the beginning of the third trimester, you probably will notice the baby's movements becoming more frequent and vigorous. You may notice a change in the movements at around 32 weeks. By that time, the growing fetus has made for crowded conditions inside the uterus. The fetus is moving around just as much, but the kicks and other movements may seem less forceful.

To keep track of the baby's activity, your doctor may ask you to keep a record of when you feel your baby moving. A sudden drop-off or decrease in movement could signal a problem and should be reported to your doctor. She or he may want to perform tests to monitor the heart rate or observe the movements of the fetus. (See page 138 for more information about monitoring the fetus.)

Many factors seem to affect the baby's movements in late pregnancy. How much and when you eat, what position you are in and sounds from the outside world have all been shown to affect fetal activity.

Many pregnant women who are busy and active don't always notice the baby's movements. You may want to check on your baby's movements from time to time, especially if you think you may have noticed a slowdown in activity. To do this, lie on your left side for 30 to 60 minutes and note how often you feel the baby move. If you are recording your baby's movements, your doctor will tell you what should prompt you to contact her or him. A commonly used figure is fewer than 10 movements in two hours.

Along with the usual sensations of kicks and rolls, you may also occasionally notice a slight twitching, like little spasms. These are probably hiccups. Fetuses get them too. There is no danger to the baby from hiccups.

Decisions to Make

The reality of being responsible for a new baby is likely to start sinking in during the third trimester. Especially if this is your first child, it's not unusual to feel overwhelmed by the prospect of caring for a new human being. Taking stock of the decisions that need to be made now, before your baby is born, may help make the new responsibilities seem less formidable once your baby is here.

Choosing Your Baby's Medical Caregiver

It's not too early to start thinking about the person who will provide health care for your child. If you already have a family physician—a doctor who provides general health care to both adults and children—she or he can provide this care. If this is not the case, you'll want to explore the options.

Your child's health care provider could be a family doctor, a pediatrician (a doctor specializing in the care of children) or a pediatric nurse-practitioner. A pediatric nurse-practitioner is a registered nurse who has special training in caring for children and who often practices with a physician.

Your child's medical caregiver will become an important person to you and your family as your baby grows up. Having a plan in place now, before your baby is born, will benefit you, your partner and your child. Once you are caring for an infant, with the around-the-clock schedule this requires, it will be harder to find the time to look for a health care provider. It will be easier to know in advance when to bring your baby in for a first checkup, and it's good to be familiar with the caregiver and the office staff.

Meeting your baby's medical caregiver before delivery will also give you and your partner a chance to ask questions about any special concerns you may have. You may want to know, for instance, how often to bring in your child for "well-baby" checkups, what procedures to follow in an emergency and who will see your baby if your regular caregiver is not available. (See Part Three for information about health care for your child throughout her or his first year.)

In choosing your baby's medical caregiver, here are some of the things that you and your partner may want to consider:

- "Philosophy" of health care—the caregiver's attitude about preventive care, nutrition and the caregiver–patient relationship
- Professional qualifications
- Accessibility—how easy or difficult it will be to contact the caregiver on the phone, or how far in advance you will have to schedule an appointment
- Location and convenience of the caregiver's office
- Attitudes and helpfulness of the office staff and nurses
- Costs to you and your insurance company

You may want to get recommendations from persons you know who have health care providers they like. But you and your partner are the ones who must be satisfied with the doctor or nurse-practitioner you choose. In addition to the above-listed factors, one of the most important requirements is that you are able to develop mutual trust and good rapport with the person.

To Breastfeed or Bottle Feed?

Breastfeeding is becoming much more common today than when you were a baby. Nearly two-thirds of mothers breastfeed today, in contrast to less than one-third 25 years ago. Several factors need to be considered when making this decision.

Breastfeeding. **Benefits and drawbacks**. Breast milk is the ideal nutrition for a newborn. It contains just the right balance of nutrients such as protein, carbohydrates and fat. It also provides the infant with antibodies to fight off some common childhood illnesses, and it helps create a protective environment in the gastrointestinal tract to ward off infection. Breast milk is also easier to digest than commercial formulas.

Breastfeeding has advantages for your own health as well as your baby's. Stimulation of your nipples triggers the release of oxytocin, a hormone that causes the uterus to contract and return to its normal size. And breastfeeding helps you return to your normal pre-pregnancy weight.

Breastfeeding has some practical advantages too. It's less expensive than bottle feeding, because there is no equipment to buy. Many women find breastfeeding to be more convenient than bottle feeding. There are no formulas to prepare, and no need to fuss with bottles, nipples and other equipment. It can be done anywhere, at any time, whenever your baby shows signs of being hungry. If modesty is a concern, a towel or baby blanket can be draped over your shoulder and breast, or you can find a quiet, private spot away from others.

Finally, breastfeeding creates intimacy and closeness with your baby. It can be extremely rewarding for both of you.

For some women, a major drawback of breastfeeding is the diminished freedom for the mother. Women who breastfeed exclusively must be with their baby for most feedings, although expressing milk with a breast pump can enable others to take over some feedings. (See page 484 for details on pumping breast milk.)

Who can and cannot breastfeed. Almost any woman can breastfeed her baby. The ability to do so has nothing to do with the size or shape of your breasts or nipples. Small breasts do not produce less milk than large breasts.

If you tried to breastfeed a previous child and weren't able to, most likely you can still breastfeed this baby. You may simply need to learn more about the proper technique. Breastfeeding is a natural process, but it still requires patience and practice. A lactation specialist can help with any problems you may have in trying to breastfeed.

Reasons why some women are advised not to breastfeed have to do with the mother's or the baby's health:

- Serious infections, such as tuberculosis, HIV infection, AIDS or hepatitis, in the mother
- Serious illnesses such as kidney or heart problems in the mother
- Certain medications taken by the mother for chronic conditions
- Rarely, disorders in the newborn make it impossible to digest breast milk
- Abnormal shape of the newborn's mouth (such as cleft lip or cleft palate) which makes it difficult for her or him to nurse

Talk with your doctor about making this decision. She or he can tell you about any factors that might prevent you from breastfeeding.

Preparing to breastfeed. For most women, there is no special preparation that needs to be done for breastfeeding. You may have heard of "toughening" your nipples to keep them from getting sore during nursing, but this is generally not necessary. Sore nipples can usually be alleviated by changing the baby's position at the breast.

However, if your nipples are flat or depressed inward, instead of protruding outward, you do need to prepare them for breastfeeding so that the baby's mouth will be able to latch on. You can help push retracted nipples outward by massaging the area around them, gently pushing them outward with your thumb and forefinger. Breast shells, which can be found in some maternity stores and pharmacies, can also be used for this purpose. These are flexible, dome-shaped devices with a small hole in the center. Worn under a bra, they help pull retracted nipples outward.

Even if you do have nipples that normally protrude, it is a good idea to check to see whether they will stay that way when the baby nurses. To do this, place your thumb and forefinger above and below the nipple on the areola—the pigmented skin surrounding the nipple—and squeeze gently. The nipple should move outward, lifting away from the tissue underneath. If instead it sinks inward, massaging the nipples or wearing breast shells should help.

Bottle feeding. If you cannot or choose not to breastfeed, your baby can be well nourished with bottle feeding. A chief advantage of bottle feeding is that it frees you from the responsibility of all of the feedings. With bottle feeding, too, your partner can share in the closeness of feeding his new baby. And some women feel more comfortable bottle feeding their babies in public.

The main drawback of bottle feeding is that it can be a nuisance. Careful preparation is required for each feeding. Nipples and bottles must be cleaned thoroughly, and formula must be stored carefully.

If you don't nurse at all after your baby is born, your breasts will eventually stop producing milk. Until this happens, they may become swollen and painful. It may be necessary to use ice packs or pain relievers for a few days after delivery. A well-fitted support bra will make you feel more comfortable.

The choice is yours. You don't have to opt exclusively for either the breast or the bottle alone. It's important that your milk supply is well established before you introduce a bottle. Many parents find that a combination of both methods works well and lets them enjoy the advantages of each.

Whatever your decision, you and your partner must be comfortable with it. Time, and support from helpful professionals, will help you find an approach that works best for you.

Circumcision

Circumcision is a procedure in which the foreskin—the sheath of tissue covering the head of the penis—is removed. The practice has been known since ancient times, when it was performed as a religious rite or as an initiation of boys into adulthood. Many parents today still have their sons circumcised, for religious or other reasons. In the United States overall, the practice is somewhat less common today than it was 50 years ago.

If you know ahead of time that you are carrying a boy, or even if you are unsure of the sex of your baby, give some thought before delivery as to whether you will have your son circumcised. If you are undecided about this option, it will help to be aware of what is currently known about the risks and benefits of this procedure, as well as some of the reasons why parents opt for or against it.

Health issues. Researchers have attempted to learn more about whether circumcision prevents infection and certain types of cancer, but more studies need to be done to answer some of these questions. It is known that circumcision prevents infection and inflammation of the foreskin. And it seems to decrease the risk of cancer of the penis. This disease occurs in fewer than one of every 100,000 men in the United States.

Some studies have shown a greater risk of cervical cancer in female sexual partners of uncircumcised men who are infected with human papillomavirus. Circumcision might also have a role in reducing the risk of sexually transmitted diseases. Practicing safe sex is a far more important factor in preventing these diseases than whether a man is circumcised.

Recent studies suggest that infants who are not circumcised may be more likely to develop urinary tract infections. These infections early in life may lead to kidney problems later in life. Infants who have abnormalities of the kidney or bladder are at higher risk for urinary tract infections, so circumcision may be advised for these babies.

Occasionally, problems can occur with the uncircumcised penis which require circumcision at an older age. These problems include inflammation of the foreskin or adherence of the foreskin to the tip of the penis. These problems occur in about 2 to 6 percent of uncircumcised males. Circumcision during infancy eliminates the possible need for the procedure at an older age.

Cleanliness. Circumcision makes it easy to keep the end of the penis clean. However, the shedding skin cells that naturally accumulate on the glans of an uncircumcised boy are not harmful. Do not try to force the foreskin back to clean the penis of an infant or young boy. Washing externally with soap and water is all that's necessary.

After your son's foreskin is fully retractable, then washing under the foreskin during a bath or shower is part of good hygiene habits. The risk of penile cancer appears to be linked to personal hygiene. Uncircumcised males with poor hygiene have a higher risk, whereas uncircumcised males with good hygiene have a lower risk.

Other factors. Many Jewish and Muslim parents throughout the world continue to have their sons circumcised for religious and cultural reasons, as they have done for many centuries. One reason why some parents choose circumcision is so their son will be like his father or his peers. Some parents prefer to have their sons make this decision later in childhood or as an adult. All of these are issues that depend on personal preferences.

Circumcision does not prevent masturbation or increase fertility. The belief that circumcision enhances the sexual experience for men or their sexual partners may not necessarily be true, either.

Risks. Like any minor surgery, circumcision poses some risk to the newborn. Excessive bleeding or infection occurs in fewer than one in 1,000 cases.

Circumcision does cause pain for the baby. Local anesthesia is frequently used. If you decide to have your son circumcised, you may want to talk with your doctor about whether local anesthesia will be used.

Reasons to postpone circumcision. Sometimes circumcision must be delayed. In premature boys, for example, the procedure is usually delayed until the baby weighs about 6 pounds. Babies born with birth defects of the penis, such as hypospadias, usually should not have circumcision done until the time that corrective surgery is planned. Other reasons to delay circumcision include illness or bleeding problems, such as hemophilia. If your baby is hospitalized or requires special care after birth, your doctor will advise you as to when circumcision might be done.

Making your decision. In deciding whether to have your son circumcised, it may help to talk to other parents of boys about what they decided and why. Health and hygiene issues, personal preferences and religious beliefs all must be weighed when deciding for or against this procedure.

If you choose circumcision, it usually will be done within days after delivery. Your consent must be obtained, either orally or in writing, before the procedure is performed. (See page 443 for details about how the procedure is done.)

Whatever your decision concerning circumcision of your son, it should be based on what is currently known about its risks and benefits. Your personal views and beliefs play an important role in making this decision.

Some Common Questions

Q: *How will I know when the baby "drops"? Will labor start right away afterward?*

A: The common term for this event, "lightening," doesn't quite convey what actually happens: the descent of the baby's head into the pelvis sometime during the last weeks of pregnancy. Because of decreased pressure on the diaphragm and stomach, you will indeed feel "lightened," as breathing and digestion become easier. If this is your first baby, lightening may occur weeks in advance of labor. In women who have had children, it usually doesn't happen until labor begins.

When lightening does occur, you'll notice a change in the shape of your abdomen as it shifts down and forward. In addition to being able to breathe more deeply when the baby drops down into your pelvis, you'll probably feel the need to urinate more often, much as you did in the first trimester, because of the increased pressure on your bladder. Some women also feel pressure or aches and pains in their pelvic joints and perineum. It is also not unusual to feel sharp twinges in the perineal area as the baby's head presses on the pelvic floor.

Lightening is usually a sign that the baby's head is engaged—that it has dropped below the upper part of the pelvis in preparation for birth. Your doctor will examine you during the last weeks of pregnancy to find whether engagement has occurred.

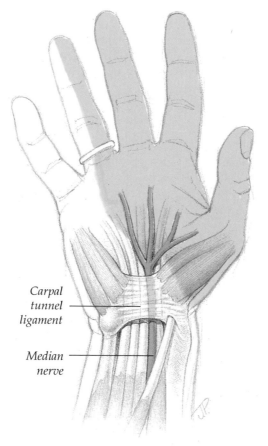

Carpal tunnel ligament

Median nerve

Q: *Lately I've been having burning and numbness in my hands. These sensations are starting to wake me up during the night. Is this something serious?*

A: You may be having symptoms of carpal tunnel syndrome. This condition occurs most commonly in women between 40 and 60 years of age, often as a result of repetitive movements of the wrists and hands. It is also common in up to 25 percent of all pregnant women. In pregnancy, hormonal effects, swelling and weight gain can compress the nerve inside the carpal tunnel. This is a sheath of tissue surrounding the median nerve that supplies the ball of the thumb, the first two fingers and half of the ring finger.

The symptoms of this syndrome are numbness, tingling and pain, often a burning sensation, in these areas. In 80 percent of pregnant women with this syndrome, the symptoms occur in both hands.

Rarely are medications or surgery needed during pregnancy. Rather, treatment includes wearing a wrist splint at night and during activities that make the symptoms worse, such as driving a car or holding a book. You may be able to relieve the discomfort by rubbing or shaking your hands.

The effects of carpal tunnel syndrome can be disturbing, but they almost always disappear after delivery. In the rare cases when they don't, or when they are severe, steroid injections can be given or minor surgery can be done to correct the problem.

Office Visits

You'll continue receiving routine exams at your visits to your doctor in late pregnancy. In addition, if you have a condition that makes your pregnancy high-risk, special tests may be performed on a regular basis to check the baby's health.

Routine Exams

During late pregnancy, your doctor will continue to monitor your blood pressure and weight, as well as the activity and movements of the fetus. You'll continue to have the size of your uterus measured and to be asked about any symptoms you may be having. As your due date draws near, your doctor will check the position of the baby. She or he may also perform a vaginal exam to check for dilation of the cervix.

Presenting part. By a few weeks before birth, most babies have moved into the head-down position in the uterus. Your doctor will check the baby's presenting part—the part of the body that is farthest down in your pelvis, ready to be born first. This is usually the baby's head, and it can be felt by the doctor in your lower abdomen just above the pubic bone, or at the top of the birth canal, during a vaginal exam.

Close to the due date, some doctors may also determine the "station" of the presenting part. This refers to how far down in the pelvis the presenting part is.

Fetal position. Babies who are positioned with their feet or buttocks down, in position to be born first, close to the time of delivery are said to be in breech presentation. By checking the presenting part, your doctor can determine the position of the fetus. (See page 318 for more about breech babies.)

Cervical changes. The condition of your cervix may be checked by a vaginal exam as you near your due date. Your doctor may check to see how much it is beginning to soften, as well as how much it has dilated (opened) and effaced (thinned out).

It is not possible for your doctor to tell you when you will go into labor on the basis of a cervical exam. Many women can go for weeks dilated at 3 centimeters, and others go into labor without any dilation or effacement beforehand. Because the cervical exam can't predict when labor will start, many doctors prefer to forgo it unless induction of labor is being considered. (See page 291 for information on induced labor.)

Monitoring the Baby's Health

Several conditions may increase the risks posed to your baby during pregnancy, as well as during labor and delivery. In a high-risk pregnancy, tests are done to determine how the fetus is doing and how well it may be able to tolerate the physical stress of birth.

Non-stress test. The non-stress test (NST) helps your doctor evaluate the condition of the fetus. This test measures the baby's heart rate in response to its own movements. Normally, the heart beats faster when the baby moves.

For the non-stress test, you'll lie on an examining table or sit in a lounge chair. A belt with ultrasound transducers attached to it will be placed around your abdomen. The baby's heart rate is recorded continuously on a tracing for about 20 minutes. The doctor is looking for accelerations of the baby's heartbeat.

If the fetus appears to be sleeping, the test may need to run longer. To get a sleeping fetus to wake up and move, you may be asked to press gently on your abdomen. Sometimes a loud sound, such as a buzzer, may be used to awaken the baby.

The results of a non-stress test are considered normal if the test is reactive—that is, if the baby's heart rate accelerated normally in response to its own movements. A non-reactive test means that the baby's heart rate did not respond normally to its own movements.

Follow-up tests are needed when a non-reactive non-stress test is obtained. This is not necessarily a cause for concern, though—normal babies occasionally have a non-reactive test.

Contraction stress test. The contraction stress test (CST) is another test used to help evaluate the condition of the fetus. It is often done when a non-stress test is non-reactive, or in some high-risk pregnancies to check whether the blood flow to the fetus is adequate.

The contraction stress test measures the baby's heart rate in response to contractions of the mother's uterus. As in the non-stress test, a belt with ultrasound transducers is used to record the fetus's heart rate in the contraction stress test. The difference is that your doctor will be looking at the heart rate during uterine contractions, rather than in response to fetal movements.

If contractions don't occur on their own during the test, they can be brought on by giving you an intravenous dose of oxytocin, or by having you stimulate your nipples, causing a natural release of oxytocin.

The recording of the baby's heart rate is watched until there are three contractions of moderate strength within a 10-minute period. The contraction stress test is said to be negative (meaning normal) if there are no decelerations (slowdowns) in the baby's heart rate in response to the contractions. A positive (meaning abnormal) test means that the baby's heart rate decreased in response to contractions. After a positive (abnormal) contraction stress test, your doctor will discuss further plans with you.

Biophysical profile. The biophysical profile is a test in which points are assigned to measurements or movements of the baby as observed during an ultrasound exam.

There are five components of the biophysical profile. Each is assigned 2 points, to yield a total of 10 possible points. The components of the test are as follows:

1. A non-stress test
2. Observation of movements of the baby's trunk
3. Observation of the baby's muscle tone (seeing the baby extend the arms or legs and then bring them back in toward the body)
4. Observation of the baby's breathing movements (although the baby isn't actually breathing inside the uterus, small amounts of fluid are moved in and out of the lungs with these movements)
5. Measurement of the amount of amniotic fluid in the sac that surrounds the baby

The total biophysical score will give your doctor an idea of the overall well-being of your baby.

Doppler Ultrasound. Doppler ultrasound is a relatively new technique in which sound waves are used to evaluate fetal blood flow. The procedure is much like an ultrasound exam. Doppler can be used to evaluate the blood flow through the fetus's umbilical artery. This technique may be used in high-risk pregnancies to determine the well-being of the fetus.

Complications

Many of the potential problems that can arise in the third trimester are best managed when they are detected early. The routine exams and tests done during late pregnancy are intended to detect the early signs of complications.

Gestational Diabetes

What causes it and who's at risk? Diabetes is a condition in which the levels of blood sugar, or glucose, are not properly regulated. It is related to a hormone called insulin, which controls glucose levels.

In one type of diabetes, the body does not produce enough insulin. This is the case in juvenile-onset diabetes, or diabetes that develops before adulthood. In another form of diabetes, the insulin that is produced is not used effectively by the body. This is the case in both diabetes that develops during pregnancy and in adult-onset diabetes (diabetes that develops during adulthood).

Diabetes that develops during pregnancy in a woman who did not have the condition before pregnancy is called gestational diabetes. Gestational diabetes is thought to result from metabolic changes brought about by the effects of hormones in pregnancy. About 1 to 5 percent of women whose glucose levels are tested during pregnancy are found to have gestational diabetes. (See page 166 for a description of how glucose testing is done.)

Women with gestational diabetes usually do not have glucose levels that are high enough to pose risks to their own health. In most cases, gestational diabetes causes no symptoms in the mother and poses no immediate threat to her health. Even so, it is an early warning sign that she has a greater risk of developing diabetes later in her life.

Although gestational diabetes is usually not a threat to the mother's health, doctors test for it because it poses some real risks for the baby. If gestational diabetes goes undetected, the baby has an increased risk of stillbirth or death as a newborn. But when the problem is properly diagnosed and managed, your baby is at no greater risk than a baby whose mother does not have diabetes.

The major risk for babies of women with gestational diabetes is macrosomia, or excessive weight at birth. Most doctors define macrosomia as a birth weight of 4,500 grams (9 pounds 14 ounces) or more. A baby as large as this may have difficulty being born. Both the likelihood of cesarean birth and the risk of birth injuries are increased when the baby is macrosomic. Keeping the glucose level of a mother who has gestational diabetes within the normal range is thought to decrease this risk.

Other problems that may develop as a result of gestational diabetes include hypoglycemia, or low blood sugar, in the baby shortly after birth. This may occur because the baby has been accustomed to receiving high levels of blood sugar across the placenta, and the supply is abruptly stopped when the umbilical cord is cut at birth.

Babies born to mothers with diabetes should have their glucose levels checked regularly after delivery. They frequently need early feeding or, occasionally, a glucose solution through an intravenous line to prevent low blood sugar.

If you have been diagnosed with gestational diabetes, you may be concerned about the possibility of your baby developing diabetes as an older child. Fortunately, there is no increased risk of juvenile-onset diabetes in babies born to mothers with gestational diabetes.

Risk factors for diabetes in pregnancy include age older than 30, a family history of adult-onset diabetes, a previous large baby, a previous stillborn baby and obesity. But nearly half of women with gestational diabetes have no risk factors. Because heredity plays a major role in the development of gestational diabetes, there is nothing a pregnant woman can do to avoid or cause it. If you have gestational diabetes, there is no need to feel guilty, or to worry about whether it was caused by something you did or didn't do. Although a balanced diet is important during your pregnancy, you cannot make yourself diabetic by gaining too much weight or by eating too much sugar.

What are the symptoms? Generally, gestational diabetes does not cause any symptoms. Subtle signs, such as fatigue or excessive thirst and urination, may sometimes occur, but many women without gestational diabetes also experience these changes late in pregnancy. Because the condition cannot be diagnosed on the basis of the mother's symptoms, glucose testing must be done to detect it.

How is it diagnosed? Gestational diabetes is detected through glucose tolerance testing. This test is generally performed at 26 to 28 weeks of pregnancy, but it may be performed earlier if your doctor feels you are at high risk for developing this condition. Because about half of women who develop diabetes during pregnancy have no risk factors for the condition, many doctors, though not all, choose to check all women for gestational diabetes, regardless of their age or risk factors. (See page 166 for more information about how glucose tolerance testing is done.)

How is it managed during pregnancy? The key to managing gestational diabetes is controlling your blood sugar level. In most cases, this can be done through a carefully planned diet, plenty of exercise and regular testing of the blood glucose level.

Once gestational diabetes is diagnosed, many doctors will obtain a set of glucose test results each week until you deliver. The set consists of testing your glucose levels in the morning before you have eaten breakfast and again two hours after you have eaten breakfast. Some doctors also include a mid-afternoon blood sugar level in the set.

To keep track of how well you are controlling your diabetes, your doctor may recommend that you use a home testing kit to check your blood glucose more often than once a week. Test strips for testing sugar in the urine are not useful for monitoring glucose levels in pregnancy because there is little correlation between the sugar levels in the blood and in the urine.

In almost all women with gestational diabetes, the condition can be controlled through diet and careful monitoring of glucose level. If, despite diet and exercise, a woman's blood glucose level remains too high, daily insulin injections may be required to lower it to a safe level. Insulin does not cross the placenta to reach the baby. Medication taken by mouth to lower the blood glucose level is not given during pregnancy.

In addition to helping you maintain a normal blood glucose level, your doctor may also advise weekly monitoring of the baby during the last weeks of pregnancy. This may be done by non-stress testing, contraction stress testing or biophysical profiles. (See page 188 for information on these tests.)

An ultrasound exam may also be done to measure the size and weight of the baby in the last weeks before your due date. This test can help your doctor decide whether a cesarean birth will be needed. She or he may also ask you to keep a "kick count," a record of how often you feel your baby moving.

Because of the higher likelihood of large babies in mothers who have diabetes, cesarean birth is more common. The need for a cesarean birth is difficult to predict before labor, however, unless the baby is very large or the mother's pelvis is very small. Most often, a cesarean procedure becomes necessary because of "failure to progress" in labor. This happens when the cervix stops dilating or the baby does not descend in the birth canal. The risk of birth injuries due to an overly large infant is also increased in pregnancies complicated by gestational diabetes.

In most women with gestational diabetes, the baby usually does not have to be delivered before term. If labor has not begun on its own by 40 to 41 weeks, it may be induced with oxytocin. Amniocentesis might be performed beforehand to determine whether the baby's lungs are mature enough for delivery.

What about the future? Gestational diabetes almost always disappears shortly after delivery. To make sure that your glucose level has returned to normal, your doctor may check it once or twice on the day after delivery. The glucose test may be repeated six weeks after delivery.

If you have had gestational diabetes in one pregnancy, your risk of it developing again in another pregnancy is increased. You are also more likely to develop "overt" diabetes (diabetes that is present all the time, not just during pregnancy) as you get older. About half of women with gestational diabetes eventually develop overt diabetes. For this reason, it is important to follow your doctor's advice concerning diet and exercise after delivery and to have your glucose level checked at least yearly. Women who develop diabetes in pregnancy can breastfeed their babies and are encouraged to do so.

Preeclampsia

What *causes it and who's at risk?* Preeclampsia is a disease characterized by high blood pressure, swelling of the face and hands and protein in the urine after the 20th week of pregnancy. It is a potentially serious condition that, if left untreated, can lead to complications or death in the mother or the baby.

Preeclampsia used to be called "toxemia," and this term is still familiar to many people. The term was used because the disease was once thought to be caused by a toxin in a pregnant woman's bloodstream. It is now known that preeclampsia is not caused by a toxin, although its true cause remains largely unknown. Because its cause is not known, there is no specific treatment for preeclampsia, nor is it known how to prevent it. The only sure way to end the preeclampsia is to deliver the baby, sometimes despite the fact that the baby may be premature.

Premature delivery may be necessary because of the serious risks posed by preeclampsia to the mother and the baby. Possible problems for the mother include liver damage, kidney damage, bleeding problems or seizures. Problems for the baby include not getting enough oxygen or nutrients from the placenta. This problem can lead to growth retardation (see page 196) or fetal distress.

Preeclampsia is a relatively common disorder, affecting 6 to 8 percent of all pregnancies. Eighty-five percent of all cases occur in the first pregnancy. Other risk factors for the development of preeclampsia include multiple pregnancy (carrying two or more fetuses), diabetes, chronic high blood pressure, kidney disease, rheumatologic disease (such as lupus) and family history. Preeclampsia is also more common in teenagers and in women older than 35.

What are the symptoms? Women who develop preeclampsia often have no symptoms at first. By the time obvious symptoms appear, the condition is often advanced. This is one important reason why your blood pressure is checked at every visit to your doctor during pregnancy.

In some women, the first sign of preeclampsia may be a sudden weight gain—more than 2 pounds in a week or 6 pounds in a month. This weight gain is due to the abnormal retention of fluids, rather than the accumulation of fat. Swelling of the face and hands, headaches, vision problems and pain in the upper abdomen may also occur.

How is it diagnosed? The diagnosis of preeclampsia begins when your blood pressure is consistently elevated over a period of time. A single high blood pressure reading does not mean you have preeclampsia.

The blood pressure readings your health care provider took during the first trimester of your pregnancy are compared with the ones taken now. Your blood pressure is considered to be elevated if the systolic pressure (the first number) has increased by 30 mm Hg or more, or if the diastolic pressure (the second number) has increased by 15 mm Hg or more, above the pressure in your first trimester. Generally, a blood pressure of 140/90 mm Hg or more is considered above the normal range.

There are various degrees of severity of preeclampsia. If the only sign you have is elevated blood pressure, your doctor may call your condition pregnancy-induced hypertension (PIH).

In addition to high blood pressure, preeclampsia is also diagnosed by detecting large amounts of protein in the urine. This is determined in one of two ways. It can be done by using a test strip that is dipped into a sample of urine.

A more accurate method is to collect all your urine over a 24-hour period and then analyze it for protein in a laboratory. Your doctor may also want to do some blood tests to see how well your liver and kidneys are functioning. Blood tests can also confirm that the number of platelets (which are necessary for blood to clot) in your blood is normal.

A syndrome called "HELLP syndrome" is a severe form of preeclampsia, distinguished from other milder forms of the condition by elevated liver enzyme values and a low blood platelet level.

How is it managed? The only "cure" for preeclampsia is delivery. Medications to treat high blood pressure in pregnancy are sometimes used, but other measures are usually preferred.

A mild case of preeclampsia may be managed at home with bed rest. How much bed rest you should have depends on your particular case. You will be asked to lie on your left or right side to allow blood to flow more freely to the placenta, and to call your doctor if any symptoms develop. Your doctor may want to see you twice a week to check your blood pressure and urine and to do blood tests, as well as to check on the status of the baby. You may also be asked to take your blood pressure on a regular basis at home.

A more severe case of preeclampsia requires a stay in the hospital. Testing of the baby's well-being, with non-stress tests, contraction stress tests or biophysical profiles, will be done on a regular basis. In addition to these tests, an ultrasound exam is often used to measure the volume of amniotic fluid. If the amount of amniotic fluid is too low, it is a sign that the blood supply to the baby has been inadequate, and delivery of the baby may be necessary.

When this occurs, the risks of early birth must be weighed against those of the less hospitable conditions inside the uterus. Before this decision is made, amniocentesis may be performed to determine whether the baby's lungs are fully mature. If the health of the mother is thought to be at significant risk, delivery may be necessary before the baby's lungs are fully mature.

Many cases of preeclampsia are mild enough, and arise close enough to the mother's due date, that they can be managed with rest and monitoring until labor starts on its own. In more severe cases, though, labor may have to be induced or a cesarean delivery performed. Magnesium sulfate is a drug that may be given intravenously to the mother with preeclampsia to increase uterine blood flow and to prevent seizures.

A pregnancy complicated by preeclampsia is rarely allowed to go beyond 40 weeks because of the increased risks to the fetus. The "ripeness" of the cervix (whether it is beginning to dilate, efface and soften) may also be a factor in determining whether labor will be induced.

What about the future? After delivery, the blood pressure usually returns to normal within several days to several weeks. Blood pressure medication may be prescribed when you are dismissed from the hospital. If blood pressure medication is necessary, its use can usually be gradually stopped a month or two after delivery. Your doctor will want to see you frequently after you go home from the hospital in order to monitor your blood pressure.

The risk that preeclampsia will recur in a subsequent pregnancy depends on how severe it was during the first pregnancy. With mild preeclampsia, the risk of recurrence is low, but it may be as high as 25 to 45 percent when preeclampsia was severe in a first pregnancy.

Problems With the Placenta

The placenta is an organ unique to pregnancy. Throughout pregnancy, it acts as a transport service between the mother and the baby. The placenta transfers oxygen and nutrients from the mother's bloodstream to the baby and carries fetal waste products in the opposite direction.

In the third trimester, the two main problems that can occur with the placenta are often signaled by the same symptom: vaginal bleeding. Any amount of bleeding in late pregnancy should be reported to your doctor immediately.

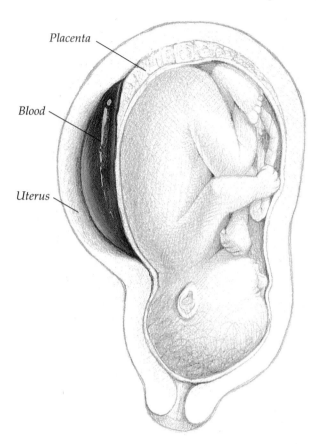

Placenta

Blood

Uterus

Placental abruption, a separa-tion of the placenta from the uterus, is a rare but serious complication. A pocket of blood can form between the placenta and the uterus. Symptoms that warrant an immediate call to your doctor include vaginal bleeding, abdominal pain, uterine ten-derness and rapid contractions.

Placental abruption. **Causes and risk factors.** Abruption, or separation, of the placenta refers to the separation of the placenta from the inner wall of the uterus before labor begins. It can decrease or interrupt the flow of oxygen-rich blood to the baby.

Placental abruption is one of the leading causes of fetal death in the third trimester. It can also cause the mother to go into shock as a result of hemorrhage or to have severe circula-tory problems. Fortunately, with close monitoring of the mother and baby and prompt delivery at signs of trouble, the outlook for both is good.

Separation of the placenta may be partial, involving only a part of the placenta, such as an edge. Or it may be complete, in which the entire placenta is separated from the inside of the uterus. Although placental abruption always causes some bleeding, the blood may not always be apparent. Sometimes the middle portion of the placenta pulls away from the uterine wall, leaving the outer margins and membranes attached. Blood can thus be trapped and concealed in a "pocket." At other times, the baby's head or another body part may be so tightly pressed against the wall of the uterus that the blood cannot make its way past.

Placental abruption occurs in about one of every 150 births. Its cause is unknown, but it appears to be more common in black women, in women who are older (especially those older than 40), in women who have had many children and in women who smoke.

By far, however, the most common condition associated with placental abruption is hypertension in pregnancy. Women who have high blood pressure during their pregnancy—whether the condition first developed while they were pregnant or was present before—are more prone to placental abruption.

The risk of abruption also seems to be higher with premature rupture of the membranes. This is a condition in which the membranes that surround the fetus break too early in pregnancy, before labor begins. Very rarely, trauma or injury to the mother may cause placental abruption.

Signs and symptoms. In the early stages of placental abruption, there may be no indication that it is happening. When symptoms do occur, the most common is bleeding from the vagina. The bleeding may be scant, heavy or somewhere in between, but the amount does not necessarily correspond to how much of the placenta has separated from the inside of the uterus. Other symptoms that may be caused by placental abruption include back or abdominal pain, uterine tenderness and rapid contractions. The uterus may feel hard and rigid.

Diagnosis. When a woman has vaginal bleeding in the third trimester, her doctor will usually try to exclude causes such as placenta previa (see below). Placental abruption is diagnosed through a process of elimination of other possible causes of the bleeding. An ultrasound exam may be done to try to detect a separated placenta, but often the condition is not detectable by this technique.

Management. When placental abruption is suspected, the steps taken depend largely on the condition of both the baby and the mother. Electronic monitoring is usually used to look at patterns of the baby's heart rate. If monitoring shows no signs that the baby is in immediate trouble, the mother may be hospitalized so that her condition can be monitored closely. This may be the chosen course if the pregnancy has not yet reached term.

Signs that the baby is in jeopardy will prompt immediate delivery. If there is severe bleeding, the mother may need blood transfusions. Cesarean delivery may be necessary, although in some situations vaginal birth may be possible.

Outlook for the future. Unfortunately, there is an increased risk (about one in 10) that placental abruption will recur in a woman's subsequent pregnancies. The good news is that, with close monitoring and prompt action at signs of danger to the baby, most of these mothers and babies get safely through birth with no long-term ill effects.

Placenta previa. **Causes and risk factors.** At term, the placenta normally is located high up near the top (fundus) of the uterus. But in some pregnancies, the placenta lies low in the uterus and may partly or completely cover the opening of the cervix. This condition, called placenta previa, poses a potential danger to mother and baby because of the risk of hemorrhage (excessive blood loss) before or during delivery.

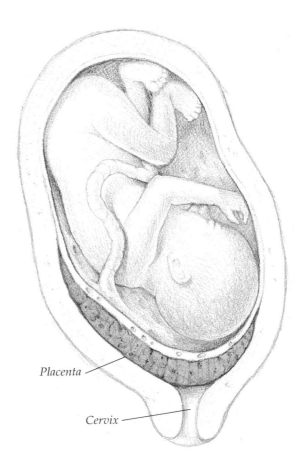

Placenta

Cervix

Painless vaginal bleeding may signal placenta previa, a partial or complete blocking of the cervix by the placenta, which normally is located near the top of the uterus. Placenta previa can lead to excessive bleeding that can harm you or your baby. Call your doctor immediately if you have any bleeding during your third trimester.

Placenta previa may take one of several forms:

1. Marginal. The edge of the placenta is at the margin of the cervical opening. As the cervix dilates during labor, more of the placenta may move upward. Vaginal delivery may be possible under certain conditions.
2. Partial. The placenta partly covers the cervical opening. Vaginal delivery is likely to result in hemorrhage as the blood vessels in the placenta rupture during labor.
3. Total. The placenta completely covers the cervical opening, making vaginal delivery impossible because of the risk of massive bleeding.

Although the placenta may lie close to the cervical opening in the second or early third trimester, it almost always migrates up toward the top of the uterus as term approaches. This is referred to as low-lying placenta.

The cause of placenta previa is not known for certain. Like placental abruption, it is more common in women who have had children before, in older women and in women who smoke. A previous cesarean birth or induced abortion also seems to increase the risk of placenta previa. And when there's a large placenta, the risk of placenta previa is increased because it is more likely for the edge of the placenta to lie near or over the cervical opening.

Signs and symptoms. The main symptom of placenta previa is painless vaginal bleeding. Most often this occurs near the end of the second trimester or the beginning of the third. The blood from placenta previa is usually bright red, and the amount may range from scant to heavy. The bleeding may stop on its own at some point after it starts, but it nearly always recurs days or weeks later.

If you notice bleeding in late pregnancy, don't assume it's harmless, even if it goes away on its own. Any bleeding in the third trimester should be reported to your doctor right away.

Diagnosis. An ultrasound exam is effective for detecting the location of the placenta. Up to 98 percent of cases of placenta previa may be detected in this way. A cervical exam, in which the entrance of the cervix is gently probed, is done only under certain circumstances when placenta previa is suspected. Because even the gentlest cervical exam can cause hemorrhage, it is done only when delivery is planned, and only when an immediate cesarean delivery can be performed.

Management. How placenta previa is managed depends on two factors: 1) whether the fetus is mature enough to be born and 2) whether there is active bleeding from the mother's vagina.

If the placenta is found to be close to, but not covering, the cervix and the woman has no bleeding, she may be allowed to rest at home—with instructions to call the doctor or hospital immediately if bleeding starts. Alternatively, bleeding that cannot be controlled will probably necessitate an immediate cesarean birth for the sake of the baby, even if the birth is preterm. Such a baby is probably better off in the hands of the skilled caregivers and the sophisticated equipment of a modern neonatal intensive care unit than inside the mother's uterus, where a bleeding placenta is no longer able to support it.

Outlook for the future. Because in most cases placenta previa can be detected accurately before the fetus is in significant danger, it no longer poses the threat to babies and their mothers that it once did. Advances in technology such as the ultrasound test and other potentially life-saving measures, however, are useless without the prompt recognition of potential problems by the pregnant woman. Bleeding in the third trimester may not necessarily lead to serious problems if it is acted on, but it should never be ignored.

Intrauterine Growth Retardation

What causes it and who's at risk? Each year in the United States, as many as 40,000 babies are born at term with a birth weight of less than 2,500 grams (less than 5½ pounds). Because of less-than-optimal conditions inside the uterus, these babies did not grow as rapidly as they should have during pregnancy, a problem known as intrauterine growth retardation (IUGR).

Advances in medicine have greatly reduced the risks for growth-retarded infants, but they are still at risk for numerous problems. These babies have low stores of body fat and glycogen (a type of carbohydrate that is readily transformed into glucose, an energy source). As a consequence, they are unable to conserve heat and may develop hypothermia. Stillbirth and fetal distress are also more common in growth-retarded fetuses. Because of their lower energy stores, these fetuses are less able to tolerate the stress of labor than an infant of normal size.

Possible causes of IUGR include problems with the placenta that prevent it from delivering enough oxygen and nutrients to the fetus. This may occur as the result of high blood pressure in the mother, but it can also occur without a known cause. Other causes of IUGR include the following:

- Cigarette smoking
- Certain infections (such as rubella, cytomegalovirus or toxoplasmosis)
- Birth defects or chromosome abnormalities
- Severe malnutrition
- Drug or alcohol use
- Juvenile diabetes
- Rheumatologic diseases
- Other chronic diseases in the mother

Women who have had a growth-retarded infant in a previous pregnancy are at an increased risk to have another undersized baby. Fortunately, careful monitoring and early intervention often can help lessen some of the dangers posed to growth-retarded infants. In some cases, growth retardation can even be reversed.

How is it diagnosed? A woman carrying a growth-retarded fetus usually has few, if any, symptoms to alert her to the problem. The careful measurements your doctor makes at each of your prenatal visits are partly intended to detect IUGR at an early stage.

This is one reason your doctor measures the fundal height of your uterus—the distance between your pubic bone and the fundus, or top, of your uterus. Between 18 and 34 weeks, this measurement in centimeters corresponds roughly to the number of weeks of pregnancy. By looking at how this measurement increases over time, the doctor may be alerted to IUGR if the size of the uterus does not seem to be increasing as it should.

Accurate dating of your pregnancy is important for making the diagnosis of IUGR. If this date is off by even one or two weeks, it may be impossible to diagnose the condition correctly. Before about 20 weeks of pregnancy, an ultrasound exam can be used to determine the gestational age as precisely as possible.

If IUGR is suspected because of low fundal height measurements, an ultrasound exam likely will be done to confirm the diagnosis. This test can be used to measure some of the physical features of the fetus. The circumference of the head and abdomen, and the ratio of one to the other, is one of the most useful of these measurements. Other measurements that may be taken include the width of the baby's head (called the biparietal diameter, or the distance between the two side bones of the skull), the length of the thigh bone (femur) and the amount of amniotic fluid.

How is it managed? First steps in the management of a woman with a growth-retarded fetus consist of reversing any factors, such as smoking, drug use or poor nutrition, that may be contributing to the problem. Sometimes the mother is admitted to the hospital for bed rest. Non-stress tests, contraction stress tests or biophysical profiles are often done to check on the baby's condition. The expectant mother may be asked to keep a daily record of the baby's movements. Ultrasound exams are generally done every two weeks to track the baby's growth and the volume of amniotic fluid.

Amniocentesis might be performed to check for chromosome abnormalities or infection, two of the causes of IUGR. (See page 75 for a description of how amniocentesis is done.) However, because it often takes about 10 days to obtain the results of amniocentesis, PUBS (percutaneous umbilical blood sampling) may be offered instead. In this procedure, ultrasound is used to guide a needle into the umbilical cord, and blood is withdrawn for analysis. (For more details on the PUBS procedure, see page 79.) Although the results are obtained more quickly with PUBS, there is a greater risk to the baby than with amniocentesis. Your doctor will discuss the pros and cons of these techniques with you if these tests are being considered.

If tests continue to show no evidence that the baby is in danger, and if the ultrasound exam shows that the baby is growing, the pregnancy may be continued until labor begins on its own. But signs that the fetus may be in danger or is not growing appropriately will prompt your doctor to consider early delivery. In weighing this decision, two questions are asked:

1. How mature is the baby?
2. How safe (or dangerous) is the uterine environment?

To answer the first question, amniocentesis may be performed to find out if the baby's lungs are fully mature. But some conditions may make it safer for the baby to be outside rather than inside the uterus, even if the baby is born early or the lungs are not mature. The expert care that can be given in a neonatal intensive care unit may be a better option for the baby than remaining inside the uterus under unfavorable conditions.

Depending on individual circumstances, birth may be accomplished by inducing labor and having the baby born vaginally or by cesarean. During labor, the baby will be monitored closely. If the fetal heart rate pattern or other tests indicate that the baby is not tolerating labor, a cesarean birth might be necessary.

Whether a growth-retarded infant is born vaginally or by cesarean, there are still risks posed to the infant's health. You may be temporarily separated from your baby soon after birth so that she or he can be watched carefully for any complications, such as low blood sugar. A growth-retarded baby may need fluid with glucose (sugar) soon after birth. This may be given by bottle or through an intravenous line. The baby's temperature will also be monitored to make sure she or he remains warm enough.

What about the future? Despite the many risks posed to the growth-retarded newborn, almost all of these babies go on to develop normally. The size of your baby at birth may not necessarily be an indication of how well she or he will grow and develop.

Most growth-retarded babies tend to catch up with their normal counterparts by 18 to 24 months. Unless there are serious birth defects, the chances are good for most of these babies to have normal intellectual and physical development in the long term.

If you have had one growth-retarded baby, you are more likely to have another baby with this problem in a future pregnancy. Good prenatal care, excellent nutrition and elimination of smoking and alcohol and drug use will increase your chances of having a healthy baby.

What causes it and who's at risk? In about 80 percent of all pregnancies, birth takes place between 38 and 42 weeks. About half of the remainder, or 10 percent, are preterm (end before 37 weeks), and the other 10 percent or so last beyond 42 weeks. These latter pregnancies—those lasting beyond the end of the 42nd week—are considered to be post-term.

Many of these pregnancies, however, may turn out not to be post-term after all. Often, a miscalculated due date is responsible for a pregnancy being considered post-term. When early ultrasound testing is used to confirm the due date, the actual frequency of post-term pregnancy turns out to be about 2 percent of all pregnancies.

The causes of post-term pregnancy are largely unknown. Heredity and hormonal factors may play a role.

Concerns in a post-term pregnancy center on the risks posed to the baby. After 41 weeks, the amount of amniotic fluid inside the uterus may decrease dramatically. This can increase the risk that the umbilical cord will become compressed during labor or delivery, interrupting the flow of oxygen to the baby.

Post-term pregnancies also increase the risk of meconium in the amniotic fluid. Meconium is the fetus's stool, and its presence means that the baby has had its first bowel movement while in the uterus. A type of pneumonia may develop if the baby inhales the meconium into the lungs while still in the uterus. For this reason, your doctor will suction the nose, mouth and back of the baby's throat as soon as the head is delivered. A pediatrician or other caregiver will then immediately pass a tube into the baby's windpipe to quickly suction out the meconium before it has a chance to reach the baby's lungs. You might not hear your baby cry until after this suctioning has been completed.

Another concern in a post-term pregnancy is macrosomia, or a baby weighing more than 4,500 grams (9 pounds 14 ounces). Such large babies may have a hard time getting safely through the birth canal during delivery. This is one of the reasons why cesarean birth is more common in post-term pregnancies. But despite the increased risks to the baby in a post-term pregnancy, most of these babies are born safely with careful management.

How is it managed? If your pregnancy progresses beyond 41 or 42 weeks, one of your doctor's first concerns will be to find out whether the due date is accurate. Going back over the findings of previous exams and tests will help her or him pin down the true length of gestation. Knowing when you first felt the baby move, when the first fetal heart sounds were heard, how well the size of the baby correlated with the date of the pregnancy, the height of the uterus at 20 weeks (normally at the level of the mother's navel) and the results of early ultrasound exams all provide measures of how far along gestation was at various points during the pregnancy.

If your doctor determines that your pregnancy is truly post-term, the approach she or he takes will depend on your individual circumstances. Tests to find out the condition of the fetus, such as non-stress tests, contraction stress tests or biophysical profiles, will yield useful information. An ultrasound exam will be used to determine how much amniotic fluid surrounds the fetus. At signs that the baby's condition may be worsening, or that the amniotic fluid volume is low, the decision will be made to deliver the baby.

In addition, the cervix may be checked weekly after 40 weeks to find out whether it is beginning to dilate. Many doctors decide to induce labor when the cervix becomes "ripe" (softened, effaced and starting to dilate) after 41 weeks.

In a woman whose cervix has not yet begun to dilate, but in whom delivery is the best course, agents can be used to ripen the cervix. These include gels containing the hormone prostaglandin or small inserts called laminaria, which are placed inside the cervix and expand as they absorb moisture.

Many doctors may adopt a wait-and-see attitude if the cervix is not dilated and there are no signs that the baby is in danger. Others feel it's best to deliver a post-term baby if labor has not begun by the end of 42 weeks, regardless of the condition of the cervix. Generally, a pregnancy will not be allowed to go beyond 43 or 44 weeks, because the risks to the baby are significantly increased after that time.

If delivery is decided on, how the baby is born—vaginally or by cesarean—will depend on many factors. A baby who is too large to pass through the mother's pelvis must be born by cesarean. A woman whose cervix is ripe and whose baby has shown no signs of problems is a candidate for vaginal delivery. The baby's heart rate, as well as contractions of the mother's uterus, will be monitored closely during a vaginal birth of a post-term infant. A cesarean birth may be necessary if there are signs that the baby is not tolerating the stress of labor.

Post-term babies may have long, thin bodies, without the whitish coating of vernix found on normal newborns. Because of the longer time they've spent in the uterus, they are frequently born with long fingernails, lots of hair and wrinkled palms and soles.

What about the future? Even with the risks of post-term pregnancy, most post-term babies come safely into the world. How to best handle your own post-term pregnancy and birth is best decided by you and your doctor, weighing the benefits and risks of the available options. Despite the risks to the baby in a post-term pregnancy, the long-term outlook for most post-term babies is excellent.

CHAPTER THIRTEEN

Expecting Twins, Triplets or More

Discovering that you and your partner are expecting more than one baby can be an overwhelming experience. Although a certain prestige and sense of being special accompany a pregnancy of multiples, most expectant parents also have fears and ambivalence about the prospect of having more than one baby. Educating yourself about the special needs and expectations associated with twin or triplet pregnancies can help you and your doctor plan a healthy pregnancy and safe births for your babies.

When the uterus contains more than one baby, doctors refer to it as a "multiple pregnancy" or "multiple gestation." Most multiple pregnancies consist of twins, although triplets and even quadruplets are becoming more frequent as a result of advances in the treatment of infertility. Twins naturally occur in about one in 100 pregnancies, triplets occur in one in 8,000 pregnancies and quadruplets occur once in every 500,000 pregnancies.

The likelihood of becoming pregnant with more than one baby increases until about age 40, after which it declines. The odds of having a multiple pregnancy also increase if you've had previous pregnancies, or if your mother had fraternal (non-identical) twins.

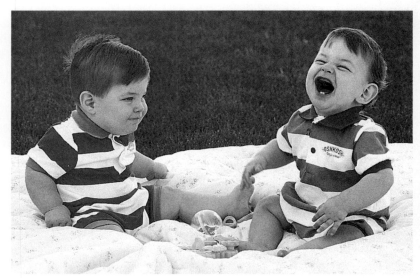

These 10-month-old fraternal twins already know what it's like to have a best friend.

The development of assisted reproductive technology and the increased use of fertility medications such as menotropins and clomiphene have artificially increased the number of pregnancies that involve more than one baby. Specialists, using newer techniques of in vitro fertilization, can harvest eggs from the mother, inseminate them with sperm from the father and implant the fertilized egg into the mother's uterus. Often three to six fertilized eggs are implanted simultaneously into the uterus. Usually one or two of the eggs survive and grow into fetuses, but occasionally three or more fetuses result.

Diagnosing Twins

Physical signs early in your pregnancy may lead your doctor to the diagnosis of twins. Your uterus may be larger than normal, or your caregiver may hear more than one fetal heartbeat during a routine prenatal exam. The results of a common blood test to check for neural tube defects may suggest twins. (See "Maternal serum alpha-fetoprotein testing," page 68.)

Your doctor may become suspicious of a twin pregnancy if you seem to be experiencing the common symptoms of pregnancy to a greater degree than is normal. In particular, morning sickness, insomnia, heartburn and fatigue may be more pronounced if you are pregnant with twins. Later in your pregnancy, you may experience more than the usual problems expectant moms might have with back pain, varicose veins, hemorrhoids and constipation.

Because of the increased space required by growing twins, you might have more discomfort in the abdomen, and you might experience shortness of breath. As your abdomen continues to increase in size, you might feel pressure on your pubic bone, which is located over the lowest part of the front of your pelvis. Sometimes health care providers prescribe special support belts to alleviate this discomfort.

In the years before the availability of ultrasound testing, twins were frequently not discovered until a woman reached the delivery room. Today, however, with increased use of prenatal ultrasound exams, more than 90 percent of twin pregnancies are diagnosed earlier in the pregnancy. During an ultrasound exam, sound waves are used to create a television-like picture of your uterus. Early diagnosis of twins enables you to better prepare for two infants. Also, your obstetrician can provide specialized care and anticipate potential problems before they occur.

If the number of fetuses is greater than three, survival of any of the babies decreases. Specialists sometimes consider reducing the number of fetuses to give at least some a chance of surviving. This technique, called selective reduction, also may be considered if one of the fetuses has a serious or potentially fatal malformation. This procedure is controversial, and it should be done only by experienced specialists who are trained in this technique, and only after a thorough discussion of the potential risks to your pregnancy and the other fetus. Couples should also thoroughly discuss their feelings before deciding for or against selective fetal reduction. It may be helpful to discuss your circumstances with your primary health care provider, social worker or religious counselor before making a decision.

Identical Versus Fraternal (Non-Identical) Twins

Of great interest to the parents of twins is the question, "Are my twins identical?" Most often the answer is "no."

Identical twins are called monozygotic twins (*mono* means "one"; *zygote* means "developing baby"). They occur when a single fertilized egg splits early in its development and forms two separate, genetically identical individuals.

The rate of identical twins is constant worldwide, at about one in 250 pregnancies, and is not influenced by race, age, family history or number of past pregnancies. Identical twins are the subject of much study and speculation about the influence of genetic and environmental factors on behavior.

Identical twins usually develop with each twin growing in its own amniotic sac, although rarely they may share a sac. When they occupy the same sac, their umbilical cords can become tangled, which can be fatal. Fortunately, only 3 percent of identical twins share a single amniotic sac.

Twins that develop from two separate eggs are twice as common as identical twins. They are called fraternal, or dizygotic, twins. There are two zygotes.

Because fraternal twins form from two separate eggs fertilized by two separate sperm, they are not genetically identical and, medically speaking, are no more closely related than are other brothers and sisters in the family. The occurrence of fraternal twins is influenced by race, age, family history, number of past pregnancies and, especially, by fertility medications.

Whether twins are identical or fraternal can sometimes be determined by examining the membranes of their placentas at the time of birth. Also, fraternal twins may have individual placentas, whereas identical twins may share the same placenta. Blood typing and sometimes genetic tests can be used to determine whether the twins are identical or fraternal.

The origins of twins

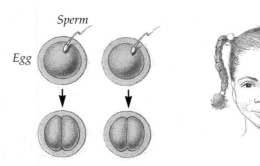
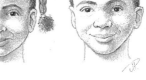

Fraternal twins, the most common kind, occur when two eggs are fertilized by two different sperm, leading to two individuals who are no more closely related than other brothers or sisters in the family.

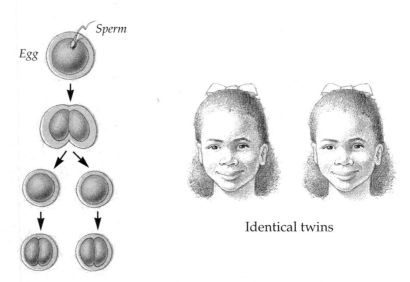

Identical twins occur when a single fertilized egg, for reasons that are unclear, splits and develops into two fetuses that are genetically identical.

Preparing for Twins

Early diagnosis of a twin or triplet pregnancy allows you and your family time to adjust to the prospect of having more than one infant in your home. Along with obtaining two (or three) sets of cribs, car seats, clothes and the like, you will need time to prepare emotionally for the arrival of more than one baby. The idea may seem overwhelming at first, but most parents of multiples seem to rally their energy and resources and rise to the occasion. Parents of twins report that they find ways to do things more efficiently around the house, and they emphasize the need to work as a team to accomplish daily tasks.

If you are pregnant with twins and work outside your home, your doctor may recommend limitation of your work hours or activities. Sometimes obstetricians recommend stopping work in the third trimester and resting in bed at home to help prevent preterm labor.

Help Is Available

You may find that talking to other parents of multiples may be especially helpful in planning for and raising twins. Some communities have special resources available for parents of multiples, including child care or financial planning information.

You may also want to contact the National Organization of Mothers of Twins Clubs, Inc. (NOMOTC) at P.O. Box 23188, Albuquerque, NM 87192-1188. This organization has local chapters in many cities and offers literature and a quarterly newsletter that contains useful advice on caring for twins. For a free copy of "Your Twins and You" and the phone number of the local chapter nearest you, phone NOMOTC at (505) 275-0955.

Eat Nutritious Foods

Your nutritional needs are especially important if you are pregnant with twins or triplets. Registered dietitians recommend increasing your daily calorie intake by 300 calories and making sure that you have adequate protein and calcium in your diet. If you are pregnant with twins, your weight gain should probably be about 35 to 45 pounds above your pre-pregnancy weight. You may notice that it is difficult to eat meals of normal size because of your enlarging abdomen. Some women find that eating six or more small meals throughout the day is more tolerable. (For more information on nutrition during pregnancy, see page 85.)

Vitamin supplements. Because a lowered blood cell count (anemia) is more common in multiple gestations, you'll need to take a prenatal vitamin that contains an adequate amount of iron. Doctors generally recommend a daily vitamin with 60 to 100 milligrams of elemental iron for women with multiple gestations.

Labor and Birth

You may look forward to the labor and birth of your babies with a mixture of excitement and apprehension. These are common emotions among women expecting single babies and are perhaps intensified in those expecting more than one baby.

Approximately half of all women who have twins have cesarean births. However, twins can often be born vaginally depending on their positions, estimated weights and gestational age. Each multiple pregnancy is unique, so discuss with your doctor the options to be considered, then decide together what's best for you.

M ost single babies are born at about 40 weeks of gestation, but twins generally arrive earlier. The average gestational age of twins is 37 weeks. Triplets frequently arrive by 35 weeks. The differences are due, in part, to preterm labor. Approximately 10 to 15 percent of twins are born by 28 weeks.

Twins Often Arrive Early

With recent advances in the care of premature babies and the availability of specialized nurseries (newborn intensive care units) they often need, premature babies are now able to survive and grow as healthy babies. Specifically, medications have been developed to enhance the maturity of the lungs of premature babies and help prevent respiratory distress syndrome, which accounts for much of the increased risk of prematurity. (For more on prematurity, see page 353.)

Your health care provider will monitor the growth and development of your twins closely. Twins appear to grow at the same rate as single babies until about 30 or 32 weeks of gestation. At this point, they seem to grow more slowly. The slowdown could be due to crowded quarters within the uterus, decreased nutritional supply of the placentas or abnormal placement of the placentas. A decrease in the rate of growth occurs even earlier in triplet pregnancies.

Feeding Your Babies

Breastfeeding twins or triplets may seem more challenging, but it's definitely possible. It does require special effort. Breast milk is the best nutrition available for infants, and many pediatricians recommend breastfeeding for at least the first six months after birth.

If you choose to breastfeed your infants, you may want to contact a lactation consultant or breastfeeding support organization in your area for advice about breastfeeding more than one infant.

Many moms of twins opt for a combination of breastfeeding and bottle feeding with formula, or bottle feeding with breast milk expressed with the help of a breast pump. In any case, you may initially want to keep a record of feeding times for each baby and approximate quantities or nursing duration to ensure that each baby is receiving adequate amounts of nutrition.

You may wonder if you'll have enough milk to provide for more than one infant. The amount of breast milk that you produce will increase in response to the demands of more than one hungry baby. You'll need to drink plenty of fluids, usually eight to 12 cups daily, and continue to take your prenatal vitamins for as long as you breastfeed. In addition, you will need to increase your calorie intake by about 400 to 500 calories a day to keep up with the demands on your body.

If you choose to bottle feed with infant formula, a helpful partner can be indispensable. Sharing the feeding responsibilities for the babies can allow you to get some rest and give your partner an opportunity to help with the babies. No matter which feeding method you choose, remember that even identical twins have distinct personalities and may have different feeding patterns. (For more information on infant feeding, see page 471.)

Risks and Complications

Carrying more than one fetus presents a challenge to both the parents and doctor. Obstetricians view twin and triplet pregnancies as high-risk pregnancies. Some of the complications of pregnancy, such as preterm labor, preeclampsia and birth defects, are more likely to occur in multiple pregnancies.

If you're expecting twins, your doctor will likely recommend more frequent prenatal visits and ultrasound exams, and may consult a perinatologist, a specialist who has had extra training and experience in dealing with complicated pregnancies. Some of the risks and potential complications of multiple pregnancies are described below.

Preterm Labor

Preterm labor occurs in about 97 percent of twin pregnancies. Preterm labor means uterine contractions that cause dilation of the cervix before 37 weeks of gestation. These contractions might or might not be uncomfortable.

Left untreated, preterm labor can result in birth of one or both babies, sometimes so premature that they are unable to survive. Occasional contractions of the uterus occur normally during the second and third trimesters, but they can be difficult to distinguish from preterm labor. If you begin having contractions that seem to become more frequent or are becoming stronger, alert your doctor immediately.

Depending on the gestational age of your babies, preterm labor can sometimes be managed with oral medications and bed rest at home. Your doctor might recommend admission to the hospital and intravenous medications, or he or she might recommend transfer to a medical center where more specialized care is available.

Medications called tocolytics sometimes can stop the contractions and halt preterm labor. (For more on preterm labor, bed rest and tocolytic medications, see pages 247 to 256.)

Preeclampsia

Another relatively common condition that occurs in multiple (as well as single-baby) pregnancies is preeclampsia. This type of high blood pressure generally occurs in the latter half of pregnancy, but it tends to occur earlier and more frequently in mothers who are carrying more than one baby.

In addition to high blood pressure, common early signs of preeclampsia include rapid weight gain, swelling (edema) of the hands and feet and protein in the urine.

Your doctor will need to watch closely for signs of these conditions, so plan on more frequent prenatal visits toward the end of your pregnancy. Health care providers sometimes treat preeclampsia with bed rest at home or in the hospital and sometimes with medications. If your condition worsens, your obstetrician may recommend inducing your labor early to avoid complications associated with preeclampsia.

Decreased growth of the fetuses within the uterus is often called intrauterine growth retardation (IUGR). This process can affect both twins to the same degree, or it may affect one twin more than the other. The difference in rate of growth is significant if the estimated fetal weights differ by more than 15 to 25 percent. Certain behaviors of the mother, including cigarette smoking and drug use, can contribute to the development of IUGR. If your pregnancy is affected by IUGR, your physician may use frequent ultrasound measurements to estimate how well your babies are growing. (For more on IUGR, see page 196.)

Intrauterine Growth Retardation

Another cause of impaired growth is a condition called twin-twin transfusion syndrome. This occurs only in identical twins, when there can be a blood vessel in the placenta connecting the circulatory systems of both babies.

If the twins share the blood supply unequally, one twin may grow larger and develop an overload of blood in its circulatory system, and the twin lacking blood grows more slowly and becomes anemic. Doctors can sometimes diagnose the condition prenatally, using ultrasound evaluations. If the degree of growth variation is great, or if it appears that the health of one of the twins may be in jeopardy, early delivery of the twins may be necessary.

Twin-Twin Transfusion Syndrome

Twins have about twice the risk of having a birth defect as single babies. Identical twins are affected more frequently than fraternal twins. Although chromosome abnormalities, such as Down syndrome, occur at the same rate per fetus in twin pregnancies as in single pregnancies, other developmental anomalies, such as clubfoot, are more common in twins. Abnormalities in the development of the digestive, cardiac and neurologic systems tend to occur more frequently in twins.

Birth Defects

Conjoined twins. "Siamese twins" is a term you may have heard about because the famous twins Chang and Eng Bunker of Thailand (formerly Siam) were displayed in the traveling circus of P.T. Barnum. The medical term for this uncommon condition is "conjoined twins."

Conjoined twins are the rarest type of twins, occurring once in every 60,000 pregnancies. They result when there is incomplete division of identical twins. These twins are most frequently joined at the chest, although some are joined at the pelvis or the head. Sometimes internal organs such as the liver or heart are shared. The success of the surgical separation of conjoined twins depends on where they are joined and the extent of organ sharing.

Vanishing twin syndrome. When an ultrasound exam is used in the first trimester of pregnancy, twins can be diagnosed as early as six or seven weeks past your last menstrual period. However, succeeding exams sometimes reveal that one of the twins has died and virtually disappeared. This phenomenon is sometimes called the vanishing twin syndrome. Up to one-half of all pregnancies that begin as twins result in a single fetus that is carried to term.

The cause of vanishing twin syndrome is unclear, but there might have been a problem with the genetic material or early development of the fetus. If you are diagnosed as having vanishing twin syndrome, it may leave you feeling frustrated and grief-stricken. You might also feel guilty, perhaps believing you must have done something wrong to cause this event. However, vanishing twin syndrome appears to be a spontaneous event, and there is no evidence to indicate that the mother has any control of this outcome.

The Good News

Fortunately, more than 90 percent of established twin pregnancies result in healthy babies, and early diagnosis and preventive care often eliminate or minimize complications. Once your babies are born, the joys and challenges of parenting twins begin. Some parents of twins say that twins are double trouble, and others proclaim them to be twice as nice. To one degree or the other, both sentiments are probably true. Either way, there's little doubt that the arrival of twins spells extra work and responsibility for both partners.

Here's a summary of helpful hints from other parents as you and your partner begin the journey of parenting twins or other multiples:

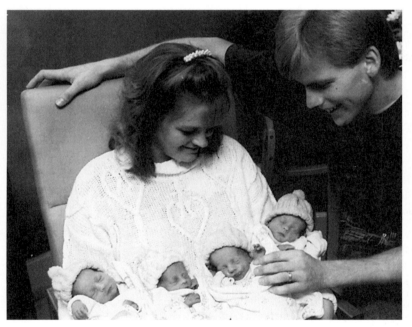

With months of anxious waiting and the challenges of lengthy bed rest, careful medical monitoring and birth behind them, these parents pause to enjoy a quiet moment together with their healthy quadruplets.

- Enlist the support of other parents of multiples. You'll have much to learn, and experienced parents are often excellent sources of practical information.

- Don't hesitate to ask for help from family and friends.

- Give serious consideration to breast-feeding. Breast milk is the most nutritious food for your babies. It's also more convenient and saves on the cost of formula. Some mothers also supplement breastfeeding with formula feeding.

- Consider using a diaper service. You may find it's cheaper than using disposable diapers. Request a discount for multiple babies.

- Relax your standards for household cleanliness.

- Unplug the phone during rest periods or when your babies are napping, or buy an answering machine.

- Don't neglect your personal need for rest, relaxation and good nutrition.

- Establish a weekly "date" with your partner, and make it happen.

- Be realistic about what you can accomplish in a given amount of time.

- Find ways to maintain a positive attitude and sense of humor. Multiples and the chaos they inevitably create are a wonderful source of delight.

CHAPTER FOURTEEN

Pregnancy and Ongoing Medical Conditions

A pregnancy without any complications or risk factors can be stressful, both physically and emotionally. When a woman has or develops a chronic medical condition or illness, the anxiety can intensify considerably. How might pregnancy affect your condition or treatment plans? Will your pregnancy develop problems, or might the baby be harmed? Will labor or birth be different because of your medical condition?

In this chapter, we have chosen to review some of the concerns that might be termed chronic medical conditions (those that existed before your pregnancy). The conditions we selected to focus on are those that are more frequently encountered by pregnant women and those that women commonly ask their doctors about. We have tried to concentrate on the key points that relate to pregnancy and have not attempted to give a comprehensive description of each condition. Women who are not yet pregnant but whose pregnancy will pose special needs should also turn to page 4, where we discuss preconception care.

We intend this chapter to provide background information for conditions that you might read about or have been previously diagnosed to have. This material is not intended to suggest the diagnosis of these conditions. Don't assume that you have a condition described here (no matter how closely the comments seem to apply to your circumstances) until your condition has been diagnosed by your doctor.

Similarly, this chapter is not meant to review these conditions in depth or discuss the management of non-pregnant women. Readers interested in additional information should consult their doctor or check a general medical reference, such as *Mayo Clinic Family Health Book*.

For variety and ease of reading, we'll occasionally use the familiar word "baby" in this chapter as a substitute for the more technically correct terms "embryo" and "fetus."

Medical conditions caused by pregnancy

Being pregnant can lead to health conditions requiring special care. For example, if you've never had high blood pressure but during pregnancy your pressure is discovered to be elevated, you may have a condition called pregnancy-induced hypertension. Pregnancy-related conditions are discussed in other chapters, especially those describing the trimesters—Chapters 10 (page 129), 11 (page 153) and 12 (page 175).

This chapter does not address such conditions. Instead, it offers a quick reference to chronic (ongoing) health conditions that may pose a special challenge and thus require special care. This chapter also discusses infections that can affect pregnancy.

Where to find it

Can I Still Have a Baby?

A common anxiety of women with chronic health conditions is that they might be told by their physician, "You should not become pregnant." This dramatic admonition highlights the dilemma faced by parents, especially mothers: What is the proper balance of responsibility we have for ourselves and for our children? Is my desire to have healthy children more important than my health, even if having children poses a risk to my life?

Today, it is exceedingly rare that a woman would be advised not to become pregnant, and it is also rare that pregnancy poses a life-threatening risk. Now, women with chronic medical conditions are likely to be given the good news that pregnancy can be managed safely for both mother and baby. The questions from women today are rarely, "Can I have a baby?" or "Would pregnancy be life-threatening to me?" Prospective mothers are more likely to ask, "How can we work to have the healthiest pregnancy for both my baby and me despite my medical condition?" or "Can I still plan to breastfeed my baby?"

Conditions that can still prompt the recommendation to avoid pregnancy include:

- Human immunodeficiency virus (HIV) infection or AIDS
- Heart failure severe enough to cause symptoms even when resting
- Cyanotic congenital heart disease, pulmonary hypertension, severe aortic stenosis or Marfan syndrome
- Cancer requiring radiation therapy or intensive chemotherapy

A Team Approach

Women with medical problems generally require a team approach to pregnancy. You likely will work with several specialists who consult together to find the best ways to keep you and your baby safe and healthy. During your pregnancy or at birth your doctor might recommend that you see some of the following:

- One or more doctors who specialize in your medical condition
- An obstetrician experienced in managing women with your medical condition
- A perinatologist—an obstetrician who specializes in high-risk pregnancies including medical problems in pregnant women, complications of pregnancy and problems occurring in an unborn baby
- A neonatologist—a pediatrician trained in the care of high-risk newborns and newborns with medical problems
- An anesthesiologist with experience in pain management and anesthesia for high-risk pregnancies
- A genetic counselor, if your condition raises issues of specialized testing or assessment of risks that your condition might pose to your children
- A dietitian, who will assess your particular nutritional needs and advise you on healthful eating during your pregnancy

Many medical conditions require extensive testing and monitoring of both you and the baby, which can make pregnancy more expensive. At home, you might need to plan for extra help. You may need extra support from your partner, family and friends. You also might choose to seek counsel from a social worker or from other women who have had pregnancies under similar circumstances; many cities have support groups for women with various conditions.

Dealing With Risks

Some chronic medical conditions may become worse as a result of pregnancy, and others may improve. The testing and treatment of many medical conditions may require modification during pregnancy and breastfeeding. A consultation with your doctor is the best way to learn of any increased risks, how management of your condition might change during this important time and ways to optimize your prospects for a successful and healthy pregnancy.

Sometimes when a woman has an underlying medical problem, the risks for the baby increase. Some conditions create a greater chance of birth defects unless your disease is carefully managed both before and during pregnancy. Many medications cross the placenta to the baby; a few can adversely affect the baby's development. If genetic counseling is suggested, it is often best to receive this before you become pregnant so you have time to use this information in planning your pregnancy.

You will likely have more frequent checkups than women without complications. If you are prepared for the possibility of more extensive tests and procedures, you may be less anxious when they are scheduled. Some conditions may result in longer hospital stays at birth, and some might require hospitalization during the pregnancy.

Family concerns. If the added stress of pregnancy requires changes in your activity level, your family routines are bound to be affected. Other family members may need to assume more responsibility for home management. Children might have to adjust to someone else helping to care for them. Your partner may worry more about your health, yet also might be resentful of an increased workload and the stress on the family's finances.

Talk openly with your family. Use this special pregnancy to improve communication skills such as sharing feelings and negotiating. Everyone will have to make adjustments, but the long-term result can be greater independence and coping skills for everyone.

Asking for or accepting help from friends and extended family members isn't always easy. Unless you offer them some guidance, they may be uncertain about what to do. Suggest specific ways they can help you: cook a meal, vacuum, do the laundry, take the kids to the park. Or make a list and let them choose items from it. You can participate by planning meals, then letting others shop and cook.

Adjust your expectations of yourself. Give yourself permission to take things slower than you normally do. This pace will prevent not only exhaustion but also much frustration. Some tasks may be done with less than your usual thoroughness. Other projects may have to be postponed until a time when you're better able to complete them; take care of yourself first.

Infections

Acquired Immunodeficiency Syndrome (AIDS)

Acquired immunodeficiency syndrome (AIDS) is caused by a virus called the human immunodeficiency virus (HIV). When HIV infects a person, the virus lies dormant for several years, during which time the person shows few or no symptoms of disease. It is not until the virus becomes active and weakens the body's immune system that the condition becomes known as AIDS. After diagnosis, 50 percent of people with AIDS die within one year, 85 percent within five years.

People with AIDS require emotional support, but the stigma still associated with the virus often isolates them from the contact they need. The emotional toll can be overwhelming for a woman who knows she has a fatal disease, who is pregnant with a baby who may also become infected and whose friends might avoid her when she needs them most.

How will my pregnancy affect my condition? Pregnancy doesn't seem to directly affect the course of HIV infection or AIDS.

How will my condition affect my pregnancy? HIV infection or AIDS doesn't directly influence pregnancy, although debilitation or infection in advanced AIDS would pose additional risks for the mother in late pregnancy, during labor and at birth. Certain antibiotics (for example, tetracycline) used to treat infections in people with AIDS may pose risks to the fetus.

The biggest risk in pregnancy for women with HIV or AIDS is the risk of passing the infection to their baby. About 20 to 50 percent of HIV-positive women pass the virus to their babies; the risk increases to 60 to 70 percent when women have active AIDS. Cesarean birth does not lower the risk. Currently, studies are being conducted which attempt to lower the risk to the fetus when the mother has HIV infection. When the virus is passed on to the baby, though, the effects are catastrophic. Babies who show active signs of AIDS during their first year of life often die before their second birthday, and none live more than a few years.

Can I breastfeed? If an HIV-positive woman has a baby who is born HIV-negative, breastfeeding is not recommended because the virus has been found in breast milk. Other possible feeding options, such as using sterilized breast milk or using breast milk from another woman known to be HIV-negative, are not common in the United States today.

Recommendations for women with this condition

- Talk to your doctor about avoiding pregnancy by the most effective contraceptive or sterilization methods.
- Talk to your doctor about responsible ways to avoid passing on HIV infection to others.
- If you are HIV-positive and are now pregnant, you need to have a serious discussion with your doctor about decisions you will need to make. You may also need to meet with infectious disease specialists and social workers.

Herpes

The herpes simplex virus comes in two forms. Herpes simplex type 1 (HSV-1) causes "cold sores" around the mouth or nose, but it may also involve the genital area. Herpes simplex type 2 (HSV-2) causes painful genital blisters that rupture and become open sores. Both are transmitted through direct contact. Herpes is not transmitted in hot tubs or swimming pools.

The initial infection, called the primary infection, tends to last longer and is more severe than later episodes. After the initial outbreak, the virus remains dormant in the infected areas, periodically reactivating. Reactivation may start with tingling, itching or pain before the sores are visible. Reactivation, or nonprimary herpes, lasts about 10 days. Herpes is contagious whenever sores are present.

How will my pregnancy affect my condition? Infections during pregnancy tend to last longer and are more severe.

How will my condition affect my pregnancy? The baby is usually safe while in your uterus, but can become infected with the virus on the way through the birth canal if you have genital herpes or can become infected by direct contact if you have oral herpes. The most serious risk for a newborn exists when the mother has a primary infection just before labor. Reactivation, or non-primary infection, poses less risk to the baby. Herpes infection can be life-threatening for a newborn. Many babies who develop herpes as a newborn can have serious complications, despite prompt and intensive treatment.

Preventing newborn herpes infection is difficult because in more than half of the newborn infections the mother has no signs suggesting herpes during labor or birth.

If you have a history of genital herpes and no sores are evident within the week before birth, the baby can usually be born vaginally with little risk of infection. If sores are present, cesarean birth will lessen the risk of newborn infection.

If you have a cold sore when you give birth, you should wash your hands frequently, keep them away from your face and wear a mask over your mouth until the cold sore heals.

Can I breastfeed? Breastfeeding is permissible, provided that the baby is protected against direct contact with the herpes sores. Hand washing before handling the baby is important. If you have mouth sores, wear a surgical-type face mask and don't kiss the baby until the sores have healed.

Recommendations for women with this condition

- Be sure that your doctor knows that you have a history of herpes.
- Ask for recommendations to minimize the risk of passing herpes to your partner or your baby.
- Always notify your physician if you sense that symptoms of herpes are developing during your pregnancy, especially if you are in labor.

Fifth Disease

Fifth disease is an infection common among school-age children. Sometimes it's called "slapped cheeks"; physicians refer to it as parvovirus infection (erythema infectiosum).

In winter and spring months, localized outbreaks occur, and large numbers of cases are reported. Most children with fifth disease feel well but occasionally may have a mild fever or mild gastrointestinal upset. The most noticeable part of the infection is the bright red rash prominent on the cheeks, giving an impression of "slapped cheeks." A lacy red rash may also be seen on the legs, trunk and neck.

In adults, the most prominent symptom is soreness of the joints, lasting days to weeks. In people with sickle cell anemia, or other types of hemolytic anemia, fifth disease can lead to severe anemia. Infection can also occur without symptoms in either children or adults.

Fifth disease is contagious for up to a week before the onset of the facial rash. Therefore, it's impractical to isolate someone with suspected fifth disease in an attempt to prevent its spread. The duration between exposure and development of the disease ranges from four to 14 days. There are no current or soon-to-be-expected vaccines available to prevent fifth disease. Antiviral therapy has not yet been of proven benefit in women with fifth disease.

How will my pregnancy affect my condition? Fifth disease seems to be unaffected by pregnancy.

How will my condition affect my pregnancy? Between one-quarter and one-half of pregnant women are susceptible to develop fifth disease. In pregnant women with proven fifth disease, about one-third of their fetuses also show evidence of infection. More than 80 percent of women who experience fifth disease during pregnancy will have a normal, healthy baby. The severity of illness in the mother does not predict the likely severity of illness in the fetus. Fifth disease does not seem to increase the risk for birth defects.

However, fifth disease in the mother can sometimes cause severe, even fatal, anemia in the fetus. The anemia can cause congestive heart failure in the fetus, manifested by a severe form of edema termed hydrops fetalis. The anemia, heart failure and edema can resolve over several weeks. It might be possible, in selected cases, to try to correct the anemia or heart failure. Possible approaches include fetal blood transfusion or administration of medication to the mother, which then passes through the placenta to the fetus.

If a woman is known to have been exposed to fifth disease or is suspected to have fifth disease, blood tests can be helpful in determining immunity or confirming infection. The blood tests commonly used are tests for antibodies that are specific for fifth disease. If the blood tests show that a woman has immunity from fifth disease, there is no cause for concern. If the tests confirm evidence of recent fifth disease, additional testing might be done for up to six weeks to watch for possible signs of anemia and congestive heart failure in the fetus.

Can I breastfeed? Fifth disease infection is unlikely to affect plans for breastfeeding.

Recommendation for women with this condition

- If you suspect you've been exposed to fifth disease, contact your physician to decide whether further investigation is needed.

Lyme Disease

Lyme disease is a tick-borne infection that can cause various symptoms, including chronic arthritis. The infection begins with a tick bite that leads to a rash, typically persisting over three to four weeks if not treated. This may be accompanied by a flu-like illness, irregular heartbeat, meningitis or other neurological symptoms in the first few months. Later, arthritis may develop in one to a few joints. Experience with Lyme disease during pregnancy is limited.

The diagnosis is clinical, often with confirmation by laboratory tests, usually of a blood sample. Treatment usually requires antibiotic medication.

How will my pregnancy affect my condition? The course of Lyme disease doesn't seem to be affected by pregnancy.

How will my condition affect my pregnancy? Most pregnancies seem to be unaffected by Lyme disease. There are case reports of fetal infection, prematurity, intrauterine growth retardation and birth defects in babies born to mothers with documented Lyme disease. It is still unclear to what degree Lyme disease might affect the risk of these problems occurring in pregnancy, but studies so far are reassuring.

Some antibiotics used for the treatment of Lyme disease should be avoided during pregnancy. Decisions for a particular pregnancy depend on the gestational age of the fetus and the severity of illness in the mother.

Can I breastfeed? Lyme disease is unlikely to alter plans for breastfeeding.

Recommendation for women with this condition

- Notify your physician if a rash develops after a tick bite.

Rubella

Rubella is a viral infection that causes fever, swollen lymph nodes, arthritis and a rash. The importance of rubella is its potential for causing serious birth defects if it develops in the mother during the early months of pregnancy. At least 75 percent of women in the childbearing years have immunity from rubella, from either vaccination or naturally occurring illness during childhood. After vaccination, long-term, possibly life-long, immunity develops in at least 95 percent of individuals. There is no effective treatment of rubella.

How will my pregnancy affect my condition? Rubella itself is not likely to be affected by pregnancy.

How will my condition affect my pregnancy? If a pregnant woman is known to be exposed to someone with a definite diagnosis of rubella, a blood test can determine whether she has protective antibodies. If she already has antibodies against rubella, the disease is unlikely to develop, and the fetus is unlikely to be at increased risk.

There appears to be no risk to pregnant women from contact with children or adults who have recently received rubella vaccination.

Recommendations for care of a pregnant woman who has rubella depend greatly on the timing of the infection during the pregnancy. Decisions regarding testing for possible birth defects (or whether to proceed with the pregnancy) are individualized for each person.

Can I breastfeed? Decisions regarding breastfeeding are unlikely to be affected by rubella concerns. There appears to be no harm to the baby if a woman receives rubella vaccine while breastfeeding.

Recommendations for women with this condition

- Check whether you received rubella vaccination as a child (usually given at 12 to 15 months of age).
- If you suspect you may have been exposed to rubella and you are uncertain of rubella immunity, contact your physician.

Cytomegalovirus (CMV)

CMV is a common viral infection that causes serious illness only in the fetus or in women who have suppressed immune systems. Almost all CMV illness in adults is unrecognized. Symptoms of CMV are sometimes similar to those of infectious mononucleosis: fever, aching muscles, chills and abnormal results of liver function tests. CMV can also recur, but recurrences are also likely to go unnoticed. After CMV infection, the virus can be intermittently shed in saliva, breast milk or urine for years.

How will my pregnancy affect my condition? CMV appears to be unaffected by pregnancy.

How will my condition affect my pregnancy? Between 15 and 50 percent of pregnant women are susceptible to CMV. In approximately 2 percent of pregnant women, CMV develops during pregnancy.

CMV is the most common cause of congenital infection. CMV can be found in 0.5 to 2.5 percent of all newborns; these newborn infections are also usually inapparent. Yet CMV can have serious effects. One in 400 to 4,000 children may have neurological problems such as deafness as a result.

Severe manifestations of congenital CMV apparent during pregnancy or at birth are rare, approximately 1 in 10,000 births. They include severe liver dysfunction, seizures, blindness, deafness and pneumonia. The risk of severe congenital CMV is highest if the mother's infection first occurs in early pregnancy.

There is currently no effective treatment for congenital CMV. Until an effective treatment is available, it is not practical or even possible to screen all pregnant women for CMV infection. Currently, development of an effective vaccine does not appear feasible.

Can I breastfeed? Breastfeeding is unlikely to be altered by CMV. It is possible for a newborn to acquire CMV infection through milk from a mother with a known history of CMV. However, most of these newborns have a higher likelihood of acquiring CMV from their mother during pregnancy or at birth, so breast milk is not regarded as a significant risk.

Recommendation for women with this condition

- Talk with your physician if you have concerns about CMV infection or CMV risk factors.

Syphilis

Syphilis is an infection caused by an organism called a spirochete, specifically termed *Treponema pallidum*. It is less common than other sexually transmitted diseases such as gonorrhea or chlamydia. The initial stage of syphilis is usually the development of painless sores on the genitals 10 days to 6 weeks after exposure. Later, skin rashes and additional serious medical problems can occur. If recognized, syphilis is easily treated with antibiotics. The diagnosis is usually made by a blood test and confirmed by further tests, possibly including a lumbar puncture. All pregnant women receiving prenatal care are given a blood test for syphilis early in pregnancy.

How will my pregnancy affect my condition? The course of syphilis seems to be unaffected by pregnancy.

How will my condition affect my pregnancy? Syphilis easily passes to the fetus and is likely to cause serious fetal infection, often fatal. In untreated infants, problems develop in multiple organs: eyes, ears, liver, bone marrow, bones, skin and heart. Prematurity and stillbirth are more common in babies born to mothers with syphilis. If promptly detected and treated, these problems can be averted.

Can I breastfeed? Plans for breastfeeding should be unaffected in women treated for syphilis.

Recommendations for women with this condition

- Promptly notify your physician if you suspect that you or your partner might have had sexual contact with someone known to have syphilis.
- Remember that your partner also needs testing and treatment, otherwise the infection is likely to recur.
- Be sure to follow through on recommended testing and treatment for syphilis.

Gonorrhea

Gonorrhea is a common sexually transmitted disease; about 3 million cases occur in the United States each year. Gonorrhea occurs in both men and women, but because women often have no symptoms for weeks to months, they are more likely to be carriers. Often the only suggestion that a woman may have gonorrhea is that her male partner is diagnosed with the infection.

Gonorrhea is usually easily treated when recognized. Late diagnosis can result in scarring of the fallopian tubes and ovaries, sometimes causing infertility.

How will my pregnancy affect my condition? Pregnancy is unlikely to affect the course of gonorrhea.

How will my condition affect my pregnancy? Gonorrhea in the mother can cause fever, skin sores and infection in her joints and bloodstream. The fetus is usually unaffected, but if a baby is born while the mother has gonorrhea, a severe eye infection can result. Because gonorrhea may have no symptoms yet poses a serious risk to a newborn's eyes, all newborns are given medication at birth to prevent development of this eye infection.

Can I breastfeed? Plans for breastfeeding are not likely to be affected by gonorrhea or its treatment.

Recommendations for women with this condition

- Promptly notify your physician if you suspect that you or your partner might have had sexual contact with someone known to have gonorrhea.
- Remember that your partner also needs testing and treatment, otherwise the infection may recur.
- Be sure to follow through on recommended testing and treatment for gonorrhea.

Chlamydia

Chlamydia is an organism transmitted by sexual contact. Chlamydial conjunctivitis, an eye infection, can be caused by contact with secretions containing *Chlamydia*. Worldwide, chlamydial eye infection is one of the leading causes of blindness in children. Chlamydia can also lead to the development of pneumonia in young infants.

Like gonorrhea, chlamydial infection is more likely to cause symptoms in men than in women.

How will my pregnancy affect my condition? Chlamydia is unlikely to be affected by pregnancy.

How will my condition affect my pregnancy? It appears that pregnancy is essentially unaffected by chlamydia. Previous concerns that chlamydia increases the risk of preterm labor or intrauterine growth retardation don't seem to be borne out in recent studies.

However, as noted above, chlamydia can cause conjunctivitis and pneumonia in young infants.

Can I breastfeed? Plans for breastfeeding are unlikely to be affected by chlamydia.

Recommendations for women with this condition

- Promptly notify your physician if you suspect that you or your partner might have had sexual contact with someone known to have chlamydia.
- Follow recommendations from your physician for testing and treatment for chlamydia.
- Remember that your partner also needs testing and treatment, otherwise the infection is likely to recur.

Toxoplasmosis ("Toxo")

Toxoplasmosis is a disease due to contact with the parasite *Toxoplasma gondii*. It is contracted by eating infected, undercooked meat. It can also be acquired from contact with feces from cats infected with toxoplasmosis. It can be passed from an infected pregnant woman to her baby. In most cases, toxoplasmosis causes no symptoms or only fatigue and muscle pain similar to what you experience with the flu.

Prevention is important in minimizing the risks of acquiring toxoplasmosis. Pregnant women should avoid eating raw or undercooked meat, emptying cat litter boxes or handling garden soil contaminated with cat feces.

How will my pregnancy affect my condition? Toxoplasmosis is unlikely to be affected by pregnancy.

How will my condition affect my pregnancy? Severe infection in the mother can lead to miscarriage, intrauterine growth retardation and preterm labor. Risks of toxoplasmosis affecting the fetus are highest if the initial infection in the mother occurs in the first trimester. Your doctor will recommend plans for diagnosis and possible treatment depending on your specific circumstances.

Can I breastfeed? Plans for breastfeeding are unlikely to be affected by toxoplasmosis.

Recommendation for women with this condition

- Discuss with your physician any concerns you have regarding toxoplasmosis.

Trichomonas

Trichomonas is a common cause of vaginal infections. It is caused by a parasite and often results in intense itching, a vaginal discharge with a bad odor and discomfort while urinating.

How will my pregnancy affect my condition? Trichomonas is unlikely to be affected by pregnancy.

How will my condition affect my pregnancy? A pregnancy affected by trichomonas may be at somewhat higher risk of preterm rupture of membranes and a baby with low birth weight. Metronidazole is a medication commonly used for treatment of trichomonas. Your doctor will decide whether to recommend its use during pregnancy.

Can I breastfeed? Treatment of trichomonas might require temporary interruption of breastfeeding if metronidazole is used.

Recommendation for women with this condition

- Notify your doctor if you suspect you have a vaginal infection or have previously had trichomonas vaginitis.

Hepatitis B

Hepatitis B is a liver infection caused by the hepatitis B virus. It is transmitted through sexual contact in much the same manner as the AIDS virus. If a pregnant woman has this virus, it can be transmitted through the placenta to her fetus. Also, her newborn baby can become infected by the virus from contact with her. The hepatitis B virus can cause liver failure and increases the risk of developing liver cancer. Most pregnant women receiving prenatal care in the United States are now screened for the possible presence of hepatitis B infection.

Vaccination against hepatitis B is now available and is commonly recommended as part of the series of immunizations given during infancy. The hepatitis B vaccination may be given to newborns, even premature babies.

How will my pregnancy affect my condition? The course of hepatitis B is usually not altered by pregnancy.

How will my condition affect my pregnancy? Women with hepatitis B infection have a higher risk of having a premature birth. The greatest concern for pregnancies complicated by hepatitis B is the risk of infecting the baby. If you have evidence of hepatitis B infection, your newborn will be given an injection of antibodies against the virus after birth.

Can I breastfeed? Because the hepatitis B virus may be found in breast milk, you should discuss with your doctor the specific risk to your baby.

Recommendations for women with this condition

- Follow the recommendations of your physician regarding testing for hepatitis B infection.
- If your work exposes you to contact with human blood, ask your doctor whether you should receive a vaccination to prevent hepatitis B.

Chickenpox (Varicella)

Most adults had chickenpox as a child; therefore, most pregnant women are immune.

How will my pregnancy affect my condition? Chickenpox is unlikely to be affected by pregnancy. Occasionally, pneumonia develops in adults with chickenpox; this appears to occur more commonly in pregnancy.

How will my condition affect my pregnancy? Chickenpox early in pregnancy can result in birth defects. The greatest threat to the baby, though, is when the mother has chickenpox the week before birth. Then it can cause serious, even life-threatening, infection in the newborn. An injection of anti-chickenpox antibodies (varicella-zoster immune globulin, VZIG) may be protective.

Can I breastfeed? Plans for breastfeeding are unlikely to be affected by chickenpox. Breastfeeding does not provide sufficient antibodies to prevent a newborn from developing chickenpox if exposed.

Recommendation for women with this condition

- Notify your physician if you have never had chickenpox and you suspect that you've recently been exposed.

Measles (Rubeola)

Measles is a very contagious viral disease that used to occur in large epidemics. Fortunately, childhood vaccination programs have resulted in low numbers of cases in the United States today.

How will my pregnancy affect my condition? Measles is unlikely to be affected by pregnancy.

How will my condition affect my pregnancy? Pregnancy is unlikely to be affected by measles infection, except for an increased risk of preterm births. Usually measles vaccinations are not given during pregnancy.

Babies born with measles or premature babies who develop measles have a high risk of serious illness. Measles occurring in older infants tends to be less severe.

Can I breastfeed? Plans for breastfeeding are unlikely to be affected by measles.

Recommendations for women with this condition

- Alert your physician if you have never been immunized against measles (usually measles vaccination is part of the "MMR," the measles, mumps, rubella vaccination given at 12 to 15 months).
- Notify your physician if you suspect that you have been exposed to someone who has measles.

Genital Warts

Genital warts are caused by the papillomavirus. They are tiny pink or red swellings in the genital area that are often painful and grow quickly. Usually you get them from direct contact with someone who has them. Genital warts can grow on the vaginal lips, inside the vagina, on the cervix or around the anus.

Ten to 20 percent of the sexually active American population carries this highly infectious disease, and the incidence increases each year. Pregnant women are particularly susceptible.

How will my pregnancy affect my condition? Genital warts can be inactive for decades. Pregnancy often activates the condition or increases the number and size of the warts.

How will my condition affect my pregnancy? A large collection of genital warts can bleed profusely or even obstruct the birth canal. Cautery, laser and surgical removal are the most common treatments used during pregnancy. If an outbreak is extensive, removal may require repeated treatments because the warts grow back quickly. Your doctor most likely will treat your genital warts only if they bleed, obstruct the birth canal or bother you unduly. Keeping them clean and dry will minimize discomfort. Genital warts generally clear up on their own within six weeks after birth.

Even in the inactive phase, the papillomavirus can be transmitted to the baby. Perhaps one in 1,000 babies born to mothers with genital warts will eventually develop juvenile laryngeal respiratory papillomatosis, in which warts grow on the vocal cords.

Can I breastfeed? Genital warts would be unlikely to affect plans for breast-feeding.

Recommendation for women with this condition

- Notify your physician if you suspect that genital warts have developed in you or your partner.

Blood Disorders

Blood Group Incompatibilities

The blood of mother and baby remain separate during pregnancy and birth. However, some of your baby's blood can escape into your bloodstream during childbirth and, less commonly, during pregnancy. If you and your child have similar blood types, this is not a problem. However, if your blood types are incompatible, you can develop antibodies that could create problems during subsequent pregnancies.

Blood groups are determined by whether a person has certain protein - molecules on the surface of the blood cells. Everyone's blood belongs to one of four major groups: A, B, AB or O. There are many additional types of minor blood groups, often with unusual names such as Kell, Lutheran and Duffy. Some major and minor blood group incompatibilities can result in increased risks to the fetus or newborn.

How will my pregnancy affect my condition? If the baby inherits the mother's exact blood type, there is no problem. But if the baby's blood type doesn't match the mother's and any fetal blood escapes into the mother's circulation, the mother may develop antibodies against that blood type. This usually occurs during birth or if there is any bleeding in the third trimester.

How will my condition affect my pregnancy? A blood group incompatibility generally does not cause significant complications for the mother. However, if she needs a blood transfusion, arranging for compatible blood could be more complex or time-consuming.

If a woman has developed antibodies from a previous blood group incompatibility, the fetal red blood cells are broken down at a rate faster than normal, sometimes causing serious fetal anemia. After birth, a baby affected by blood group incompatibility may have anemia and could develop significant jaundice requiring medical treatment.

Can I breastfeed? Occasionally, nursing is temporarily interrupted in newborns with severe jaundice, but generally a blood group incompatibility does not affect nursing.

Recommendations for women with this condition

- If you know that you have a blood group incompatibility, tell your doctor so that the blood bank in the hospital where you plan to give birth can be alerted.
- Ask your doctor whether your blood group incompatibility poses a risk of anemia and jaundice for the baby. If the risk is high, be prepared for additional testing to monitor the degree of fetal anemia.

Rh (Rhesus) Incompatibility

Rh is the term for a group of proteins (antigens) found on the surface of blood cells. Eighty-five percent of whites are Rh-positive, which means they have the Rh antigen present on their red blood cells. Among blacks, the percentage is slightly higher, and virtually all American Indians and Asians are Rh-positive. About 15 percent of whites and 7 percent of blacks are Rh-negative, which means their blood cells lack the Rh antigen. When you become pregnant, your doctor will test your blood's Rh factor. If you are Rh-negative and the father is Rh-positive, your children could be either Rh-negative or Rh-positive. When the mother is Rh-negative and the fetus is Rh-positive, this condition is termed Rh incompatibility.

How will my pregnancy affect my condition? If you are Rh-negative and your fetus is Rh-positive, you might develop antibodies that will cause loss of fetal red blood cells (fetal anemia). In most cases, your first pregnancy is not at risk even if the fetus is Rh-positive, because you have not yet developed the Rh antibodies. If you become pregnant with another Rh-positive baby, your antibodies can pass through the placenta and cause fetal anemia. The risk increases with each Rh-incompatible pregnancy.

How will my condition affect my pregnancy? If you are Rh-negative, blood tests will likely be done to determine whether you have Rh antibodies. Your doctor will determine whether it might be beneficial for you to receive Rh immune globulin (RhIg) during or after any of your pregnancies. Rh injections are used to prevent the development of high levels of antibodies that could lead to fetal anemia.

Further testing may also be recommended to assess whether the fetus has developed anemia. These tests may include amniocentesis (see page 75). In selected circumstances, early birth of the baby or even giving the fetus a blood transfusion while still in the uterus may be recommended. After birth, the baby may have anemia and may develop significant jaundice requiring medical treatment.

Can I breastfeed? Rh incompatibility is unlikely to affect plans for breast-feeding. Occasionally, nursing is temporarily interrupted in newborns with severe jaundice.

Recommendations for women with this condition

- Notify your physician as soon as you think you might be pregnant.
- Ask your doctor whether your Rh blood group incompatibility poses a risk of anemia and jaundice for the baby. If the risk is high, be prepared for additional testing to monitor the degree of fetal anemia.

Sickle Cell Anemia

Sickle cell anemia is an inherited, chronic anemia caused by a tendency of red blood cells to assume an abnormal crescent, or sickle, shape. It occurs almost exclusively in black populations.

Until about 20 years ago, pregnancy was not considered safe for women with sickle cell anemia. Good outcomes are possible today, but these women should be followed by a team of medical specialists, which will likely include an obstetrician, a perinatologist experienced in care of women with sickle cell anemia, a hematologist and a neonatologist.

How will my pregnancy affect my condition? Sickle cell crises can be caused by infections that occur more frequently in pregnancy, such as urinary tract infection, pneumonia and uterine infection.

How will my condition affect my pregnancy? Pregnant women with sickle cell anemia have a higher risk of pregnancy-induced hypertension. Women with sickle cell anemia may also have previously existing lung and kidney disease as well as sickle cell crises that might require additional management. Sometimes it is difficult to distinguish painful conditions arising in pregnancy (such as ectopic pregnancy, preterm labor or placental abruption) from sickle cell crises. Fever and increased white blood cell counts occur with infection and also during sickle cell crisis.

It is important to monitor pregnant women for complications of sickle cell anemia, such as seizures, congestive heart failure and severe anemia. During the final two months of pregnancy, the anemia is likely to be most severe, possibly requiring blood transfusions.

If cesarean birth or other obstetrical intervention is needed, decisions regarding anesthesia will likely favor use of epidural rather than general anesthesia.

Monitoring the health of the fetus is important during sickle cell crises. Intrauterine growth of the fetus may be impaired in women with sickle cell disease.

Can I breastfeed? Sickle cell anemia should not affect plans for breastfeeding.

Recommendations for women with this condition

- Seek a team of specialists experienced in managing pregnancies in women with sickle cell anemia.
- Work closely with your physicians to determine the causes and best management of concerns that arise during your pregnancy.
- If you are pregnant in the fall or winter, ask your physician whether you should receive influenza vaccine.

Immune Thrombocytopenic Purpura (ITP)

ITP is a condition that results in an abnormally low number of platelets in the body. Platelets are an important means for stopping bleeding from cuts or bruises. Extremely low platelet levels can result in bleeding after minor injury.

How will my pregnancy affect my condition? Pregnancy itself doesn't affect the course or severity of ITP. However, some pregnancy-related conditions such as preeclampsia or HELLP syndrome (see page 193) can result in lowered platelet counts.

How will my condition affect my pregnancy? Women with very low platelet counts will have various tests to determine the cause. If it is determined to be ITP, treatment options include prednisone or similar medications, intravenous medication known as immunoglobulin and, rarely, an operation to remove the spleen.

ITP can sometimes decrease the platelet counts in the fetus. The fetal platelet count can't be predicted by the mother's platelet count or even by the length of time she's had a low platelet level. Near the time of birth or during labor, tests might be done to determine the fetal platelet count. If it is extremely low, cesarean birth may be advised to lessen risks of bleeding for the baby. Also, the use of forceps or vacuum extraction might be avoided.

If the mother's platelet count is very low, it is less likely that spinal or epidural anesthesia would be offered during labor and birth. If cesarean birth is necessary, sometimes platelet transfusions are given.

Can I breastfeed? ITP is unlikely to alter plans for breastfeeding.

Recommendation for women with this condition

- Unless specifically recommended by your physician, do not use aspirin or ibuprofen because these medicines inhibit platelet function. Acetaminophen is safe.

Cancer

One in 1,000 pregnancies is complicated by cancer. There is no evidence that there is an increased cancer risk during pregnancy or that pregnancy directly affects the course of cancer. If cancer is discovered after you already are pregnant, you might have to make the difficult decision about whether to continue the pregnancy. This will depend on the type of cancer, how advanced it is, what the best treatment would be and how far along your pregnancy is. During the first trimester, you might be advised to terminate the pregnancy and begin immediate treatment for the cancer. If you are further along, it sometimes is possible to put off treatment until after the baby is born. You and your doctors will work together to make a decision.

Treatment

Cancer treatments are individualized for each person. Pregnancy adds a complication, because what is best for you is not necessarily good for the baby. A balance must be struck between your therapy and the baby's safety.

Chemotherapy. This is the most dangerous during the first trimester because it has a risk of inducing birth defects. Therefore, you should avoid becoming pregnant while you are undergoing treatment with these powerful medications.

If cancer is diagnosed when you already are pregnant, chemotherapy during the second and third trimesters may lower your baby's birth weight, but the degree of risk for other complications varies according to the medications used.

If you are still having chemotherapy at the time of the baby's birth, breast-feeding is not recommended. There is no evidence that chemotherapy will cause chromosome damage to future babies.

Radiation therapy. This might or might not affect the baby, depending on the strength of exposure, the location of the radiation site and the gestational age of the baby. Radiation applied to your head and neck, for instance, can be relatively safe, but radiation applied to your chest or abdominal area is almost certain to affect the baby. Effects of large-dose radiation exposure on the baby range from organ abnormalities and mental retardation as a result of early exposure to fetal growth retardation as a result of late exposure. The most vulnerable period is between eight and 15 weeks gestational age. If X-ray studies are necessary for diagnosis, magnetic resonance imaging (MRI) can often be substituted.

Surgery. This is usually possible while you are pregnant. Most pregnancies will even tolerate removal of the ovaries, should that be necessary, as long as supplemental progesterone is given. Surgery does not seem to increase the risk of preterm labor, but inflammation or infection in the abdomen after surgery can.

Breast Cancer

How will my pregnancy affect my condition? One of the greatest hazards of breast cancer is late diagnosis. Because the breasts undergo normal hormonal changes during pregnancy, the signs of developing cancer can be missed so that the disease might be advanced before it is discovered. The chance of the cancer spreading also is increased. Therefore, it is especially important to continue regular breast self-exams all the way through your pregnancy.

If you have been diagnosed with breast cancer, it is not advisable to become pregnant until you have completed treatment. If breast cancer is discovered while you already are pregnant, your prognosis is the same as that for non-pregnant women. Advanced disease, though, must be treated promptly, exposing the fetus to possible risk from radiation or chemotherapy.

If you've had breast cancer in the past, you are not necessarily discouraged from becoming pregnant. The greatest risk for recurrence, though, is during the first two or three years after treatment. It's advisable to wait until this period has passed and to consult with your doctor first.

Pregnancy does not lessen your chances of a disease cure unless it prevents diagnosis or interferes with treatment. Radiation, for example, is not generally used because it might affect the baby when directed near the uterus. Depending on the extent of the disease, surgery and chemotherapy may be recommended.

How will my condition affect my pregnancy? Pregnancy would not be directly affected by breast cancer. However, decisions about cancer treatment may involve the question of whether to continue the pregnancy because of serious risks to the fetus.

Can I breastfeed? Once the baby is born, breastfeeding seems to be safe as long as you are not receiving chemotherapy.

Recommendation for women with this condition

- Seek a team of specialists experienced in managing pregnancies in women with breast cancer.

Cervical Cancer

Cervical cancer often progresses through its early stages without producing any symptoms. In fact, it is usually discovered when a routine Pap smear shows abnormal cells. Then your doctor might suggest a biopsy, which involves using an instrument (colposcope) equipped with a magnifying lens and a light to examine your cervix and remove a tiny piece of tissue to be evaluated by a pathologist. The biopsy is minor surgery, for which you might or might not need a local anesthetic. During pregnancy, it is done in a way that reduces the risk of bleeding or miscarriage.

The treatment for cervical cancer depends on the extent of the problem. In a non-pregnant woman, if a biopsy shows cancerous or pre-cancerous cells that are just on the surface of the cervix, they can be destroyed by laser surgery, freezing or cauterization. For a deeper invasion, the doctor can remove a cone-shaped slice of tissue in an attempt to remove all the cancerous tissue. If the borders of the cone contain cancer cells, a second conization can be done or the uterus can be irradiated or removed.

How will my pregnancy affect my condition? Pregnancy does not directly affect the prognosis for cervical cancer, but it does complicate treatment. Sometimes treatment is kept to a minimum until after the baby is born. If the baby is close to maturity, it might be possible to wait until after the birth before beginning treatment.

How will my condition affect my pregnancy? The more tissue that must be removed from the cervix, the greater the risk of bleeding, membrane rupture or miscarriage. For an invasive cancer that involves a large part of the cervix and extends into the uterus, prompt surgery or radiation might be necessary, even though this could mean the loss of the baby.

Can I breastfeed? The safety of breastfeeding depends largely on the specific medications planned for use in treatment.

Recommendation for women with this condition

- Seek a team of specialists experienced in managing pregnancies in women with cervical cancer.

Ovarian Cancer

Ovarian cancer seldom causes symptoms in the early stages; as a result, it is one of the leading causes of death from cancer in American women. Nevertheless, the incidence during pregnancy is low because ovarian cancer is more common among older women. When a tumor is discovered during pregnancy, it is usually in the early stages.

How will my pregnancy affect my condition? Pregnancy does not seem to affect the disease. Treatment is the same as that for non-pregnant women and requires surgery to remove the diseased ovary.

How will my condition affect my pregnancy? If the cancer is advanced, the other ovary might also have to be removed, as well as the uterus, but, if possible, this procedure will be delayed until the baby can be born.

Can I breastfeed? The safety of breastfeeding depends largely on the specific medications planned for use in treatment.

Recommendation for women with this condition

- Seek a team of specialists experienced in managing pregnancies in women with ovarian cancer.

Malignant Melanoma

Malignant melanoma, a form of skin cancer, is more common in pregnancy than either breast or ovarian cancer. A key factor in prognosis is the size of the lesion. Prompt investigation of new or abnormal-appearing moles is important for improving outcome.

How will my pregnancy affect my condition? Survival in malignant melanoma depends on the location and size of the lesion. Pregnancy does not appear to influence the progress of the disease.

How will my condition affect my pregnancy? Because the treatment of malignant melanoma is primarily surgical, operation on the region affected by the lesion will likely be recommended. It is possible, though uncommon, for malignant melanoma to metastasize to the placenta or the fetus.

Can I breastfeed? Plans for breastfeeding will be affected primarily by the overall health of the mother and chemotherapy, if any is used.

Recommendation for women with this condition

- Seek a team of specialists experienced in managing pregnancies in women with malignant melanoma.

Most cases of lymphoma during pregnancy are Hodgkin's lymphoma. The typical symptom is enlargement of lymph nodes.

Lymphoma

How will my pregnancy affect my condition? Pregnancy doesn't appear to directly affect the course of lymphoma.

How will my condition affect my pregnancy? Therapy for lymphoma must be individualized, but it often involves surgery followed by chemotherapy or radiation. Treatment decisions for pregnant women depend on the stage of disease as well as circumstances of the pregnancy.

Can I breastfeed? Breastfeeding plans will depend on the specific recommendations for treatment of the lymphoma.

Recommendation for women with this condition

- Seek a team of specialists experienced in managing pregnancies in women with lymphoma.

Arthritis

Rheumatoid arthritis is a condition causing chronic inflammation of the joints. It usually doesn't begin until women are in their 30s to 40s.

Rheumatoid Arthritis

How will my pregnancy affect my condition? About three-fourths of women with rheumatoid arthritis improve during pregnancy, but almost all will have their symptoms return after pregnancy.

How will my condition affect my pregnancy? Pregnancy itself seems to be unaffected by rheumatoid arthritis, but medications used in treatment may require adjustment. Aspirin is helpful and widely used in the treatment of rheumatoid arthritis. However, aspirin can cause bleeding or other problems in the fetus. Therefore, during pregnancy, prednisone or similar anti-inflammatory medications might be recommended instead.

Can I breastfeed? Aspirin can be used by breastfeeding women, but the dose used might be lower and the baby might require monitoring for aspirin effects.

Recommendations for women with this condition

- Work closely with your doctor to monitor your symptoms and medication use.

- Don't adjust your medications except on the recommendation of your physician.

Lupus

Lupus (systemic lupus erythematosus) is a condition resulting in chronic inflammation of many organ systems, especially skin, joints and kidneys. It commonly results in a characteristic rash and arthritis of varying severity. Other, more serious problems can arise, such as kidney failure or seizures.

How will my pregnancy affect my condition? Women who have lupus often experience a worsening of their symptoms during pregnancy. If lupus symptoms have been quiet for more than six months, the condition will worsen in about one-third of women. If lupus is active at the beginning of pregnancy, there is a much higher risk of worsening during pregnancy. Fortunately, the deterioration during pregnancy improves after birth in 90 percent of affected women.

How will my condition affect my pregnancy? Pregnant women with lupus must be observed closely for worsening of their condition. In addition, there is a higher risk of high blood pressure or preeclampsia developing, especially in women whose lupus has affected their kidneys. Women with active lupus also have a higher risk of miscarriage.

During pregnancy in women with lupus, the fetus may not grow as well as expected. Poor fetal growth is called intrauterine growth retardation (see page 196). The fetus might also develop an unusually low heart rate, termed fetal heart block. Both of these conditions can be identified through monitoring during the pregnancy. In addition, an unusual rash sometimes develops in the newborn or in the first two months.

Medications used by the mother for improvement of lupus may require adjustment during pregnancy. Aspirin-like medications (NSAIDs—nonsteroidal anti-inflammatory drugs) may either be reduced in dosage or switched to prednisone or similar medications.

Can I breastfeed? For most women with lupus, plans for breastfeeding are not likely to be affected.

Recommendations for women with this condition

- Work closely with your physician to monitor the severity of your lupus during pregnancy.
- Be prepared for worsening of your lupus during pregnancy; anticipate a possible need to decrease your activity.
- Be prepared for additional testing and possible hospitalization(s) during your pregnancy.
- Be prepared for close observation of your baby, during and after pregnancy.

Metabolic Conditions

Maternal PKU

Phenylketonuria, or PKU, is an inherited abnormality in the metabolism of the amino acid phenylalanine. In untreated persons, levels of phenylalanine can increase enough to cause brain injury. Careful dietary restriction of phenylalanine can prevent or minimize brain injury.

How will my pregnancy affect my condition? The dietary restrictions of phenylketonuria can be more difficult to manage during pregnancy.

How will my condition affect my pregnancy? Close regulation of phenylalanine levels, beginning before conception, is crucial for the health of the baby. With careful control it is possible that the infant can be unaffected by the mother's PKU. However, if maternal levels of phenylalanine are not well regulated, the infant is likely to have mild to severe mental retardation. Additional abnormalities possible in affected infants include an abnormally small head and congenital heart disease.

Can I breastfeed? Decisions regarding breastfeeding should be discussed with your physician. Whether it's safe to breastfeed may be determined by results of newborn screening for PKU in your infant.

Recommendations for women with this condition

- Discuss plans for management of your PKU before pregnancy if possible.
- Notify your physician if you think you may be pregnant.
- Seek a team of specialists experienced in managing pregnancies in women with PKU.

Endocrine Disorders

Diabetes

A key fuel for our bodies is glucose. Insulin is a hormone produced by the pancreas to enable glucose to move from the bloodstream into the muscles and fat. Your body needs to produce just the right amount of insulin to deal with the amount of glucose in the bloodstream at any one time. Diabetes is a condition in which there is an insufficiency of insulin produced to meet the body's needs. This alters the normal balance of glucose and insulin.

Hormones produced by the placenta decrease the normal utilization of insulin (insulin resistance); the pancreas compensates by increasing the amount of insulin it produces. These changes affect the normal control of blood glucose. It is important to monitor pregnant women for the potential development of a diabetic condition.

Until recently, women with diabetes were commonly advised not to become pregnant. The effects of diabetes on pregnancy used to be devastating, for both mother and baby; in fact, diabetes used to be the most common cause of stillbirth. Miscarriage, heart defects, spina bifida and brain deformity were additional possible complications. Such dramatic progress has been made in the management of diabetes during pregnancy that now fetal death is a rarity. This is one of the great success stories of obstetrics in the past 20 years.

During pregnancy, there are two diabetic conditions to consider: overt diabetes mellitus and gestational diabetes. Diabetes mellitus (type I diabetes) is a condition, usually diagnosed in late childhood, that requires insulin injections for control of blood glucose. Gestational diabetes is a condition unique to pregnancy in which altered control of glucose becomes evident during pregnancy. Gestational diabetes is often managed by careful attention to diet, but it might also require insulin injections. (For more information on gestational diabetes, see page 189.)

Both diabetes mellitus and gestational diabetes require medical management that is complex and often necessitates a team of medical specialists, including obstetricians, endocrinologists, ophthalmologists and neonatologists. Proper management of your diabetes requires the detailed knowledge of your unique health history.

In this section, we provide an overview of important aspects of diabetes mellitus and pregnancy.

Diabetes Mellitus (Type I Diabetes)

How will my pregnancy affect my condition? Insulin requirements tend to increase during pregnancy because hormones from the placenta impair the normal response to insulin (insulin resistance). Some women require two to three times their usual dose of insulin during pregnancy. Many women also require multiple daily doses for optimal control. Adjustments in insulin dosing might be needed weekly. The risk of ketoacidosis is higher. The diet changes of pregnancy pose a further challenge.

Diabetes complications such as retinopathy (eye abnormalities due to diabetes) can worsen during pregnancy. This worsening seems to be related to control of diabetes and blood pressure rather than to pregnancy itself. Retinopathy can require intensive treatment before, during and after pregnancy. Repeated examinations by an ophthalmologist experienced in the management of diabetic retinopathy are important to minimize complications with vision.

Women with diabetic nephropathy (kidney problems related to diabetes) need careful monitoring during pregnancy. Potential problems include hypertension and deterioration in kidney function. Complications for the fetus include greater risk of birth defects and intrauterine growth retardation. Women with diabetic nephropathy may need to deliver early if risks in the pregnancy outweigh risks to the baby from premature birth.

How will my condition affect my pregnancy? Normal glucose control

at the time of conception appears to be important. If diabetes is not in good control at the time of conception, the fetus has a higher risk of congenital birth defects.

Insulin doesn't cross the placenta, but glucose does. If your glucose level becomes high, the baby will receive a higher-than-normal glucose load. The baby must then produce extra insulin to metabolize this extra glucose. The glucose is stored as fat and accounts for the large size (macrosomia) of some babies born to mothers with diabetes.

Diabetes produces premature aging of the blood vessels of the uterus and placenta, causing a three times greater-than-normal risk of stillbirth. Because of this and a tendency for large babies, doctors sometimes induce labor three or four weeks early. Early birth poses another risk, though, because babies of women who have diabetes are particularly susceptible to respiratory distress syndrome and jaundice. The decision of whether to allow you to continue the pregnancy to full term or to induce labor is not an easy one; if possible, tests are done to make sure the baby's lungs are mature.

Can I breastfeed? Breastfeeding will be unaffected because insulin does not enter breast milk. However, your insulin needs will decrease because you utilize more of your glucose to produce milk.

Newborns of mothers with diabetes may have low blood glucose levels during the first hours and days after birth. These infants may initially have difficulty with feeding, and they sometimes require intravenous glucose or tube feedings.

Recommendations for women with this condition

- Even if you are experienced with and educated about diabetes, look on pregnancy as a new challenge in managing your diabetes—it is important to work closely with your medical team for the well-being of you and your baby.
- Work carefully for tight control of your diabetes, beginning before conception if possible.
- Avoid ketoacidosis.
- Work closely with your registered dietitian for best control of blood glucose levels.
- Exercise during and after pregnancy.

Hyperthyroidism

Hyperthyroidism occurs when the thyroid produces too much thyroid hormone. An enlarged thyroid and other symptoms suggest the condition, which is confirmed by laboratory tests. The most common condition causing hyperthyroidism during pregnancy is Graves' disease. It can be difficult to diagnose and treat, so your doctor might ask a specialist in endocrinology to assist.

How will my pregnancy affect my condition? Hyperthyroidism sometimes worsens during the first trimester but it can also improve during the second half of pregnancy.

Hyperthyroidism develops in some women after birth. Excessive fatigue, nervousness and heat intolerance can be signs of hyperthyroidism. Sometimes these symptoms are mistaken for postpartum blues.

How will my condition affect my pregnancy? Most pregnancies in women with hyperthyroidism proceed normally. There is a higher risk of preterm birth, intrauterine growth retardation and high maternal blood pressure if hyperthyroidism is difficult to control.

Can I breastfeed? Administration of radioactive iodine for treatment of hyperthyroidism must be avoided in pregnancy or during breastfeeding. Some medications used to treat hyperthyroidism could affect the infant's thyroid status; therefore, careful dosing is important. Two commonly used medications, propylthiouracil and methimazole, can safely be used, but dosages may require adjustment.

Recommendations for women with this condition

- Don't adjust your medications without recommendation from your physician.
- If you have a history of hyperthyroidism, notify your physician if the symptoms of hyperthyroidism seem to be returning.

Hypothyroidism (Myxedema)

An underactive thyroid occurs in about one in 200 pregnancies. Because the activity of the thyroid gland is normally altered during pregnancy, hypothyroidism can be more difficult to diagnose in a pregnant woman.

How will my pregnancy affect my condition? The course of hypothyroidism appears to be minimally affected by pregnancy. Doses of the thyroid medication thyroxine may need to be increased during pregnancy. Certain tests such as thyroid scanning must be avoided during pregnancy.

How will my condition affect my pregnancy? Women with hypothyroidism may have impaired fertility. There is a higher likelihood of high blood pressure late in pregnancy, placental abruption (see page 194) and intrauterine growth retardation (see page 196).

Can I breastfeed? Breastfeeding is not affected by hypothyroidism. It must be interrupted, however, if thyroid scanning is needed.

Recommendations for women with this condition

- If you are (or might be) pregnant, or if you are breastfeeding, notify your physician before having thyroid scanning.
- Don't adjust your medication without a recommendation from your physician.

Migraine Headaches

Migraine is a common type of headache in women in the childbearing years. Most women with migraine report that their migraines are influenced by their menstrual cycle. The headaches usually occur just before or during menstruation.

How will my pregnancy affect my condition? Migraine headaches may worsen during the first trimester, then they often improve during the second. Avoid factors that seem to cause migraines for you. Your physician may recommend changes or avoidance of some medications used for treatment of migraine, specifically aspirin, propranolol and ergotamine-containing medications.

How will my condition affect my pregnancy? Pregnancy itself should be unaffected by migraines.

Can I breastfeed? Aspirin can be used by a breastfeeding woman, but the doses used might be lowered and the baby might require monitoring for aspirin effects. Propranolol can probably be safely used by a nursing mother. The doses and possible effects in the baby should be discussed with your physician.

Ergotamine-containing medications should not be used by nursing mothers.

Recommendations for women with this condition

- Discuss plans for management of migraine with your physician.
- Don't adjust medications without checking with your physician.
- If your migraine is not improving despite your usual treatment, check with your physician.

Gastrointestinal Conditions

Inflammatory Bowel Disease

Crohn's disease (regional ileitis) and ulcerative colitis are two conditions characterized by chronic inflammation of the intestine, especially the colon (large intestine). Other parts of the body are occasionally involved by the inflammatory process, especially the eyes, joints, skin and liver. The inflammation from these conditions causes recurrent episodes of fever, diarrhea, rectal bleeding and abdominal pain. Because other medical conditions can cause the same symptoms, various tests may be necessary to establish the diagnosis. These conditions can begin during pregnancy, but the diagnosis is more likely to be made before pregnancy.

How will my pregnancy affect my condition? Most women with inactive Crohn's disease before pregnancy will continue to have inactive disease during pregnancy. For those with active disease, it is likely to remain active or even worsen during pregnancy.

In ulcerative colitis, approximately one-third of women who become pregnant while their colitis is in remission will experience a flare-up. If the colitis is active when they become pregnant, about half of the time it is likely to remain active or even worsen. A flare-up of ulcerative colitis is most likely during the first three months of pregnancy.

For most women with either Crohn's disease or ulcerative colitis, treatment is unlikely to be significantly affected by pregnancy. Medications commonly used for treatment of inflammatory bowel disease (prednisone and sulfasalazine) do not harm the fetus. In general, potential concern for effects on the fetus is likely to be outweighed by benefit to both the mother and the baby by improvement in the mother's condition.

Immunosuppressive medications such as azathioprine and 6-mercaptopurine are used in selected circumstances for inflammatory bowel disease. Because these medications might cause harm to the fetus, women who require them must discuss with their physician the risks and possible benefits as well as options for management of their pregnancies.

If an operation becomes necessary during pregnancy, this can probably be done safely, but extra precautions may be necessary to minimize risk to the fetus. The degree of possible risk depends on the mother's condition, the type of operation required and the gestational age of the fetus.

Diagnostic tests such as sigmoidoscopy, rectal biopsy or gastroscopy can be safely performed during pregnancy. Even a limited exam with a flexible colonoscope is possible if needed for management of inflammatory bowel disease. However, diagnostic X-rays are usually postponed until after birth.

How will my condition affect my pregnancy? Problems with pregnancy are no more likely to occur in women with inflammatory bowel disease than in others. There may be a higher risk of premature birth in women with active Crohn's disease.

Can I breastfeed? It is likely that you can continue taking your usual medications and safely breastfeed, but check with your physician first regarding specific medications and dosages you are taking.

Recommendations for women with this condition

- Discuss plans for pregnancy with your physician before pregnancy, if possible.
- Work closely with your physician for management of your symptoms during pregnancy.

Gallstones

The gallbladder is a pear-shaped sac about 3 to 4 inches long and an inch in diameter that lies under your liver on the right side of your upper abdomen. It stores bile, a fluid produced in your liver. Gallstones are crystalline structures that arise from bile. They can be as small as a grain of sand or as large as a golf ball; sometimes there can be several gallstones in the gallbladder at the same time. Gallstones are three times more common in women. Fortunately, most gallstones cause no symptoms or difficulties.

Gallstones can obstruct the flow of bile from the liver to the intestine (a gallbladder attack), resulting in severe and constant pain that begins suddenly and lasts several hours. Nausea and vomiting are also common. Severe or recurrent gallbladder attacks may require surgical or laparoscopic removal of the gallbladder.

How will my pregnancy affect my condition? Gallstones are more common during pregnancy, especially in women who have been pregnant several times and in those who are obese. Management of a gallstone attack is the same as in non-pregnant women. Some X-ray procedures used for evaluation of gallstones may be deferred until after pregnancy to minimize radiation exposure to the fetus.

How will my condition affect my pregnancy? Most pregnancies will be unaffected by gallbladder attacks, even in women with known gallstones. Operation to remove the gallbladder is needed in about one in 1,000 pregnancies. This operation can be done safely for both mother and fetus. Laparoscopic removal may be very difficult during pregnancy.

Can I breastfeed? Breastfeeding is unlikely to be affected by gallstones or their treatment.

Recommendations for women with this condition

- Alert your physician if you have a history of gallstones.
- Contact your physician if symptoms of a gallbladder attack develop.

Gynecological Conditions

Endometriosis occurs when bits of the endometrium (the tissue that lines the uterus) escape the uterus and become implanted on other pelvic organs. Most often, these implants develop on the ovaries, the fallopian tubes, the uterus or its supporting ligaments. During the menstrual cycle, the tissue first thickens and then begins bleeding. Because the implants are embedded within other tissue, there is nowhere for the blood to go. Blood blisters form, which can be painful. The surrounding tissue sometimes creates cysts to encapsulate the blisters. The cysts, in turn, can become scar tissue that binds organs together. This scar tissue can block the fallopian tubes, interfering with conception or preventing fertilized eggs from arriving at the uterus.

Approximately 10 to 15 percent of American women of childbearing age have endometriosis. Most have no symptoms, but for a few the disease is a progressive one that becomes more painful and debilitating over time.

How will my pregnancy affect my condition? During pregnancy, endometriosis implants generally shrink and the symptoms may disappear. This improvement may be sustained after the pregnancy.

How will my condition affect my pregnancy? Endometriosis can be a cause of infertility. If you have endometriosis in an early stage, your doctor might suggest that you become pregnant sooner rather than later, when it might be more difficult to conceive. Women with endometriosis are more likely than most to have a pregnancy outside the uterus (ectopic pregnancy, see page 141).

Can I breastfeed? Plans for breastfeeding are unlikely to be altered by endometriosis.

Recommendation for women with this condition

- Discuss with your doctor how pregnancy plans might be affected by endometriosis.

Endometriosis

Pelvic inflammatory disease (PID), also called acute salpingitis, is inflammation caused by infection of the uterus, fallopian tubes and ovaries. More than two million women seek medical care each year in the United States for PID. Many bacterial organisms are involved in the infection, which seems to originate in the cervix and move upward to the uterus and fallopian tubes. The most common of these organisms include *Neisseria gonorrhoeae* (for more information about gonorrhea, see page 218) and *Chlamydia trachomatis* (for more information about chlamydia, see page 218).

A significant number of women will have problems with infertility and ectopic (tubal) pregnancies after recovering from PID. Women with multiple sexual partners are at the greatest risk for PID.

Pelvic Inflammatory Disease

How will my pregnancy affect my condition? Pregnancy doesn't seem to directly affect the treatment of or recovery from PID.

How will my condition affect my pregnancy? Let your doctor know if you have had PID previously. He or she may check for the most common organisms that cause PID at your first prenatal visit by taking a sample of cells and mucus from the cervix. Test results will determine if you need to be treated with antibiotics.

Because PID is a sexually transmitted disease, your physician may also test you and your partner for other sexually transmitted diseases in order to safeguard your pregnancy.

If PID is appropriately treated, your pregnancy will be at no more risk of complications than that of women who don't have PID.

Can I breastfeed? Because the organisms that cause PID can be tested for and treated early in pregnancy, they would pose no danger in the postpartum period when you are breastfeeding.

Recommendation for women with this condition

- If you have PID, your partner also needs to be tested and treated. As you resume sexual relations, you are at risk for infection if he has not been treated.

Uterine Fibroids

Uterine fibroids, also termed uterine leiomyomas, are found in 25 percent of women older than 35 years. A fibroid is simply a mass of tightly compacted muscle and fibrous tissue. Fibroids vary widely in size and location. They can be as small as a pea or as large as a grapefruit. Most fibroids cause no symptoms but can be felt easily on pelvic examination. They can cause symptoms of pelvic pressure and heaviness, increased urinary frequency and changes in menstrual flow.

How will my pregnancy affect my condition? Fibroids tend to enlarge during pregnancy. They can occasionally bleed or lose their blood supply, resulting in pelvic pain.

How will my condition affect my pregnancy? Increased risks attributed to uterine fibroids depend on the size and location of the fibroid mass. Fibroids can sometimes increase the risk of miscarriage during the first and second trimesters. Premature onset of labor is also more likely. Rarely, infertility can be related to the presence of uterine fibroids distorting the cervical opening or impairing the ability of the embryo to implant in the uterus.

Can I breastfeed? Uterine fibroids are unlikely to affect plans for breastfeeding.

Recommendation for women with this condition

- Discuss with your physician whether your uterine fibroids appear likely to cause concern during pregnancy. If so, ask whether there are symptoms you should report.

Cardiovascular Disorders

Pregnancy imposes major changes in the workload of the heart and circulation. (For more details of normal cardiovascular changes during pregnancy, see page 20). Until recently, many women with a history of heart problems were advised not to become pregnant. Now, most women with cardiovascular problems can have safe and successful pregnancies. Women who have congenital heart disease or cardiovascular conditions should be monitored closely during pregnancy to minimize risks to mother and baby.

Some heart problems (such as cyanotic congenital heart disease, pulmonary hypertension and severe aortic stenosis) pose a high risk to both the mother and the baby. Women with these problems are advised to avoid pregnancy unless the problem can be corrected first. The more restricted you are in your daily activities because of your heart condition, the more dangerous pregnancy would be for you.

Your physician will be familiar with the specifics of your cardiovascular condition. Management of your pregnancy may require the combined efforts of your physician, a perinatologist, neonatologist, cardiologist and anesthesiologist specializing in obstetrics.

How will my pregnancy affect my condition? The workload on your heart increases even in the first trimester of pregnancy. Abrupt changes in the circulation occur during labor, especially during pushing. Immediately after birth your heart has a major increased load due to changes in circulation from the decrease in blood flow through your uterus.

Pregnancy can pose a risk of endocarditis, a potentially life-threatening bacterial infection of the membrane that lines the interior of the heart's four chambers and valves. If you have a malformed heart or heart valves, or if your valves are scarred, infecting organisms are provided with a roughened surface inside your heart where they can congregate, multiply and potentially spread to other parts of your body. Because bacteria can easily enter your bloodstream during childbirth, women at risk for endocarditis are treated with antibiotics just before and after the birth to minimize the risk of infection.

Minor abnormalities in heart rhythm, such as occasional extra atrial or ventricular beats, are common during pregnancy and are usually not a cause for concern.

How will my condition affect my pregnancy? Some medications, such as anticoagulants, may require adjustment or substitution before or during pregnancy to minimize risks to the fetus or newborn. Others may require adjustment because of the changes in circulation during pregnancy.

Women with heart disease should be monitored closely during pregnancy for possible worsening of their underlying condition. More frequent examination and testing often will be necessary. Some of the normal changes accompanying pregnancy may be of special concern for women with cardiovascular problems. For example, anemia poses greater risks in some types of heart conditions. Fluid retention may be more difficult to manage or might indicate worsening of the underlying heart problem.

Labor may require very close monitoring and in some women will require specialized technology such as pulmonary or arterial pressure catheters and ready availability of echocardiography. During labor, pain-relief medications are used in part to decrease stress on the mother's circulation. Epidural or spinal anesthesia is commonly used. Forceps are more likely to be used during vaginal births to minimize prolonged pushing. Labor might even be avoided by planning a cesarean birth.

Because major changes in your circulation occur after birth, continued close medical supervision and intensive monitoring may be needed during the first couple of weeks after birth.

Can I breastfeed? Most medications used in the management of heart disease require no adjustment for breastfeeding. Some newborns might require monitoring for possible effects of medications.

Recommendations for women with this condition

- Seek a team of specialists experienced in managing pregnancies in women with heart disease.
- Work closely with your physician to determine the causes and best management of concerns that arise during your pregnancy.

Mitral Valve Prolapse

The mitral valve is the valve in your heart between the left atrium and the left ventricle. Mitral valve prolapse is a condition in which parts of the mitral valve called the leaflets bulge toward the left atrium during the contraction of the heart muscle. Sometimes this occurs because the leaflets are generously sized for your heart; in other cases the mitral valve has formed abnormally. Sometimes this ballooning motion results in an abnormal regurgitation of blood from the left ventricle back into the left atrium. If you have mitral valve prolapse you are slightly more likely to have abnormalities of heart rhythm, such as atrial fibrillation or extra ventricular beats.

Mitral valve prolapse may be detected by listening to the heart during a physical examination. The diagnosis is often confirmed by an ultrasound exam of the heart (echocardiogram).

How will my pregnancy affect my condition? Pregnancy, labor and birth will not usually affect mitral valve prolapse. However, if high blood pressure develops during pregnancy, symptoms of mitral valve prolapse might worsen. Some women with mitral valve prolapse seem to be at higher risk of developing an infection (endocarditis) on the surface of the mitral valve, especially after birth. Your physician can assess your degree of risk and decide whether to recommend the use of antibiotics during labor to minimize the risk of endocarditis.

How will my condition affect my pregnancy? Pregnancy will usually be unaffected by mitral valve prolapse.

Can I breastfeed? Breastfeeding should be unaffected by mitral valve prolapse.

Recommendation for women with this condition
- Alert your physician if you have been told you have mitral valve prolapse.

Hypertension most commonly means an elevated pressure in blood pumping into the arteries. Blood pressure adjusts to meet the requirements of the body as it changes with position or activity. Chronic hypertension can develop for various reasons. The management of hypertension may depend greatly on the primary underlying reason, for example, chronic kidney disease. Hypertension can impose stress on the heart, kidneys and eyes.

Hypertension

How will my pregnancy affect my condition? Blood pressure normally changes during pregnancy to meet the needs of the uterus and other organs affected by pregnancy. Blood pressure does not normally become elevated during pregnancy. Preexisting hypertension may worsen during pregnancy. Except for the potentially serious complications that can arise during pregnancy, the long-term course of chronic hypertension does not seem to be affected either favorably or unfavorably by pregnancy. Pregnancy can also reveal previously unrecognized hypertension in some women and might indicate a potential for hypertension in others. The unique condition of hypertension during pregnancy is termed preeclampsia. (Preeclampsia is discussed on page 192.)

How will my condition affect my pregnancy? Hypertension during pregnancy requires close observation, especially during the last trimester. Chronic hypertension can worsen markedly, leading to problems for both mother and baby.

Possible maternal problems can include swelling, congestive heart failure, seizures, impairment of kidney or liver function, vision changes and bleeding. Severe hypertension in pregnancy can become life-threatening. Some women with hypertension will develop problems during subsequent pregnancies.

Possible fetal problems include impairment of growth (intrauterine growth retardation), greater risk of asphyxia before or during labor, greater risk of placental abruption and possible effects from medications used to treat maternal hypertension.

Can I breastfeed? Breastfeeding will likely be unaffected by hypertension. Most hypertension medications will not affect the newborn; check with your physician for specific recommendations.

Recommendations for women with this condition

- Follow the recommendation of your physician for evaluating high blood pressure.
- If you have hypertension, anticipate more frequent exams and testing, especially during the last trimester and during labor.

Asthma

Asthma is a chronic respiratory disease that causes periodic tightness in the chest, cough, wheezing and difficulty in breathing.

How will my pregnancy affect my condition? Pregnancy does not have a predictable effect on asthma. Asthma might be unaffected, worsen or improve. Asthma sometimes worsens in the third trimester or during labor.

The treatment of asthma is largely unaffected by pregnancy.

How will my condition affect my pregnancy? In general, treatment that is beneficial for the mother is also best for the fetus. Severe episodes of asthma which cause low oxygen levels in the mother will lower the oxygen available for the fetus. This condition could be harmful for the baby.

Because of this concern, you may be somewhat more likely to be treated with oxygen, have pulmonary function tests or have arterial blood gas studies if you have a severe asthma attack while pregnant. In addition, your physician may observe you more closely for anemia, which would pose an added stress for women with asthma. Recurrent severe asthma attacks could result in a slower weight gain in the fetus (intrauterine growth retardation, see page 196).

After your first trimester, your physician might recommend that you receive influenza vaccine. Expectorants that contain iodides should be avoided during pregnancy and breastfeeding because they could cause serious thyroid enlargement in the baby. Iodide-containing expectorants are available only by prescription.

Can I breastfeed? Asthma or its treatment will usually not affect plans for breastfeeding.

Recommendations for women with this condition

- Take prescribed medications as directed.
- Notify your physician if your asthma is worsening despite medication.
- Don't treat yourself with non-prescription asthma medications unless recommended by your physician.
- Avoid activities that may trigger an asthma attack.
- If you are pregnant in the fall or winter, ask your physician whether you should receive influenza vaccine.

Psychiatric Disorders

Disorders relating to mental health include variations in responses to the normal stresses of life, for example, anxiety, situational depression and grief responses. More serious and chronic mental health disorders include personality disorders, depression and mood disorders, and thought disorders (psychosis) such as schizophrenia.

How will my pregnancy affect my condition? Pregnancy brings many physical, emotional and social changes. Women with psychiatric disorders may have widely varying responses to pregnancy, especially pregnancies that are unexpected. Even an uncomplicated pregnancy poses new concerns for women with psychiatric disorders. Abortion, miscarriage or stillbirth also can pose greater difficulties for these women. A woman's psychiatric condition might change during the differing circumstances of pregnancy, labor and after birth. It is especially important for these women to receive continued support during the demanding months after birth.

Psychotic disorders are not necessarily affected by pregnancy, and psychosis during one pregnancy doesn't mean that future pregnancies will be affected.

Management of psychiatric disorders is generally the same as in non-pregnant women. Many medications used in treatment of psychiatric disorders can be used safely in pregnant women.

How will my condition affect my pregnancy? Assuming that you are receiving regular prenatal and psychiatric care, your pregnancy should be similar to that of women without a psychiatric condition.

Can I breastfeed? Breastfeeding is possible for most women with psychiatric conditions. Possible effects from medications should be discussed with your physician.

Recommendations for women with this condition

- Alert your physician if you have had a history of a psychiatric, emotional or mental condition.
- Work closely with physicians experienced in managing pregnancies in women with your particular condition.
- Check with your physician before changing doses or starting or stopping use of any medications.

Epilepsy

Epilepsy is a seizure disorder that results from abnormal electrical activity in the brain.

How will my pregnancy affect my condition? The frequency of seizures in women with epilepsy varies unpredictably during pregnancy. About half of the time, seizure frequency is unaffected. About one-quarter of pregnant women with epilepsy have a decrease in seizures, but another quarter have an increase in seizures. The increase is mostly during the first trimester and is thought to be due to changes in body chemistry. In addition, severe nausea and vomiting during early pregnancy may interfere with your ability to take anticonvulsant medication. This can increase the risk of seizures.

The blood levels of some of the medications used in the treatment of epilepsy tend to decrease during pregnancy. This means that you may require more frequent adjustment of your medications and more frequent blood tests to check levels.

How will my condition affect my pregnancy? More than 90 percent of women with epilepsy have successful pregnancy outcomes. Most women continue to take the same medications for epilepsy that they used before becoming pregnant. Supplements of folic acid are commonly added during pregnancy for women taking anticonvulsant medications.

Epilepsy appears to cause an increased risk of vaginal bleeding and an increased risk of placental abruption. There may also be a higher-than-expected rate of premature rupture of membranes and pregnancy-induced hypertension.

There are three main risks for the fetus, including the effects of epilepsy itself during pregnancy, such as possible effects from maternal seizures. Also, there is an increased risk that epilepsy will be inherited by the baby. Third, there is an increased risk of birth defects in babies born to women with epilepsy. The degree of each of these risks varies widely in individuals and is too complex to summarize.

In general, if your epilepsy is well controlled with medications, it is probably best for you to continue taking the same medications during pregnancy.

Can I breastfeed? Breastfeeding is usually safe while taking medication for epilepsy. The specific medicines you take should be reviewed by your doctor.

Recommendations for women with this condition

- Do not make changes in your medications without first checking with your physician.
- Be prepared for more frequent testing of medication levels during your pregnancy.
- Ask your physician about folic acid supplementation during pregnancy.

Urinary Tract Infection (UTI)

Many of the normal body changes during pregnancy increase the risk of bladder and kidney infections.

How will my pregnancy affect my condition? Bladder infections (cystitis) are more likely to result in kidney infection (pyelonephritis) during pregnancy.

How will my condition affect my pregnancy? UTI, especially kidney infection, can lead to premature onset of labor. Because UTIs during pregnancy are more likely to be severe, several methods of screening are used to detect early evidence of infection. Kidney infection may require admission to the hospital for intravenous antibiotics. After an episode of UTI has resolved, antibiotic medication might be continued to lessen the possibility of recurrence.

Can I breastfeed? A UTI and most medications used in treatment are unlikely to affect plans for nursing.

Recommendations for women with this condition

- Increase your fluid intake until the infection has resolved.
- Avoid long periods without urination; specifically, don't try to "hold it." Frequent urination is helpful in clearing up a UTI.
- Urinate after intercourse to lessen the likelihood of developing a new infection.

Maternal Death

An often unspoken concern for couples is the risk of death during pregnancy or childbirth. This concern partly arises from the known risks associated with pregnancy. Worry about maternal death also reflects the sense of responsibility many new parents face. Common questions are, "What would happen to my baby if I should die?" or "How would my partner manage if I were to die?"

The overall risk of maternal death in the United States is low. With earlier and better prenatal care, advanced technology, specialized training of medical personnel and the refinement of anesthesia techniques, the rates have decreased markedly during the past 50 years. Currently in the United States, the risk of maternal death from causes directly related to pregnancy is one in approximately 12,500 live births.

The major causes of maternal death are hypertension, bleeding, pulmonary embolism (a blood clot that goes to the lungs), ectopic pregnancy and infection. Less common causes are stroke, problems associated with anesthesia, damaged heart muscle (cardiomyopathy) and abortion or miscarriage complications.

If you have a chronic medical condition, you can decrease the risk of maternal death during pregnancy and childbirth by taking the following precautions:

- Have preconception and prenatal health care.

- See physicians experienced in the management of pregnant women with your medical condition.

- Labor and give birth in a medical facility equipped to respond to emergencies promptly, rather than depending on emergency medical transport if problems arise. For example, a woman with preeclampsia should labor and give birth in a facility equipped to handle emergency complications, such as seizures, rather than depending on an ambulance or helicopter for emergency medical transport.

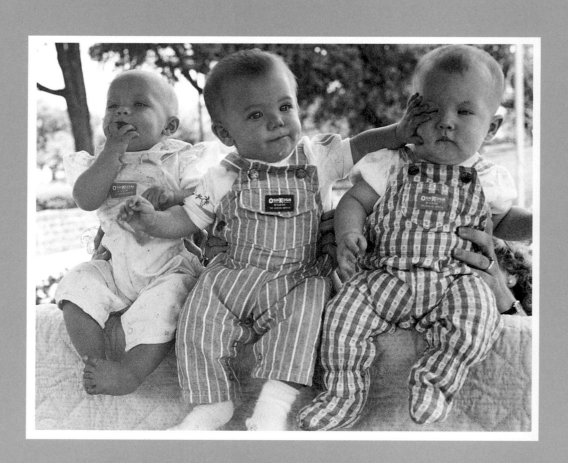

CHAPTER FIFTEEN

Stopping or Delaying Preterm Birth

Making bed rest more comfortable

Your due date...it comes up in most conversations with family and friends. Even strangers ask you about it. You excitedly plan your life around it, especially because you're now past the halfway point of 20 weeks. But suddenly, still weeks before that much anticipated date, you begin to have problems—bleeding, cramping, contractions. Your doctor tells you that your baby is at risk for preterm delivery and recommends immediate bed rest or medical treatment.

The unexpected physical problems and the disruption of normal living may, understandably, set off a chain reaction of worries: Am I going to have my baby early? Will she or he be all right? Will I be all right? Who will care for my other children? How can I pay the bills when I'm not working? How can I do housework? Will I still be able to take as much leave as I planned after the baby arrives?

About 6 to 7 percent of all pregnant women go into preterm labor, sometimes in the second but more often in the third trimester. Sometimes, there is no explanation for why the preterm labor (contractions that start opening the cervix before the 37th week of pregnancy) occurs. Generally, however, women who are at higher risk for preterm birth have one or more complications, including:

- Expecting twins, triplets or more (see page 201)
- Dilated cervix
- Problems with an abnormally shaped uterus
- Previous preterm birth
- Problems with the amniotic fluid or amniotic sac
- Previous preterm labor
- Previous miscarriages or abortions
- Infections, including urinary tract infections
- Problems with the placenta (see page 194)
- Preexisting medical conditions
- Preeclampsia (see page 192)

Whether or not preterm labor is anticipated, its onset must be addressed immediately to prevent a problem from becoming a life-threatening crisis. Treatment will depend, in part, on the severity of any high-risk conditions, the development of your baby, your living circumstances and your doctor's recommendations given the risks and benefits of various alternatives to help stop or delay preterm labor and birth.

Even if you have several risk factors, they usually can be overcome. You may have to make some temporary changes in your lifestyle, perhaps even spend several months on bed rest. But the odds are high that between modern medical technology and your own efforts, you can carry and give birth to a healthy baby.

In this chapter, we focus on the treatments most doctors recommend for preterm labor, including bed rest at home or in a hospital and medications to stop labor. We also recommend ways to help you better cope with the emotional whirlwind you may experience given the restrictions that bed rest poses, as well as practical suggestions to handle the lifestyle changes these limitations may impose.

Remember, you do have choices about how you spend your time, even when confined to bed. And each day away from the delivery room means a day closer to your real due date.

Why Bed Rest?

If you develop a high-risk complication and signs of possible preterm labor, such as a dilated cervix, your doctor may request that you stay in bed. Sometimes he or she may tell you to reduce activity, to take it easy and to avoid stressful situations. But often doctors will recommend total, or what is called therapeutic, bed rest. Total bed rest has several specific benefits. It:

- Decreases pressure of the baby on your cervix and reduces cervical stretching, which may cause premature contractions and miscarriage.
- Increases blood flow to the placenta, helping your baby to receive maximal nutrition and oxygen. This is particularly important if the baby is not growing as rapidly as he or she should.
- Helps your organs, particularly your heart and kidneys, to function more efficiently, improving problems with high blood pressure.

Although you may not feel like you need bed rest, it's important to try it—even at the risk of feeling lousy once restricted to bed. Although no one treatment works for every expectant mom at risk for preterm labor, your doctor will want to help you do everything possible to maintain your pregnancy and avoid having to deliver your baby before he or she is ready to be born. Assuming a positive attitude about staying in bed may make the difference in how effectively bed rest helps you and your baby.

Choosing the Best Positions

If your doctor advises that you stay in bed, you will be much more comfortable lying on your side, very often your left side. Lying on your side increases blood flow returning to your heart, thus increasing the blood and oxygen supply to your growing baby. It also eases the occasional development of low blood pressure, which may be caused by pressure of your baby and your uterus on the blood vessels in your abdomen (particularly when on your back or standing).

If your membranes have ruptured or you have changes in your cervix, your doctor may also recommend that while on your side, you rest with your hips higher than your shoulders. A hospital bed can be adjusted to accomplish this position, but at home you can raise the foot of the bed or mattress in several ways (see page 254). This position, known as the Trendelenburg position, also helps decrease pressure on the cervix. It may, however, cause heartburn and problems with eating. Headaches and stuffy nose and ears may also occur.

Relieving Discomfort

When you are on bed rest, your muscles will lose tone and your joints may begin to ache. Try to change position, from one side to the other, every hour or two. This will help decrease discomfort in your hips and lower back. You may find it more comfortable using pillows to support your abdomen, back, head and shoulders. Do not lie flat on your back, except for short stretches to ease cramped muscles. Have your partner, support person or nurse massage your back with a soothing lotion, and use lotion on your heels and elbows to decrease the soreness from constant rubbing against bed sheets. Socks and long sleeves may also help.

Limited exercise in bed will help your muscle tone and circulation, but don't start doing sit-ups or stretches before checking with your doctor. You may be able to do isometric exercises, but ask first. They could cause contractions. Some exercises that you can probably do, even in bed, include:

- Moving your head, hands and feet in circles
- Tensing and relaxing arm and leg muscles without tightening abdominal muscles
- Pressing hands and feet against the bed's headboard or footboard

Getting Out of Bed Properly

If you are allowed to get up to go to the bathroom, getting out of bed properly is just as important as how you lie in bed. After pushing yourself up into a seated position, sit still for a few seconds. When you put your feet on the floor and stand up, have someone help support you or lean on a sturdy chair before you begin to walk. If you feel light-headed or dizzy at any time, stop and rest.

Which Is Better—Bed Rest at Home or in the Hospital?

This decision depends on what you need—and what works best for you. There is no single best approach to treating expectant moms at risk for preterm birth. Your needs may change from one hour to the next, from one day to the next, from one week to the next. Several considerations will help you and your doctor make the decision: the cause of your preterm labor, if known, the number of high-risk factors you may have, your ability to truly rest at home, the care and support you can receive at home versus that in a hospital, your stress and comfort levels and the effectiveness of any medication treatment.

For example, if your membranes have ruptured and your doctor recommends that you use the Trendelenburg position, you and your baby will probably be better off in the hospital. But if you have borderline-high blood pressure, you may remain at home if you can assure your doctor that you will primarily rest and get help with child care and other domestic duties. Even if you need to take medication to lower your blood pressure and make arrangments to have your blood pressure monitored, you may be more comfortable and less stressed by remaining at home with your family. If you simply can't rest comfortably at home, however, or if your hypertension is severe, you may need bed rest in the hospital. If emergency complications arise, you'll be in a place where help is readily available.

Monitoring Contractions

Even if you're facing the risk of preterm delivery and need total bed rest for several months, treatment at home may work well. However, if your symptoms suggest preterm labor is imminent, your doctor will advise you to stay in the hospital to determine the condition of your cervix and to monitor contractions. You may receive intravenous fluids and medications to help slow or stop the labor. Your doctor may also want you to stay at the hospital to monitor your baby's heart rate and to make sure your baby is okay. If after a few hours your cervix has not dilated more and the contractions do not exceed four per hour, you may be able to continue bed rest at home, possibly using a monitor to check your contractions yourself. Alternatively, you may be able to communicate by telephone with a nurse who can help follow your condition.

Delaying Delivery With Medication

If bed rest and fluids are not enough to halt your contractions at home or in the hospital, your doctor will probably recommend medication. If an infection is causing the problems, antibiotics may be sufficient. With other complications, a medication to stop uterine contractions, called a tocolytic, may be necessary. Some tocolytics may be administered intravenously or by injection; others are taken as pills or suppositories. The specific tocolytic prescribed for you will depend in part on high-risk factors you may have. And the choice of medication may also determine whether it should be administered in the hospital or at home.

One of the most commonly used tocolytics is magnesium sulfate, particularly if you have preterm labor complicated by hypertension, diabetes, heart disease or bleeding. It is given intravenously in the hospital, where your doctor can keep a close watch on you and your baby. Magnesium sulfate is effective, but it can cause side effects for expectant mothers and babies. You may feel weakness in your muscles or be unusually tired or sleepy. Your baby may initially be sleepy or uninterested in nursing at birth.

Two other medications, ritodrine and terbutaline, also are available to halt contractions. Generally, they are not recommended if you have hypertension, heart disease, diabetes or hyperthyroidism (excessive secretion of the thyroid glands). If your doctor selects one of these medications, you'll likely receive it by injection or intravenously. Once the contractions have been controlled for 12 to 24 hours, you might begin taking these medications as pills. These medications have possible side effects too. They may increase your heart rate and cause jitters or nausea or vomiting; in rare cases, they cause fluid to accumulate in your lungs. The side effects do, however, tend to subside as your body becomes accustomed to the medications. These medications also enter your baby's blood circulation and may cause a temporarily faster heartbeat.

If none of these medications are effective, your doctor may recommend one of two other medications, indomethacin or nifedipine. Indomethacin, however, is usually not used for more than 48 hours because prolonged use could cause potential problems for your baby.

Obstetricians, especially those specializing in high-risk obstetrics (perinatologists), are continuing to look for medications that will more effectively stop preterm labor with fewer side effects. Usually, however, the sooner you begin taking any tocolytic treatment—preferably before your cervix has dilated too much—the more effective it can be in stopping any preterm labor and delaying the birth of your baby.

Keeping Your Unborn Baby Healthy With Medication

While using one medication to halt your contractions, your doctor may use another to improve the condition of your baby. Generally, because the doctor will need to monitor your baby closely, you will receive these medications at the hospital.

For example, concentrations of the steroid hormone called cortisone normally increase in a baby just before birth. This is nature's way of preparing your baby's lungs to function independently after birth. If preterm labor persists, your doctor may give you an injection of betamethasone or dexamethasone for your baby. These medications, forms of cortisone, can help speed up the maturation of your baby's lungs. (For more information on respiratory distress syndrome, see page 364.)

If you are less than 32 weeks pregnant and are having preterm labor, your doctor may also give you phenobarbital. This may help decrease the risk of bleeding in your baby's brain after birth. (For more information on intracranial hemorrhage, see page 366.)

Unless fetal monitoring or other tests indicate that your baby is in distress, or you have complications that indicate you may need to have a cesarean birth—such as a heart condition, placental abruption (see page 194) or placenta previa (see page 195)—your baby can probably be born vaginally. Two of three babies born after preterm labor are born vaginally.

How to Beat the Bed Rest Blues

Days, weeks or months of enforced inactivity—ranging from limiting your activity to total bed rest—can be difficult. To better accept the restrictions and develop strategies to cope with them, you'll do well to prepare yourself emotionally. Here are some suggestions from women who've had the experience.

Psyching Yourself Up

Many expectant mothers blame themselves when they consider the possibility of losing their babies or when their own health is at risk. They often ask: Could I have done anything differently? Probably not. Often, the reasons for high-risk pregnancies are either unknown or unavoidable. Many pregnant women at risk for premature birth find it difficult to let go of plans for a full-term pregnancy and birth and to accept the possibility that they or their baby will require special care after birth. You can help yourself accept these realities if you:

- Expect to have angry, negative feelings at times. Try not to feel as if you have been singled out. Many women have ambivalent feelings about their pregnancy even if it is going normally—loving and accepting it at one moment, bored and wishing for it to be over the next. This ambivalence sharpens dramatically when pregnancy problems arise.

- Understand the problem. Ask your health care provider to explain and recommend materials to help you learn more about expectant mothers and babies in your situation. Knowing what lies ahead can help you adjust and set realistic expectations.

- Ask your doctor, in advance, how a preterm birth and your baby will be handled. Facing the problem is easier if you can minimize surprises. Ask under what circumstances you or your baby might be transferred to another hospital or to special care units—a newborn intensive care unit for your baby and a perinatal care unit for yourself.

- Raise your concerns with your doctor as well as with your family. You will need all the support you can get. Don't hold back. The act of ventilating your worries with your health care provider and with someone close to you (your partner, your mother, another mother who has had similar problems) may help relieve your frustration, fears and stress.

- Be involved in your care. Learn what will help your own and your baby's health. If preterm labor threatens, learn how to recognize your contractions and the sensations that may signal them. If you are taking medications, learn about possible side effects and measures you can take to prevent or alleviate them. Find out if there are alternatives to the treatment you are receiving. If the treatment plan changes, find out why.

- Discover whether there are support groups in your area providing emotional and informational support to women and families dealing with complicated pregnancies. Write or call Sidelines National Support Network, 2805 Park Place, Laguna Beach, CA 92651; telephone (714) 497-2265. If the group holds meetings and you can't attend, send your partner or a friend, if possible. Gather literature from the group to read. If you need outside assistance that is beyond your means, a hospital or a religious or community social service organization may be able to provide help. Call the public health department to speak with a visiting nurse or a social worker who helps mothers who have high-risk pregnancies.

- Avoid dwelling on how much longer your pregnancy and bed rest will persist. Take it one day at a time. Recognize that each day longer gives your baby more time to mature, for his or her lungs and other organs to become stronger. Set short-term goals and mark them off on a calendar: first reaching 24 weeks, then 28, 32 and 36 weeks. Celebrate when you reach each goal.

Y our other children may find your extended bed rest frightening and disruptive. They may become angry, whining and uncooperative and demand more attention. Try to reassure them, first of all, that you are staying in bed to help protect your health and that of their younger brother or sister. Your bed rest may actually provide opportunities to give them even more attention than usual. You can:

Staying Attentive to Your Other Children

- Cuddle and talk.
- Play bedside games and puzzles.
- Read to them and help with homework.
- Let them help you—massage your back or feet, read to you, prepare or serve meals, do small housekeeping duties—but don't make requests too demanding.

Arrange for someone to help with their care, to take them to school and play groups, to prepare meals and to welcome them when they return. Try not to allow them to feel that their care is an additional burden on you or the family. If you need outside assistance, find out about child care, latchkey and baby-sitting facilities in your area. Financial assistance may be available to help pay for child care while you are on bed rest. Ask a social worker, public health nurse or visiting nurse.

Tips for expectant fathers

As hard as it may be for your partner to accept the reality that her pregnancy is in danger, her bed rest and health and that of your unborn child do not negate the stress and difficulties you may be facing. You may have feelings of guilt, asking yourself: Did I do something wrong during, or even before, her pregnancy? As much as you both long for a healthy baby, you may find that you are hearing most of the reports about your partner's pregnancy secondhand. You may feel as if you are merely an observer. Saddled with new responsibilities, you're probably juggling job concerns along with caring for your partner and perhaps other children. And as much as you try to hide your reactions, you may find yourself becoming angry and resentful.

Here are suggestions to help you better cope with the abrupt changes in your family's life which accompany bed rest during pregnancy:

- Share your partner's concerns. Go to the doctor's appointments together so that you fully understand the health problems she faces and the measures she must take to protect herself and your baby.

- Avoid blaming your partner if she forgets to follow her doctor's instructions. She may already feel guilty about the problems with her pregnancy, and further blame can compound her feelings of inadequacy.

- Help with domestic responsibilities, or arrange for help from other family members or outside assistance.

- Don't resent the time your partner has to lie in bed. Bed rest, although it may sound like a luxury, is hard work.

- Do take time to relax and take care of yourself. Your burnout will only add to the stress.

- Spend as much time as you can with your family. The fact that you are there, giving support, will help relieve the stress your partner inevitably feels.

Keeping Your Household Going

To help relieve you of anxiety, try to get some reliable household help on a regular basis. You may get assistance from relatives, friends and neighbors, but avoid relying on catch-as-catch-can help. Above all, try not to saddle your partner with the sole responsibility for keeping the household going. Burnout is likely to occur sooner than you expect. Commercial agencies experienced in providing such help may be available in your area. If you can't afford the expense, talk to a social worker or public health visiting nurse about getting assistance.

If you can't get enough help and your home is not as neat as you like, try to relax your standards. Focus on what's most important—your health and your unborn baby's health.

Managing Finances

If you take care of family finances, set aside a particular part of your day to handle money matters—balancing your checkbook, paying bills and budgeting expenses. Keep track of all expenses for medical care and child care because many may be deductible when filing your annual income taxes. If you use an accountant or tax advisor, ask what deductions are allowed.

Be sure to check your health insurance policy to see if special care for you or your baby is covered. For example, will expenses be covered if you or your baby needs care in an intensive care unit? If problems arise and you need information, talk to your health care provider or hospital social worker. If you anticipate problems with uncovered expenses, you may be able to work out a payment plan with the hospital in advance.

If you work outside the home, check your company's leave policy and make sure it adheres to new laws regarding maternity leave versus sick leave. Notify your employer about how long you anticipate being absent, if possible. Depending on your job responsibilities, you may want to arrange with your supervisor a specific time each day when you would be willing to discuss ongoing projects. If job worries add stress to your life at this time, it may be better to take a leave.

Entertaining Visitors, Taking Outings

If you're up to it, encourage visitors to stop by. But don't hesitate to discourage drop-ins, even by friends, or to avoid visitors who may make you uncomfortable. Plan shared activities with your friends, such as mealtime parties, if they bring the food, serve themselves and clean up afterward.

Depending on how your pregnancy progresses, your doctor may approve of an occasional outing. If you are not having any contractions, for example, you may be able to go to a movie or visit friends. Or, closer to home, perhaps you can relax on a lawn chair. Even if you're feeling fine, don't stop your bed rest, as tempting as it may be, unless you've checked with your doctor first. Talk with your doctor about how frequently you'll have doctor's appointments and any limitations on traveling to and from your appointments.

Setting Up Your Bedroom

Whether you are restricted to bed rest at home or in the hospital, you should arrange your room so that all your necessities and amenities are within arm's length. If at home, set up one room where you can rest undisturbed for as long as you are restricted or confined to your bed. For some expectant moms, the best location is the bedroom. However, you may find you prefer to be in a den, a sunporch or another room where you don't feel as isolated from family life.

If you need to raise the foot of your bed and you're not in a hospital bed, place a dense foam wedge or pillows under the end of the mattress. Or place cinder blocks or patio flagstones under the foot of the bed. Don't use books or small bricks, because they don't provide stable support.

It's also helpful to position a table at mattress height next to your bed. Consider using a wheeled cart with a shelf or two and a utility basket on wheels for soiled towels, handkerchiefs and linen. Attach plastic bags to dispose of used tissues. Organize other everyday necessities you will want within reach as well as amenities that will keep you occupied and help make your days more pleasant. Here are some suggestions:

- A bell or buzzer to summon assistance
- A wireless intercom set (you might borrow one to see how much you use it)
- Telephone, address book, telephone directories
- Pen, pencils, paper
- Water pitcher, cups, straws
- Tissues, moist disposable towels
- Hair brush, comb, mirror
- Body, face and hand lotion
- Books, catalogs, magazines, newspapers
- Television, remote control, VCR, videos
- Radio, cassette or compact disc player
- Cosmetics
- Nail files, scissors
- Thermos for hot water, tea bags
- Hobby materials
- Laptop computer

Making Time Fly

Just attending to your regular daily needs may well occupy more of your time than you expect. And organizing a daily schedule, without being too rigid, may also help you feel psychologically and physically better. Divide each day into scheduled periods: a time for telephoning your office, speaking to friends or relatives, reading, watching television, paying bills, being with your other children.

Still, you probably will find time on your hands. One way to fill those empty hours is to take up new activities that you didn't have time for before in your hectic day-to-day schedule. For example:

- Start receiving a publication or newspaper you don't ordinarily read— a business magazine, say, and become financially savvy.
- Take up a hobby—knitting, embroidery, drawing.
- Enroll in a correspondence course.
- Learn a foreign language through a home-study program via mail, video or audio cassettes or computer.
- Learn to use new computer software.
- Volunteer your services. Many organizations, including social service agencies, charities, museums and theaters, need volunteers to help with telephone solicitations or mailings.

If you fill each day with activity and order, you will likely feel less bored and depressed. You'll also probably sleep better at night and awake refreshed the next day.

As difficult as bed rest can be, the more you focus positive efforts on taking care of yourself and your baby, the more likely you will be able to reach your due date as planned. The challenges of a high-risk pregnancy can be uniquely rewarding and enriching for you and your partner. It can be a time of sharing and a special sense of closeness. Family life can take on new meaning. Take pictures and consider keeping a diary; someday you'll want to retell the story of this incredible pregnancy when a certain special little one is old enough to understand.

About Beginnings

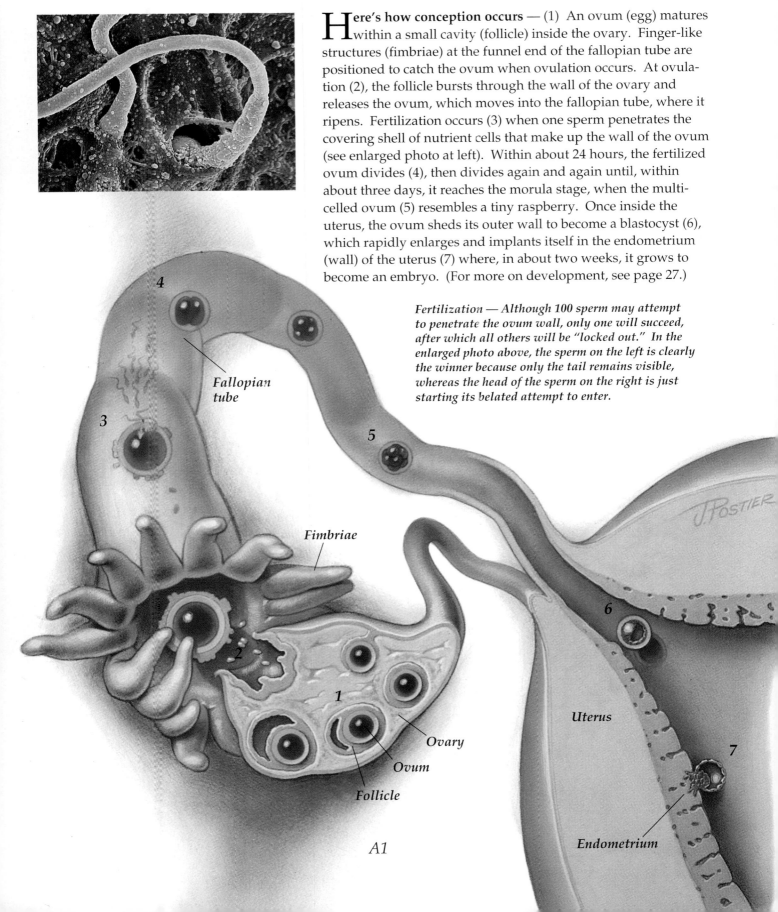

Here's how conception occurs — (1) An ovum (egg) matures within a small cavity (follicle) inside the ovary. Finger-like structures (fimbriae) at the funnel end of the fallopian tube are positioned to catch the ovum when ovulation occurs. At ovulation (2), the follicle bursts through the wall of the ovary and releases the ovum, which moves into the fallopian tube, where it ripens. Fertilization occurs (3) when one sperm penetrates the covering shell of nutrient cells that make up the wall of the ovum (see enlarged photo at left). Within about 24 hours, the fertilized ovum divides (4), then divides again and again until, within about three days, it reaches the morula stage, when the multi-celled ovum (5) resembles a tiny raspberry. Once inside the uterus, the ovum sheds its outer wall to become a blastocyst (6), which rapidly enlarges and implants itself in the endometrium (wall) of the uterus (7) where, in about two weeks, it grows to become an embryo. (For more on development, see page 27.)

Fertilization — Although 100 sperm may attempt to penetrate the ovum wall, only one will succeed, after which all others will be "locked out." In the enlarged photo above, the sperm on the left is clearly the winner because only the tail remains visible, whereas the head of the sperm on the right is just starting its belated attempt to enter.

Fallopian tube

Fimbriae

J. POSTIER

Ovary

Ovum

Follicle

Uterus

Endometrium

A1

The Baby Within You

Once conceived, your baby develops rapidly, changing in the first several weeks from a cluster of cells the size of a pinhead to an embryo that's beginning to resemble a baby. The embryo at **immediate right** is 5 weeks old. Although less than half an inch long, the brain, eyes, heart, liver and backbone are forming. The placenta, upper right

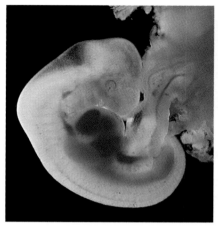

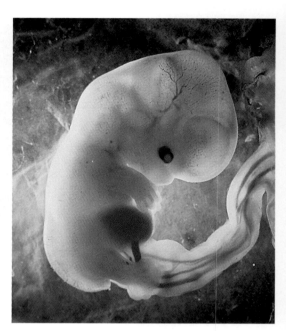

corner of photo, provides nourishment and eliminates wastes. At **far right** is a 6-week-old embryo. A tiny arm has formed, and finger-like structures are apparent on a paddle-shaped hand. The eyelids are taking shape. The embryo is about half an inch long, and the heart is beating about 150 times a minute.

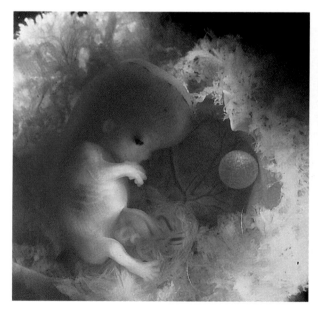

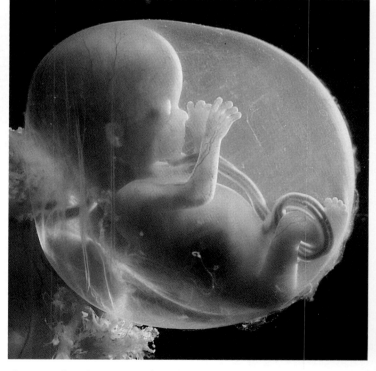

At 9 weeks after conception, your embryo has developed sufficiently to be called a fetus, and at about 11 weeks, your fetus might resemble the one shown __above__. Comfortably nestled within the lacy interior of your uterus, your baby still has plenty of room because she or he is less than 3 inches long. Eyes and ears are clearly identifiable. Arms, legs, fingers and toes are developing quickly, and all organs, nerves and muscles are formed and beginning to function. Your fetus can flex the arms and kick the legs; you won't feel movements until your baby grows larger.

At 17 weeks, __above__, your fetus has a baby-like appearance that includes thin eyebrows, scalp hair and rather well-developed limbs. Head-to-rump length is about 7½ inches. Weight is about a pound. At this age, the typical fetus is becoming increasingly active, moving head, arms and legs vigorously about and making breathing movements. Your baby's hearing is well developed. She or he probably is hearing your conversations.

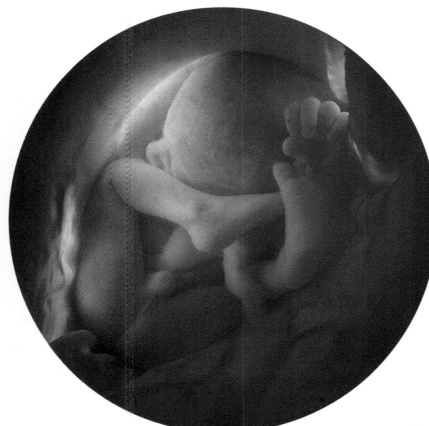

At 28 weeks after conception, your baby is 12 to 15 inches long, weighs about 3 pounds and is beginning to fill the available space in your uterus. Eyelids can open and close. Sex organs are developing. And although still immature, your baby's lungs are capable of sustaining life in the event of premature birth, with help from a ventilator and other special equipment and assistance available in a hospital newborn intensive care unit. (For more on premature birth, see page 353.)

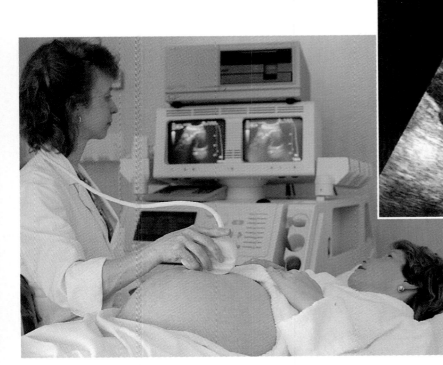

An ultrasound test can offer live-action viewing of your baby. During this safe and painless test, high-frequency sound waves penetrate your abdomen. As they bounce off bones and tissues of your baby, they are converted into a black-and-white image you can view, in motion, on a television screen. Your doctor can use this test to confirm the dating of your pregnancy, to check for structural variations and for other purposes relating to your baby's health and development. <u>Inset</u>: This typical ultrasound photograph (scan) shows a healthy, normal fetus that is 16 weeks gestational age. (For more on ultrasound testing, see page 72.)

Preparing for Birth

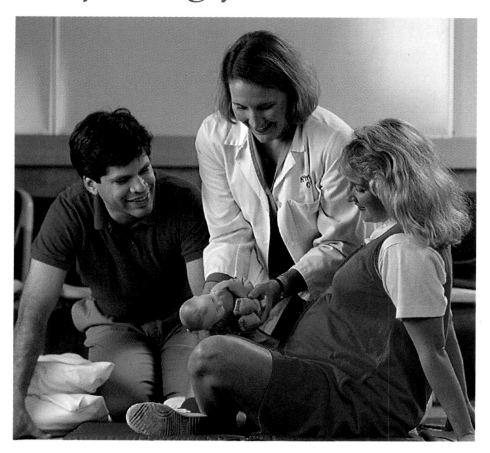

Childbirth education classes can make the birthing process easier, possibly even shorter. You'll learn relaxation and breathing techniques to help relieve fear, tension and pain. Your partner will learn how best to assist you during labor and birth and at home. Classes include a wide range of practical topics aimed at helping families plan, prepare for and celebrate the birth of a baby. (For more on childbirth education, see page 264.)

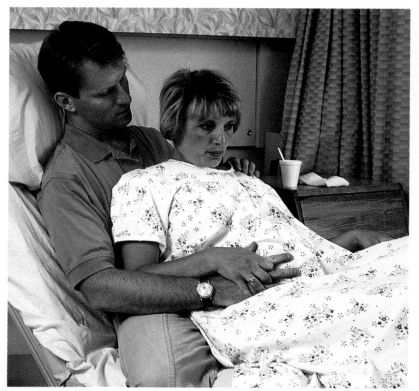

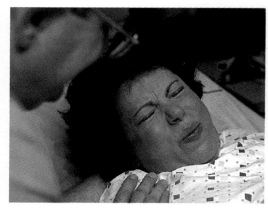

Labor is physically and emotionally demanding. Your partner can help by giving you support and encouragement and with specific techniques you'll both learn in childbirth education classes. For example, by timing the length of your contractions and the intervals between them and by encouraging rhythmic breathing in early labor (__left__) and during the more trying transition phase (__above__), your partner can help keep you focused on the task of pushing your baby out. (For more on labor, see page 277.)

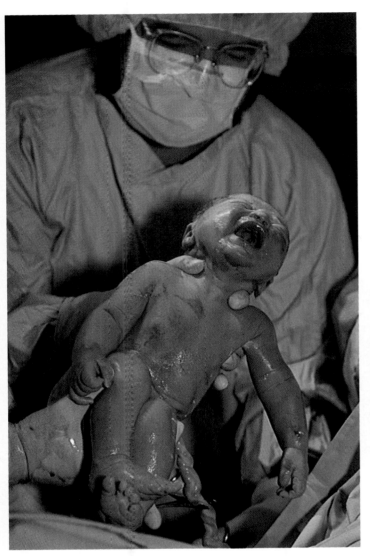

Moments old and slippery from amniotic fluid and blood, a newborn greets the world with a hearty cry, a sign of good health. Newborns usually have bluish or dusky-colored skin and "pink up" within a few minutes. (For more on birth, see page 305.)

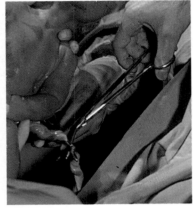

Sometimes fathers help cut the umbilical cord. For the baby, it's painless. For a new dad, it can be a memorable experience. (For more on fatherhood, see page 669.)

Ears — Babies have good hearing. Quiet music may soothe your baby, but she or he may be startled by a loud noise.

Eyes — Your newborn's eyes can focus on, and follow, slowly moving objects. Eyelids may be puffy for the first day or two.

Head — Your baby's head may be temporarily misshapen from passage through the narrow birth canal, a condition that generally lasts only a day or two before the head assumes a more rounded, normal appearance.

Hands — Babies arrive with dimpled knuckles and pudgy hands. Fingernails may need trimming to prevent scratches.

Umbilical cord — A plastic clamp secures the umbilical cord. The cord will dry up and darken in a few days and fall off within three weeks.

Genitals — Your daughter may arrive with labia that are swollen. There may be a small mucous discharge or a little bleeding. Your son's scrotum may be swollen. All of these appearances are normal.

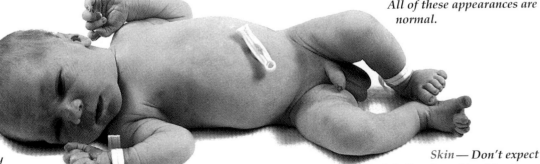

Bracelet — Your baby's identification band will be in place before she or he leaves the delivery room.

Skin — Don't expect pink, flawless skin. Most babies arrive with a few bruises from the birth process and blotchy patches or discolorations that may disappear in a few days or during the first year.

The First Year

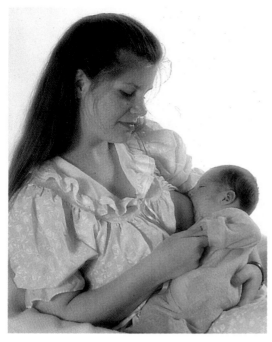

Joys of parenthood — Bringing your baby home marks a new beginning filled with hope, joy and fulfillment. It's also a lot of work. The juggling act begins when you're home with a newborn who is completely dependent on you and your partner. During that important first year, try to keep your lifestyle as simple as possible. Sleep when your baby sleeps. Simplify meal planning and preparation. Settle for a messy house. And accept help offered by family and friends. Enjoy your baby's remarkable growth and development during this first year.

Two weeks — Long before your baby understands the meaning of words, she or he learns about trust by your prompt response to the hunger cry. Whether you breastfeed or bottle feed, take time to enjoy this special closeness with your baby. (For more on feeding, see page 471.)

Two months — Babies begin "bunching" their sleeping times in the first two months of life, staying awake longer during the day and sleeping longer at night. They still take frequent naps but are awake and alert for longer periods. By two months, some babies can sleep six to eight hours at a time. Most likely, your goal is to make those hours nighttime hours. (For tips on how to encourage your baby to "sleep through" the night, see page 523.)

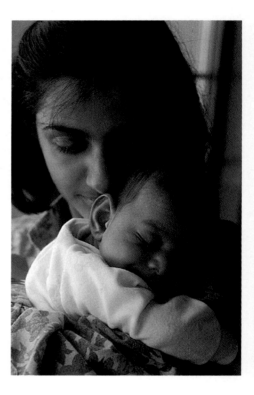

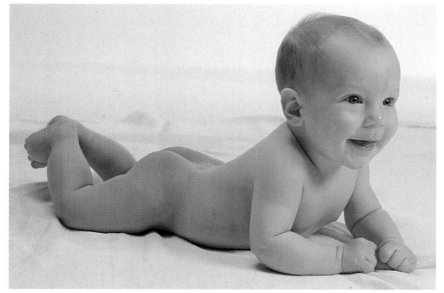

Four months — Muscles in your baby's arms and neck are gaining strength. Place your baby down and she or he most likely will use those newfound muscles to rise up for a better look. At this point, your baby discovers that playing on the floor can be fun. About half of 4-month-old babies can roll over under their own power. Don't leave your baby alone on an elevated surface. (For more on baby from four to six months, see page 545.)

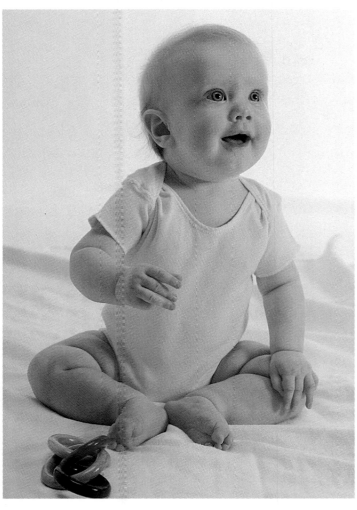

Six months — Your baby is learning to sit up without help, but despite the grin, the maneuver may sap all of her or his energy, and tipping over remains a distinct possibility. In a few more weeks your baby's balance and strength will improve to the point that movement and play can be included in the sitting-up position. (For more on baby from six to nine months, see page 559.)

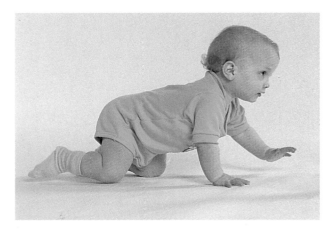

Nine months — Crawling requires all four limbs. Some babies begin by using only their arms, scooting along like a soldier in basic training. It will take perseverance and practice for your baby to figure out how to coordinate arms with legs. But it won't take long. Soon, if you look away for a minute, you may wonder where your little explorer went.

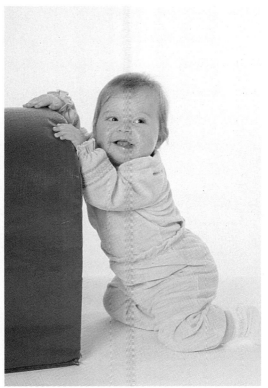

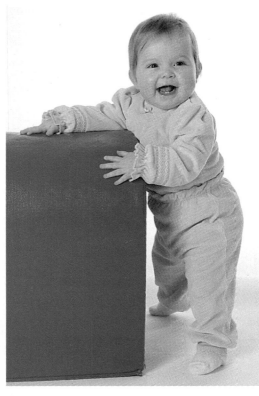

Twelve months — At one year, your baby probably can pull up into a standing position by grasping and holding furniture or anything else available for support. Standing helps your baby develop the muscle strength and control she or he will need for "cruising" — walking sideways while hanging onto furniture. (For more on baby from nine to 12 months, see page 575.)

Your Baby's Health

Because of your baby's fear of strangers and unwillingness to be away from you, the checkup at nine months may differ somewhat from previous health checks. For example, your baby's doctor or nurse-practitioner may choose to do the exam while you hold your baby in your arms or on your lap. As your baby becomes better acquainted with her or his health care provider, fears will fade and trust will prevail at future visits. Your health care provider will be interested in your observations of, and opinions about, your baby's health, so don't hesitate to speak up. Your remarks are just as important as the clinical exam your baby will receive.

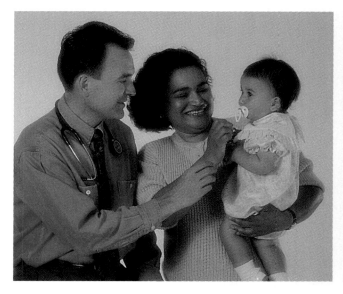

When Your Baby Is Ill (For more on medical problems, see page 603.)

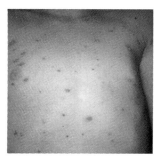

Chickenpox — Itchy, red rash that breaks out on the face, scalp, chest, back and, to a lesser extent, arms and legs.

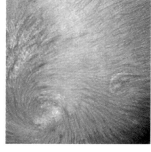

Cradle cap — Dry, scaly patches give scalp a dirty appearance. A yellow crust may form over the scales.

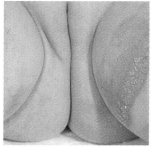

Diaper rash — Red rash caused by continually moist skin that becomes irritated, or by an infection.

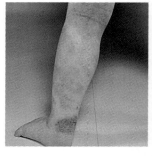

Eczema — Itchy, red, sometimes oozing, scaly, brownish, crusty patches of skin on scalp, face, arms or legs.

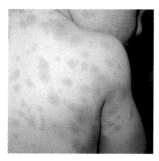

Hives — Allergic disorder that produces splotchy, red, raised rash with pale centers and itching.

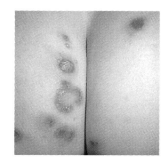

Impetigo — Honey-colored, crusty infection. Begins with a single red bump and develops rapidly into pimple-like blisters with crusted tops.

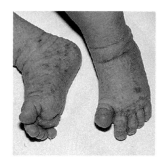

Scabies — Blistery, pink rash on feet, hands or skin folds. It can lead to severe itching. It is caused by a tiny mite.

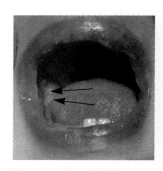

Thrush — Looks like patches of milk on the inside of your baby's cheeks and tongue, but they won't wash off.

Part Two

Childbirth

CHAPTER SIXTEEN

Preparing for Childbirth

Each laboring woman is an individual; each labor and birth are unique. You could compare childbirth to a journey to a new place—made more challenging because of many twists and turns and unmarked crossroads. The start is the first labor pain, and the end is the arrival of the baby, but you can't tell from a distance which path will take you there or what you'll encounter along the way. This chapter describes some of the routes you may choose, and helps prepare you for unexpected detours you might encounter along the way.

Labor goes more smoothly when the mind and body cooperate. The premise behind prepared childbirth is that anxiety about childbirth causes muscular tension that increases pain. The anxiety can be diminished by learning what is happening to your body, and the tension can be dealt with by learning techniques that will help you relax.

In doing so you will better cope with the stresses of labor and birth. The road you are traveling may be a new one, but by learning all you can about what lies ahead it should not be bewildering or scary.

Hospital, Birthing Center or Home?

Where you choose to bring your baby into the world is one of the many decisions facing you. Your choice will depend closely on your health care provider and where he or she has hospital privileges (see Chapter 4). Other factors to consider are costs, the amount and type of medical insurance you have, the range of facilities available to you and the ability of their staff to adapt to your needs and wishes. The most important considerations are your health and the health of your baby.

Talk to your doctor about how your labor and delivery will be handled. What do you have in mind for your birthing experience? Will you be more comfortable in a home setting or a high-tech medical setting? Or do you want something in between—a home-like environment with medical equipment and personnel immediately available?

Developing a relationship of trust and confidence with your caregiver as your pregnancy progresses is crucial. Medical professionals who explain why things are done and what your options are, in an atmosphere of caring support, give you peace of mind and promote a more enjoyable birth experience.

The Hospital

In the early years of the United States, birth was a social event, attended by midwives as well as neighbors and relatives. By the beginning of the 19th century, physicians with formal medical training began delivering babies. For the next hundred years, a quiet changeover took place, in which traditional midwifery was replaced by the new "medical obstetrics."

By the 1930s and 1940s, most women were coming to hospitals for an event that formerly had taken place at home. The newly available science and technology made hospitals the safest place to have babies, but birth, which was once considered a natural process, had become a medical procedure. In those days, doctors "delivered" babies from women who lay flat on their backs in operating rooms, without family members present.

Since the 1960s, expectations have shifted, a change led by women who wanted more control of their birthing experiences. The result has been family-centered maternity care in many hospitals. Birthing rooms provide relaxed surroundings where women choose their own most comfortable positions for laboring, and where partners, and often other family members, are welcome to share in the experience. Birth is again becoming a natural process—guided by sensitive professionals—rather than a medical procedure.

Today, 98.8 percent of U.S. women give birth in hospitals. The overriding advantage of hospital birth is that experienced personnel, sophisticated equipment and blood supplies are available for any emergency. Monitoring ensures greater safety margins. You have many pain management options and can change your mind about these as labor progresses. And as hospitals have become more in tune with women's wishes, their policies have changed to be more family-oriented.

There are some disadvantages to hospital birth. You might have more medical interventions than in a birthing center. Unless you choose rooming-in, you will be periodically separated from your baby. Births in hospitals are typically more costly than other options because of the staff and equipment.

But hospitals should be the only choice for anyone who is considered high-risk. Women who are high-risk are those who have preexisting medical conditions, who had complications during previous pregnancies or have had complications during the current pregnancy.

Today's hospitals offer various options to provide families with labor experiences that meet their expectations.

Birthing rooms. Women used to labor in a pre-op room, give birth in a surgical suite, wake up in a recovery room, and then go to a maternity ward for their recuperation period. This traditional arrangement is still available in some hospitals, but increasingly more common are birthing rooms, referred to as LDRs (labor/delivery/recovery rooms) or LDRPs (labor/delivery/recovery/postpartum rooms).

Birthing rooms are typically decorated to resemble bedrooms rather than hospital rooms, but medical equipment is at hand should it be needed, and operating rooms for cesarean births are nearby. Labor and delivery take place in the same room, and the father or other labor companion is an integral part of the team.

If this arrangement is what you want, make sure the hospital you are considering has this option. A visit might be worthwhile (if your childbirth preparation class is at the hospital, a tour might be included in the curriculum). Don't be wowed, though, by superficial things such as the decor in the rooms. Ask about hospital policies concerning items in your birthing plan (a list of preferences you may have about medical procedures). (For more details on developing a birthing plan, see page 273.) Find out how many birthing rooms are available and what the alternatives are should they all be in use when you arrive.

Rooming-in. In an effort to create a more home-like atmosphere, some hospitals have introduced the rooming-in plan. Instead of being taken to a nursery, the baby stays with the mother virtually 24 hours a day. Family members are encouraged to care for the baby as soon as possible by holding, feeding, diapering and bathing.

Rooming-in is a good option for first-time parents, who can benefit from the guidance of experienced nurses during the hospital stay. However, the 24-hour-a-day responsibility can be overwhelming, especially if you've had a long and exhausting labor. For women who've had a cesarean birth, in particular, rooming-in can be difficult because you may not be able to get needed rest.

It's important to check ahead of time on the flexibility of your hospital's rooming-in policy, in case you change your mind during your hospital stay. Also find out what the rooming-in policy is regarding visitors.

Nursery. Some women, particularly those who have older children or other demands waiting for them when they get home, might choose to have their baby stay in the hospital nursery. They can still have the baby in the room as much as they want, but can return him or her to the nursery when they want to rest or entertain visitors. If they are not breastfeeding, they have the option of leaving the night feedings to the nurses.

If you decide it's best if your baby stays in the nursery, don't be worried that you're not spending enough time with your child. The two of you will still have plenty of time together, and this arrangement may give you a necessary chance to rest before you go home.

Mother-baby care. Another option in some hospitals is making the decision between rooming-in vs. the nursery unnecessary. It is called "mother-baby care." Instead of certain nurses looking after mothers and others responsible for babies in the nursery, a single nurse is assigned to each mother and baby as a unit. Whether the baby stays with the mother or goes to the nursery at night, the mother is encouraged to have the baby in the room during the day so that the nurse can teach baby care. Another name for this approach is family-centered maternity care.

Length of stay. In the past, long hospital stays were necessary because of widespread use of sedative medications during childbirth and the view that birth was a medical procedure. There was also an expectation among parents that the hospital stay after birth was a retreat, a time of recuperation before returning home. Today, postpartum stays of 24 hours are common after a vaginal birth, three to five days after a cesarean birth.

The following factors can affect length of stay:

- Mother's rate of recovery from labor and birth
- Success of infant feeding
- Accessibility of follow-up pediatric care
- Availability of help at home
- Extent of insurance coverage

If the mother's condition necessitates extended care, the baby is welcome also. However, if an infant is required to stay an extra day or two, whether the mother can stay as well depends on the hospital's policy. Some have "sleep-over" arrangements, at a reduced rate or even free, which allow use of the hospital room as long as the mother is responsible for her own meals and care. In addition, some hospitals have a room set aside for parents who are returning to bring home a baby who has required extended care. They can spend a couple of days learning to care for their baby, assisted by an experienced nurse.

Birthing Center

The idea of free-standing birthing centers developed as an alternative to hospital birth for women who couldn't afford the cost of high-tech medical care. The first one in the United States opened in 1944 in New Mexico. Now such facilities are growing in popularity as women have begun asking for more control over their birthing experiences. In 1991, nearly 15,000 women gave birth in birthing centers.

Birthing centers encourage natural childbirth. Their philosophy is that birth is not a medical procedure but rather a natural process. They usually are run by certified nurse-midwives, and may or may not be overseen by a physician. It's important, however, that they have backup arrangements with a hospital for access to obstetric skills and equipment in case of an emergency.

Women who choose birthing centers do so for various reasons. Those without insurance are attracted by the lower costs. Others prefer the less structured, more home-like atmosphere. Labor and birth occur in the same room, which often is decorated with plants, wallpaper and soft lighting. Entire families, including children, are encouraged to take an active part. Women go home as soon as they wish, usually several hours after delivery.

Birthing centers must screen pregnant women very carefully because they can handle only low-risk deliveries. Complications still occur, however, and if the doctor or midwife considers it necessary to get you to a hospital, you might be required to move to another facility altogether. Sometimes they move you "just in case."

If you are considering delivering at a birthing center, find out about its policies. Is there on-site medical backup in case you or your baby needs it? What determines whether you or your baby needs to be moved to the hospital? How far away is the hospital from the birthing center? Does the doctor or midwife accompany you, or are you assigned to a completely new team once you get there? How soon after birth will you be expected to leave? And will your insurance company cover the cost of care at a birthing center?

Home Birth

In some rural areas and religious communities, the practice of having babies at home is still popular. Today, home birthing also is a growing but controversial trend among women who can afford hospital care but choose not to deliver there. In the United States, more than 20,000 women a year are having their babies at home.

The advantages of home birth are obvious. The environment is familiar and comfortable. You can make your own decisions and give birth in your own way. The birth includes the entire family in its own home. The cost is minimal, involving only the fee for the doctor or midwife.

The disadvantages of home birth are what make it so controversial. If you require medical intervention you have to be moved to a hospital; one study showed this happened in 16 percent of cases, 2 percent of which were emergency transfers. Sometimes, emergency care is more complicated under circumstances where the woman hasn't seen a doctor for prenatal care.

Parents choosing home birth have added responsibilities. Many physicians will not attend home births because they believe their ability to give appropriate care is restricted and because they are not always covered by malpractice insurance if they aid in home births. The usual choices for caregivers are therefore certified nurse-midwives or lay midwives. Parent education, then, is even more vital than for other situations. Prenatal care, as well, is of the utmost importance; you must be carefully screened throughout your pregnancy for risks to you or the baby. Also, you must rely on your own methods of coping with pain.

Considering the availability of hospital birthing rooms, which provide most of the comforts of home, medication if desired and medical care to promptly respond to an emergency, home birth is usually not the best option.

Preparing Your Body and Mind

The prospect of pain during childbirth often raises the most looming questions for a woman during her first pregnancy: How bad will it be? How long will it last? How will I cope? Will I want medication? Will I lose control?

The pain of labor is different from anything you've ever felt, except perhaps menstrual cramps. "It feels like really, really bad cramps," said one woman. Another described it as "a belt around my lower abdomen, squeezing down and hurting." The sensation is a new one because for the first time your uterus is working really hard. All your life you've known what it feels like to contract your other body muscles, but this is the first time you're feeling your uterus powering up for a major effort. The contractions are involuntary; they begin on their own and continue, at their own pace, without any conscious input from you.

Medical relief of pain during childbirth first appeared in England when chloroform, quickly dubbed "the royal gas," was used by Queen Victoria. Scopolamine, morphine and ether followed, but while women's pain was lessened, infant mortality rose. Despite the risks, though, women were reluctant to give up the anesthetics and face pain again once they had experienced the alternative.

In the 1930s, Dr. Grantly Dick-Read, an English obstetrician, began educating women about what he called "natural childbirth." Dick-Read believed that pain is enhanced by fear and ignorance, and reduced by relaxation and knowledge. He described a fear-tension-pain cycle that could be broken if women were active participants during birth and practiced progressive relaxation techniques and breathing exercises.

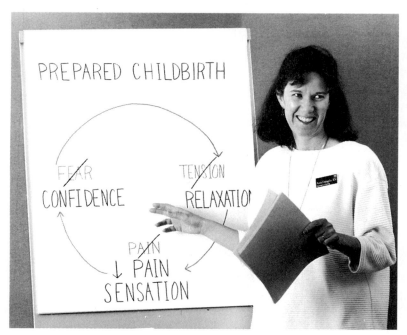

In childbirth education classes, you'll learn ways to deal with one of the most common fears of expectant mothers—pain of childbirth. You'll learn how fear can make you tense, and how tension and pain are related. You'll also receive practical tips on relaxation, breathing techniques and visualization skills that can help overcome or reduce pain.

But what really changed childbirth was the Lamaze method, which swept through the United States in the 1960s. Dr. Fernand Lamaze was a French obstetrician who also believed in the importance of education and training. He taught breathing, relaxation and massage techniques, but in addition he encouraged couples to work together as a team.

Dr. Robert Bradley of Colorado is known for having promoted husband-coached childbirth. For decades fathers had been excluded from the labor room, left to pace the hospital halls for hours while the mothers gave birth attended by strangers. Both Bradley and Lamaze believed that fathers who were present throughout labor and delivery could significantly reduce fear and pain.

While these "natural childbirth" methods were successful to a certain degree, they sometimes left women feeling they had failed if they couldn't make it through without pain medication. Today, women are realizing that childbirth is not a test you pass or fail. Each delivery is different, each person's needs unique. If medication can help you, that is only one of many choices you can make about your own birthing experience. And by learning techniques that will help you relax, you can minimize the amount of medication needed.

The philosophies of childbirth preparation classes vary, but they all have common elements. All involve education to reduce fear. All teach relaxation and breathing techniques to relieve tension and direct the woman's concentration away from her pain. All educate a partner to give the woman praise, support and accurate information on her progress. Studies show that these methods make the birthing process easier and shorten the length of labor.

Why Take Childbirth Education Classes?

Childbirth classes teach you what's happening to your body during pregnancy, labor and birth so that you feel positive rather than fearful. They also educate you about birthing options, birthing positions and developing a birthing plan. They offer a forum where you can share your concerns with other couples who are experiencing the same life event as you. You will talk about cesarean births, when and why they are done, who can be present, choice of anesthetic and emotional concerns. It is better to be prepared than taken by surprise.

When Should You Enroll?

First-trimester classes discuss topics such as nutrition and exercise, fetal development, effects of alcohol and cigarettes on the baby, and sexuality during pregnancy. Childbirth preparation classes usually start between the sixth and seventh months of pregnancy. Most are a couple hours per session and last six to eight weeks, although intense, all-day or weekend courses sometimes are available as an alternative. You take these with your chosen labor companion, and you should time your enrollment so that you finish your prepa-

rations at least a couple of weeks before your baby is due. If your baby is premature you may miss some of the classes, but if you begin too early you and
your partner probably won't be motivated enough to practice the techniques.

Classes usually are available through the hospital where you plan to deliver,
or your caregiver may refer you to a class. Check with your health-care provider
about where and how to enroll. Talk to friends about the classes they took, and
find out how they liked them. Then call the organizations that interest you.

Find out how long the classes have been running and what certification or
training the instructors have. Inquire about the course content to make sure
your needs will be covered. Find out how many couples will be in the
class—more than 10 or 12 will not allow for enough personal instruction.

In other words, make sure you are signing up for a legitimate, worthwhile
course led by experienced, well-trained professionals.

Other classes offer everything from preparation for breastfeeding and newborn care to sibling rivalry and becoming a grandparent. Some might cover subjects such as circumcision, tubal ligation while you are still in the hospital and
other issues that you should think about before the birth of your baby. Many of
these classes can be taken early in your pregnancy.

Facing Your Fears

All men and women have some fears as they head toward the birth experience.
The biggest fear is of the unknown. Even if a woman is delivering her fifth
baby, she knows that this experience will be different. Will my labor be long or
short, tolerable or terrible? Will I want epidural anesthesia? Will I need an
episiotomy? Will I tear? Will I need a cesarean section?

Talking about your fears can lighten an unnecessarily heavy emotional load.
Childbirth preparation classes give you a unique opportunity to share, because
the other couples there probably have the same worries and the instructor is
skilled at addressing them.

What if we don't make it to the hospital? Although first-time parents
commonly worry about the baby being born on the way to the hospital, this
rarely happens. It is of more concern to women who have already had a baby,
particularly if their labor went rapidly. In that case, the doctor might decide to
induce them a little early or will have them come in a few days before their due
date if they live far away. Although babies occasionally are born in cars, this is
rare, and the outcome usually is good.

If this fear continues to plague you despite knowing that it is a rare occurrence, discuss with your doctor the idea of coming to the hospital earlier in
labor—when your contractions are five to seven minutes apart, perhaps, rather
than the customary three to five.

I can't stand the thought of baring myself to strangers. Many
women worry about this, but few voice it. Childbirth instructors often show
videos of actual births, and some doctors have childbirth videos you can
watch in the office. These can be enormously helpful in getting you used to
what the process looks like. Birth is a messy experience: it would be impossible for a naked, wet baby to emerge from a dry, fully clothed mother. The
professionals in the room see this every day, so they aren't shocked by anything. A century or two ago you would have had your relatives and neighbors in the room instead!

What if I lose control in labor? Loss of control, to many people, means making noise. Some women have a big fear of making noise. But have you ever watched a pro tennis player grunt with each swing of her racquet? Have you heard Olympic weight lifters, with their neck veins bulging out, groaning with the strain? You hear those noises in basketball, in volleyball and in track and field. One man said, when his wife expressed embarrassment about her grunts, "I hear worse noises than that at the Y."

Birth is a physical, participatory event. "You don't just come in, take your pantyhose off and let the doctor deliver you of your baby," a childbirth educator tells her classes. "It's the athletic event of your year and you can't do it without your mascara running. It's exhausting and messy—and wonderful and awesome." It is labor.

This childbirth educator shows a movie that has birth noises. Afterward she gets down on the floor and shows everyone how to push the baby out. "I moan and groan and make birth noises," she says. "I'm old and I'm heavy and it's hysterical, but I use humor to show them that noise is a normal part of the birthing process."

The underlying fear of losing control is that your body is going to take you somewhere you're not sure you want to go, as though you're stepping on board a train whose speed and destination you can't control. The sensations of birth are sensations you've never felt before, and until you experience them you won't know how you'll respond. It's not a big deal to lose control, but it does waste energy. This is why you need to learn coping skills ahead of time that will help you refocus.

What if something happens to my wife? Women don't seem as concerned as men about the possibility of maternal death because their focus is on getting the baby out. But fear that the mother might die can be a big one for the labor companion, even though maternal death is extremely rare these days. Most men don't easily admit this type of concern to their partners. Nevertheless, the best remedy is to share the anxiety ahead of time. Who knows? She might be relieved to talk about it, too. And during labor, when the partner's fear can be compounded by a feeling of helplessness, the remedy is to get actively involved by participating in breathing, relaxation techniques and sensitive support.

What if something is wrong with the baby? Every pregnant woman worries about whether her baby will be perfect. That the baby might die is another universal fear. It sometimes manifests itself in dreams, which are common for both mothers and fathers toward the end of a pregnancy. One man dreamed that the first time he was caring for the baby alone, he "lost" the baby. His wife was due home and he was running all around their apartment, desperately trying to find the baby.

Sometimes babies are born with problems, and sometimes babies die (see page 391), but death occurs in only a small percentage of cases. The numbers are on your side.

Sit down and make a list of your fears. Share them with your labor companion. Prospective parents have the same concerns but are often reluctant to admit them, each thinking he or she must be stoic in order to prop up the other. Sharing helps. Share with each other, with the instructor and the other couples in your class and with your doctor. When you voice your fears they have less power over you.

The Value of Exercise

Just as important as fitness of mind is fitness of body. The value of exercise during pregnancy was discovered during the 1930s when a British study showed that working-class women had easier births than women in the upper classes who lived a sedentary lifestyle.

Many women today are physically active and remain so throughout their pregnancies. Those who do, and those who want to begin a conditioning program, should consult their doctors for recommendations (see page 108). Whether you carry on with your current fitness program or want to begin getting in shape by starting a walking program, you will be working toward a healthier body and, possibly, an easier birth.

When you are pregnant, many changes occur in your body. One change is that the ligaments in your joints relax, particularly in your pelvis, because of the increase in levels of estrogen and progesterone. You can take advantage of these changes by performing exercises that will make your body ready for labor. These exercises are often taught in childbirth classes, and they concentrate on the muscle groups receiving the most stress during the third trimester, labor and birth.

Tailor sitting. This exercise strengthens and stretches muscles in your back, thighs and pelvis and improves your posture. It can help keep your pelvic joints flexible, improve blood flow to your lower body and ease delivery.

Tailor sitting features outstretched knees with heels in toward your groin. If it's difficult for you, try using a wall to support your back, put cushions under each thigh or just sit with your legs crossed, changing the front leg occasionally. Keep your back straight.

You may be pleasantly surprised to find that the exercise is not as difficult in practice as it looks. Pregnancy tends to make your body a bit more supple.

Tailor Sitting. Sit on the floor with your back straight, the bottoms of your feet together and your knees dropped comfortably. You should feel a stretch in your inner thighs, but don't bounce your knees up and down rapidly.

Kegel exercises. The pelvic floor muscles help support the pelvic organs: the uterus, bladder and bowel. Toning them will ease the discomfort of late pregnancy, and also will minimize two common problems that can begin during pregnancy and continue afterward: leakage of urine and hemorrhoids. (The technique for Kegel exercises is explained on page 180.)

Squatting. Only in Western cultures did the flat-on-the-back position (doctors refer to it as "supine") become popular for birth. In other cultures, upright positions have always been preferred, and for good reason. The baby is lined up correctly for passage down the birth canal, and gravity might help the process along. Contractions are stronger, more efficient and less painful.

Sitting and squatting are beneficial because they open the pelvic outlet an extra quarter to half inch, allowing more room for the baby to descend. You will probably spend much of your time in labor walking and sitting. Squatting for a few minutes every so often will help open your pelvis. Sitting is easy enough, but squatting is tiring, so you should practice it frequently during pregnancy to strengthen the muscles needed. An exercise called a wall slide may be especially helpful.

Wall Slide. Position your feet about shoulder width apart and support your back against a wall. Slide your back down the wall until you are in a position similar to sitting on a chair (only there's no chair under you). Rest your hands on your thighs for better balance. Don't slide down far enough to let your knees extend over your toes. Keep your knees and feet pointing forward. Hold the position for a few seconds. Slide back up. Repeat the slide three to five times, working up gradually to 10 repetitions.

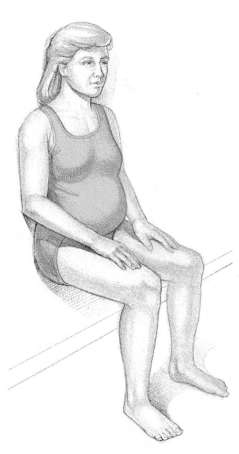

Pelvic tilt.

This exercise strengthens abdominal muscles, helps relieve backache during pregnancy and labor and eases delivery. It can also improve the flexibility of your back and ward off back pain.

As with tailor sitting, squatting and Kegel exercises, the pelvic tilt can yield considerable benefits with minimal effort. You can do pelvic tilts standing or sitting. The exercise requires no special equipment beyond reasonably comfortable clothes.

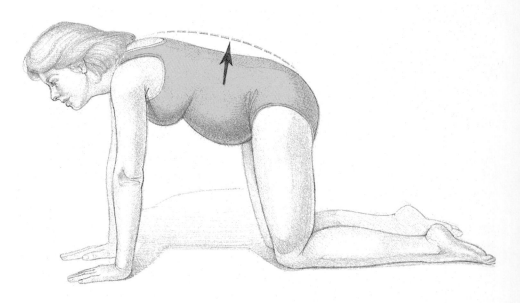

Pelvic Tilt. You can do pelvic tilt in various positions, but down on your hands and knees is one of the easiest ways to learn it. Rest comfortably on your hands and knees with your head in line with your back. Pull in your abdomen, arching your back upward. Hold the position for several seconds. Relax your abdomen and back, but keep your back flat (don't let your abdomen sag). Repeat three to five times, working up gradually to 10 repetitions.

Relaxation is the release of tension from the mind and body through conscious effort. It is the main ingredient of all childbirth education programs. By reducing muscle tension you short-circuit the fear-tension-pain cycle, allowing your body to work naturally. This means that you conserve energy for the labor ahead.

Relaxation doesn't mean fighting the pain, which would actually create more tension. It means allowing the pain to "roll over" you while you concentrate on tension-relieving and distracting exercises.

Relaxation is a learned skill, and one that must be practiced to be effective. The more proficient you become at it, the more self-confident you will be during labor.

Progressive relaxation. Beginning with your head or your feet, relax one muscle group at a time, moving toward the other end of your body. If you have trouble isolating the muscles, first tense each group for a few seconds, then release and feel the tension ebb away. Come back to your jaw now and then, because if your jaw is loose, you are too.

Touch relaxation. This is similar to progressive relaxation, but your cue for releasing each muscle group is when your partner presses, strokes or massages in tiny circles. He or she should apply pressure for five to 10 seconds, then move on to the next spot. Practice together until your response to the touch becomes automatic.

Relaxation Techniques

> ### Tips for mastering relaxation skills
>
> - Choose a quiet environment.
> - Turn on soft music, if desired.
> - Assume a comfortable position, with pillows to support you. Try a variety: sitting, semi-reclining, side-lying.
> - Use slow, deep abdominal breathing. Feel the coolness of the air as you breathe in, feel the tension carried away as you breathe out.
> - Become aware of areas of tension in your body and concentrate on relaxing them.
>
> With any of these techniques, the more you practice ahead of time, the better they will work when you really need them.

Tips for practicing touch relaxation skills:

- Pick a private, quiet place to practice touch relaxation. Ask your partner to begin at your head and work down.
- Temples: Press temples gently but firmly with fingertips.
- Base of skull: Press firmly with thumbs or fingertips on either side of the spine, just below the skull.
- Shoulders: Use firm fingertip pressure on top of the shoulders, midway between the neck and arms.
- Back: Rest hands on shoulder blades and move thumbs to either side of spine. Apply pressure for three to five seconds and then move thumbs down an inch. Repeat this step every inch to the level of the waist, then move outward, applying pressure every inch along the hip bones.
- Arms: Beginning at the shoulder, firmly press massage points that extend down the top of the arms to within about two inches of the wrists.
- Hands: Use thumbs to apply pressure to the three massage points on the palms of the hands—the center of the base of the hands (near the wrists), the center of the palms and the base of the middle finger.
- Legs: Apply thumb pressure in a firm, stroking action down the middle of the backs of the thighs and lower legs. Avoid pressure to the areas behind the knees.
- Feet: Apply firm pressure with the thumbs, beginning at the heel and moving toward the toes.

Not everyone likes to be touched during labor. If you don't want to be touched, your labor partner can still be involved by giving you verbal rather than tactile cues.

Massage. Massage helps muscles relax and causes the brain to release endorphins, which enhance the sense of well-being. Shoulder massage, sweeping strokes down the arms and legs and small circular movements on brow and temples all help relax muscles. Use oil or lotion, if you like, to reduce friction against the skin. Your partner can massage you while you are in practically any position: standing, sitting, kneeling or lying on your side.

Here are some common back massage techniques your partner might try:

- Begin on the lower back, with hands on either side of the spine, and slowly move up to the shoulders. Slide hands across the shoulders, then down along the sides of the back. Gradually increase pressure, at the direction of the recipient.
- Move your hands to the lower back. With fingers pointing outward and wrists about an inch apart, inhale. As you exhale, gently press down. Inhale again and move the hands slightly lower on the back; repeat, pressing with the exhale. Continue moving down the back.
- Place your thumbs about ½ inch to either side of the spine, at the small of the back. Press firmly, making small, slow, circular motions. Slowly move up the back to the neck. Then place your index fingers at either side of the spine and draw a firm line down the back to the buttocks. Repeat.
- To massage the neck and shoulders, rest your hands on the shoulders. Make circular motions (not squeezing or grasping motions) with the thumbs in the area between the upper back and lower neck. Then use gentle sweeping motions, hand over hand, from the arm to the neck.

Note: Moving your hands totally off and then back on the body may cause tension. Try to keep one hand resting on the mother, even while changing massage techniques or while reaching for more lotion.

Guided imagery. Used in other disciplines such as yoga and biofeedback, this technique allows you to create an environment that gives you a feeling of relaxation and well-being. It has been called "daydreaming with a purpose." We all have a special, peaceful place we can go in our imagination. Choose what makes you most relaxed: sit on a desert island, climb a mountain, watch a flower open. Your chosen place can be real or imaginary. Concentrate on details such as smells, colors or the wind against your skin. Feel your body growing heavier and enjoy the sensation. Sometimes you can enhance the imagery by playing tapes of surf, rain, waterfalls, birds in the woods or any soft music you enjoy.

Meditation. Focus on a single point. This can be something external in the room, such as a picture or a stuffed animal you have brought along, or it can be a mental image or a word you repeat to yourself over and over. When distracting thoughts come into your consciousness, allow them to pass by, without dwelling on them, and bring your focus back to your chosen focal point.

Nerves that transmit sensations of heat, cold and pressure fire faster than pain nerves, reaching the spinal column earlier and closing off the gateway that the pain impulses use. This mechanism stops or weakens sensations of pain. Many pain-blocking techniques are available, but you must change them every quarter to half hour to maintain their effectiveness.

Massage. In addition to encouraging relaxation (as described on page 270), massage blocks pain sensations. Some women feel most of the pain of labor in their backs, and for them a back massage given by the labor companion is particularly useful. It's not unusual for mothers to request that labor companions "push as hard as they can," because this counter-pressure can be especially effective during labor.

Heat or cold. Changes of temperature can block pain impulses and encourage relaxation. They can be applied in the form of ice packs, heat packs, warm showers or baths.

Sound. Music can focus your attention on something other than pain and help you relax. If you've been practicing breathing techniques or relaxation to music at home, bring the same tapes or compact discs with you to the hospital. Hearing them may help you relax automatically, and your perception of the pain will likely decrease. Many hospitals have cassette or compact disc players available; if not, bring your own. But if music doesn't work for you during labor, don't worry about it. Just as some women don't like to be touched during labor, others may not want the distraction of music to interrupt their concentration.

Pain-Blocking Techniques

Many relaxation exercises involve breathing techniques. This approach goes back to the old principle that if something hurts, think about something else to take your mind off it. By focusing on your breathing, your concentration is focused away from pain and anxiety. You relax, and so conserve energy. You feel in control.

Lamaze instructors teach expectant mothers to take a deep breath to begin and end each contraction. Inhale through your nose, imagining cool, pure air. Exhale slowly through your mouth, imagining tension blowing away. The deep breath signals to everyone in the room that a contraction is beginning or ending and is a cue for your body to relax.

Start with the first breathing technique and use it as long as it works for you, then move on to the next level.

Lamaze first level: slow-pace breathing. This is the type of breathing you use when you are relaxed or sleeping. Take in slow, deep breaths through your nose, and exhale through your mouth at about half the speed of your normal rate. If you like, repeat a phrase over and over with the breathing: "I am" (inhale) "relaxed" (exhale). Or count "In one-two-three, out one-two-three." Or breathe in rhythm with walking or rocking.

Lamaze second level: modified-pace breathing. Breathe faster than your normal rate but shallowly enough to prevent hyperventilation: "in one-two, out one-two, in one-two, out one-two." Keep your body, particularly

Breathing Techniques for Labor

your jaw, relaxed. Concentrate on the rhythm, which may be faster at the height of the contraction, then slower as it fades.

Lamaze third level: pattern-pace breathing. Use this type near the end of labor, or at the height of strong contractions. The rate is a little faster than normal, as with modified-pace breathing, but now you use a pant-blow rhythm, "ha-ha-ha-hoo" or "hee-hee-hee-hoo," that forces you to focus on the breathing rather than the pain. Repeat this pattern over and over again. Start out slowly, increase the speed as each contraction peaks, and decrease it as it fades. Keep in mind that when you increase the rate, the breathing should become shallower so that you don't hyperventilate—if your hands or feet tingle, slow down. There is some concern that hyperventilation can decrease oxygen supply to the baby. If moaning or making other noises helps, go ahead. Keep your eyes open and focused and your muscles relaxed.

Breathing to prevent pushing. If you feel the urge to push but the doctor says your cervix is not fully dilated and you must hold back, blow out tiny puffs with your cheeks until the urge to push passes.

Breathing for pushing. When your cervix is fully dilated and the doctor tells you to go ahead and push, it's time for your final effort. Relax your pelvis. Take a couple of deep breaths and bear down when you feel the urge, which may be overwhelming. Push for five or six seconds. Quickly exhale, then take in another breath and push again. Contractions at this stage will last for a minute or more, so it's important that you inhale at regular intervals and don't hold your breath. Your partner can keep time.

Pace-breathing techniques:

- Lessen fatigue and conserve energy
- Provide oxygen to your body and your baby
- Help you and your labor companion relax, remain calm and feel more "in control"
- Help reduce discomfort and pain

Your personal preferences and the nature of your contractions will guide you in deciding when to use pace-breathing patterns in your labor. Also, your nurses and doctor can help remind you to use breathing and relaxation techniques. Practicing these techniques helps you learn what you are comfortable with and what works best for you. It also increases your ability to use the techniques effectively in labor.

Unless you have a cesarean birth scheduled in advance, you will experience at least some labor. Even if you already know that you want epidural anesthesia, your cervix must be dilated 3 to 5 centimeters before it can be given, otherwise it is likely to slow down or even stop your progress. So it's still important to learn breathing and relaxation techniques.

Planning Labor Support

Bradley and Lamaze brought fathers back into the delivery room and made them a vital part of the team. Now female companions are coming back also. Some women choose a woman—mother, sister or friend—to be their primary labor companion, or to help the baby's father with his role.

Specially trained labor assistants, or doulas, are another option. These have been common in Europe for many years, but only recently have they become available in the United States. In some communities a doula can be hired to help with labor, either in the absence of a regular companion or as someone extra to serve as the mother's assistant. Some can be hired to help out at home, too, before or after the birth, when the new mother needs mothering herself. So far, only about 400 doulas are available in the United States, but their numbers are growing.

Whomever you choose as your birth partner, the presence and touch of a support person can have a dramatic effect. Women who have a partner experience less pain and fewer complications, use fewer medications and have shorter labors.

The role of your labor companion might be to:

- Provide emotional support. You'll want to be reassured of your partner's love. You'll need to be reminded that there's no pass or fail, just a wonderful prize for you both at the end of the journey.
- Go to classes with you, to learn relaxation and breathing techniques.
- Help decide when it's time to call the doctor and go to the hospital.
- Handle hospital admission procedures.
- Keep family and friends updated. Help provide the level of privacy you want.
- In the early stages, keep you supplied with liquids and ice, or light food if you're allowed it. Walk with you and keep you company.
- Serve as your labor coach by reminding you to breathe normally and use guided imagery.
- Assess your degree of relaxation and suggest new measures whenever the current one no longer is working. Help you to change positions often and encourage you to go to the bathroom hourly.
- Relieve physical discomfort with touch, massage, cold or heat. Even small things, such as lip ointment or a wet washcloth for your face, can help.
- Take pictures.

Developing a Birthing Plan

Many women are letting doctors know that they prefer "low-tech, high-touch care," as long as there is no risk to baby or mother. It is this desire that has led to recent changes in obstetrics.

There are many issues to discuss with your doctor if you want to make a birthing plan based on informed choices. Some women want a minimum of medical intervention; others choose some medical form of pain relief. Childbirth preparation classes can help you learn about the various options. (Read Chapters 17 and 18 for more detail about some of the procedures.) Talk with your doctor ahead of time, during some of your prenatal visits. But remember, this is a discussion, not an interrogation. The purpose is to promote understanding, develop trust and foster teamwork. Neither you nor the doctor should dictate ahead of time what has to be done, because you may not know what you want or what is needed until you are actually in labor.

Points for discussion when forming a birthing plan:

- Who will be allowed in the labor room? My chosen partner only, or family members, friends and my other children, if I so desire?
- Will I be free to make use of the hallways for walking during labor?
- Will I be allowed to eat and drink during labor?
- Is shaving pubic hair a standard procedure? If so, will it be total or partial?
- Is an enema required or an option?
- Do you use IVs (intravenous fluids) routinely, or only to accompany epidural anesthesia or in case of complications?
- Is artificial rupturing of membranes routine or done only when necessary to speed things up or when internal fetal monitoring must be done?
- Is continuous electronic fetal monitoring routine?
- What options for pain will be available?
- Under what conditions do you use medications to augment labor?
- Do you encourage mothers to give birth in positions other than the traditional one of lying on the back?
- Who cuts the umbilical cord? The doctor in all cases, or may my baby's father or I have the opportunity?
- Under what circumstances do you perform an episiotomy (a cut to enlarge the vaginal opening)?
- How long do mother and baby stay together after birth?
- Can I nurse my baby right away after birth?
- How often will I be able to see my baby? If I choose the nursery rather than rooming-in, may I see my baby whenever I wish, or do you have a schedule that must be followed?

The best advice for making a birthing plan is this: be realistic. Not all birthing plans work out, but most realistic ones do. For instance, declaring "I'm not going to use an anesthetic, regardless; I'm going to be natural the whole way" is not realistic because it's common to change your mind about what you want as things progress. A more rational plan would be this: "I'm going to try to avoid medication and procedures. If I run into trouble I'll consider some of the options I've already discussed with my doctor, maybe a narcotic or an epidural."

Being realistic means being flexible. Then you won't be disappointed if things don't go according to plan—and they rarely do. Most women giving birth for the first time don't have an accurate perception of what it will be like, and they think they're going to be in more control than they will be. They might be more concerned about peripheral things before labor than they will be while they are actually in labor. Or they may have unrealistic expectations of what they can do or of how they will compare to friends and relatives. These can set them up for a feeling of failure even before they've gotten started.

Also, not every labor goes according to plan because no labor is like any other. Even women who have given birth many times report that each experience was different. Variations in the position of the baby and the strength of the contractions are things over which you have no control.

Sometimes problems occur that nobody expected. That's when the medical staff needs to respond promptly. If that happens, remember that you chose your doctor because you trusted him or her. So let the doctor now take over. Your goal is bringing into the world a healthy baby. The details of how your baby gets here are not as important as that he or she gets here safely.

Control what you can and let go of what you can't. If you are prepared, educated and open-minded, if you regard your birthing plan as a guide rather than an ultimatum and if you build in plenty of flexibility, your labor and delivery can be a rewarding, exhilarating experience.

B ecause your baby's birth can come as many as several weeks before or after your due date, it is hard to schedule your life around it. You just have to prepare and then wait for the day to arrive. Three weeks before your due date is a good target for having the following plans in place.

Getting Ready for the Hospital

Pre-register. If you are planning to give birth in a hospital, inquire about advance registration. If you fill out paperwork and sort out insurance matters before the big day, when you arrive in labor you can go straight to your room.

Get an infant car seat. Some hospitals provide new parents with infant car seats for a nominal rental fee. If yours doesn't, research the various kinds and buy the one of your choice. Install it in the car or have it readily available for your coming-home day (see page 447). Car seats are required by law in every state.

Plan your departure. As your due date approaches, keep the gas tank full and make a practice run or two to the hospital or birthing center. Make arrangements for your other children, including an emergency plan for a friend or neighbor to help out in case you have to leave in the middle of the night or if someone from out of town hasn't yet arrived.

Pack a suitcase. If you don't want to put everything into it yet—your cosmetics, for example—make a list so that you can gather items easily when you prepare to leave. Normally, you don't have to rush (you might even have time to shower and do your hair and makeup before going to the hospital), but it's best to be organized. You can pack everything into one suitcase, or just take a small one for the labor and have someone bring you the other things later.

Leave your jewelry and other valuables at home, or send them home with your labor companion. If you are thinking about bringing your own nightgown for labor, be aware that it might get stains on it. You might want to wear a hospital gown instead.

Here's a checklist of things you might want to pack for use during the labor phase of your hospitalization:

- Bathrobe and slippers
- Warm socks (labor rooms are often kept cool)
- Lip salve (lips often become dry during breathing techniques)
- Hard candy to suck on
- Toiletries (for both mom and dad)
- Glasses (you may have to remove contact lenses)
- Reading material
- Tapes or compact discs, with a player if necessary
- This book
- Snacks for the birthing partner
- A watch for timing contractions, notepad and pencil
- Camera, with fresh batteries and plenty of film

- Video camera, with battery fully charged
- List of telephone numbers to call when the baby arrives
- Telephone credit card

For after you give birth:

- Pajamas or nightgown, with front openings if you plan to breastfeed
- Nursing bra if you plan to breastfeed
- Supportive bra if you plan to bottle feed
- Underwear
- Toiletries, cosmetics and hair dryer
- Address book
- Baby book
- Presents "from the baby" to your other children
- Small amount of money for snacks or for items you forgot to bring

For going home:

- Loose clothing (probably a mid-pregnancy maternity outfit)
- Baby outfit, including a hat
- Baby blanket
- Car seat for the baby

You're now ready. All that's left is your body's signal that it's time for your new baby to enter the world and join the family.

CHAPTER SEVENTEEN

Labor

Some women breeze right through to the end of pregnancy, whereas others become increasingly uncomfortable as the pregnancy progresses. For example, as your due date approaches, your sleep may be disturbed because you can't find a comfortable position, and once you do drift off your bladder may wake you. Or, after you return to bed, the baby may get the hiccups—which at least gives you reason to smile.

Time seems to stand still. You've packed your suitcase, set up the crib and laid out the baby clothes, and even though your due date has come and gone, still nothing happens. But remember, this calculated date is nothing more than an estimate of when your baby will be born. So, try to keep busy. Work as long as you can, indulge in a favorite hobby, read some good books and visit with friends and family. An active mind will help the days move along until the big day finally arrives and you're in labor!

How Labor Begins

Despite almost miraculous advances in modern medicine, no one knows exactly how labor begins. Certainly you have no say over when it starts, but somehow your body knows—accurately, most of the time—when your baby has matured enough to live outside your womb.

Our current understanding of how labor begins involves the chemical signals produced by your body, called prostaglandins, which shorten, soften and dilate your cervix. At term, something triggers your body to produce prostaglandins in large amounts, which cause the uterine contractions you may have felt throughout your pregnancy to become stronger. These contractions, in turn, cause even more production of prostaglandins, and the cycle accelerates into labor.

Whatever the cause, the grand finale to the nine long months of pregnancy finally begins. You're in labor.

Signs of Labor

On TV and in the movies, a pregnant woman may suddenly double over with a cry of pain. "The baby's coming!" she gasps, and everyone around her jumps into panicked action, as if the baby is about to drop onto the floor. In reality, this situation seldom occurs. Instead, more subtle signals herald the beginning of labor. You may have some or all of these signs and symptoms:

Lightening. As you approach your due date, you may feel that the baby has "dropped," settling deeper into your pelvis. This position lowers your center of gravity and relieves some of the pressure on your diaphragm. You feel lighter. You can breathe again. At the same time you may feel increased pressure on your bladder, which causes more trips to the bathroom. Lightening can occur weeks before the onset of labor, or anytime right up until the day labor begins. It may be noticeable enough that your friends comment on your changed appearance, or you might not be aware of it at all.

Effacement (ripening of the cervix). Your softening cervix prepares for birth by thinning, or effacing, going from an inch or more in thickness to paper thinness. However, you won't be aware of this thinning process unless your cervix is checked during a pelvic exam. Effacement is measured in percentages, and if your doctor says, "You are 50 percent effaced," it means your cervix is half its original thickness. When your cervix is 100 percent effaced, it is completely thinned out.

If you think of the cervix as the neck of a turtleneck sweater, you can visualize it stretching and pulling over the baby's head. The three insets show that during labor, the cervix progressively thins out (effacement) and opens (dilation) to allow the baby to pass through to the vagina. Doctors describe effacement in percentages of completion, and dilation in centimeters of openness.

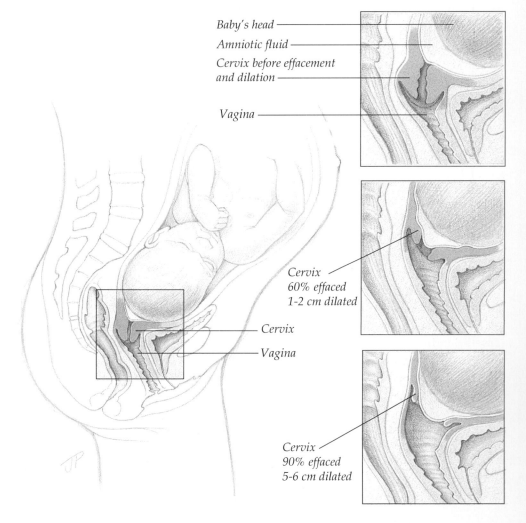

Baby's head
Amniotic fluid
Cervix before effacement and dilation
Vagina

Cervix
Vagina

*Cervix
60% effaced
1-2 cm dilated*

*Cervix
90% effaced
5-6 cm dilated*

Dilation (opening of the cervix). The doctor might also tell you that your cervix is beginning to open up, or dilate. With a first pregnancy, effacement usually begins before dilation; with subsequent pregnancies, the opposite is generally true. Dilation is measured in centimeters, the cervix opening from zero to 10 centimeters. The illustration below shows the actual sizes of different dilations.

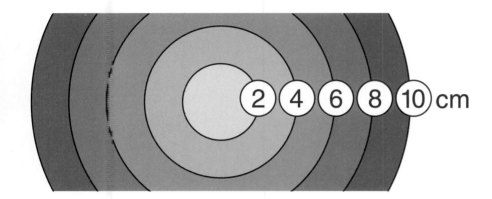

The cervix dilates (opens) gradually to approximately 10 centimeters. The doctor estimates dilation by feeling the opening cervix during a pelvic exam.

Bloody show (loss of mucus plug). During pregnancy, the cervical opening becomes blocked with a thick plug of mucus that prevents bacteria from entering the uterus. When the cervix begins to thin and relax, this plug is sometimes discharged, a sign that things could happen soon, although labor might still be up to a week away. The plug does not look like a cork, as some women expect, but more like stringy mucus or thick discharge. It can be clear, pink or blood-tinged and can appear minutes, hours or even days before actual labor begins. Some women, however, don't notice it at all.

Rupture of membranes (breaking of waters). Sometimes, the amniotic sac breaks or leaks before labor begins, and the fluid that has cushioned the baby comes out in a trickle or gush. In reality, only 10 percent of women experience such dramatic "breaking of the waters," and even then it usually happens at home, often in bed. (Some women, in preparation for this possibility, cover their mattresses with plastic.) Most frequently, however, your membranes rupture sometime during labor, often during the second stage.

Your doctor will probably discuss what you should do if your membranes rupture. Most doctors want to evaluate you and your baby as soon as the membranes rupture. There is a risk of infection if labor hasn't started within 24 hours. If more than 24 hours elapses, your doctor might intervene to help get your labor going. If you are uncertain about whether the leaking fluid is amniotic fluid or urine (many pregnant women leak urine in the later stages of pregnancy), be sure to have it checked. Meanwhile, don't do anything that could introduce bacteria into your vagina: no baths, tampons or sexual intercourse. Let your doctor know if the fluid is anything other than clear and odorless, particularly if it is greenish or foul-smelling, because this could be a sign of uterine infection.

Digestive disturbances. Many women experience diarrhea or nausea at the onset of labor. This is also probably another response to increased levels of prostaglandin.

Spurt of energy (nesting behavior). You might wake up one morning feeling energetic, raring to clean and anxious to do a million things you've been putting off. This behavior is commonly known as "nesting."

> *"I felt an overwhelming need to polish things. I had it in my head that I wouldn't have another chance for years, that it was now or never. I don't know what came over me—I even tackled some old brass planters that were stored in the basement."*

Even though the thought of coming home to a clean house may be tempting, try not to wear yourself out. You'll need your energy for the hard work ahead.

Contractions (labor pains). Although other signs may or may not indicate the beginning of labor, contractions are the real thing...or are they?

For some time you may have been aware of some occasional painless contractions. When you put your hands on your abdomen you can sometimes feel your uterus tighten and relax. Your uterus is warming up, exercising its muscle mass to build strength for the big job ahead. As you approach your due date, these contractions become stronger, even painful at times. It can be easy to mistake them for the real thing. How can you tell the difference?

How frequent are they? Using a watch or clock, measure the frequency of your contractions by timing them from the beginning of one to the beginning of the next. True labor will develop into a regular pattern, with contractions growing closer together, but in false labor they remain irregular.

How long does each one last? Measure the duration of each contraction by timing when it begins and when it stops. True contractions last about 15 to 30 seconds at the onset and get progressively longer (up to 60 seconds) and stronger. False labor contractions vary in length and intensity.

Are the contractions influenced by your activity? The contractions in true labor won't go away regardless of activity and may grow stronger with increased activity such as walking. False labor will often stop regardless of activity.

Where do you feel the contractions? In true labor the pain tends to be high up on your abdomen, radiating throughout your abdomen and lower back. In false labor the contractions are often concentrated in the lower abdomen and groin.

Even after trying to monitor all these signs of labor, you may not know whether you are truly in labor. Some women have painful contractions for days with no cervical changes, whereas others may feel only a little pressure and backache. Sometimes a woman may even discount what she's feeling because her due date is weeks away, and then when she comes in for her regular check-up finds she is almost fully dilated!

You might leave for the hospital with regular contractions that are three minutes apart, and after you arrive, they simply stop. If this happens, try not to feel embarrassed or frustrated. Instead, think positively and regard it as a good practice run. The scenario is different for everyone. If in doubt, call your doctor, because sometimes the only way to be sure is to have a vaginal exam to assess whether your cervix is dilating.

Remember, though, if your contractions continue to get longer, stronger and closer together, you're on your way!

The Hospital

Instructions regarding when to go to the hospital after the onset of labor vary from doctor to doctor. One might tell you to wait until your contractions are three to five minutes apart for a period of one hour, another might tell you to come in when you can no longer walk or talk through them and a third might have you wait until the pain moves from low down in the front of your abdomen to higher up, above the navel. Your doctor will individualize the instructions for each of your pregnancies. All doctors agree, however, that if you're unsure or anxious, you should go to the hospital for evaluation.

If your labor seems to be progressing very rapidly, you should go to the hospital sooner rather than later. Some of the impending signs of a rapid, or precipitous, delivery are frequent contractions and a history of fast labor; you may also have a rapid delivery if your baby is smaller than average.

Listed below are other important signs that require immediate medical attention.

Preterm labor—If you are having contractions or have a sudden release of fluid from your vagina three or more weeks before your due date, you should seek medical attention because you could be in preterm labor. Remember, you may not experience contractions even if your water has broken.

Vaginal bleeding—Bright red bleeding at any time during your pregnancy demands immediate attention. It could be a sign of a serious problem such as an abruption, which occurs when the placenta separates from the uterine wall, or placenta previa, in which the placenta partially or completely covers the inside opening of the cervix and tears away from the cervix as the uterus expands. Both of these conditions are medical emergencies. At times, however, especially after a recent pelvic exam, you may notice some scant blood mixed with mucus. This is normal and should not be cause for alarm.

Constant, severe abdominal pain—Although uncommon, this can be another indication of placental separation. In combination with a fever and vaginal discharge, it may also signal an infection. If you have these symptoms, call your doctor immediately.

Umbilical cord prolapse—A rare but dangerous situation can occur after the bag of waters has broken. It's possible that a loop of umbilical cord can slip through the opening cervix and protrude from the vagina before the baby is born. As the baby presses against the cervix, the pressure on the cord can block the baby's blood supply. This situation is an emergency. Call an ambulance, and do not attempt to push the cord back in. Instead, immediately get on your hands and knees with your chest lowered to the floor and your bottom in the air. Gravity will help keep the baby from pressing against the cord. If possible, have someone place a warm wet cloth over the cord to keep it warm and moist.

Decreased fetal movement—A baby's activity level often slows during the last few days before birth. It's almost as if the baby is resting, storing energy for the big day. But a baby might also move less when something is wrong. If you are worried about your baby's decreased movement, don't hesitate to call your doctor. The use of a fetal activity chart is becoming increasingly common to track your baby's movements throughout the last few weeks of pregnancy.

Admission Procedures

Because admission procedures can be time-consuming, pre-registering before you go into labor can greatly cut down on how long it takes to be admitted to the hospital. If you want to become more familiar with the hospital you'll be in during your childbirth experience, many hospitals offer tours of the labor rooms, delivery rooms and postpartum units either during childbirth classes or at other designated times. Your doctor or childbirth educator will tell you where to check in on your arrival. From there you will be taken to your room, often a labor room, where the admission procedures will be completed and you'll have a chance to get settled.

Review of records. If your medical records are filed at an office that is separate from the hospital, they will probably have been sent to the hospital as you neared term. Your records will inform the hospital staff of the particulars of your pregnancy as soon as you are admitted.

Vital signs. Your pulse, blood pressure and temperature will be taken on admission and at intervals throughout your labor and delivery.

Lab tests. Lab work is tailored to each particular pregnancy. Some of the more commonly ordered tests are a CBC (complete blood cell count), which screens for anemia, a condition in which iron reserves in the blood are low; a urinalysis, which can help detect the condition of preeclampsia (see page 192); and a cervical culture, which may detect infection, sometimes related to prematurely ruptured membranes.

Vaginal exam. Effacement and dilation of your cervix will be assessed through vaginal exams. The "presenting part," or the part of the baby pressing against the cervix, can also be determined through a vaginal exam. When the head is the presenting part, as is most commonly the case, it is said to be a vertex presentation. When the baby's bottom is the presenting part, it is a breech presentation. Exams at various stages of labor will monitor your progress. If you have had prolonged ruptured membranes, you may have fewer vaginal exams to decrease the risk of infection.

Enemas. In the past, it was the norm for a woman to have an enema when she went into labor, the theory being that emptying the bowel reduced the risk of infection to mother and baby and stimulated stronger contractions. The bowel usually will empty without intervention during the course of labor, and occasionally a small amount of stool is expelled during the birth. This is perfectly normal and nothing to be worried about.

Shaving. Shaving the entire pubic area also used to be standard practice, to prepare a clean site for an episiotomy. The procedure was then reduced to a partial prep—shaving just the perineum (the area between the vagina and anus)—to remove hair from the episiotomy site. Now it is known that hair doesn't contribute to infection, so even partial shaving is being phased out.

Notifying friends and relatives

When you first suspect you're in labor you're bound to be excited. You may even want to call everyone and tell them that this is the day! But what if it's a false alarm? It's probably better to wait to make your calls until you know for sure that you're in labor.

As you consider those who need to be notified when you go to the hospital, be sure to include those responsible for the care of your other children, persons who will care for any pets you may have and the appropriate people from your workplace.

Labor doesn't really start until the cervix begins to dilate. It's possible to have contractions for hours before you are actually "in labor." The average duration of labor is about 14 hours, but because every labor is unique, it could take less than six hours or up to 24 or more. Even though every labor is different, the sequence of events remains the same.

Course of Events

Effacement. The cervix may begin thinning days ahead of labor or not until the first contractions have begun. If this is your first baby, effacement is more likely to occur before labor begins.

Dilation. The contractions gradually dilate the cervix until it is wide enough—10 centimeters (4 inches)—for the baby to pass through.

Engagement. When the largest diameter of the baby's head has moved into the midpelvis, it is said to be engaged. The baby can settle in this position as early as a couple of weeks before term (lightening) or not until labor has begun.

Stages. Labor is divided into three stages:

- First stage: early and active labor. The cervix opens so the baby can leave the uterus.
- Second stage: the actual birth. Working along with your contractions, the baby is pushed out through your expanding vagina.
- Third stage: the placenta detaches from the wall of the uterus and is expelled through the vagina.

This chapter deals with only the first stage of labor. The second and third stages are discussed in the next chapter.

A multitude of factors can affect how your labor will progress. The infinite combinations of these factors make each labor unique.

Factors That Affect Labor

Size of the baby's head. Because the bones of the cranium, or skull, are not yet fused together, the baby's head molds itself to the shape and size of the mother's pelvis as it moves through the birth canal. If the head moves through at an awkward angle, it can affect the location and intensity of the mother's discomfort and also the length of labor.

Position of the baby. Birth is easiest if the baby comes head first through the birth canal, with its chin tucked down on the chest so that the smallest diameter leads the way. But babies aren't always so accommodating; sometimes their heads aren't in the best position, and sometimes they are breech, with their buttocks or feet coming first. They may even lie sideways in the uterus (transverse lie) or come shoulder first. (For more information on the positions the baby can be in, see page 317.)

Shape and diameter of the mother's pelvis. The pelvis has a rather complex shape. In assessing the pelvis for childbirth, three measurements are important: the inlet, or top; the midpelvis; and the outlet, or bottom. All three diameters must be wide enough to accommodate the baby's head as it passes through. The hormone relaxin, produced by the placenta, relaxes the binding ligaments that hold the three pelvic bones together, allowing the pelvis to open wider. This widening, along with the molding of the baby's skull, usually allows the head enough room to move through the pelvis. This relaxing effect of the ligaments also contributes to the "clumsiness" you may feel or the "waddling" gait you might have during pregnancy.

Ability of the cervix to efface and dilate. In rare cases, the cervix may be unable to efface and dilate. But for the vast majority of labors, the cervix opens as expected.

Ability for effective pushing. Because a woman uses her abdominal muscles to help push the baby out, the better physical shape she's in, the more she can assist. However, if she's had a long labor and is tired, her pushing may be less effective.

Mother's physical state. If a mother is well rested when she goes into active labor, she has more strength to work with her contractions. If she is ill or tired when she goes into labor, or if the early phases of labor are particularly long, she may enter the active phase already exhausted. This can affect how well she copes with pain and may diminish her ability to concentrate on relaxation.

Mother's mental preparation. A mother who has a positive outlook, who knows generally what to expect, who has trust in her medical team and who has thought through the choices available to her will be ready to take an active part in labor. Those who are frightened, anxious and know little about labor and birth will have a harder time. Stress starts in motion a whole range of physiological reactions that can ultimately interfere with labor.

Support from staff and birth partner. Medical personnel and labor partners work together as a team to help a mother stay relaxed during her labor. Through their support and presence, they can enhance the coping skills necessary for labor and birth.

Medication. Certain medications for pain relief can both help and hinder labor. Some obstetricians believe that if medications relieve pain early on, they can leave a woman rested and better equipped for the hard work ahead, and if they help her relax, she can concentrate on getting the baby out. If, however, they slow down labor or interfere with her ability to push, they can undo some of their usefulness. The key is to find a balance, to relieve pain without hindering birth. Medications should be used only when needed and only with very close observation by experienced nurses and physicians.

First-Stage Labor

The first stage of labor takes the longest because the cervical opening must stretch from being closed to being "complete," or 10 centimeters (4 inches) in diameter. For first deliveries the average duration is about 12 hours, and for subsequent deliveries about half that time. But "average" is approximate, and each pregnancy is unique. First-stage labor is divided into three phases: early (latent) labor, active labor and transition.

Early Labor

"As I was reading in bed that night, I was aware of some mild contractions but turned the light out and went to sleep. Only a couple of hours went by before I woke up. 'This might be it,' I told my husband. We seemed to have plenty of time, so I showered and put on makeup. At four in the morning I was blow-drying my hair. I suppose that sounds silly, especially when I knew I wouldn't be too glamorous later on, but I at least wanted to start out looking as clean and attractive as possible."

Contractions. During this early phase of labor, contractions may vary tremendously from woman to woman. For some, they might last about 15 to 30 seconds at the beginning and be irregularly spaced, perhaps 15 to 30 minutes apart. For others, they may start out fast and then slow down. But the frequency and intensity continue to increase as the cervix dilates to about 3 or 4 centimeters (1½ inches). By that time, contractions often last 30 to 40 seconds, occur every three to five minutes and take on a more regular pattern.

Pain. The pain felt during this early phase is caused by uterine contractions and cervical dilation. It's been described as an aching feeling, pressure, fullness, cramping and backache. In addition, it's not uncommon to have loose stools during this phase, which may be nature's way of emptying your bowel to give the baby more room to move down the birth canal.

Activity. Some medical personnel humorously refer to the early phase as the "entertainment phase." You may feel like watching TV or videos, playing games or making phone calls. Many women prefer to remain at home during this time to rest and nap, while they still can, to conserve energy for the work ahead. Choose activities you find most comfortable. You may want to relax in a chair or get up and move around. Walking is a great activity because it may actually help your labor along.

"I tried to sleep, but I was too excited. I got out of bed around 2:00 a.m., folded laundry, washed dishes, read my childbirth book. I hit the shower about 4:00 a.m., and called the doctor around 5:30. and then we headed in. We stopped by my mom's first to drop off the keys, and I had to get out of the car and pace."

Keep up your fluid intake, but restrict what you eat to easily digestible foods: toast, fruit and other carbohydrates, rather than meats and fatty foods, because digestion slows down during labor.

Emotions. As the first contractions begin, you may be giddy with excitement and full of relief that after nine long months of waiting your baby is soon to be born. At the same time, though, you may be scared about the unknown.

Early labor—tips for the labor companion

"What's this really going to be like?" "What's my role?" "What am I supposed to be doing?" "I can't remember a thing they told me in class!"

These thoughts, more than thoughts of babies, may be running through your head during the early phase of labor. You may be more apprehensive than your partner, worrying more about her well-being and whether you will be a good support for her.

You can help in early labor by:

- Timing contractions
    (Frequency is measured from the beginning of one to the beginning of the next.)
    (Duration is measured from the beginning to the end of one contraction.)
- Encouraging activities such as walking
- Practicing relaxation techniques during early contractions
- Supporting and affirming your partner

Duration of early labor. Eight hours is the average length of early labor for first babies, and five hours is the average for subsequent births. Any length of time between one and 20 hours is considered normal.

Active Labor: When the Work Begins

Contractions. For the cervix to dilate to about 7 centimeters (2.8 inches), contractions must grow stronger and progressively longer—going from 45 seconds to a minute in length. They also begin to occur closer together. At the onset of active labor, contractions may be about five minutes apart, but as labor progresses they change to two- to three-minute intervals.

Pain. "It felt like a tight belt around my lower abdomen," said one woman. During active labor, you may have a tightening feeling in your pubic area and increasing pressure in your back. When the discomfort reaches this level, the breathing techniques used in combination with the relaxation and concentration exercises taught in childbirth preparation classes may be very beneficial. Also, pain medication is often requested during active labor, and if an epidural anesthetic is chosen, it is usually placed at this phase. In addition to pain, common symptoms as you approach the end of active labor are nausea and loose stools.

Activity. Between contractions, you will still be able to talk, listen to music or watch TV, at least during the early part of the process. If walking feels comfortable, continue with it, stopping to breathe through contractions. Walking may even help your labor progress because of the motion and the influence of gravity. Some women find that as the pain intensifies, rocking in a rocking chair or taking a warm shower helps them relax between contractions. Emptying your bladder every hour or so is important during this stage. It is often difficult to feel the urge to urinate, even with a full bladder, because of the pressure from the descending baby.

Once you're in the hospital you may be asked to stop eating altogether and to drink only clear liquids. Withholding food and liquids from women in labor began in the 1940s, when general anesthesia was commonly used for cesarean and difficult births. The anesthetic can cause nausea, and if one vomits while unconscious, food particles can obstruct breathing or inhaled gastric acid can cause a dangerous form of pneumonia.

Now that general anesthesia is less commonly used, eating isn't quite the concern it used to be. Still, there's a chance that anything you eat will come back up again during active labor. You may want to avoid this possibility by keeping what you eat to a minimum. Many doctors still prefer that you don't eat or drink anything in case you require general anesthesia on short notice. The hospital personnel will inform you of your doctor's recommendations. To keep your mouth and throat from becoming dry, you can suck on ice chips, ice pops or hard candy. Applying lip balm or petroleum jelly to your lips can help keep them moist.

Emotions. The initial excitement of early labor gives way to seriousness as labor progresses and the pain intensifies. Your smile fades. You may become inwardly focused, highly sensitive and irritable.

Active labor—tips for the labor companion

During this intense time, labor companions may feel increasingly helpless. You may try to be supportive and helpful, using massage and relaxation techniques learned in class, and end up on the receiving end of an outburst. "Don't touch me!" and "Leave me alone!" could be the messages during one contraction and "Rub harder!" "Don't leave me!" during the next. It can be difficult to know when to lead and when to follow. The important thing is to see it through; your physical presence is what counts. If you become too frustrated, however, or physically exhausted, it may be important to ask for help so you can take a break.

Encourage and praise her

"You did a great job with that contraction!"

Accept her irritability without taking it personally

Remind her to:
- Relax between contractions and to take each contraction one at a time
- Empty her bladder every one to two hours
- Change positions frequently, discourage her from lying flat on her back

Provide:
- A calm, quiet environment
- Lip balm for dry lips
- Ice chips, mouthwash and hard candy for dry mouth
- Cold washcloth for face, arms, legs, back
  (keep two or three washcloths in a basin filled with ice water)
- Socks for cold feet
- Small paper bag as needed for hyperventilation
- Touch relaxation for relief of tension
- Massage and back rubs as needed
  (use counterpressure with the heel of your hand or tennis balls for back labor)

How to recognize relaxation:
- Look at her forehead—Is it smooth or furrowed?
- Look at her eyes—Are they calm or panicked?
- Look at her jaw—Is it slack or are her teeth clenched?
- Look at her hands and feet—Are they loose or tensed?
- Listen to her breathing—Is it rhythmically paced or strained and uneven?

When you're encouraging your partner to relax, use additional descriptions such as:
- "Let your muscles go limp."
- "Let go of your tension."
- "Loosen up your hands, jaw, etc."
- "Allow your body to melt between contractions."

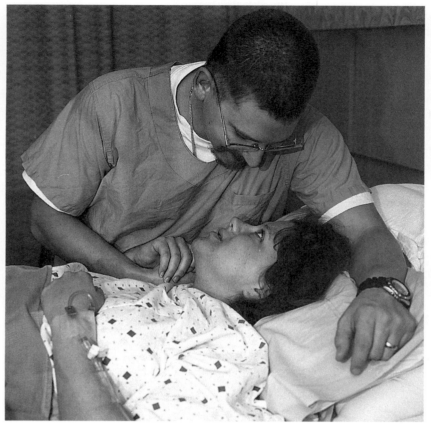

As the tone in the room changes, you may begin to realize the importance of your childbirth classes and that you may actually need to use the breathing and relaxation techniques to get through your contractions. "Am I really going to be able to do this?" you may wonder. "I thought I was ready, but now I'm not so sure. It's more work than I thought it was going to be. Can we stop now?"

You might withdraw within yourself to find the strength to deal with what your body is going through. You may even need to have the room quiet and the lights dimmed so that you are totally free to concentrate on the job at hand.

"For me, this was a time to turn off the TV and put on some relaxing music, although I got to the point where I didn't even want the music. Everything seemed to irritate me."

You've been sharing this pregnancy. Now, your partnership takes on another dimension, that of you providing the support and comfort she needs during labor.

During active labor, many women become more reliant on their labor companions. But others may resist relying on their labor companions in an attempt to stay "in control."

Duration of active phase. For most women, the active phase of labor lasts about half as long as the time spent in early labor. Four hours is considered average.

The Transition Phase: Difficult but Brief

The most difficult phase of labor is transition. But fortunately, it's also the shortest, often lasting less than 30 minutes. It's during transition that the cervix stretches open those last few centimeters, dilating from 7 to 10 centimeters.

How do you know when you're in transition? Sometimes, doctors and nurses can tell that a woman is in transition simply by noting the changing character of her contractions and her reaction to them. For other women, the changes are more subtle, and they gradually intensify.

Contractions. Your contractions during transition increase in strength and frequency, with little reprieve between them. There may be time for only a hurried breath before the next one hits. Maximal intensity is reached almost immediately, and contractions now last up to 60 seconds. The best way to make it through transition is to let your uterus do its work and not fight it. Concentrate on getting through just the first half of each contraction; after it peaks, the second half is easier. If your contractions are being monitored, your labor companion can watch their progress, letting you know when they've peaked, so you know the hardest part is over.

If you feel the urge to push, try to hold back until you've been told you're fully dilated, to prevent your cervix from tearing or becoming swollen. Resisting this sensation can be difficult when your body is telling you to bear down, but using a puff-breath breathing pattern can help decrease this strong urge. (See page 271 for a description of breathing techniques.)

Pain. The birth canal is beginning to stretch and hurt now, and the pain may be intense. You may feel nauseated and even vomit, or you may get the hiccups. If your legs begin to shake or cramp, change position or have your partner massage them. If you haven't had any medication for pain relief, your discomfort will probably be at its maximal intensity.

Remember, the pain of contractions is a sign that your body is working as it was designed to. The hardest part of transition is to concentrate on allowing your uterus to do its job while letting the rest of your body remain as relaxed as possible.

Activity. During transition, every bit of concentration needs to be focused on making it through each contraction. You may not want anything distracting you such as radio or TV. Changing positions, a cool cloth placed on the forehead, massage between contractions, and breathing, relaxation and focusing techniques learned in class can be important tools for making it through this challenging phase. Don't think about the contraction you just had or the contractions to come, just take each one as it comes.

Emotions. For some women, transition goes quickly, and they're suddenly past it and ready to push. But others may feel if they had a choice they'd rather pack up and leave town on the next bus. You may be tired, fed up, scared and discouraged; you may even become angry—at the pain, your partner or your doctor. "How long is this going to go on?" you may want to know. You might even lose sight of why you're really there.

This combination of pain and fear can make you feel out of control, and you may end up thinking there's nothing that can stop the pain and that your baby is never going to be born. Also, the intense pressure and stretching in combination with the discomfort of contractions can be very frightening, and in your innermost thoughts you may think that there's a possibility you could even die. You might cry, "I can't take this anymore!" But remember, your body was designed to give birth, and you are capable of making it through this tough time.

At this point, the medical staff may discourage you from having intravenous pain medication, because it could slow down labor and possibly affect your baby's breathing once he or she is born. It may still be possible for an epidural or spinal anesthetic. Trust the staff to help you make decisions about pain medication, and remember to try to stay focused on making it through each contraction, taking each one as it comes.

As difficult as transition can be, remember that it means you're almost finished. Soon it will be time to push!

Duration of transition. The average length of time for transition is about 30 to 90 minutes.

Transition—tips for the labor companion

Transition is not only the hardest time for the mother but also the greatest challenge for the labor companion. Contractions are relentless, and your presence is of utmost importance despite what she may say or how she may act. Breathing with her, helping her focus and giving her constant reassurance that she's doing a good job will help her through this time of transition. Keep in mind, however, that when asked what the most important role of the labor companion was during labor, most mothers say that the partner's physical presence was more important than anything.

- Remind her that this is the shortest part of labor and to take one contraction at a time.
- Because your voice is familiar, she may listen better to instructions from you. A firm, positive voice can give her confidence.
- Ask what you can do to help. Never criticize.
- If she is having difficulty staying focused, try taking her face in your hands and making direct eye contact. If necessary, tell her to open her eyes and to look at you.
- Breathe with her, maintaining eye contact.
- Talk to her between contractions; tell her she's doing a good job.
- If she tells you to leave her alone, respect her wishes. But stay close by.
- Don't take everything she says personally. She is likely to say things she doesn't mean and won't even remember later on.
- Try distractions such as massage or music, but don't be surprised if she rejects them. The same things that may be of help to her at one moment may irritate her at another.
- Suggest a position change.
- Remember to ask the staff for help and ideas.
- Don't give up on her. Your confidence and strength will give her confidence and strength.
- Remind her that this is pain with a purpose, and that she will have a baby to show for her hard work.

Medical Intervention

Today's technology allows for successful pregnancy outcomes that in your grandmother's and great-grandmother's eras would not have been possible. There are medications to help stop premature labor, surgical techniques to assist in difficult deliveries and many medical interventions that can aid in the healthy and safe care of mothers and their unborn babies.

Despite the best-laid plans and preparation for your pregnancy and labor, medical intervention is sometimes needed. Your pregnancy may be going along in textbook fashion when suddenly an unexpected problem develops. In addition, there are interventions that are commonly and consistently used, depending on your physician and the hospital you're in. It's important to be familiar with some of these interventions because even though you may never have need of most of them, being knowledgeable about them and knowing that their use is for the well-being of you and your baby can be comforting.

"I see myself as an insurance provider, " explains one obstetrician. "If things go well, I'm hardly needed; but if there's trouble, I can step in and help." When your welfare and that of your baby are at stake, it is good to know that the medical staff has the tools and expertise to help.

Some of the interventions used most commonly during labor and birth are described on the following pages.

It is common for a woman in labor to have an IV (short for "intravenous," or "within the vein") placed into a vein, usually on the back of her hand or arm. When an IV is used, a needle is inserted into a vein and is attached, by means of a plastic tube, to a bag holding fluid that slowly drips into your body. This fluid helps keep you hydrated throughout your labor and assures access for the administration of medications, if they are needed. Many doctors routinely request an IV. This is a topic you may want to discuss with your physician, keeping in mind that the circumstances of your particular labor will influence the doctor's decision.

IV's

Advantages

- Labor is hard physical work, and, as in any exercise, your need for fluids increases. If you are unable to take fluids or to keep them down, an IV will help keep you hydrated.
- Access is available for the administration of medications such as oxytocin, which helps stimulate contractions.
- If you want a narcotic for pain relief, it is more comfortable and effective to receive it through the IV than through injection into a muscle.
- In an emergency, access is available for the administration of anesthetics, life-supporting medications or blood transfusions.

Concerns

- You may experience minor discomfort during insertion of the needle, although more and more frequently an injection is given at the insertion site to numb the area.
- Movement and activity are limited by the IV pole and tubing; however, the availability of a heparin lock has created more freedom of movement. A heparin lock is a short piece of tubing connected to the IV needle; the lock is injected periodically with heparin to prevent the IV needle from clotting. If you don't need continuous IV fluid, a heparin lock can be used instead of a regular IV setup to provide access to the vein, should the need arise. Use of a heparin lock should be discussed with your doctor before labor
- Changing positions can be cumbersome.

To induce labor means to give it an artificial start, through medical interventions. The decision to induce is made because of concerns for the mother or baby or when contractions have not yet begun on their own and the baby is ready to be born. To augment labor means to speed up labor when it is progressing so slowly that problems might arise for the mother or baby. It is necessary for the cervix to be "ripe," or soft, as determined through a vaginal exam, before the induction can occur.

Induced and Augmented Labor

Possible reasons for inducing labor

- Membranes have ruptured but labor hasn't started
- Rh complications (isoimmunization)
- Infection inside the uterus (chorioamnionitis)
- Baby is small for gestational age (fetal growth retardation)
- Baby is past term (more than 42 weeks of gestation)

- Decrease in amniotic fluid
- Development of complications, such as high blood pressure and preeclampsia, that could lead to eclampsia
- Complications of existing maternal medical problems, such as kidney or lung disease or diabetes

Because induction is not always effective, there is a possibility that you will be sent home. Your doctor may want you to return later to attempt the induction again.

Methods of inducing or augmenting labor. There are three ways to induce or augment labor: nipple stimulation, artificial rupture of membranes, and administration of oxytocin.

Nipple stimulation. This natural form of inducing labor goes back centuries in many parts of the world. In the United States, however, it is less commonly used, especially in more traditional medical settings. Nipple stimulation can be done manually or with an electric breastfeeding pump. The concept is the same as what happens when a baby nurses right after birth, stimulating contractions, which in turn clamp down the uterus to help stop bleeding. The naturally occurring hormone oxytocin is responsible for causing the uterine contractions. Drawbacks to this method include a mother's feelings of modesty and lack of control over the intended effects.

Artificial rupture of membranes (amniotomy). When the bag of waters (amniotic sac) breaks or ruptures, production of the hormone prostaglandin increases, speeding up contractions. Sometimes a doctor may choose to rupture the amniotic membrane artificially. This membrane, with a bulge of fluid behind it, precedes the baby's head through the open cervix. The doctor guides a sterile tool, which resembles a long crochet hook, into the sac and painlessly withdraws it, leaving a tear. This procedure, which feels much like a vaginal exam, releases a gush of warm amniotic fluid from the vagina. Doctors vary widely on its use, some allowing the rupture of membranes to occur naturally, usually during the second stage of labor. Others routinely rupture the membranes early in labor to get

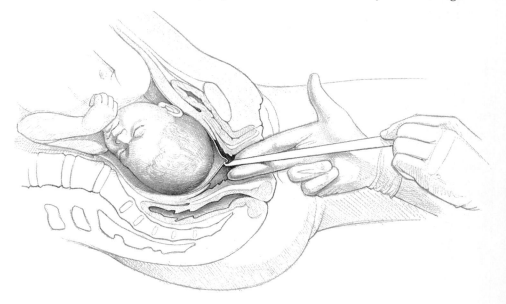

Artificially rupturing the membranes of the amniotic sac can sometimes start or speed up contractions.

contractions going and shorten the first stage. Rupturing the membranes can also be done later in the first stage if labor is progressing slowly.

Advantages

- Labor may be shortened by about an hour.
- The procedure allows for the amniotic fluid to be examined for the presence of meconium, which may be a sign of fetal distress.
- With direct access to the baby's scalp, the doctor is able to attach a fetal scalp monitor to measure the baby's heart rate or, if necessary, to take a blood sample to measure the level of oxygen in the blood. Also, the procedure allows for insertion of an internal pressure monitor, which can accurately record uterine contractions.

Concerns

- If the membranes are ruptured before the baby's head is engaged in the pelvis, the baby may turn to a breech or other unfavorable position, making birth more difficult.
- It's also possible for the umbilical cord to slip out first (prolapsed cord).
- Infection can occur if too much time elapses between rupture and birth.

Administration of oxytocin. The body naturally produces the hormone oxytocin to stimulate contractions. Synthetic forms of oxytocin are available to help stimulate labor and are marketed under several brand names (Pitocin and Syntocinon are examples).

Doctors administer synthetic forms of oxytocin to bring the amount of oxytocin to a level the body should be producing naturally. An infusion pump connected to the IV delivers the hormone in tiny, well-regulated increments until adequate response by the uterus is achieved.

The risk of complications is reduced by constantly monitoring uterine activity and the baby's heart rate through internal monitoring or, if one-to-one nursing care is available, through external, intermittent monitoring.

Advantages

- Oxytocin can initiate labor that otherwise may not have started on its own.
- If labor has leveled off and progress is not being made, oxytocin can speed the pace of labor.

Concerns

- Because of the necessity to have an IV and monitors, it's harder to change positions, and you are confined to your bed.
- Sometimes labor progresses too quickly and contractions are so strong that it becomes difficult to manage the contractions without pain medication.
- Contractions can become so powerful and close together that it may become necessary to discontinue administering the oxytocin.

When things aren't going as planned

Don't be afraid to ask for information when interventions are suggested that you don't understand or are not comfortable with. Either you or your partner can ask the following questions to help gain insight and clarification:

- Why do I need this procedure?
- How will it help me and my baby?
- Are other options available? If so, what are they? What are the risks?
- What might happen if the procedure isn't done?
- What will happen if we wait an hour?

Electronic Fetal Monitoring (EFM)

The baby's reaction to uterine contractions can be monitored by observing the baby's heart rate. The heart can respond to contractions with both increased and decreased rates, but a significant drop in the baby's heart rate just after a contraction can suggest that the placental blood supply is inadequate.

Two methods of electronic fetal monitoring are used: external and internal. In external monitoring, two wide straps are placed around the mother's abdomen. The one high on the uterus holds a pressure gauge to measure and record the strength and frequency of contractions. The other strap, placed lower on the abdomen, holds a transducer that records the baby's heart rate. They are connected to a monitor that displays and prints out both tracings simultaneously, so that their interaction can be observed.

Internal monitoring, the more accurate form of monitoring, can be done only after membranes have spontaneously or artificially been ruptured. To monitor the baby's heart rate, the doctor attaches a tiny coiled wire to the baby's scalp where it protrudes through the cervix. To measure the strength of contractions, the doctor inserts a narrow, pressure-sensitive, fluid-filled tube between the wall of the uterus and the baby. The tube responds to the pressure of each contraction. As in external monitoring, these devices are connected to a monitor that displays and records the tracings as well as amplifies the sound of the baby's heartbeat.

Advantages

- The doctor can more carefully monitor labor, especially if problems arise.
- It is reassuring to see and hear the baby's heartbeat.
- You can follow the progression of contractions.
- Earlier intervention is possible for true emergencies because of earlier detection of problems.

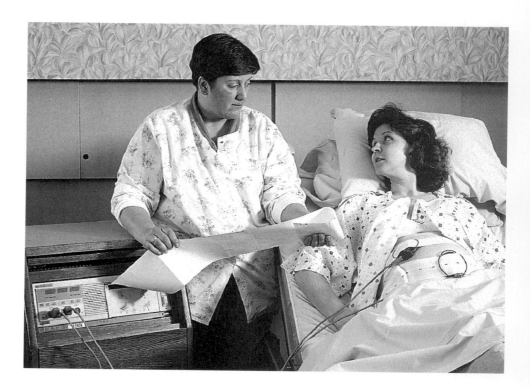

External fetal monitoring detects and records the baby's heart rate and the strength and frequency of contractions during labor.

Concerns

- In low-risk pregnancies, routine, continuous monitoring hasn't been shown to improve outcomes any more than intermittent monitoring.
- Freedom of movement is limited because of dependence on needed equipment.
- Routine use has been associated with an increase in cesarean births because of the increase in diagnosis of possible fetal distress.

Fetal Stimulation Tests

A fetal stimulation test is a noninvasive test used to assess the baby's well-being. Ordinarily, when a baby's scalp is stimulated, the baby will move around and his or her heart rate will go up. Some doctors use a clamp to pinch the scalp gently, and others tickle or press it with a finger to elicit a response. A baby who doesn't respond by moving or having an increase in heart rate may not be getting enough oxygen.

Fetal Blood Sampling

A more precise test to assess the well-being of the baby can be done by checking the baby's pH through fetal blood sampling. If the pH is low, it may mean that blood flow through the uterus and placenta isn't sufficient or that the baby isn't tolerating labor very well.

How do you get a blood sample from a baby who hasn't yet been born? The procedure is similar to the finger-prick blood test you have probably had many times in your life. A funnel-shaped tube called an endoscope is inserted into the dilated cervix and pressed against the baby's head. Using a tiny blade on a long handle, the doctor gently nicks the scalp to obtain a drop of blood, which is sent to the lab and analyzed.

Positions for Labor

The positions a woman chooses for labor and birth are, in many ways, cultural. In non-Western societies, upright positions are the most common: standing, kneeling, sitting and squatting. These positions were used throughout most of the world until lying on the back (supine position) became popular about the 17th century. With the greater involvement of medical birth attendants in later years, the supine position became even more popular because it made it easier for them to assist in the birth.

Lying on your back, however, can cause the weight of your uterus to press against an important blood vessel, the inferior vena cava, which can decrease the placental blood supply. In this position, the uterus can also push against your diaphragm at a time when your breathing is very important. In addition, the baby may not be aligned as well with the birth canal, causing contractions to actually push the baby against your pubic bone rather than through your pelvic outlet. Many medical practitioners are now encouraging women to labor on their sides or to use more upright positions because lying on the back has few advantages, other than when the need for a vacuum or forceps delivery arises.

Most women, when given the freedom to move around, will try many different positions. Labor is a process of movement. If you "listen" to your body to discover the positions that feel good, you will keep labor progressing by allowing the baby to find the best way to fit through your pelvis. Think of how you get a snug-fitting ring off your finger. Do you pull it straight off, or do you twist and turn it until you slowly work it off? Twisting and turning—changing positions— works for labor too. There is no "best" position.

Upright Positions

Laboring in upright positions has the advantage of widening your pelvic opening. Because of the effects of gravity, contractions are stronger and more efficient, and your uterus relaxes more completely between them. Gravity may even assist in pressing the baby's head against your cervix so that it dilates more rapidly.

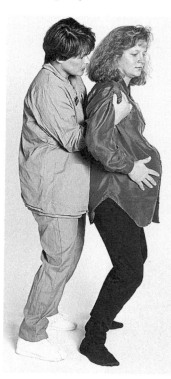

It's helpful to have someone support you during contractions while you're walking during early labor.

Standing or walking. This is most comfortable during the early part of labor. Some women are able to walk right up until the time of transition if they aren't anesthetized or on continuous monitoring. It is helpful if they have someone to physically lean on during contractions.

Sitting. When you sit, your uterus drops forward, improving the blood supply to the contracting muscles and removing pressure from your diaphragm.

Squatting. Squatting can open your pelvis a little wider, giving the baby more room to rotate as he or she moves through the birth canal. Unless your birthing bed has a specially designed squatting bar, you probably won't be able to maintain this position for long. With the help of a couple of support people, however, it is still possible to sustain this position if you find it works for you.

Upright kneeling. If you want to remain upright but no longer feel comfortable walking, try kneeling on a pillow and leaning forward against your bed or a chair. This gives you the advantages of an upright position without putting strain on your back.

Horizontal and Semihorizontal Positions

Hands and knees (down on "all fours"). For the smallest diameter of the baby's skull to pass through the pelvis, most babies move through the birth canal face down, toward your back (the anterior position). But about 30 percent of the time, babies are turned face-up (the posterior position). This position slows the progression of labor and can cause severe "back labor." A hands-and-knees position allows the baby to fall forward, taking the pressure off your spine and giving the baby more room to rotate into a more favorable position.

Reclining. Lying flat on your back is often the most uncomfortable position during labor. Your pelvis doesn't open up as much, and in this position the baby is not directed toward the birth canal. Instead of lying flat, try a semi-

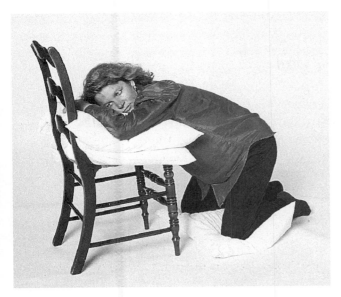

Use a chair and pillows to get in a comfortable position that allows you to concentrate on relaxing and breathing.

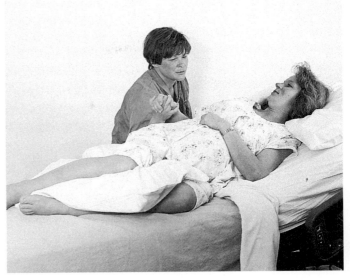

Lying on your side instead of flat on your back helps maximize blood flow to the uterus and baby. A pillow between your knees usually feels comfortable.

reclining position, with your upper body elevated. It may feel good to place a pillow under your knees, bending them slightly. If you curl forward during each contraction, the baby will be better aligned in the direction of the birth canal.

Side-lying (lateral). If you find yourself restricted to bed because of medical equipment, anesthesia or evidence of stress to your baby, you may be asked to stay on your side. This position keeps the weight of your uterus off the vena cava, maximizing blood flow to your uterus and baby.

Changing positions. Experiment to find the positions most comfortable to you as your labor progresses. If at first the baby isn't in the best position to move down the birth canal, changing position often can help to get the baby turned around and heading in the right direction.

Listen to what your body is telling you, using pain as a stimulus to change positions. After each position change, however, wait a few minutes, to give the new position a chance before assessing how well it is working; the first couple of contractions may be a little stronger until you get used to a new position.

Labor Pain

You've mastered breathing and relaxation techniques, practiced various labor positions and are relatively free from fear. Does this mean you'll also be free from pain?

No. Labor is the only natural process that has pain as a normal component. It is not the kind of pain that damages, but is pain with a purpose. Keep in mind that the intervals between contractions are relatively free of discomfort. Most women report that the pain, at times, can be severe. Those who are not prepared for this have a harder time coping with the pain than those who know it is coming. But, as we'll discuss, there are ways of dealing with it.

What Causes the Pain?

The sources of pain in labor and birth are essentially twofold. The most familiar are contractions, or "tightenings," which are created by the uterine fibers as they squeeze together. The uterine muscle is composed of circular, longitudinal and "figure-eight" fibers, tightening the muscle in every possible direction. However, the uterus doesn't actually squeeze the baby out; rather, it slowly draws the cervix up over the baby's head, not unlike the image of pulling on a turtleneck sweater. The second, and more significant, source of pain occurs as the cervix and vagina are gradually stretched to allow the baby to pass through the birth canal.

How Bad Will It Be?

Although some women have only mild to moderate discomfort, most, at some point, experience severe pain during childbirth. The degree of pain is influenced by many factors.

Attitude. How you view pain is important. If your attitude is one of wondering how you can possibly endure it, rather than one of dealing with each contraction as it comes, you will likely have a more difficult time coping.

Physical state. If you are tired and sleep-deprived before you reach active labor, it could make labor harder to cope with. As your due date approaches, try to curtail activities and rest as much as possible to be in the best condition for the work to come.

Physiological factors. The size and position of the baby, the size and shape of your pelvis, the intensity of your contractions, the length of your labor and whether you've given birth before can all affect the degree of pain you will experience.

Personal expectations. Don't try to "do as well as" a friend or relative, but simply do the best you can with your particular circumstances and strengths. Try not to have fixed ideas about whether you will use pain medication, because until you are in labor you will not know what your needs will be.

Cultural expectations. Pain is viewed differently from culture to culture. It may be expected in one part of the world for a woman to writhe and moan during childbirth, whereas in another she may be expected to endure in silence. This difference does not necessarily mean that one experiences more pain than the other, only that it is expressed in different ways.

Keeping pain in perspective is important. Remember that the pain is temporary and that it is pain with a purpose. Don't lose sight of the fact that the result will be your long-awaited baby.

Medication-Free Methods of Pain Relief

Natural methods of pain relief take many forms, some dating back centuries. They can help decrease anxiety, making pain more manageable through relaxation, and can block pain pathways by keeping nerves busy with competing signals. A few of the many ways of dealing with pain without medication are discussed on the following page.

Education. A woman who knows what is to take place, has seen where it will take place and has a relationship with a doctor she trusts will not be as afraid and, in all likelihood, will have less pain than someone who is tense and terrified. The education and experience gained in childbirth preparation classes can greatly help to decrease anxiety for both the mother and the labor companion.

Labor support. A loving and knowledgeable labor partner can enhance the birthing experience and decrease the need for pain medications through encouragement and diversionary activities, such as walking, standing or sitting, and by simply being there.

Diversion. Relaxation, positive imagery, massage and music are some of the techniques used to focus attention away from the pain of labor. The key is to use various tools and techniques. Let your body be as relaxed and loose as possible while your uterus does the work.

Heat and cold. If you are experiencing back labor, the use of heat, through either a warm compress or a heating pad to your lower back, can help. It can also feel good on your abdomen and in your groin area. Warm compresses on the perineum, the area between the vagina and anus, can help soothe and relax it for ease in delivery.

If you become too warm, which is common during labor, a cool, wet cloth to your face and neck often feels good. Sucking on ice chips can also help to cool you and at the same time create a distracting sensation in your mouth.

Positioning. Change positions frequently, experimenting to find the most comfortable positions as your labor progresses. Some women find that rhythmic movements, such as rocking in a rocking chair or rocking back and forth on their hands and knees, can be soothing and a distraction from pain.

Hydrotherapy. Many hospitals have showers in the labor rooms and some even have bathtubs or whirlpool baths to help ease the discomforts of labor. The soothing, warm water can alleviate discomfort by blocking certain pain impulses to the brain. If you're using a shower, your partner might even want to bring a swimsuit and get in the shower with you to help support you during contractions. It's important to remember that if your membranes have already ruptured, your doctor may recommend that you not take a tub or whirlpool bath because of the possibility of water entering the uterus.

Other methods. Research is under way for methods of pain relief that don't involve medication and have no side effects on the mother or baby. Some have involved hypnosis, acupuncture and a procedure called transcutaneous electrical nerve stimulation (or TENS), which sends small pulses of electricity to electrodes attached to the skin on either side of the spine, theoretically blocking the pain impulses coming from the uterus. All three of these methods have been tried in recent years, but their success rates are not high nor are they consistent. In addition, not much scientific information regarding them is available.

Medications That Relieve Pain During Childbirth

The majority of women choose to use some type of pain medication during the birthing process. What you decide to use, if anything, depends on your informed preferences, your doctor's recommendations, what is available at your medical facility and the specific character of your labor. It's important to learn about the different options ahead of time. Then you can make knowledgeable choices regarding pain medication. Be sure that you remain flexible, however, because you may need to change your mind if things don't go as intended.

All medications involve some element of risk. The risks must be weighed against the desire to relieve pain.

Tranquilizers, sedatives and barbiturates. Even though these medications have no specific pain-relieving properties, their relaxing effect may make pain more manageable by decreasing anxiety. The primary benefit is to allow you to rest or sleep during the very early part of labor, conserving energy for the second stage. Some may also relieve nausea. One drawback is that they can sometimes make it difficult for the mother to remember details of the labor experience.

Narcotics. Narcotics offer reasonable pain relief, do not interfere with pushing ability and can be given as an injection or intravenously. However, they do have a sedative effect, are often not as effective as expected and can cause nausea and vomiting, dizziness, itching and occasionally respiratory problems. Because they can slow the baby's respirations at birth, narcotics aren't given too close to the time of delivery. However, should the baby be affected by the narcotics, medications are available that can be given immediately after birth which counteract these effects.

Local anesthetic. A "local" is a medication that is injected directly into tissue, much as a dentist numbs your mouth before drilling. The simplest local used during the birthing process is one that numbs the perineum before an episiotomy is made or repaired. Given at this site, a local has no effect on the baby, nor does it provide pain relief for labor. Injections at other sites have more widespread effects.

Paracervical block. This is another method of local pain relief. An injection into the tissues around the cervix relieves the pain of uterine contractions and cervical stretching during first-stage labor. Today, because of the increased use of epidural or spinal anesthetics (see below), paracervical blocks are not often used.

Regional anesthetics. A regional anesthetic is injected into the space surrounding the spinal nerves. Several medications are used for regional anesthesia. Depending on the medications chosen by the anesthesiologist, regional anesthesia can block nerve signals, causing temporary pain relief or loss of sensation from the chest level down.

Epidural and spinal blocks. These types of regional anesthetic are becoming increasingly popular. They are used in labor and can be used as anesthesia for episiotomies and cesarean birth. The use of epidural and spinal blocks is directly related to the availability of anesthesiologists. In hospitals with 24-hour anesthesia coverage, the rates vary from 30 to 90 percent of all laboring women.

During the administration of an epidural anesthetic, you are asked to lie curled on your side or to sit up in bed with your back rounded (which can be uncomfortable during contractions) so that there will be more space between the vertebrae. Your back is scrubbed with an antiseptic solution, and an anesthetic is injected to numb the site, after which a needle is inserted between two vertebrae and through the tough tissue beside the spinal column. Anesthetic is sometimes given as a single dose through the needle, which is then removed. However, it is increasingly common to place a plastic catheter (a thin, flexible tube) that allows repeat doses of anesthetic. In this case, the anesthesiologist then threads a catheter through the needle, slides the needle out and tapes the catheter to your back to keep it in place. After a test dose of the medication is administered, it is intermittently replenished or administered continuously by an infusion pump. (For more information on spinal block, see page 335.)

Advantages

- Epidural and spinal anesthesia are the most effective forms of anesthesia for childbirth. You can receive almost total pain relief but still be awake and alert, and able to enjoy your baby's birth.
- Because you can relax, and sometimes even sleep, with an epidural or spinal, energy can be conserved during labor.
- It can increase blood flow to the uterus.
- It's possible to regulate the concentration of medication so that the effect can wear off as you get closer to the time to push, although the effect is not always easy to regulate.

Concerns

- If the medication used causes numbness in your legs, you must remain in bed. Some medications used for epidural or spinal anesthesia provide pain relief, yet do not numb your legs. This is called a "walking epidural" or a "narcotic spinal."
- It is necessary to have both an IV and a fetal monitor.
- An epidural can be hard to place effectively. If this is the case, a spinal needle or catheter may be placed successfully.
- If you have an epidural and if you can't feel the urge to bear down when it's time to push, the concentration can be changed or the rate of infusion can be reduced.
- Because it can take up to 20 minutes or more before you feel the effects of the pain relief, an epidural may be given too late to be of any help. Spinal analgesia may be an effective alternative—pain relief is almost immediate.
- If the epidural needle punctures the dura (membrane around the spinal cord and spinal fluid), a headache may develop, but this is easily treated.
- Any regional anesthetic can be an additional expense.

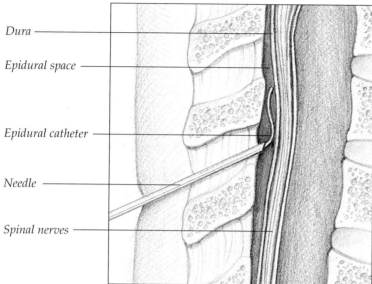

Dura
Epidural space
Epidural catheter
Needle
Spinal nerves

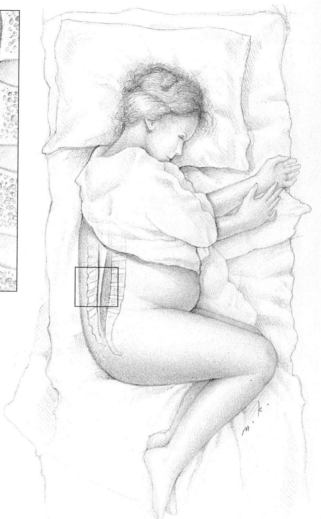

To receive an epidural block, you lie on your side in a curled-up position or sit on the bed with your back rounded. The doctor first numbs an area of your back with a local anesthetic and then inserts a needle into the epidural space just outside the membrane (dura) that encloses the spinal fluid and spinal nerves. A tiny catheter can be inserted through the needle, and the catheter is taped in place. The medication flows (as shown in the colored area) through the catheter to surround the nerves, blocking the pain.

When Problems Develop During Labor

Because some type of complication occurs about 30 percent of the time, it is very important to keep a positive and flexible attitude regarding your labor. Described below are some of the problems that can arise.

Difficult Labor

Doctors refer to labor that doesn't follow the normal progression as dystocia. This can take several forms.

Off-and-on labor. If you arrive at the hospital and your cervix is still fairly closed, and your contractions are not very strong, you might be asked to walk around, sit for a while and then walk some more to help stimulate contractions and dilate the cervix. If your cervix doesn't change after three or four hours, you will probably be sent home. Sometimes it could be a day or two before your labor becomes effective.

Hypotonic labor. Labor may start out effectively with the cervix dilating normally, but it can halt if contractions begin to dwindle to less than two every 10 minutes. Walking, position changes and an amniotomy (see page 292) or oxytocin (see page 293) are interventions that can help start labor again.

Hypertonic labor. Contractions are painful and come too quickly in hypertonic labor. The uterus doesn't relax completely between them and they aren't strong enough to be effective. If you receive pain medication, which can also help you relax, a normal pattern of contractions can often be established. Your partner can help by encouraging relaxation and pain-relieving activities.

Prolonged labor. If labor drags on for 24 hours without much progress, it is labeled prolonged labor. This might occur when contractions are poorly coordinated or not strong enough or because the baby can't fit through the birth canal. A century ago a woman may have labored for days, exhausted and at risk for infection, but now options are available such as oxytocin augmentation, forceps- or vacuum-assisted birth (see page 312) or cesarean birth (see page 327).

Rapid (precipitous) labor. Precipitous labor is defined as labor that lasts for less than three hours. The pain can be frightening because the contractions are so relentless that you can't keep up with them. The reaction of the staff, as they hurry to collect the needed equipment and assemble the necessary personnel, can make you feel even more terrified and out of control, although it's important to know that each person there knows exactly what to do. Someone will support you through contractions to help you avoid the urge to push before preparations are complete.

Failure to progress. The cervix, on average, should dilate at least 1 centimeter during every two hours of active labor. If this dilation doesn't occur, or if your cervix dilates as it should but the baby doesn't begin to descend, your doctor will discuss with you possible interventions such as amniotomy or administration of oxytocin.

Although any deviation from the norm increases fear and anxiety, abnormal labor does not indicate that you or your baby will have a bad outcome. Rather, try to think of it as a detour on that unpredictable path toward birth.

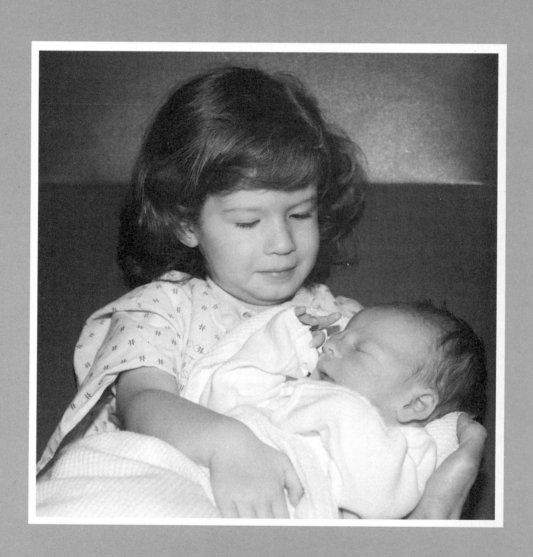

CHAPTER EIGHTEEN

Birth

*Birth is something no one else can do for
the mother, but something no woman
should have to do alone.*

As labor progresses and the cervix is nearly fully dilated, the contractions become more frequent and more intense. This transition time can be the hardest part of labor; you may feel nauseated, shaky and sometimes panicked because the contractions seem beyond your control.

"You are fully dilated and can now begin to push" is a welcome announcement. This is the time you've prepared for. Now that you are more in charge, you can actively push your baby toward birth. Soon your baby will be born! In hospitals or birth facilities where mothers are moved to a separate room for birth, being completely dilated also means that it is time to move to the delivery room. If you've taken your glasses off during labor, don't forget to bring them to the delivery room!

Pushing the Baby Out

The human pelvis is a challenging route for babies to negotiate. They slowly bend and rotate, corkscrewing down through a bony passageway. The baby doesn't have far to go, but pushing can last anywhere from minutes to hours. First-time mothers may need two to three hours, whereas women who have previously given birth usually complete the second stage more quickly. Remember, every birth is different.

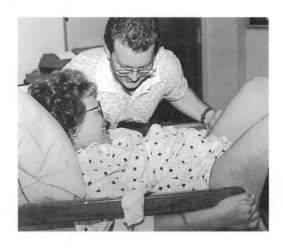

A labor companion can help in many ways, not the least of which is simply being there to comfort, coach, encourage and share the experience.

Contractions

Each contraction will last a minute or more. If you have an epidural, you might not feel the pushing urge and will have to rely on your nurse or doctor to tell you when to bear down. Pushing is most effective when you are having a contraction because two forces—the involuntary contraction of your uterus and the voluntary contraction of your abdominal muscles—combine to move the baby.

When a contraction begins, take a deep breath and push for a count of 10. Ask your nurse or partner to count for you. Then grab a quick breath without letting go of the push, and go straight back into it. The best progress is achieved by exerting constant pressure all the way through each contraction. The baby will slide back up the birth canal a little after each contraction (one step back for each two steps forward), but if you can build on the pushes you will minimize this.

Pain

The baby's head stretches your vagina and perineum (the skin between the vagina and rectum); this stretching causes a burning and stretching sensation. "It feels like I'm going to split!" is a common description. Others say it feels like an urgent need for a bowel movement. Your legs might cramp and shake from pressure of the baby's head on nerves in your pelvis. Changing positions or having your partner massage your legs may help.

"Pushing does hurt, but if you push with the pain it becomes more tolerable, and that's progress," says a Mayo doctor. "The mistake women sometimes make at first is to back off from the pain, and that makes it worse. If you let yourself head right into the pain, it actually gets better."

Feelings

When given the go-ahead to push, some women find renewed motivation, energy, commitment and excitement. They are relieved that they can finally work with their body and push with the contractions. One laboring woman said, "It felt so much better when I pushed. Actually, it didn't even hurt—it felt good. And my gosh, it was such a natural thing!" Another said, "I felt like an Olympic athlete when I was pushing him out."

Other women may be frightened by the intensity of the contractions and other sensations. Maybe the panic of transition isn't there, but if they can't quite coordinate the breathing and the pushing with the contractions, they feel overwhelmed.

This reaction develops because pushing doesn't necessarily come naturally. Even though the urge is there, you must master the technique before your pushing becomes effective. "There are so many things to think about, it's hard to relax some things and work others."

You must put all of your energy into bearing down with your abdominal muscles—pushing toward your rectum. At the same time you have to relax your pelvic floor muscles, and the feeling is awkward. You won't do it perfectly on the first push, but soon you'll be pushing effectively. It even feels good. "It's hard work you like to do," says an obstetrics nurse.

Pushing—tips for the labor companion

Fathers or partners are sometimes discouraged at this point, and often a little fearful. You can't seem to do anything to help because only the mother can push the baby out. But you can be encouraging as a coach. You can count during the pushes, giving enthusiastic feedback about how well the mom is doing. Perhaps she needs to hold your hand, maybe she needs a cool washcloth on her forehead. She may need support for her legs or back during the pushes. Most important of all, you are there with her, going through this incredible experience together.

S ome women tend to hold back. Laboring women might feel embarrassed because they're half naked, grunting and straining in front of other people and worried that they might even urinate or move their bowels a little. This embarrassment can hamper their ability to give an all-out effort; they need to accept that noises and bodily functions are all a normal part of childbirth.

It's easy to get discouraged if the baby doesn't move down as fast as you'd like. Then you might need help from your partner and a nurse's or doctor's suggestions for position changes, breathing techniques and when and how to push. Sometimes there is a whole roomful of people cheering, grunting and pushing along with you!

How Babies Come Out

The mother's pelvis is widest from side to side at the inlet (top) and from front to back at the outlet (bottom). The baby's head is widest from front to back, and the shoulders are widest from side to side. As a result, the baby must twist and turn on the way through the birth canal.

Unless the baby begins from an unusual starting position, all babies perform roughly the same choreographed routine on their way out. The head turns to one side. The chin is forced down onto the chest so that the back of the head leads the way. At the outlet to the pelvis, the baby's face usually turns toward the mother's back. The perineum begins to bulge, the labia part and the baby's head appears in the vaginal opening during contractions.

When the head starts to appear, the first sight of that wrinkled scalp inspires renewed energy for everyone in the room. It won't be long now until the baby is born.

"Crowning" occurs when the head is completely emerging from the vaginal opening. The back of the head presents first, then the brow and face. The baby turns toward your thigh to line its head up with its shoulders again. There is often a brief pause at this point to suction the baby's nose and mouth, wipe the face clean and sometimes slip a loop of umbilical cord over the baby's head. Next comes a push and a tug to let the first shoulder out. Then the other shoulder and the rest of the baby quickly slip out. Congratulations, your baby is born!

"I started pushing around 11:10, and at 12:01 he arrived! It was the most amazing and wonderful experience I've ever had—and every day gets better. Thank you, Alex, for being you and for coming into our lives!"

Cutting the Umbilical Cord

Immediately after the birth, the baby is still connected to the placenta by the umbilical cord. Often the parents can assist with the clamping and cutting of the cord. If you'd like to assist, make your wishes known, and you'll be shown what to do.

There is usually no particular urgency to cut the umbilical cord. Two clamps are placed on the cord, and then a scissors is used to snip painlessly between the clamps. (Occasionally, if the umbilical cord has looped snugly around the baby's neck, the cord is clamped and cut before the shoulders are delivered.)

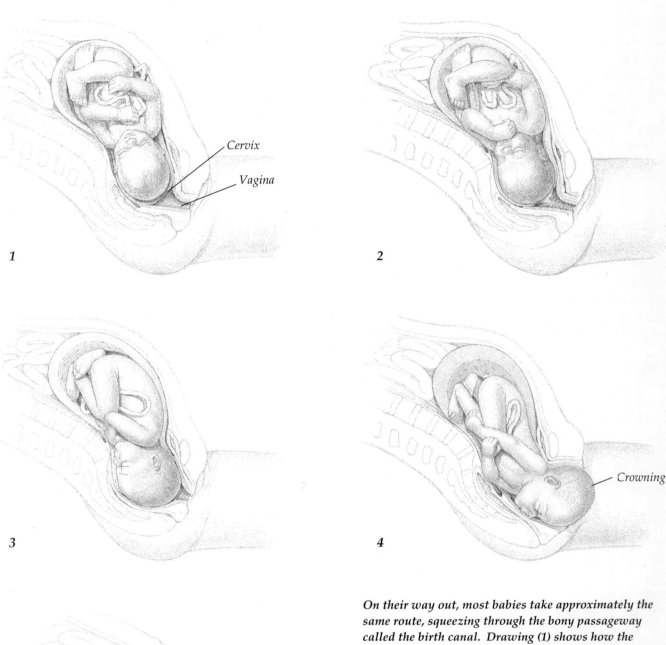

Cervix

Vagina

1

2

3

4

Crowning

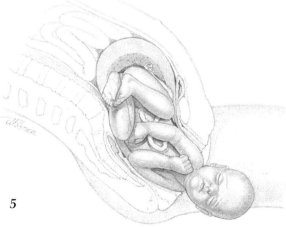

5

On their way out, most babies take approximately the same route, squeezing through the bony passageway called the birth canal. Drawing (1) shows how the cervix thins and spreads as the baby is descending facing the mother's side. In this position, the widest part of the baby's head is positioned in the widest part of the mother's pelvis. Next, (2) the cervix is almost completely open (dilated). With chin on chest, the back of the baby's head leads the way as the head and torso begin to twist to face the mother's back. With the cervix completely open (3), the baby has completed the 90-degree rotation and, facing the mother's back, begins to enter the vagina. (4) "Crowning"—the appearance of the baby's head—is an exciting time for everyone. Once the head is born, the baby's head and shoulders again twist to face the mother's side (5); this positioning enables the baby to slip through the lower pelvis, which is widest from front to back.

Recording the event

It's common to celebrate a birth by taking pictures or video or tape recordings. They can help you share the excitement with close friends and relatives. You can relive the experience in future years. But it's wise to think through your plans ahead of time.

Here are points to consider:

- The most important aspects of labor and birth may be what you feel, not what you see.
- Some women don't feel very photogenic during labor and birth. They may also object to being "on stage." Giving birth isn't a performance, and some women are distracted by having recordings or pictures taken.
- Similarly, medical personnel may be self-conscious and uncomfortable about photos or recordings, especially if they are expected to provide a continuous "play-by-play" narration of the event. It's polite to ask in advance.
- Concentrating on taking photos or recordings can be distracting for the labor companion. It's more important to be a partner than a recorder.
- The most memorable photos are those that include the baby.
- The hospital or birthing facility may have guidelines concerning taking photos or recordings. For example, the privacy of others must be protected.

Memories of birth are enhanced by telling and retelling the story from the perspective of both parents. There is more going on than either can take in alone. Sharing your experiences helps each understand the birth from the other's view. It's important to take time, in the hours and days after the birth, to relive the events and emotions you've just gone through.

Birthing Positions

Labor and birth can occur in various positions. During the past 200 years, women in Western cultures have most commonly given birth while lying on their backs. This position allows the woman to be assisted easily during birth. However, various positions are effective for birth. Once you are in labor, you may find that certain positions are more comfortable than others. In fact, there may be times that you will be asked not to lie on your back so that blood flow to the uterus will be more efficient.

Practices in labor and delivery vary from one setting to another, so talk to your doctor and nurses about different possibilities before labor begins.

Lying Positions

On your back. In the traditional Western position, the woman lies flat on her back with her legs in stirrups. A more comfortable and natural modification of this position is a semireclining position—that is, you lie back but not all the way. The head of the bed is elevated, and your head and shoulders rest against pillows. During each contraction you grab your legs behind the knees or handles near the stirrups and pull back toward your body. Or, you may pull your body forward into a more upright position.

Side-lying. A side-lying position is good if you're tired or if you have an epidural. Your partner can hold your upper leg, which will widen the pelvic outlet, or you might be able to rest it on a special shelf attached to the bed. This position helps support the weight of the baby. It is easy for you to rest between contractions, and the pressure is off your perineum.

Leg supports. The stirrups used during birth are different from those you rest your feet on when you have a pelvic exam. They are higher than the bed, they hold your entire leg rather than just your feet, and they may come equipped with straps to keep your legs secure.

The use of leg supports in birthing rooms varies, but they are common if you have an epidural anesthetic. Leg supports are also used during forceps-assisted births because your legs must be up and out of the way.

Upright Positions

Some women find upright positions more comfortable. A labor that has not been progressing might gain some momentum if the mother assumes an upright position. The pelvic opening will widen in this position. The length of second-stage labor may even be shortened.

Kneeling. This is a popular upright position because it relieves backache by directing the baby's weight away from the spine. Many birthing beds are constructed in two sections; one can be lowered and the other raised. You can kneel on the foot portion of the bed and rest your arms and upper body on or against the upper section.

All fours (hands and knees). Getting down on all fours is another way to ease backache. It may also be good for someone who has had significant tearing in the past or who wants to avoid an episiotomy, because the baby's head presses less directly on the perineum. If the baby appears to be stressed and develops a slow heart rate, this position is sometimes used because it maximizes blood flow to the uterus and placenta. Another advantage is that it may give an improperly positioned baby a better chance of turning the right way around. A variation on this position is to lie chest-down on a stack of pillows.

Squatting. If you have begun pushing but the baby is not moving down through the birth canal, you can squat to open your pelvis a little more. Squatting also allows you to bear down more effectively. Unless you have prepared for it you may not have the strength to sustain a squat for very long. Lean against the bed or chair—or squat right on the bed—and ask someone to help support your weight. Some birthing beds have a special squatting bar. Squat only during contractions; sit or go onto your hands and knees between them.

Birthing chair or stool. A less strenuous variation of squatting is the birthing chair. If you find squatting helpful but tiring, try a birthing stool. Women who have used birthing stools report that they felt more in control of their birth experience, and they particularly liked being able to see the baby at the moment of birth. Perhaps the greatest benefit of the birthing stool, however, is that your partner can sit in front of or behind you for a close, shared experience.

Pain Medications

Some of the same anesthetics used during first-stage labor can be continued through the pushing stage until the baby is born.

A pudendal block is a local anesthetic injected into the vaginal wall and the ligaments supporting the pelvic floor. Because it affects only the vagina and rectum, it is used only for second-stage labor and for episiotomy (snipping the perineum to enlarge the vaginal opening). It is the most popular form of pain relief, used by more than half of all delivering women.

Pudendal Block

Advantages

- Pain relief is good and you still maintain the urge to push.
- It is one of the safest forms of pain management.

Concerns

- It is not always effective.

An epidural block given early in labor can be continued for episiotomy and birth. It is safe and lasts as long as necessary, and it allows you to remain awake and alert. (For a complete description of epidural block anesthesia, see page 300.)

Epidural Block

Assisted Vaginal Births

During second-stage labor, various situations can require medical intervention. If the baby's head is turned so that the smallest dimensions aren't leading the way, the passage through the pelvis can be an especially tight fit. Distress could develop in the baby, necessitating a speedy birth.

Perhaps the mother has heart or lung disease, infection or some other medical condition that prevents her from exerting herself. Or, more commonly, maybe she has been pushing for hours and is simply too exhausted for the final effort required to push the baby out. If conditions are likely to be improved by quick delivery, the doctor might advise an assisted birth.

Doctors have several methods to choose from: episiotomy, forceps-assisted birth and vacuum-assisted birth. Because these procedures can increase pain, many women need additional anesthesia. Some of the available options are spinal or epidural blocks or local anesthetics. (For details on epidural and spinal blocks and on local anesthetics, see page 300.)

An episiotomy is an incision made into the perineum toward the rectum (midline episiotomy), or a little to the side (mediolateral episiotomy), to enlarge the vaginal opening. The doctor makes the cut with a scissors when the baby is crowning and the perineum is stretched taut. If you haven't had an

Episiotomy

epidural or a pudendal block, the doctor gives you a local anesthetic so that you won't feel the cut or the repair. Once the snip is made, the baby is born with a few pushes.

For decades, doctors usually performed episiotomies fairly routinely. Their reasoning was that this shortened the second stage of labor, limited trauma to the baby, prevented tearing of the mother's vagina and perineum and decreased the risk of pelvic relaxation, which may cause bladder and rectal problems later.

Recently, the need for routine episiotomies has been questioned because performing them for the reasons listed above may not always be valid. As a result, many doctors are waiting longer before performing an episiotomy, and are doing it only if necessary.

Advantages

- A straight, clean cut goes where the doctor wants it to go and is easier to repair than a tear.
- Procedure can speed up delivery.
- Premature and other fragile babies come out faster and are spared some of the pressure of stretching the perineum.
- Certain birth situations (large babies, breech babies and others) require an episiotomy for the safety of the baby.

Concerns

- Tears can occur despite an episiotomy.
- An episiotomy can delay recovery from birth more than if there is no episiotomy and no tear.

Most first-time mothers in the United States have episiotomies. The more babies you have, the less need you have for an episiotomy because your perineum stretches a little more during each birth, decreasing the likelihood of tearing. You also become more experienced at pushing, and skillful pushing is less likely to result in an episiotomy. Episiotomy is no longer routine; many doctors wait until the baby's head is crowning before they decide whether one will be necessary.

If you have concerns about having an episiotomy, discuss them with your doctor before delivery. If you want to avoid one, ask the doctor to work with you toward this goal. When you are in labor, warm, moist cloths placed on your perineum can help soothe and relax it, and the doctor can massage and stretch it during contractions. It is important to control the strength of your pushes, sometimes avoiding them altogether to give your perineum time to stretch.

Forceps-Assisted Birth

Forceps are shaped like a pair of spoons that, when hooked together, resemble a set of salad tongs. The doctor gently slides one "spoon" at a time into your vagina and around the side of the baby's head. The two pieces lock together at their shanks and safely and snugly cup the baby's cheeks. While your uterus contracts and you push, the doctor skillfully pulls on the forceps to help the baby through the birth canal, sometimes on the very next push.

Your doctor will offer a pain medication or anesthesia, such as an epidural or a pudendal block, before placing the forceps. Sometimes a catheter is used to empty your bladder first, and your perineal area is cleansed with soapy water. Episiotomy is frequently done before a forceps birth, but despite this, tears can occur.

The use of forceps varies among hospitals, depending on maternal circumstances, the experience of the staff and the types of anesthesia available. The most common reason for using forceps is maternal exhaustion.

Sometimes a woman is so tired by the time the doctor suggests forceps that she's happy for any suggestion. "Whatever you need to do to get this baby out, do it," is a typical comment.

Forceps have prevented many mothers from requiring a cesarean birth. And forceps have helped deliver many babies quickly when needed. The possibility of using forceps to assist a vaginal birth is an important option for many obstetrical services. Many other obstetrical services do not use forceps at all.

Occasionally a doctor might suggest forceps to hasten birth even though you feel capable of pushing for a while longer and the baby seems to be tolerating labor well. If this happens, you might want to ask what other options you have.

Vacuum-Assisted Birth

An instrument known as a vacuum extractor is sometimes used instead of forceps. The doctor presses a large rubber or plastic cup against the baby's head, creates suction with a pump and then gently pulls on the instrument to help ease the baby down the birth canal. The force of the suction may cause a bruise.

The vacuum extractor is less likely than forceps to injure the mother, and it leaves more room in the pelvis for the baby to pass through. But if speed is an issue, forceps may be a better choice for getting the baby out faster because there can be difficulty maintaining the suction during vacuum-assisted birth.

After the Birth

Many events are happening simultaneously after your baby is born: parents are celebrating the excitement of birth, the mother is relieved that labor is done and someone is keeping a watchful eye as the baby is beginning to breathe.

For most couples, the placenta is of little significance. For the medical personnel attending the birth, delivering the placenta and ensuring that the mother doesn't have excessive blood loss are very important.

Delivering the Placenta

After your baby is born, contractions may stop for a while, then resume to deliver the placenta. This is the third stage of labor.

Usually the placenta separates from the wall of the uterus within five to 10 minutes, but sometimes it takes as long as half an hour. Periodically your doctor or one of the birth attendants will massage your lower abdomen to both check on and encourage the uterus to continue to squeeze down and shrink in size. Often, having someone check your uterus is only a minor interruption. Sometimes, though, the uterine contractions or the massaging of your abdomen definitely hurts. These uterine contractions are important to close off blood vessels and minimize bleeding after birth.

The uterus becomes firm and bulges noticeably in your abdomen as the placenta moves downward. Massaging your lower abdomen helps move the placenta along. Often you'll be asked to give a small push to assist in delivering the placenta. If the placenta is slow to come down, it's sometimes necessary for the doctor to reach inside to remove it directly. The placenta is inspected to make sure it looks normal and that no remnants, which could cause bleeding, have been left behind. If you'd like a closer look, be sure to ask.

Episiotomy Repair

Once the placenta has been delivered, the episiotomy and any significant tears can be repaired. If your anesthetic has worn off, you will be given a local anesthetic to numb the area. Closing an episiotomy takes 10 to 20 minutes, but significant tears take a little longer because the various layers of tissue must be separately stitched. The stitches gradually dissolve, and you won't need to have them removed.

"The hospital invited new parents to a candlelight dinner. We moms came in our bathrobes, and as soon as each woman entered the room you could tell how she delivered. Those who'd had cesareans hunched over in what we called the "cesarean shuffle," and those who'd had vaginal births with episiotomies carried pillows to sit on."

Episiotomies and tears can take up to several weeks to heal. At first you will be uncomfortable. Ice can help reduce swelling, and heat lamps are sometimes used to dry and soothe the wound. Soaking in a warm bath feels good, and anesthetic sprays also help.

Care of the New Mother

You'll be checked frequently during the first several hours after your baby is born. The firmness of your uterus is checked, and your lower abdomen probably will be massaged. The amount of vaginal bleeding you have is monitored; sometimes medication is given to ensure that the uterus stays firm. Your temperature and blood pressure will also be monitored.

It's important to be aware that mothers often have shaking or strong shivering in the first few hours after birth. It doesn't mean that your body is chilled, but a warm blanket often helps.

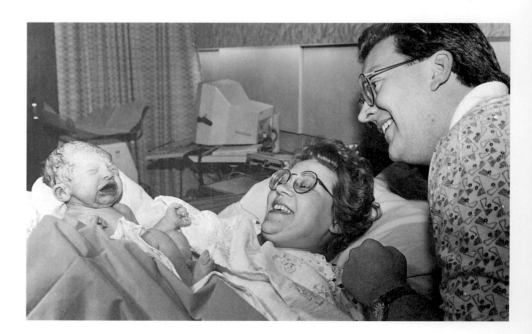

Parents of newborn babies react to the miracle of birth in many ways, including elation.

Your feelings after delivery. You can't predict how you will feel after the birth. Some new mothers are overjoyed, wanting to cuddle the new baby immediately. "I'm not tired anymore!" exclaimed one who had been ready to give up from exhaustion and frustration just moments before. Others remain consumed with fatigue; they want to rest and to wait for the placenta to be delivered and to be cleaned up before they hold the baby. Some new mothers are even afraid to hold their babies at first.

> *"I was overly aware of the height of the bed, the huge gap under the railings and the hardness of the floor. I had the shakes and was sure I'd drop the baby! My husband stacked pillows against the railings and stood right there so that I didn't feel so nervous."*

It's not uncommon to experience a confusing mixture of emotions. You might need to compare notes with your partner and relate the details to friends and relatives before you can assimilate what you've been through and the miracle that has taken place. You might feel reluctant to show your feelings in front of the people bustling around the room. What do they expect you to do and say?

If you feel no emotion at first, don't worry that there's something wrong with you, because this, too, is a normal reaction. Perhaps you expected to be overwhelmed by love for the tiny baby you've waited so long for, but what you see is a stranger who may bear no resemblance to the image you've had in your mind.

> *"I'd walk down to the nursery and stand at the window with the other parents. I'd say to myself, 'I can see why that baby belongs to the couple next to me —*
> *he looks just like them. And the one over there obviously belongs to this other couple. But does mine really belong to me? She looks like a total stranger!'*
> *Now that she's 3 she looks like my clone, but when she was born I saw no resemblance at all."*

Just as it takes time to fall in love with a grown-up, it can take time to fall in love with a baby. As you come to know this new little person, your feelings will deepen. There is no right or wrong way to experience these emotions; every new parent will react differently to one of life's most intense and wonderful experiences.

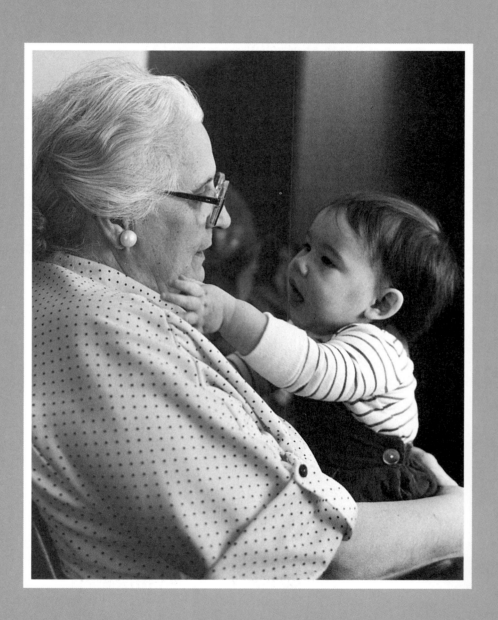

CHAPTER NINETEEN

Complications of Childbirth

Every woman wants a problem-free birth, but in many labors and deliveries an obstetrical or medical complication develops. The major problems for the baby are premature birth (see page 353), abnormal position during labor and problems with the placenta or umbilical cord. The major problems in the mother include abnormal bleeding, infection, eclampsia, premature labor and obstructions to the normal course of labor or delivery. Because these complications can occur suddenly in an otherwise normal pregnancy, you should be familiar with them in case they happen to you or your baby.

Complications With the Baby

For months you've been probing your abdomen, trying to figure out what the various lumps and bumps are. Are you patting the baby's bottom, or is it the head? The protrusion that's so fascinating to watch when it glides back and forth—is it an elbow or a heel?

Doctors are skilled at answering these questions, but they can be difficult even for them. As a result, they often use an ultrasound examination to determine the position of the baby. (For more information on ultrasound exams, see page 72.) Knowing how the baby is positioned helps them determine how to manage the birth. Unless the baby is in the best and most common position—head down and facing to one side or the other—the trip through the pelvis can be difficult, and sometimes impossible.

Abnormal Fetal Position

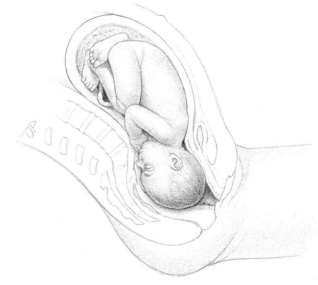

Compare the positions of the other babies in this chapter with the position of the baby shown here, who is in the ideal and most common position for birth. The smallest dimension of the baby's head leads the way through the birth canal.

317

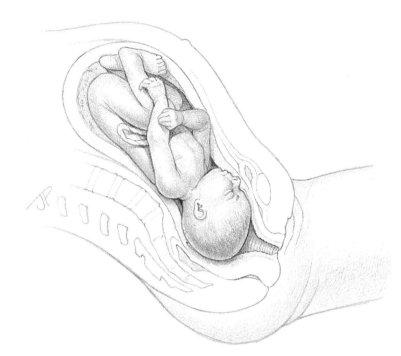

A baby who is in the occiput posterior position has the face toward the mother's abdomen, and therefore a larger dimension of the baby's head tries to lead through the birth canal.

Occiput posterior. The most common variation of the normal position is when the baby is "sunny-side up," facing its mother's abdomen. Intense back labor often accompanies this position, along with prolonged labor and increased tearing during birth. Some babies will turn if they have enough room. Sometimes changing positions can help rotate the baby. Your doctor might have you get on your hands and knees with your buttocks in the air, a position that causes the uterus to drop forward.

If this doesn't work, your doctor might try to rotate the baby by reaching through the vagina, grasping the head with either a hand or forceps and simply rotating it. If that technique doesn't work, your doctor will decide whether the baby is likely to fit through at all or whether a cesarean birth would be safer.

Malpresentation of the head. When the baby enters the pelvis, its chin should be pressed down to its chest so that the back of the head, which has the smallest diameter, leads the way. If the chin is not down, a larger diameter of the head has to fit through the pelvis. In about one in 500 births, babies can "present" with the top of the head, the forehead or even the face. Once again, your doctor will decide the best method for delivery.

Cephalopelvic disproportion. This term means that the baby's head won't fit through the mother's pelvis. The disproportion can be absolute, in which the head is too big or the pelvis is too small. This is true cephalopelvic disproportion. More commonly, the condition is "relative"—the baby's head is not properly aligned and the smallest diameter isn't leading the way. This is called secondary arrest of labor, and it is much more common than true cephalopelvic disproportion. In either case, labor will progress to a certain point and then the cerivx will not dilate further.

Women frequently expect doctors to know ahead of time whether the baby will fit through the pelvis. With an ultrasound exam, the size of the baby can be estimated. X-rays or magnetic resonance imaging (MRI) can be used to measure the bones of the mother's pelvis. Unfortunately, these measurements are poor predictors of whether the baby will fit through the pelvis. The forces of labor can temporarily "mold" a baby's head to fit through the pelvis, and loosened ligaments allow the bones in the mother's pelvis to move. Because of both of these variables, the best way to find out whether cephalopelvic disproportion is going to be a problem is by monitoring what happens as labor progresses.

Breech presentation. A baby is breech when it is not in a head-down position on entering the birth canal. The buttocks or one or both feet might enter the pelvis first. Three to 4 percent of full-term births are breech, and the rate increases with premature babies.

Unless the baby can be repositioned, the mother faces an increased chance of tears, episiotomy extension, cesarean birth and postpartum infection. The baby

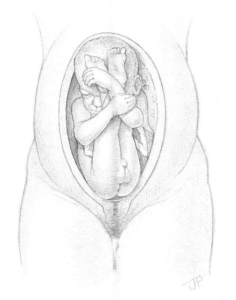
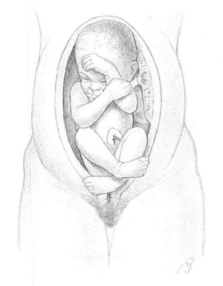
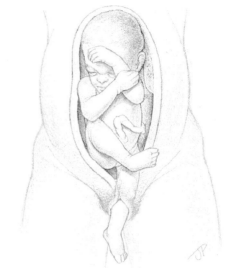

When the baby's buttocks or feet enter the birth canal before the head, the baby is in a breech position. Three types of breech positions are shown above, a frank breech on the left, a complete breech in the center, and a footling breech on the right.

also has significant risks. A prolapsed umbilical cord is serious and more common in breech births (see page 320). In addition, it is impossible to be certain whether the head will fit through the pelvis. The head is the largest and least compressible part of the baby to travel through the birth canal and may become trapped even though the body was born easily.

The doctor may try to turn the baby into the proper position, sometimes a couple of weeks before the due date. This technique is called an "external version." If the baby is not too far down in the pelvis, the doctor might be able to move the baby into a head-down position simply by pushing on the baby through the mother's abdomen. Medication is often given to relax the uterus, to relieve pain or both. A hospital setting is best in case the umbilical cord becomes compressed, in which case an immediate cesarean birth is required.

If an external version doesn't work, the doctor will try to determine whether vaginal birth will be possible and what the risk factors are. The chances of having a successful vaginal birth are increased by a small baby, a previous vaginal delivery, a previous breech delivery, good progress of cervical dilation and carrying the baby low in the pelvis so that the risk of cord prolapse is minimal.

The doctor will weigh many factors before making a decision. Without a complete evaluation (possibly including ultrasound exam of the baby and MRI scan of the mother's pelvis), vaginal birth may be more of a risk for the baby. Cesarean birth presents more risk for the mother. Because of the severity of the possible complications for the newborn, however, the vast majority of breech babies today are born by cesarean.

Transverse lie. If the baby is lying crosswise in the uterus, this position is called a transverse lie. This occurs in about one in 300 pregnancies. Often the shoulder is the presenting part. This position almost always calls for cesarean birth.

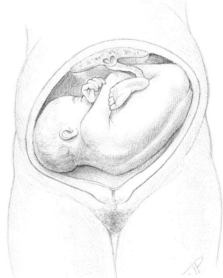

A baby who is positioned horizontally across the uterus, rather than vertically, is in a transverse lie position. Most babies in this position have a cesarean birth.

Placenta and Cord Complications

P*lacenta previa.* When the placenta is attached too low to the uterine wall, where cervical dilation will dislodge it, both the mother and baby are at greater risk of serious bleeding. This condition occurs in about one in 200 births. (See page 195 for a complete discussion.)

Placental abruption. When the placenta detaches from the uterine wall before the baby is born, the mother's life is threatened by blood loss, and the baby's source of oxygen is cut off. This occurs in less than 1 to 2 percent of all births. (See page 194 for more information.)

Aging placenta. When a pregnancy continues beyond 42 weeks, the placenta often fails to provide adequate oxygen or nutrition. Fetal growth may be halted altogether by the increasingly harmful womb environment, and the baby may become malnourished. As a result, the stillbirth rate of postmaturity is twice that of infants born after a pregnancy of normal length. To minimize the risk to the baby, doctors may induce labor in pregnancies that continue one to two weeks beyond the due date.

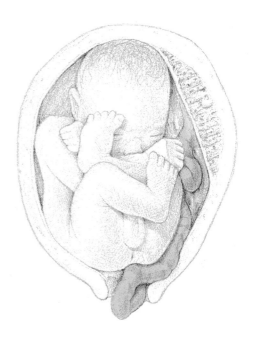

Cord prolapse is a serious complication in which a portion of the umbilical cord comes through the cervix before the baby, blocking off blood flow to the baby when the uterus contracts.

Cord prolapse. If the umbilical cord slips out through the cervix, the baby is in grave danger because the blood flow can be blocked each time the uterus contracts (this also can occur in the absence of contractions—in other words, before labor begins). Cord prolapse is most likely to occur with a small or premature baby, with a baby in a breech position or when the amniotic sac breaks before the baby is down far enough in the pelvis. If the cord slips out after complete cervical dilation has already taken place, and if birth is imminent, vaginal birth might still be possible. Otherwise, cesarean birth is the usual option. Umbilical cord prolapse occurs in approximately one in 300 births.

Cord compression. If the cord is wrapped around the baby's neck, if the cord is in a position between the baby's head and the mother's pelvic bones or if there is decreased amniotic fluid, each contraction will squeeze the cord and slow down the blood flow. This problem usually develops when the baby is well down in the birth canal, close to the time of birth. Cord compression occurs in roughly 10 percent of births. If cord compression is prolonged or severe, the baby may show signs of distress. If your baby is in distress, the heart rate will slow, the blood pH will decrease and the baby may pass meconium (first bowel movement). To maximize blood flow to your placenta, the best position is on your side or in a knee-chest position. You may be given oxygen to increase the amount the baby gets. Then your doctor will make a decision about what steps to take next. These could include forceps or vacuum assistance (if birth is imminent) or cesarean birth.

Complications With the Mother

A woman who has lost sleep for several days before the birth, or who has had a particularly long and difficult labor, may be exhausted. This is the time to limit visitors, rest as much as possible and perhaps send the baby to the nursery. Your doctor might even prescribe a sleeping pill to help you get a full night's sleep.

Serious bleeding (hemorrhage) occurs in about 5 percent of all births. It usually occurs during or within 24 hours of childbirth, but it can happen up to six weeks later. Overall, the likelihood of a woman needing a blood transfusion after childbirth is less than 2 percent. Even cesarean births necessitate a transfusion only 3 percent of the time.

The body responds to hemorrhage by diverting most of its blood supply to the brain and heart. This is a survival mechanism designed to protect these most important organs, but it takes care of them at the expense of other organs. Because the oxygen supply going to body cells is greatly depleted, shock sets in.

The following symptoms can occur with heavy bleeding:

- Pale face
- Chills
- Dizziness or fainting
- Clammy hands
- Nausea or vomiting
- Racing heart

If you feel any of these blood-loss symptoms, get immediate help. If you are still in the hospital, the staff can take several simple steps to ease your discomfort: lower the head of your bed, massage your uterus and give you more fluids and oxytocin through an IV. (Pitocin and Syntocinon are synthetic forms of oxytocin, a hormone that stimulates uterine contractions.) If you're home when hemorrhaging begins, contact your doctor immediately. Blood loss is an emergency situation that requires immediate action.

The three main causes of serious bleeding after birth are uterine atony, tearing and retained placenta. In more than 90 percent of women with such bleeding, one of these is the cause.

Uterine atony. This is the most common cause. After you've given birth, your uterus must contract to control bleeding from the placental site. The reason your nurse periodically massages your abdomen is to encourage your uterus to contract. Sometimes the uterine muscle is too exhausted; then medication is administered to help the process. The doctor also can press on your abdomen with one hand and on your uterus from within your vagina with the other. If these measures aren't enough to control bleeding, surgery may be necessary.

Tearing (lacerations). If your vagina, cervix, anal sphincter or rectum tear during the birth, excessive bleeding can result. Tearing might be caused by a large baby, forceps- or vacuum-assisted birth, a too-rapid expulsion of the baby or an episiotomy that tears. Your doctor will need to find and repair the tear.

Retained placenta. If the placenta isn't expelled on its own within 30 minutes after the baby is born, excessive bleeding can result. Your doctor might have to reach into your uterus to remove the placenta from the uterine wall. If so, you will be given an anesthetic for pain.

Even when the placenta is expelled on its own, your doctor carefully examines it to make sure it is intact. If any tissue is missing, there is a risk of bleeding; your doctor will examine your uterus and attempt to remove retained placental tissue manually. If this doesn't work, the uterus can be scraped (curettage) or suctioned to clean it out.

Bruises (hematomas). Hematomas result when bleeding occurs within tissue and can't escape through the skin. In the lower genital tract, swelling can be so severe that urination becomes difficult or temporarily impossible.

Small hematomas are allowed to improve on their own, but large ones might have to be drained to decrease the discomfort. Vessels that continue to bleed can be tied off. If the loss of blood is too great, a blood transfusion may be needed. Occasionally, hematomas occur in the abdominal cavity and need to be drained surgically through an abdominal incision (laparotomy).

Hematomas, especially those that must be opened, can become infected. It is essential to keep the area clean and to change pads frequently. Antibiotics are often given to treat any infection that occurs.

Uterine rupture. In approximately one in 1,500 births, the uterus tears during pregnancy or labor. If this happens, the mother loses blood and the baby's oxygen supply is decreased. Immediate surgical intervention is required to remove the baby and repair the tear. One reason doctors like to use a monitor, especially while administering oxytocin, is to make sure that the uterus isn't contracting so hard it might tear. The doctor will try very hard to repair a rupture, but sometimes hysterectomy (removal of all or part of the uterus) is the only way to control the bleeding.

Uterine inversion. In fewer than one in 2,000 births, the uterus turns inside out after the baby and placenta are born. The usual cause is that the placenta is improperly attached and doesn't detach from the uterine wall when the doctor pulls on the umbilical cord. The doctor will try to push the uterus back through the cervix and into its proper place.

Transfusions

Less than 2 percent of women who give birth will require a blood transfusion. Women who have a cesarean birth are slightly more likely to need a transfusion.

Risks of transfusions. Up to 3 percent of blood transfusions can trigger a reaction. This might cause fever, chills, nausea and vomiting, a racing pulse or itching. The transfusion can be stopped and the symptoms treated.

Infectious disease is another risk. By far the most common is hepatitis. Blood is carefully screened, but the risk is still approximately one in 3,000 units transfused.

Before 1983, when the first case of AIDS was diagnosed in the United States, the blood supply was not tested for HIV (human immunodeficiency virus, which leads to AIDS). Since 1985, when screening was begun to detect HIV-infected blood, the number of people getting the AIDS virus from a blood transfusion has diminished greatly. The risk of contracting HIV is now estimated to be about one in 250,000 units of blood.

Autologous transfusions. Some people have become so hesitant to use the general blood supply that they want to avoid it under all circumstances. When they know they are going to have surgery, they donate their own blood for use at a later date. The need for transfusion during or after childbirth is small (less than 2 percent), but if you have had bleeding problems with past births or have a known complication such as placenta previa (see page 195), discuss the possibility of pre-donation with your doctor.

Directed donations. Women who know they are at risk for postpartum hemorrhage can ask relatives with similar blood types to donate blood to be used if needed. The donors must be healthy and usually must have a doctor's order to do this.

One drawback to this method is that blood banks need to have the donated blood at least 48 hours before the birth (and most would prefer to get it three weeks in advance) so that they can test and prepare it for use. If the blood donations have not been given in advance, the general blood supply must be used because hospitals are not able to give blood without first testing it.

Another drawback is the safety of directed donations. A family member or friend may feel pressured into agreeing to donate blood, especially in an emergency. It is very important that blood donors exclude themselves if they have any risk factors for HIV or hepatitis. The safest directed donation would be from a person who donates blood regularly and voluntarily. If you are interested in the specific questions that are asked of potential blood donors, contact your hospital blood bank or local blood donation center.

Postpartum Infection

Endometritis. The most common type of infection that occurs after childbirth is endometritis. It occurs in 1 to 8 percent of all births. Endometritis is an inflammation and infection of the mucous membrane that lines the uterus. Bacteria grow, usually at the site of the placenta, and spread through the uterus and possibly even to the ovarian and pelvic blood vessels.

The infection comes from various normal vaginal organisms that make their way up into the uterus, and it is far more common after cesarean birth than after vaginal birth. Other contributing factors are a long labor and early rupture of membranes.

Endometritis usually occurs 48 to 72 hours after delivery. When it is mild, there may be only an increase in temperature to about 101 degrees Fahrenheit for several days. More severe cases involve chills and high fever, a faster heart rate, loss of appetite, headache, backache and general discomfort.

It is not unusual for a woman with endometritis to have severe and prolonged after pains—uterine contractions after delivery. Her uterus is large and tender when her abdomen is touched. Vaginal discharge (lochia) may be less than normal and may smell foul. A serious infection like this can last anywhere from one week to many weeks, depending on how far the infection has spread.

Treatment for endometritis includes intravenous antibiotics for two to seven days in the hospital and either oral or intravenous fluids. Acetaminophen can help relieve fever. In some hospitals you may be isolated from other new mothers, although there is little likelihood that the infection can spread to other patients. Breastfeeding can continue during treatment.

Urinary tract infection. For the first 24 to 48 hours after delivery, your body produces what seems to be alarming amounts of urine—from 2 to 4 cups at a time, an amount that is two to three times more than usual. This is your body's way of getting rid of all the extra fluid it carried in your bloodstream during pregnancy. Urinating frequently also may help prevent urinary tract infections.

Sometimes after giving birth, you may be unable to empty your bladder completely. The remaining urine provides an ideal breeding ground for bacteria, which can cause a urinary tract infection. Symptoms include a frequent, almost panicky urge to go, pain on urination, mild fever and tenderness over the area of the bladder.

A urinary tract infection is diagnosed by testing a urine sample for bacteria. Your doctor might want the sample to be collected through a catheter because the results are more accurate. A catheter is a small, flexible rubber tube that is inserted into your bladder to empty it of urine. Some women say the procedure hurts, although only for a moment, but others report no discomfort at all.

Treatment for a urinary tract infection includes antibiotics, drinking plenty of fluids, emptying the bladder often and taking acetaminophen for the fever.

Deep-Vein Thrombophlebitis

The hormones of pregnancy increase the likelihood of blood clots forming. Thrombophlebitis—a clot inside a vein—used to be common after pregnancy because new mothers were kept in bed for up to two weeks. Now you will be asked to get up and walk soon after birth, even after a cesarean birth. Walking gets the blood moving and prevents clotting.

Although no longer as common, clotting still occurs in roughly one in 500 pregnancies. The symptoms are tenderness, pain or swelling in the leg, often around the calf. You may also have a fever. These symptoms are caused by an obstruction in the veins, which interferes with the return circulation of the blood so that pressure builds up in the affected limb. The condition usually appears within the first days after labor, but it can occur up to several weeks later.

The main danger with thrombophlebitis is that the blood clot can break loose and be carried by the blood through the veins into the heart and out into the pulmonary arteries, where it can lodge and obstruct blood flow to a portion of the lungs. This occurs in approximately one in 3,000 women who have recently given birth. Depending on the size of the clot (now called a pulmonary embolism), the results may range from no symptoms, to chest pain and shortness of breath, to shock and even death.

Treatment consists of bed rest with the legs elevated and medication (heparin) to "thin" the blood to prevent further clot formation. Treatment takes place in the hospital because heparin must be administered intravenously. Bed rest is essential because the more the leg moves, the more likely the clot is to break loose. Heat or ice packs on the leg will reduce discomfort, and pain medication can be taken if needed.

For the first few days in the hospital you are not allowed to leave your bed, even to walk to the bathroom, but you should be able to have your baby with you. After the heparin is discontinued, your doctor may prescribe an oral blood thinner for three to six months.

If this condition develops with one pregnancy, you are more likely to have it in a subsequent one. You may be placed on blood thinners during the pregnancy to prevent the complication. You should discuss this possibility with your doctor.

Pelvic thrombophlebitis. Clotting can also occur in the pelvic veins, more commonly after cesarean birth. Pain may be present in the lower abdomen, usually on the right side, two to four days after delivery. It might be accompanied by fever, nausea and vomiting. Treatment includes antibiotics, blood thinners (heparin) and possible surgery.

Eclampsia (Postpartum)

Preeclampsia is the combination of high blood pressure (hypertension), protein in the urine and fluid retention that makes your face and hands puffy. (See page 192 for details.) Preeclampsia usually improves after birth, but sometimes preeclampsia develops into eclampsia up to 72 hours after birth. The term eclampsia is used to describe a condition in which a woman develops seizures in a pregnancy complicated by pregnancy-induced hypertension or preeclampsia. It is often associated with lack of prenatal care. Warning signs that seizures might be imminent include pain in the upper right side of your abdomen, headache and seeing flashing lights. If the condition is untreated, convulsions follow, sometimes leading to unconsciousness. If any of these symptoms develops, get immediate medical help.

Sorting Out Your Feelings

Childbirth usually does not have complications; however, those discussed here are the most common and can occur suddenly in what has been an otherwise normal pregnancy. They can occur even if you and your doctor have been doing everything right to care for your pregnancy. If something does go wrong, you need to trust your doctor to do the best for both you and your baby. If you are uncomfortable with the advice and treatment you are receiving, don't be afraid to ask for a second opinion or to see an obstetrician who treats high-risk pregnancies (perinatologist). Most doctors will not be offended at this request and may even welcome it.

When things start to go wrong, it's easy to feel out of control. Your body, formerly an ally, seems to have betrayed you. Often, it's best to relinquish control and become as flexible as you can. Your doctor will explain concerns and discuss possible outcomes and new courses of action. Trust your caregivers; they will try to do what is best for you and your baby. The miracle of modern medicine is that conditions that used to end in tragedy can now turn out well for both mother and baby.

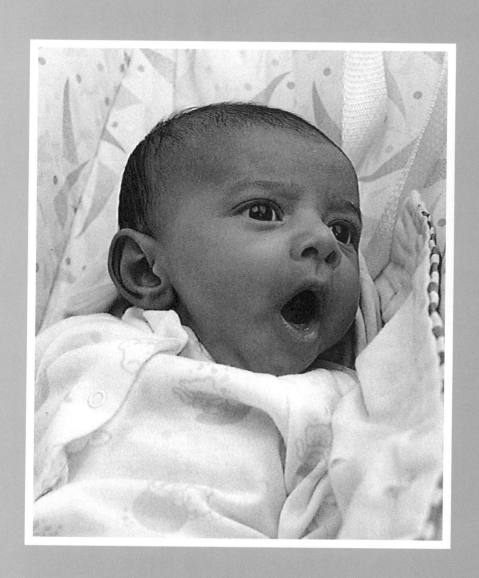

CHAPTER TWENTY

Cesarean Birth

"When my doctor cut into my uterus, the first thing to appear was my baby's head. She immediately let out a howl, and that sound was the high point of my life. I'll never forget it.

My doctor laughed and said, 'Cesarean babies hardly ever cry before we get them out. Boy! Are you in trouble!' She was right about that—this kid has been a real handful!"

It's important to educate yourself about cesarean birth before you near the end of your pregnancy. About one-quarter of American babies are born by cesarean, so it makes sense to be mentally ready for the possibility that your baby will be born this way. Here are issues you can discuss in advance with your doctor:

- Will your partner be allowed in the operating room?
- Can you have a regional anesthetic, such as an epidural, so that you will be awake to experience the birth?
- When will you both be able to see and hold the baby?
- Can you breastfeed as soon as you feel up to it, even in the recovery room?
- Can pictures be taken?

Why a Cesarean Birth Might Be Necessary

A cesarean birth may be planned for specific medical reasons or, as in most first-time cesareans, it might occur unexpectedly. First-time cesareans are seldom planned, because for most women it is assumed they will deliver vaginally. If a repeat cesarean is planned, it may be scheduled or might be done after a trial of labor.

Cesarean birth is done when the doctor decides it is safer than a vaginal birth for mother or baby. Many different considerations can contribute to such a decision.

Failure to Progress in Labor

This is one of the most frequent reasons doctors deliver a baby by cesarean. Some of the causes of failure to progress are that the cervix might not dilate completely, labor might slow down or stop altogether or sometimes the baby just won't fit through the mother's pelvis.

Repeat Cesarean

One-third of all cesareans performed are repeat cesareans. This number is decreasing, however, now that more women are electing to try vaginal birth after cesarean (VBAC). (Details on VBAC begin on page 341.)

Fetal Distress

Concerns about the baby's health during labor prompt 10 to 15 percent of cesarean births. The most common cause of fetal distress is that the baby is not getting enough oxygen, either because the umbilical cord is being compressed or because the placenta is no longer functioning effectively. The fetal heart rate is monitored in order to assess the baby's condition; sometimes other tests help indicate how well the baby is tolerating labor.

Malposition of the Baby

Breech positions (see page 318) are the cause of 15 percent of cesarean births. Sometimes the doctor is able to move a breech baby into a more favorable position by turning the baby before labor starts (a procedure called external version). If this is not successful, cesarean birth is considered. A foot-first (footling breech) or a sideways (transverse) position can also lead to cesarean birth if the doctor's attempts to turn the baby into the proper position are unsuccessful.

Not Enough Room for the Baby

It's possible for a baby to be head down but still be unable to fit through the pelvis. For example, if the baby is coming brow or face first or facing forward (in a "sunny-side up" position, occiput posterior), the smallest head circumference is not leading the way. And even though the cervix might be fully dilated, the baby simply may be unable to fit through the pelvis. In this case, cesarean birth might be necessary. Some babies are too large to safely deliver vaginally; size becomes an increased concern for women with a relatively small pelvis or when babies are estimated to weigh more than 9 to 10 pounds.

Maternal Health Conditions

If the mother has diabetes, heart or pulmonary disease or high blood pressure, cesarean birth may sometimes be the safer route for birth. If the mother has an active case of genital herpes (diagnosed by a positive culture or actual lesions), cesarean birth may be recommended to prevent the baby from picking up the virus on the way through the birth canal.

Multiple Births

When more than one baby is present, it is not unusual for one to be malpositioned. In this case, cesarean birth is often safer than vaginal birth.

Obstetrical Emergencies

When severe placental abruption (see page 194), placenta previa (see page 195), uterine rupture (see page 322) or cord prolapse (see page 320) occurs, immediate action is required, and cesarean birth is usually the fastest and safest option.

Risks of Cesarean Birth

Cesarean birth is major surgery, and, as with other surgical procedures, risks are involved. The estimated risk of a woman dying after cesarean birth is less than one in 2,500 (the risk of death after vaginal birth is less than one in 10,000). These are estimated risks for a large population of women. Individual medical conditions such as some heart problems may make the risk of vaginal birth higher than that of cesarean birth.

Other risks for the mother include the following:

- Infection. The uterus or nearby pelvic organs such as the bladder and kidneys can become infected. The risk with elective cesarean is less than that with emergency cesarean.

- Increased blood loss. Blood loss on average is about twice as much with cesarean birth as with vaginal birth. However, blood transfusions are rarely needed during cesarean births.

- Decreased bowel function. The bowel sometimes slows down for several days after surgery, resulting in distention, bloating and discomfort.

- Respiratory complications. General anesthesia can sometimes lead to pneumonia.

- Longer hospital stay and recovery time. Three to five days in the hospital is the common length of stay, whereas it is less than one to three days for vaginal birth.

- Reactions to anesthesia. The mother's health could be endangered by unexpected responses (such as blood pressure that drops quickly) to anesthesia or other medications used during surgery.

Risks for the Mother

In cesarean birth, possible risks to the baby include the following:

- Premature birth. If the due date was not accurately calculated, the baby might be delivered too early.

- Breathing problems. Babies born by cesarean are more likely to develop breathing problems such as transient tachypnea (abnormally fast breathing during the first few days after birth). (For more information about respiratory problems, see page 378.)

- Low Apgar scores. Babies born by cesarean sometimes have low Apgar scores. (For an explanation of Apgar scores, see page 349.) The low score can be an effect of anesthesia and cesarean birth, or the baby may have been in distress to begin with. Or perhaps the baby was not stimulated as much as he or she would have been by vaginal birth.

- Fetal injury. Although rare, the surgeon can accidentally nick the baby while making the uterine incision.

Risks for the Baby

Planned Cesarean Births

Some cesarean births are planned from the start. If you have certain pregnancy complications or some chronic medical conditions, for instance, cesarean birth might be your best option.

An emergency cesarean can be hectic and scary, but a planned cesarean can offer a couple of benefits: you can avoid a long labor and can organize your life around a scheduled birth date. One of the hardest things about the end of a pregnancy is that you don't know when the baby will come, so it's difficult to make plans during the last several weeks. If the birth is scheduled, you can organize your household and responsibilities at work and have your support systems in place before your hospitalization. A scheduled birth also allows you to arrange care for your other children without any middle-of-the-night panic.

If it's necessary to have a repeat cesarean, it may be a relief to be able to schedule your delivery date, but at the same time, experience may make you anxious about certain aspects of having surgery again. Talk over your fears with your doctor, childbirth instructor or partner. Tell yourself that you made it through once before and you can do it again. Think about how much more you know now: the path is more familiar and less scary, and your coping skills are probably better this time. If you had a cesarean birth after a long labor during your last delivery, you will likely be far less tired after a planned cesarean.

Unplanned but Non-Emergency Cesareans

If there is no medical urgency requiring an immediate cesarean, yet a surgical birth is recommended, you should have time to discuss the situation with your doctor and your partner to prepare for the idea of cesarean birth. Depending on the reason for the cesarean, you might even be able to take part in the decision. For example, if your baby is in the breech position, your doctor may attempt to turn the baby into a head-first position by pushing on the baby through your abdomen. This procedure is called an external version. Other alternatives include a vaginal breech birth, or you could have a cesarean. Your partner's input and emotional support can be very helpful during these decisions.

Emergency Cesareans

If an emergency arises that prompts a "stat" or emergency cesarean, things can move so rapidly that you and your partner might feel frightened, swept up in events beyond your control. The staff may suddenly jump into action and appear frenzied until you realize that everyone is rapidly accomplishing specific tasks. Speed can be critical in delivering a healthy baby.

*"I'd been getting nowhere for hours. My husband left the room and called my
family to let them know that nothing was going to happen anytime soon.
During that time the baby got into trouble, and my husband walked back into a
scene of pandemonium. Nurses were moving at top speed, my bed was being
pushed out the door and it all scared him half to death.*

*The result was pretty funny, though. Twenty minutes after he'd called
everyone to tell them not to expect any news till morning, he called back and
yelled, 'The baby's here!' We saved the phone bill to document the drama."*

Remember, it is the set of circumstances (the pelvis, uterus, mother's condition and baby's condition) that determines which route a baby takes. It is not
your fault if the baby is breech or if the head won't fit through your pelvis. If
you set your goal as the result of the birth process rather than the birth process
itself, you'll be less likely to be disappointed if you have a cesarean. After all,
your aim is to have a healthy baby, whatever it takes.

Emotional Impact of Cesarean Birth

With a national rate of cesarean births approaching 25 percent, it's important,
even if everything in your pregnancy is going well, to be prepared for the possibility of a cesarean birth. An emergency cesarean can be a frightening and sometimes disappointing experience, but it's important to remember that the vast
majority of cesarean births end well for both mother and baby.

*"My primary concern was always the baby. When his heart rate began dipping,
I just wanted him out as quickly as possible, no matter what it took. Surgery
was a small price to pay to end all that fear and anxiety."*

However, even women who initially were accepting of the surgery can later
lapse into negative feelings, and even become angry because their expectations
were unfulfilled. Some women may grieve that they weren't able to have a
vaginal birth, and then they may feel guilty about these feelings because they
think they shouldn't have them. Feelings of inadequacy and failure can occur
after a cesarean, as can doubts about femininity and self-worth. Occasionally
such thoughts can affect feelings toward the new baby, or the relationship
toward the father, and they may even interfere with plans for future pregnancies.
Well-meaning friends and family can contribute to negative feelings with
thoughtless remarks such as, "You took the easy way out," or "Are you going
to have your next baby the natural way?"

If you find yourself struggling with uncomfortable feelings, try talking about
them with your partner, a friend, nurse or doctor. Ventilating your feelings can
help put the experience in perspective and lead to acceptance. If the negative
feelings don't go away, a support group can help you realize you are not alone.
Your childbirth educator or doctor may be able to refer you to one, or check your
local phone book or newspaper for listings of such groups.

The Increasing Use of Cesarean Birth

When cesarean births were first done, they were used only to save a mother's life or when there were no other alternatives for delivering a baby. As recently as 1970, the cesarean rate in the United States was only 5.5 percent, even though the risks to both mother and baby were often high for vaginal births. Then doctors began performing cesareans when vaginal birth was possible but surgical intervention offered a better outcome for mother or baby. By 1978 the rate of cesarean birth increased to 15.3 percent, and by 1990 it was 23.5 percent, one of the highest in the world.

Nearly a million cesarean births are performed each year in the United States. Both doctors and patients have become concerned about this high rate and are looking for ways to lower it.

Factors in the Rising Cesarean Rate

The high rates of cesarean birth in the United States are a result of a combination of factors, as listed below.

The increased use of electronic fetal monitors. Monitors have had a direct impact on the number of cesarean procedures because they alert doctors to possible fetal difficulties during labor. The diagnosis of fetal distress increased 225 percent from 1980 to 1985 during a parallel increase in the use of fetal monitoring. It's difficult for a doctor to look at what appears to be an abnormal or "non-reassuring" fetal heart rate reading and be fully sure that everything is okay. Doctors have to make decisions based on their own experience, and because they have seen what can happen when things go wrong, they tend to be cautious and conservative.

Fetal distress can be more accurately diagnosed with an internal rather than an external fetal heart rate monitor, and it can be confirmed with analysis of a blood sample from the fetal scalp (a low pH indicates lack of oxygen and perhaps the need for immediate delivery). However, there isn't always time for these options.

Maternal medical conditions. Better management of chronic diseases such as diabetes and kidney or heart disease now allows women with these conditions to carry a baby, but the high risk of the pregnancy might make a cesarean birth the safer route for some mothers or babies.

Cesarean has become the preferred method of birth for most breech babies. Eighty percent of babies in the breech position are delivered by cesarean.

Cesarean deliveries have replaced many forceps deliveries. Complications that were managed by forceps-assisted birth in the past are sometimes now handled by cesarean birth. There isn't a simple right or wrong answer to which approach is best.

Age and fertility characteristics. Many women are postponing having children until they are older. Because older women tend to have an increase in complications, more of them have cesarean births. Also, cesarean rates are higher for women giving birth for the first time. As family sizes shrink, a higher proportion of all births are first births.

"Once a cesarean, always a cesarean." This statement was dogma until health care providers determined that low transverse uterine incisions (see page 337) are safe and do not increase the chance of uterine rupture during future labors. Studies now show that 60 to 80 percent of women who have previously undergone cesarean birth can successfully give birth vaginally. Despite this finding, repeat cesarean births still are the reason for nearly half of the increase in cesarean rates.

The threat of malpractice suits. The threat of being sued is a reason frequently given by physicians for the increased cesarean rate. They feel pressured into practicing "defensive medicine" at the slightest sign of something going wrong. For example, the fetal monitor may show some sign for concern and yet a woman delivers vaginally; later, if something is wrong with the baby, there has been a tendency to blame the doctor and file suit even though the baby's problem might have had nothing to do with the method of birth.

Lack of experience. Some experts believe that many teaching hospitals no longer provide sufficient opportunity for physicians in training (obstetrical residents) to learn how to manage anything other than normal labors. They may receive little practice in vaginal breech deliveries, in trying to turn breech babies (for more information on external version, see page 319) and even in the use of forceps; instead, they learn to rely on cesarean birth. The fear of lawsuits has even caused training in these special procedures to be dropped from some family medicine residency programs.

Current Recommendations

Many doctors and hospitals are trying hard to lower their rates of cesarean birth. The following recommendations may influence whether you have a cesarean birth:

- Look to friends, nurses, midwives and childbirth educators for advice on choosing a doctor who will work with you toward your goals.

- Develop good communication with your doctor, and discuss the subject of cesarean birth in advance.

- Attend childbirth education classes with your partner and become familiar with relaxation, breathing, imagery, massage and other techniques that reduce discomfort. These may help decrease your need for pain medication, which at times may affect your labor and your baby.

- If the baby is breech, ask whether an external version is possible.

- If your labor progresses slowly, walking and changing positions may speed things up.

- A supportive labor companion, even someone in addition to your partner, can be very helpful.

Cesarean birth, when it first became safe, was a medical miracle. There is no doubt that many women and babies are alive today because of this alternative to vaginal delivery. If you want to take part in the decision making, communication with your doctor is paramount. Working together as a team will help you feel more involved and satisfied with your birth experience.

What Happens During a Cesarean?

Preoperative Preparation

Whether a cesarean birth was planned or unexpected, you'll be prepared for surgery with a "preop prep." Part of the prep might be done in your room and the rest done in the operating room. Below are the standard preparations for a cesarean. In an emergency, some of these steps may be cut short or omitted altogether.

- Anesthesia options. The anesthesiologist will discuss these options with you and your doctor.

- Antacid. You may be given an antacid to neutralize stomach acids.

- Shaving. The hair on your abdomen and the upper one-third of your pubic hair may be shaved, followed by a scrub with an antiseptic wash.

- IV. An intravenous needle is inserted into your hand or arm so that fluids and medications can be given during and after surgery.

- Blood pressure cuff. The anesthesiologist or nurse anesthetist will wrap a cuff around your arm to monitor your blood pressure during surgery.

- Cardiac monitor. A monitor will allow the staff to watch your heart rate and rhythm throughout the procedure.

- Saturation monitor. A device clamped on your finger is used to monitor the oxygen level in your blood.

- Urinary catheter. A catheter will be inserted into your bladder to keep it empty.

The Operating Room

You will be wheeled to the operating room on a gurney (a narrow bed on wheels) or on the bed you've already been laboring in. The scene there is quite different from a relatively calm birthing room. Surgery is a team effort, so many more people will be present. There may be as many as a dozen people in the room if you or the baby pose complex medical problems.

From the gurney you will be transferred to the operating table. If you don't already have an IV, one will be placed now. You also might receive supplementary oxygen. If you are going to receive an epidural or spinal anesthetic, and it hasn't already been administered, you'll sit up or lie on your side while the anesthesiologist administers the anesthetic. You'll then lie on your back with your legs positioned securely in place, and your arms will be outstretched and secured on padded boards. A nurse will scrub your abdomen with an antiseptic solution and drape it with sterile cloths. A cloth drape (anesthesia screen) will be placed below your chin to protect the surgical field.

If yours is not an emergency situation, your doctor and the anesthesiologist will have already discussed the various options with you. What anesthesia is safest for the baby? What is safest for you? What is the reason for the cesarean? What options are feasible right now? All of these factors must be weighed.

Regional anesthesia. Regional anesthesia numbs your body from the chest down so that surgery can be done while you are fully awake. You feel little or no pain, and little or no medication reaches the baby. (For a description of how an epidural or spinal block is done, see page 300.)

Advantages

- You are awake for your baby's birth.
- The baby has minimal exposure to the medication.
- The procedure is simple and reliable.
- The baby's father or the labor companion can be present for the birth.
- Pain relief can be continued in the postoperative period.

Concerns

- Nausea and vomiting are possible side effects.
- General anesthesia may sometimes still be necessary.
- Postoperative headache occurs in a small number of women, but a technique called an epidural blood patch or other treatment can alleviate this.

Epidural anesthesia. With epidural anesthesia, a needle or catheter delivers pain medication just outside the fluid-filled space surrounding the spinal cord. The effect wears off in three to five hours, but additional doses of anesthetic can be given to extend the pain relief if necessary. One drawback to an epidural anesthetic is that it takes up to 20 minutes to administer, time you may not have in an emergency. An epidural anesthetic is used for about 40 percent of cesarean births.

Spinal block. A spinal block is similar to an epidural, but the needle that supplies the pain-relieving medication goes into, rather than just outside, the fluid surrounding the spinal nerves. With this anesthesia, the procedure can be performed more quickly and easily than with an epidural, but only one dose can be given, which lasts about two hours. Spinal blocks are used for about 40 percent of cesarean births.

General anesthesia. Less than 20 percent of cesarean births are done with general anesthesia, and it is usually the choice for emergency surgery if the baby needs to be delivered as quickly as possible. Combinations of medication can be given by IV and inhalation to induce muscle relaxation and sleep. Under general anesthesia, you reach complete unconsciousness, with loss of sensation, and you cannot see, feel or hear, nor will you have any memory of the surgery.

Some anesthetic does get through to the baby, but only a small amount. If needed, medications can be given to the baby to counteract the effects of the anesthetic.

Once the source of anesthesia has been removed, its major effects wear off in five to 15 minutes, but you might feel groggy for hours after surgery. This feeling might make it difficult at first to hold and enjoy your baby.

Advantage

- It can be administered quickly in emergencies.

Concerns

- You're not awake to take in the experience of your baby's birth.
- The baby might be sleepy at first from the effects of the anesthesia.
- There is a small risk of vomiting or inhaling (aspirating) any partially digested food in your stomach. This is the reason doctors recommend that you don't eat during labor.
- You will be groggy for some time afterward and may feel more nauseated than after regional anesthesia.

Incisions

The doctor will make two separate incisions: one in your abdominal wall and one in your uterus. The one you see on the outside does not necessarily indicate the type of incision on your uterus.

Abdominal incisions. The incision on your abdomen will be about six inches long. This incision goes through skin, fat and muscle to the lining of the abdominal cavity (peritoneum). Any bleeding vessels will be sealed with heat (cauterization) or tied off.

Vertical incision. A vertical incision goes from just below the navel to just above the pubic bone. It is used by some doctors when they need a large incision or when the baby must be removed quickly.

Bikini incision. A bikini incision is a horizontal cut made across the lower abdomen, near the pubic hairline. This is the preferred incision because it heals well and causes the least postoperative discomfort.

The skin incision made for a cesarean birth could be a vertical incision about the length between the navel and the pubic hair (left drawing) or a bikini incision, a more horizontal incision lower on the abdomen (right drawing).

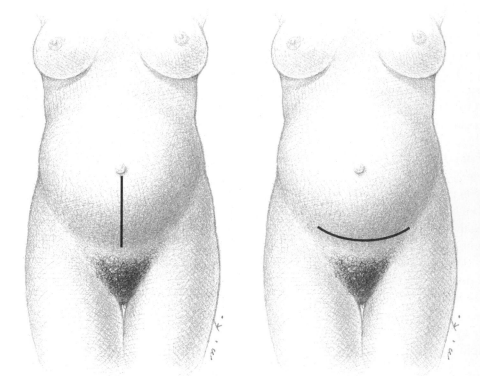

Uterine incisions. The uterine incision is usually smaller than the abdominal incision. Your doctor considers several factors, including the urgency of the delivery and the position of the baby, when choosing which type of incision to use.

Low transverse incision. Now the most common, the low transverse incision is made sideways across the lower portion of the uterus. It bleeds less than incisions higher on the uterus, forms a strong scar and presents little danger of rupturing during future labors.

Classical incision. Also called a high vertical, a classical incision was the type of incision originally done with cesareans. Because this type of incision poses the greatest risk for bleeding and for subsequent tearing (rupture) of the uterus, it now is used only when absolutely necessary.

Low vertical incision. This is similar to a classical incision, but it is lower on the uterus where the tissue is thinner. It might be used to deliver a baby who is in an awkward position, such as transverse or breech, or when there is risk that the incision will need to be extended to become a classical incision.

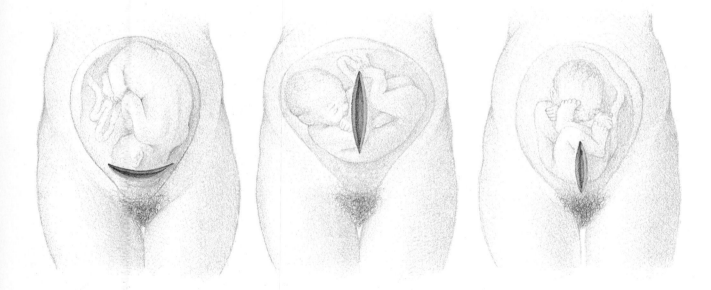

The uterine incision your doctor chooses for a cesarean birth depends on how quickly the baby needs to be delivered and the position the baby is in. The incision shown on the left, called a low transverse incision, is now the most common. The incision shown in the center, called a classical incision, *is now usually reserved for rapid delivery or for pregnancies with special problems. The incision shown on the right, called a low vertical incision, might be used to deliver a baby who is not in an ideal position, or if there is risk that the incision will need to be extended to a classical incision.*

The Baby Is Born

Because the doctor wants to keep the uterine incision as small as possible, you will feel some tugging (but no pain) as the baby is pulled out. After the baby is born, the doctor clamps the umbilical cord and hands the baby to another member of the team. Soon you will have your first look.

If your previous babies were born vaginally, you will notice some differences. For one thing, unless you were in labor for a long time before your cesarean, the baby's head won't be as molded. (The illustration on page 346 shows head molding.)

After the baby is delivered, the doctor will remove the placenta from your uterus and will begin to close the incision layer by layer. You may be feeling a little drowsy, so even though the stitching can take up to an hour, the time will probably pass quickly. The internal sutures dissolve on their own and won't need to be removed. The skin incision may be stitched or it can be "stapled" with small metal clips that bend in the middle to pull the edges of skin together. If staples are used, before you go home they will be removed with tiny pliers that straighten the bend to release the ends. All you feel, if anything, is a slight pinching.

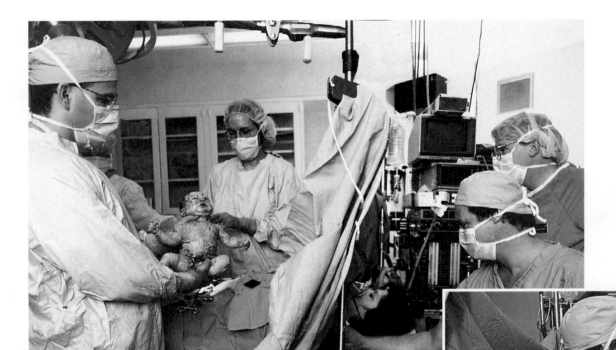

For a planned cesarean or one that is not performed under emergency circumstances, a regional anesthetic allows the mother to remain awake during the procedure. Often, the father can be present to witness the birth. Within minutes of the birth, mom and dad can greet their new baby while the surgeons finish the operation.

The labor companion during cesarean birth

If the cesarean birth is not an emergency and if the mother remains awake, many hospitals allow the labor companion to come into the operating room. Some people are thrilled by the idea. Others may be squeamish or downright scared of the drama of the operating room, especially when the procedure involves someone they know and love. Because the anesthesia screen is large enough to block your view if you sit near the mother's head, you may (or may not) watch the birth.

You will be shown where to get surgical scrubs (the clean, comfortable clothing worn in an operating room), a covering for your hair, shoe covers and a face mask.

The mother-to-be will likely be apprehensive about the surgery, so supporting her by holding her hand, talking gently and maintaining eye contact can help decrease her anxiety and make her more relaxed. Breathing and relaxation exercises may help if she is overly apprehensive. It's important to help her focus on the birth rather than the operation.

If you want to take photos or videos of the birth, first ask permission from the doctor and ask where you should sit or walk in the operating room. Most couples focus on recording their first sight of the newborn and their time together rather than on technical details of the birth. Be particularly careful to stay out of the way and to avoid tripping over any cables or touching operating room equipment.

Recovery

Immediately after surgery, you will be taken to a recovery room, where your vital signs will be monitored frequently until the anesthetic has worn off and your condition is stable. Then you will be taken to a room in the maternity section. During the next 24 hours your vital signs, urinary output, vaginal flow and abdominal dressing will continue to be monitored. Your uterus will also be checked to make sure it remains contracted to minimize the risk of bleeding.

Postoperative Pain Relief

Although everyone's pain threshold is different, it's important to be medicated for pain when the anesthetic wears off so that you can stay comfortable and in control.

Narcotics. Narcotics can be given through your IV or injected into a muscle once the IV has been removed. They also can be given through an epidural catheter before its removal. The epidural catheter can be left in place up to 24 hours after surgery. You and your doctor will decide what is best for you.

Patient-controlled analgesia pumps. Many hospitals connect a small IV pump to your IV so that you can receive small doses of narcotic by pressing a button when you feel you need it. Because the drug goes directly into your IV, pain relief is fast. The pump has a lock-out device to limit the amount of medication you can receive within a given time, which prevents you from over-medicating.

Antibiotics

To prevent a uterine infection, antibiotics may be given through your IV just after the baby is born, and possibly again later.

Breastfeeding

If you plan on nursing your baby, the sooner you start, the better. It's not too soon to try when you're still in the recovery area. Pillows situated behind you can help raise you into a comfortable position. If you've had an epidural, you will probably be comfortable for an hour or two after surgery, which should make breastfeeding more comfortable. If you have had a general anesthetic, you may be more uncomfortable, so breastfeeding may not be your first priority. You will feel much more comfortable if you are medicated for pain before you begin. Holding your baby in a football hold, under your arm, is a comfortable position for breastfeeding after a cesarean because it avoids pressure on your abdomen.

Preventing Fluid Buildup in the Lungs

If you remain lying down for long periods after surgery, it's possible for your lungs to accumulate fluid. You will be encouraged to change positions frequently, to take slow, deep breaths and to cough to help keep your lungs clear. Sometimes coughing and turning can pull on your incision, but if you hold a pillow across your stomach and apply slight pressure, you'll be more comfortable while coughing.

Eating and Drinking

Because you probably will be allowed only ice chips or sips of water for the first 12 to 24 hours, the IV line stays in until you are able to take enough fluids by mouth to prevent dehydration. When your digestive system begins to rumble back into action (you'll know because you'll begin to pass gas), you can have more fluids and probably some easily digested food. When the IV is removed, so is the patient-controlled analgesia pump; at that point you can switch to pain medication in injection or pill form.

Urinary Catheter

The catheter continues to empty your bladder until you can get out of bed and walk to the bathroom, usually the day after surgery.

Walking

About six to eight hours after surgery, or maybe the following day, you will be asked to start taking brief walks. You may prefer to lie still until your incisions heal because they hurt every time you move, but walking is good for your body. It helps clear your lungs, improves your circulation, promotes healing and gets your digestive system going. Walking also prevents blood clots, a common complication in the days when women were kept in bed for weeks after surgery. Between short excursions from your bed—probably just to the bathroom or the chair at first—you can promote circulation by flexing your feet and making circles with your ankles even while lying down.

A fter the birth, your uterus will continue to contract, which is its way of controlling bleeding. The contractions may hurt at times, especially during breastfeeding. Breastfeeding causes your body to produce oxytocin, which stimulates uterine contractions. It may be helpful to coordinate pain medication with breastfeeding. Relaxation techniques can also help. After-birth pains start anytime after surgery and may last four to five days.

After-Birth Pains

Y our abdomen begins rumbling, usually around the second or third day after surgery, as your gastrointestinal system returns to normal. Walking can help move things along.

Gas Pains

A bloody discharge called lochia (see page 417) may last anywhere from two to eight weeks, the same as with a vaginal birth.

Vaginal Flow

T he typical stay after cesarean birth is about three days, a day or two longer if you have any problems. Your body is still healing when you are home; full recovery will take four to six weeks.

Hospital Stay

Vaginal Birth After Cesarean (VBAC)

Your first baby was born by cesarean. Now you're pregnant again, facing choices of how to give birth. Should you plan for another cesarean? Or should you go through a trial of labor and see how things go this time around? But how far are you willing to go, knowing that you could be in the operating room again despite an attempt at vaginal birth? If you have such reservations, will they prevent you from giving vaginal birth the total effort needed to deliver a baby?

"The pushing seemed impossible. For a while I thought, 'I can't do this; I want a cesarean.' But now that it's over there's no comparison. It's only been 24 hours, but I feel like I could run a race."

Why Try?

Initially, doctors feared that a uterus with a cesarean scar would rupture along the scar line during the final, intense stages of labor. When a woman became pregnant a second time they automatically scheduled her for another cesarean birth. Then doctors stopped routinely using classical vertical incisions and began to use low transverse incisions. Because the lower part of the uterus doesn't stretch as much during pregnancy, the risk of rupture is less likely. Other factors also encourage trying for a vaginal birth after a cesarean.

Safety. Vaginal birth, even vaginal birth after cesarean, is generally safer for the mother and for the baby.

Shorter recovery time. Instead of three to five days in the hospital, you can go home after one or two. And you'll get back to your regular activity level far more quickly if you don't have to wait for incisions to heal.

More personal involvement. The effort of your pushing will help your baby be born. Your labor companion and others you may choose to have present can make it more of a family experience.

Lower cost. A vaginal birth costs less than a cesarean birth.

Current Recommendations

The American College of Obstetricians and Gynecologists (ACOG) makes the following recommendations:

- Vaginal birth after cesarean (VBAC) is preferred over repeat cesarean for women with low transverse uterine scars.
- There is no set limit on the number of previous cesareans that make VBAC too risky. Studies show that women who've undergone two or three cesarean births can go on to have a safe VBAC.
- Prior cephalopelvic disproportion (see page 318) is not a specific reason to rule out VBAC. A second baby might have a smaller head or be in a better position.
- Women with high vertical uterine scars should not be considered candidates for VBAC because not enough data exist to ensure safety.

Factors Affecting VBAC Rates

The large majority—perhaps as many as 90 percent—of women who have undergone cesarean are candidates for VBAC. Of those who do try to have a vaginal delivery, 60 to 80 percent are successful. Despite such positive statistics, only 20 percent of the women who qualify are choosing VBAC. Why?

Tips for women planning a VBAC

- Discuss your concerns, fears and expectations with your doctor.
- Take a class for parents who are considering VBAC.
- Build confidence by thinking positively: "My body is strong and it knows how to give birth."
- Take care of yourself during your pregnancy. If you eat properly, exercise regularly and get plenty of rest, you will improve your chance for normal labor and birth.

Women's fears. Some women are afraid of going through labor, especially if they may have had a long and difficult labor that resulted in a cesarean. Others fear failure and loss of control. Worry about uterine rupture also is still common, even though this rarely occurs.

Hospital facilities. ACOG recommends that VBAC be tried only if a hospital has continuous electronic fetal monitoring, a surgical team that can be assembled quickly and the ability to administer anesthetics and blood 24 hours a day. As a result, in many small facilities the doctor is more likely to schedule a cesarean than risk the need for an emergency procedure.

Doctors' attitudes. Some doctors have been hesitant to give up the ease of scheduling a repeat cesarean birth. Recently trained doctors who were exposed to VBACs during their residencies may be more likely to encourage them.

Because couples considering VBAC often have many concerns and questions, they may need extra information and support from their caregivers and their childbirth educators. In addition to regular childbirth classes, if possible they should attend VBAC classes. These classes allow couples to discuss birth experiences and to share feelings of anger and disappointment. If prospective parents can work through their experiences and concerns, they are often more willing to try vaginal birth. Another objective of these classes is to reinforce the safety of VBAC.

The highest rate of VBAC is in women who have experienced both kinds of births; given a choice, they opt for vaginal.

Preparation for VBAC

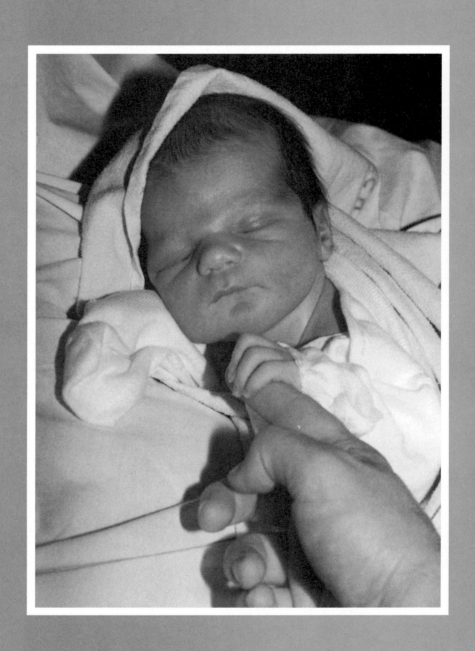

CHAPTER TWENTY-ONE

Your Baby's First Hours

From the moment you first learned you were pregnant, you've probably been eagerly anticipating two things: the first glimpse of your baby and your elation at his or her arrival.

Your mental picture, the product of thousands of advertisements, movies and television shows, is of a plump, cuddly infant announcing his or her arrival with a lusty cry. You see yourself reaching out to hold and snuggle your baby moments after birth, perhaps with your partner looking on admiringly.

The birth of your baby is truly the culmination of a miracle, a moment for celebration and relief. You've protected and nurtured this baby through pregnancy and labored to give birth. But the reality of what your baby looks like and your own feelings at this moment may not be quite what you envisioned.

This chapter gives you an overview of what your baby will really look like, the attention she or he will get from the medical staff and how your baby might respond to her or his new environment. You'll also be prepared for what to expect of yourself during the early moments when you first welcome your new baby. (For more information about the capabilities of a newborn, see page 437.)

After months of anticipation, with the emotions and physical pain of labor and delivery behind them, a new mom and dad and their minutes-old daughter pause in the birthing room to get acquainted.

What Will My Baby Look Like?

The tiny person you'll greet may not be the perfect little cherub you've imagined. The picture-perfect "newborns" you see in movies or ads are probably several months old. A newly born baby is likely to emerge somewhat messy-looking, with head a bit misshapen and larger than you imagined, eyelids puffy, legs drawn up, arms folded across the chest.

Your baby might or might not be crying at birth, and it may take several minutes before your baby starts to breathe well. Your baby must make enormous adjustments after emerging from the protective pool of amniotic fluid in your uterus to a strange, new environment where her or his body must function on its own.

At the moment of birth, however, the condition of your baby is much the same as it was in the uterus—warm, wet and slippery from amniotic fluid and traces of blood. Your baby may be covered with a whitish, waxy or cheesy coating called the vernix caseosa. Vernix will be most noticeable under the arms, behind the ears and in the groin; premature babies are liberally coated with it. Although nurses or doctors will wipe your baby's face almost immediately and quickly dry the baby with a blanket or towels, they are otherwise in no hurry to clean your baby. Making sure that breathing and circulation are normal and keeping your baby warm are their first concerns. Your baby will probably not have a bath until he or she reaches the nursery.

A baby's skin is normally somewhat plum-colored or blue-tinged during the entire time spent in the uterus, and it may seem blue-hued at birth. Parents are sometimes alarmed that this bluish color is a sign that their baby has circulatory problems. Remember, it often takes several minutes before your baby starts breathing well alone and circulating the more highly oxygenated red blood that will give your baby's skin its normal pinkish tinge. It's normal for a newborn's hands and feet to remain slightly bluish gray. But this color does not indicate that your baby is cold.

The head usually leads the way in the descent through the birth canal. Bones in the baby's skull can temporarily shift and mold to the shape of the pelvis to allow easy passage. Your baby's head may look elongated (cone-shaped) at birth, but the shape will return to normal within a few days.

A baby born to non-white parents may appear especially dusky initially. As the baby's blood becomes more highly oxygenated, the lips, tongue and nail beds will show a normal, healthy-looking, pinkish tone. In fact, doctors first check these sites in all babies to assess whether well-oxygenated blood is circulating properly.

At birth, your baby's head may seem elongated, even pointy, especially if a vacuum extractor (see

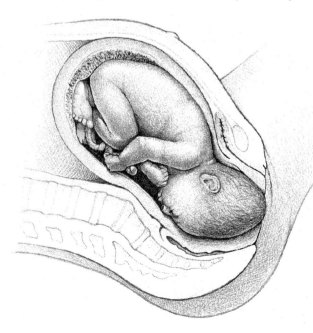

Head mold-ing at birth

24 hours after birth

page 313) was used to assist in the birth. This distortion is called molding; it results from compression of soft, not yet fully joined bones of the skull during your baby's passage through the birth canal.

Pressure of the baby's skull against the mother's pelvis may cause temporary puffiness at the scalp, called caput succedaneum (caput, for short). Pressure from the mother's pelvis can leave a bruise (a cephalhematoma) on the baby's head.

Your baby's nose may seem flattened at first, also from pressure in the birth canal, and the cheeks may have marks or bruises if forceps were used. Within several days, molding and caput will give way to a rounded, shapely head. A cephalhematoma may take several weeks to disappear.

You or your partner may have brown, gray, blue or green eyes, but your new baby's eyes will likely appear dark bluish brown, blue-black, grayish blue or slate-colored. The true eye color probably won't become definite for six to nine months. Parents and relatives sometimes play a game of guessing what color the baby's eyes will be. In fact, eye color is so uncertain that most birth announcements don't even have a blank space for this information.

Some babies are born almost bald, some have thick hair and some have a light cap of soft hair. Hair color may change some during the first year. The basic color remains the same but, for example, blond newborns may be lighter or darker blond as infants, and sometimes a reddish tinge isn't apparent at birth. Downy, fine hair called lanugo may be temporarily apparent on the back, shoulders, forehead and temples.

Mistaken identity

Don't be upset if a doctor or nurse in the birthing room refers to your baby as "he" or "she," even if you've seen otherwise with your own eyes. Staff members are usually attending to several mothers and babies at the same time. Under these busy circumstances it's easy to mis-state whether the latest baby—yours—is a boy or girl. If you think the staff member is mistaken, don't be alarmed, just look for yourself.

Your Feelings After Delivery

Your reaction to your baby's arrival might not be at all what you expected. You may be immersed in a jumble of emotions when your baby arrives.

Many new mothers are overjoyed, wanting to cuddle their new babies the moment they emerge. Many other mothers are exhausted, still recovering from exertion and pain. They prefer to rest, to wait for the placenta to be delivered and to clean up before holding their babies. Some new mothers are afraid to hold their babies for fear of dropping them.

You may have the urge to nurse your baby immediately, but don't be disappointed if your baby is disinclined at first try. Babies sometimes need an hour or two before starting to nurse. Some babies may cry for a few moments, then lie quietly, content to look around or even drop off for a quick nap. Others don't even open their eyes immediately.

Let your feelings be your guide after your baby is born. Do what you feel like doing, even if it is not what you planned to do.

Celebrate, laugh or cry from joy, if you wish. Or, perhaps you'll reserve your emotions for the moment you and your partner are first alone with your new baby.

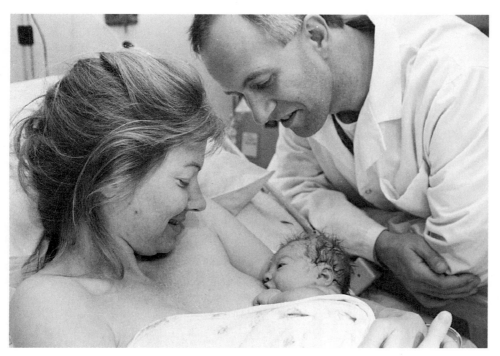

Giving birth is an incredible experience—exciting, scary at times, noisy, quiet, very private and personal, yet at the same time there is a strong urge to have others celebrating with you. In the moments after birth, don't feel inhibited by the presence of your caregivers; they are accustomed to the intimacies shared by many couples after birth as well as by the natural messiness that accompanies childbirth. So enjoy, relax, laugh, cry, kiss and hug your baby or partner or both!

Whether you breastfeed or bottle feed your baby, the first feeding will probably be a memorable moment. Dad's on hand, here, to share the experience. Don't be disappointed if your baby is not interested in nursing immediately after delivery. The birth process can leave both of you exhausted, and your baby may be more interested in napping than nursing.

Attention Your Baby Receives From the Medical Staff

When you give that final push and your baby is born, two teams take over, one to care for your baby and the other to care for you. Often, there is too much going on in the room for one person to care for both. The following is a description of what birth attendants will look for and the care your newborn baby will receive in the birthing room.

Breathing

To ensure that the baby can breathe properly, usually the doctor or nurse-midwife clears the nose and mouth of fluid as soon as the head appears—before the baby is fully delivered—and often again immediately after birth.

A baby's lungs, too, are filled with fluid before birth. Usually, this fluid is absorbed in the lymph and blood, and the lungs start filling with air almost as soon as the baby takes the first breath. But some babies are literally too tired to start breathing on their own. In this case, a nurse or doctor will stimulate breathing by rubbing the baby's body or even assist breathing with an oxygen bag and mask.

To ensure proper breathing, the doctor or nurse-midwife will suction fluids from your baby's nose and mouth just as soon as the head appears, and probably again immediately after birth.

Sometimes, babies may need further breathing assistance; in many hospitals these babies are promptly moved to a nearby room set up for further help. Premature babies may, of course, require respiratory and other assistance in a special intensive care facility. (For more information on premature babies, see page 353.)

Heart Rate and Circulation

While the baby's airway is being cleared, the heart rate and circulation will be checked. The heartbeat may have been monitored during labor, but just after birth a nurse or doctor will check the heart rate with a stethoscope or by feeling the pulse in the umbilical cord.

The baby's color—especially the color of the lips and tongue—will be observed to make sure circulation is normal. In the uterus, a fetus's blood bypasses the lungs via a detour called the ductus arteriosus. It is more important for the fetus to send blood to the placenta, which functions as the lungs before a baby is born. Shortly after birth, this detour closes off and the baby's blood starts circulating through his or her lungs to pick up oxygen and get rid of carbon dioxide. A healthy color indicates that this process is taking place.

Apgar Scores

So many parents have heard about Apgar scores that they are as anxious to learn their new baby's score as they are, later on, to read their child's first school report card. Apgar scores were devised in 1953 by an anesthesiologist, Dr. Virginia Apgar, as a quick evaluation of a newborn baby's health. Apgar scores, taken at one and five minutes after birth, rate new babies on a scale of zero to 2, for five criteria: appearance and color, pulse, reflexes, activity and respiration. The total possible score is 10.

Many doctors today, however, downplay the significance of Apgar scores. For one thing, they point out, they will not wait a full minute to take action if a baby shows breathing or circulatory problems. For another, most babies with lower scores will ultimately turn out to be perfectly healthy. Also, Apgar scores are not reliable indicators of possible neurologic problems, such as cerebral palsy.

Apgar Scores: How Healthy Is Your Newborn?

	Points		
Sign	**0**	**1**	**2**
Appearance (color)	Pale or blue	Body pink, extremities blue	Pink
Pulse (heartbeat)	Not detectable	Below 100	Above 100
Grimace (reflex irritability)	No response to stimulation	Grimace	Lusty cry, cough or sneeze
Activity (muscle tone)	Flaccid (no or weak activity)	Some movement of extremities	Active motion
Respiration	None	Slow, irregular	Good, crying

Scores determined for each sign are totaled. The highest possible score is 10. By 5 minutes of age, most healthy babies have scores of at least 7. A score less than that indicates that the baby warrants careful watching.

If your baby's Apgar score is less than 5 after five minutes, an experienced physician or labor-room nurse will probably give your baby a quick but careful overall inspection. These professionals have their own language: Is the baby breathing and beginning to "pink up"? Are the baby's lungs particularly "juicy"? Does the baby need suctioning? Is the baby "floppy"? Is the heart rate reasonably OK? Are there any other obvious physical abnormalities that might require immediate attention? (For more information on interpreting comments you may hear in the delivery room, see the box on page 358.)

Meconium Aspiration

Meconium is the dark-green, tarry substance that has been accumulating in the baby's intestinal tract since about the 16th week of gestation. Babies do not have bowel movements until after birth; however, 10 to 15 percent of babies may pass some stool just before or during labor.

Most babies who have passed a small amount of meconium into the amniotic fluid will have no difficulties. Meconium in the amniotic fluid will not be troublesome to a newborn baby's eyes, skin or throat. Even if swallowed, it won't harm the baby.

Doctors do worry about increased risk to the baby if large amounts of meconium pass into the amniotic fluid. The fluid can become thick or "pea-soupy" and may actually contain chunks of meconium.

Babies have breathing movements that are often easily demonstrated during a prenatal ultrasound test. When labor begins, babies stop these breathing movements until they are born. However, if babies are sufficiently stressed during labor, they can make gasping efforts and can inhale meconium-tainted amniotic fluid into their lungs. This is called meconium aspiration. If the baby has inhaled meconium into the lungs, immediate medical attention may be required.

Because aspiration of meconium can cause problems for newborns, the birthing room staff is always alert to recognize meconium-colored amniotic fluid and to be ready to clear it from the baby's air passages. Immediate suctioning of meconium from the baby's lungs often helps prevent or minimize the problem, but some babies can become extremely ill and require assisted ventilation.

Remember: Most babies won't pass meconium until after they are born. Of those who pass meconium before they are born, most won't aspirate meconium into their lungs. Of those who aspirate meconium, most will be fine; but the very few who develop problems because of meconium aspiration can become critically ill within the first hours of life.

Pediatric care

Most hospitals have an experienced nurse or doctor available to check and care for your baby at birth. But you may request your family doctor, pediatrician, nurse-practitioner or one of their colleagues to be present. Discuss arrangements for new baby care with your obstetrician, family physician or other professionals during your pregnancy.

Umbilical Cord

By the time your baby is handed to you, attendants will have clamped and cut the umbilical cord; sometimes the father is offered the opportunity to do this. The cord will be clamped with a metal pin or plastic clamp; the remnant (stump) may range from a very short one at the skin line to one that is an inch-and-a-half long. Before you leave the hospital, you'll be instructed on how to care for the umbilical stump.

About one in five babies is born with the umbilical cord wrapped around the neck—a so-called nuchal cord. New parents sometimes worry that the cord is strangling their baby. There's rarely cause for concern. The cord is almost always only loosely wrapped and does not harm the throat or neck, and blood flow in the cord is unimpaired. It is possible that a compressed or prolapsed cord—a loop of umbilical cord that has slid down between the baby's head and the mother's pelvis—can cause problems for a baby during labor. This is one of the reasons that the baby is watched so carefully during labor. If problems from cord compression arise, medical intervention, such as cesarean birth, can be done to help the baby. (For more information on cord compression, see page 320.)

Almost immediately after birth, an identification bracelet is attached to your baby's wrist. This is not just to ensure that you take the right baby home with you but to be certain that the correct data are entered on the baby's records and that any medical procedures and laboratory tests are performed on the right baby. Incidentally, the traditional footprint may look cute in the baby book, but it isn't equivalent to fingerprinting. Fingerprint experts explain that a baby's footprints are usually not accurate enough to be used for positive identification.

Identification Procedures

To avert the possibility of gonorrhea being passed from mother to baby, all states require that infants' eyes be protected from this infection immediately after birth. Gonorrheal eye infections were a leading cause of blindness until early in the 20th century, when postnatal treatment of babies' eyes became mandatory.

Until the 1970s, a silver nitrate solution was routinely dropped in the baby's eyes to prevent gonorrheal infection. But this solution can irritate the eyes and cause the eyelids to become puffy for a day or so. Also, it does not protect against the increasingly common infection called chlamydia. Now, soon after birth, an antibiotic ointment or solution, commonly either tetracycline or erythromycin, is placed onto the eyes. These newer preparations are gentler to the eyes, yet are still effective for preventing newborn eye infections.

Preventing Eye Disease

In the United States, virtually all babies receive an injection of vitamin K shortly after they are born. Vitamin K is necessary for normal blood coagulation (the process for stopping bleeding after a cut or a bruise). Because newborns have rather low levels of vitamin K for the first few weeks, vitamin K is given to prevent the rare possibility (one in 4,000 births) that a newborn would be so deficient in vitamin K that serious bleeding might develop, including bleeding inside the skull or in the brain. This problem is unique to babies in their first several weeks of life and is not related to hemophilia.

Vitamin K Injections

Shortly after your baby's birth, or soon after arrival in the nursery, a physician or nurse-practitioner will do a physical exam to detect any abnormalities. The doctor will check your baby's hips for possible dislocations, listen to her or his heart for possible murmurs, feel your baby's abdomen for urinary tract abnormalities and look at the eyes for cataracts or a rare eye tumor called a retinoblastoma.

All of these conditions are uncommon, but they can affect a baby's health and future development and should be detected early to help plan treatment for the babies who are affected.

Your Baby's First Exam

Problems That Can Prolong Hospitalization

Jaundice. Most newborns have a yellowish appearance to their skin called jaundice. It's caused by a buildup of a chemical called bilirubin in the baby's blood. Bilirubin is the product of spent red blood cells. Bilirubin is normally cleansed from the bloodstream, processed by the liver, sent to the kidneys and eliminated in the urine. Newborns often have more bilirubin than their immature livers can manage. Consequently, bilirubin builds up in their blood, causing the skin discoloration. The condition may last a week to 10 days. Among premature newborns, the problem is more pronounced because their livers are even less mature. The yellow tinge may persist for a couple of weeks or more.

Mild jaundice doesn't require treatment. If the bilirubin becomes moderately high, the doctor probably will place the baby under a bilirubin light. This treatment, called phototherapy, uses an ultraviolet lamp to help rid the baby's body of excess bilirubin.

Blood tests document the levels of bilirubin. When the bilirubin returns to a normal level, the phototherapy can be discontinued.

Infection. When a new baby has difficulty breathing, is unusually sleepy, eats poorly or has persistently high or low temperatures, doctors may suspect an infection (sepsis). Sepsis is suspected in about one of 25 newborns and necessitates evaluation and possible treatment with antibiotics. True infection, entailing possible risks to the baby and a prolonged hospital stay, actually occurs in only about one of every 250 babies.

Feeding difficulty. Whether you breastfeed or bottle feed, you may have difficulty in the first few days getting your newborn baby interested in taking nourishment of any kind. Some babies just seem to adopt a kind of slow-and-sleepy approach to eating. Pokey eaters occasionally require tube feedings to help them along for a few days, after which they generally catch on and bottle feed or breastfeed with enthusiasm. (For more information on feeding, see page 471.)

Physical Measurements

The average newborn weighs about 7½ pounds and is about 20 inches long. If your baby is from 5½ to 10 pounds and is 18 to 22 inches long, your baby's weight and length are in the normal range.

Shortly after delivery, your baby's height, weight and head size are checked, because the size of your baby can be an important indicator of your baby's health, or even your own health, at the time you give birth.

Your baby's health. If your baby's weight, length and head size are smaller or larger than the normal range, such findings do not necessarily indicate problems. But they do alert the nurses and doctors to watch your baby more closely to observe for problems, such as a low blood sugar level, that may need special attention.

Your own health. Women who deliver exceptionally small or large babies may also require observation and sometimes testing to see if there may be an underlying health problem. For example, an exceptionally large baby can sometimes indicate that the mother has a condition such as diabetes, which may need treatment.

CHAPTER TWENTY-TWO

If Your Baby Arrives Early

"Stunned is the term that best describes my feelings. After a moment, questions and fears came spilling out. 'Will my baby be all right?' 'Is this my fault?' 'Have I done something wrong?'"

These words, taken from a diary, record a mother's response to the news that her baby probably would be born two months too soon. We'll call the expectant mom Julie and her obstetrician Dr. Patterson. Julie wrote these words in her diary not long after Dr. Patterson admitted her to the hospital.

She had visited the doctor a week earlier, feeling just fine. Throughout her pregnancy, she'd been doing everything right—having regular checkups, eating a balanced diet, exercising and avoiding alcohol and medications. She felt healthy and remained employed full-time.

On the day that she was admitted to the hospital, Julie had noticed some fluid leakage in the morning. It was just a trickle. She thought it was urine and reasoned it was probably due to the increased pressure on her bladder that came from being seven months pregnant. But later in the day the fluid developed a reddish tinge.

Julie had no reason to believe that her trip to the doctor's office would be anything more than a routine check. But Dr. Patterson discovered that her "bag of water" had broken prematurely and was the cause of the trickle. This condition is called premature rupture of membranes (PROM).

The membranes (or, more precisely, the chorionic and amniotic membranes) contain the amniotic fluid in which babies develop in the uterus. Julie was probably going into preterm labor.

Julie had heard of and read about pregnant women whose sacs of amniotic fluid had broken. But in her mind's eye she envisioned a Niagara-like gush of fluid. Some women do have a considerable flow, but others have only a little leakage. The amount of leakage depends on where the break occurs; if it's high on the membranes, the flow may be slow.

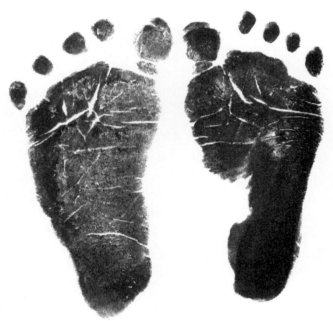

Footprints of a full-term baby girl whose birth weight was 8 pounds 4 ounces.

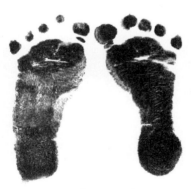

Footprints of a premature baby boy whose birth weight was 1 pound 8 ounces.

353

The shock and concern Julie noted in her diary are understandable. Like most women, she was totally unprepared for such a turn of events. After all, Julie had safely and uneventfully reached her 32nd week of pregnancy.

As with most women who receive this news, Julie's first reaction was fear for her baby, then guilt that she might somehow be at fault.

Who Has Premature Babies?

Each year, for reasons that remain unclear, about 13 percent of all black babies and 6 percent of white babies are born prematurely—that is, before they've completed 37 weeks of development. Babies born earlier than the 23rd week rarely survive, even with optimal care in the best-equipped neonatal, or newborn, intensive care unit (NICU). Today, more than two-thirds of babies born at 24 to 25 weeks can survive with the help of newborn intensive care.

The risk of complications is lower in babies whose births can be postponed for at least a few days after onset of labor. Medications given to the mother can enhance maturation of the baby's lungs and lessen the risk of bleeding within the brain in premature babies. However, these medications require a day or two before their effects can help the baby.

The vast majority of premature babies not only survive but also ultimately do well, as was the case with Julie's child. Progress in neonatal intensive care has improved the outlook for these infants dramatically.

Warning Signs of Preterm Labor

About three of four cases of preterm labor occur in women who are already known to be at high risk, such as women who've had premature babies previously or who are expecting twins or triplets. Sometimes doctors discover preterm labor during a routine prenatal examination; this situation occurs in about one in 10 pregnant women. For doctor and patient, preterm labor can be a totally unexpected event. Still, most women do have warnings, fluid leakage being just one of them. Other signs or symptoms include the following:

- Painless uterine contractions—this is a "tightening" of the uterus. Women sometimes mistakenly attribute it to gas pain, constipation or movement of the fetus, such as a kick
- Pain in the abdomen, pelvis or back
- Menstrual-like cramps
- Vaginal bleeding, or a vaginal discharge that may be red-tinged
- Pelvic pressure
- More frequent urination
- Diarrhea

If you have any of these warnings, immediately call them to the attention of your physician. But don't automatically conclude that you're going into preterm labor. Ten to 30 percent of pregnant women have some or all of these symptoms, but most will not go into preterm labor. So don't panic.

Even if you do experience preterm labor, you are not necessarily going to have a preterm birth. Depending on the circumstances of your pregnancy and the health of your fetus, your doctor might take steps to stop labor. More than half of women who have preterm labor go on to deliver their babies at full term.

Postponing Birth

"I was rushed from the doctor's office to the labor and delivery room in the hospital. There, doctors and nurses examined me, did a pelvic exam to check whether my cervix was dilating, took my blood pressure and blood samples and hooked a big belt (fetal monitor) around my middle. In some ways, the monitor is comforting because you have some indication of how the baby is doing.

"I was asked to lie still. If you move too much the monitor gets messed up. Nurses suggested I lie on my left side to somehow make it easier on the baby. They explained why this position was important. I wasn't in a frame of mind to remember. Fifteen hours of trying to lie still when you're frightened and worried seems 10 times longer."

If you experience preterm labor, the initial efforts of your doctors and nurses will focus on four considerations:

- The health and maturity of your baby
- Your health
- Your ability to deliver your baby
- The safest options for your child's birth

Unless birth seems imminent, your physician probably will make every effort to continue your pregnancy, giving your baby every opportunity to mature fully. If you're an expectant mother who's known to be at high risk, factors that might have brought on early labor will be carefully considered, as will your general physical condition.

Your doctor might begin by reviewing your medical history and doing a physical exam. During your pelvic exam, your doctor will pay particular attention to your cervix, checking to see if it's opening (dilating) or thinning (effacing).

Tests may be done to evaluate your baby's health. An ultrasound exam may be helpful in determining whether the placenta is in its normal location, especially if you've had bleeding; this is done to assess the possibility of placenta previa (see page 195). Additional, more detailed ultrasound testing may be done to look for possible abnormalities in your baby, to check on how active your baby is and to see whether the volume of amniotic fluid is normal. An ultrasound exam can also check blood flow from your baby through the placenta, giving an indication of how well the placenta is working. This test is called color flow Doppler ultrasound. For more information on this test, see page 189.

From information gained in ultrasound testing, your doctor will determine a biophysical profile (BPP) score that outlines the health status of your baby. Scores usually range from zero to 10—the higher scores being more reassuring and lower numbers more worrisome.

Additional testing may be done to determine whether a specific bacterium, group B streptococcus (also called beta-hemolytic strep), is present in the vagina.

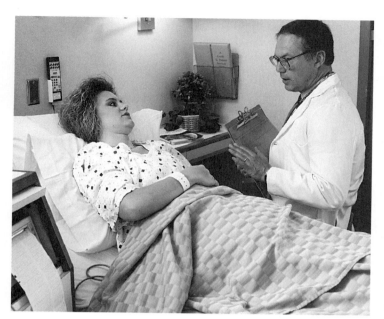

Deciding whether to attempt to stop preterm labor depends on many factors that you and your doctor will discuss.

Up to 20 percent of women may normally have this bacterium present in the vagina. Group B strep is not related to strep throat. Expectant mothers who are harboring group B strep are at increased risk of intrauterine infection. Their newborns are also at higher risk for group B strep infection. For these reasons, physicians sometimes pre-scribe antibiotics for mothers in preterm labor. In addition, because urinary tract infections can cause premature onset of labor, a urine sample is often checked.

A sample of fluid from the vagina may be tested to determine whether it contains amniotic fluid. It's sometimes difficult to tell whether fluid represents urine or amniotic fluid. Simple tests often can distinguish whether it is amniotic fluid; a test result of "positive nitrazine" or "positive ferning" indicates that the membranes have ruptured. If a woman goes into preterm labor, it is better if the membranes remain intact because there's a greater chance of stopping labor and less risk of infection.

Analysis of a sample of amniotic fluid can predict the maturity of the baby's lungs and also indicate whether there is infection in the amniotic fluid. If the membranes have not ruptured, amniotic fluid can be collected by an amniocen-tesis test. For a description of amniocentesis, see page 75.

Most women in preterm labor receive fluids intravenously and are asked to rest in bed. Sometimes these measures alone will stop preterm labor.

Your doctor may be less likely to suggest trying to stop labor if you are less than 22 weeks along, or if your cervix is dilated more than about 8 centimeters. In these circumstances, premature birth may be inevitable despite everyone's best efforts.

Decisions involved in trying to stop preterm labor are complex. Your physician will assess your health, the health of your baby, how your placenta and cervix are functioning, risks of infection and how far along you are in your pregnancy. After taking these factors into consideration, your physician will evaluate whether an attempt should be made to stop preterm labor and what these efforts should be.

If contractions decrease and your cervix is not dilating, you may simply be sent home. You may be advised to remain on bed rest to reduce the chances of another episode of preterm labor, or your activity may be unrestricted. (For more information on bed rest, see page 248.) Regardless of your level of activity, con-tinue to be alert for any increase in contractions, leakage of fluid or bleeding.

If contractions continue, especially if your cervix dilates, if you and your baby seem to be healthy and if you're less than 35 to 36 weeks along in your pregnancy, your doctor will probably recommend a medication called a tocolytic to help stop your preterm labor. For more information on tocolytic therapy, see page 250. If contractions can't be stopped, or your baby's survival is threatened, your doctor will make plans for delivery.

If your doctor determines that you are having preterm labor and if your hos-pital does not regularly care for women receiving tocolytic medication, he or she might recommend you transfer to another hospital for continuing care.

Inducing Preterm Labor

"Because the premature rupture of membranes posed a risk of infection, a sample of amniotic fluid was analyzed to see if the baby's lungs were mature. When test results showed my baby's lungs were in reasonably good condition, my doctor suggested that labor be induced. At that point, I agreed heartily.

"They added oxytocin to my IV to induce labor. It's a strange feeling to lie there, knowing that contractions should be starting. But for hours nothing happened. Nurses and doctors kept asking me if I felt contractions. I did not. After a while I think I started imagining them. But the monitor showed contractions I couldn't feel.

"The wait seemed to have no end. The staff encouraged Jack to stay by my side, but he felt rather helpless.

"Finally, seven hours later, I began to feel I was in labor, and nine hours after that David was born—all scrawny 2 pounds 14 ounces of him.

"My doctor held David up for a second. He was curled up like a ball and was not much bigger than the doctor's hand. More than the glimpse, I remember the sound. He had a good steady cry. So did I. I was just thankful he was alive."

If your baby's health is threatened before your pregnancy runs its normal full-term course, or if you develop a health problem, such as severe high blood pressure (hypertension), your physician may actually recommend that your baby be delivered early. Sometimes the baby is delivered by cesarean birth, but often physicians induce, or medically start, labor.

To induce labor, your doctor usually gives you a medication called oxytocin. Oxytocin is produced naturally when a woman goes into labor. It is available as a medication that is administered by intravenous infusion. After the medication is started, you may begin to have contractions within half an hour, but most likely it will take longer. Sometimes a medication called prostaglandin is given as a vaginal suppository or vaginal gel. The purpose is to "ripen," or soften, the cervix. This, too, helps imitate the natural onset of labor.

Because you've been expecting a normal birth, early labor and a premature baby can require major psychological adjustments. You may have been planning a low-key, relaxed, prepared childbirth in a birthing room. Even though it's not working out that way, take heart. Preterm labor will require modifications of some, but not all, of your plans. Most premature births follow a course similar to that of a normal birth.

The Birth Setting for Premature Babies

A birthing room can be a wonderful place to have a full-term baby. But the best setting for preterm labor and birth is in a standard labor and delivery room, where personnel and equipment are readily available to deal with the complications sometimes associated with premature birth.

Breech births, for example, are more common among preterm babies. Breech babies born before the 34th week of pregnancy are likely to be delivered by cesarean birth. In a standard delivery room, a cesarean birth can be performed without delay. Fetal monitoring and other equipment used to check your baby's condition are also readily available.

Forceps-assisted births are more common among premature babies than in full-term births because the forceps can protect a baby's delicate head.

When a premature baby is about to be born in a hospital or medical center, a pediatric team will be called to the delivery room to attend to the baby's needs immediately. At birth, the baby's condition will be assessed and assistance given as necessary. Often the baby will be transferred to a specially equipped facility called a neonatal (newborn) intensive care unit (NICU).

If your premature child is born in a hospital where personnel and facilities for ongoing newborn care are limited, your doctor may make arrangements to transfer your baby to a more fully equipped facility.

Immediate Care of Your Premature Baby

Although many of the procedures following the birth of a baby are standard (see page 348), special precautions are necessary after premature delivery. Immediately after birth, for example, your premature baby will be checked for abnormalities, especially difficulty with breathing, heart rate or blood pressure.

Fortunately, for many babies born after about 34 weeks, all that may be required are brief suctioning of fluids from the mouth and throat, stimulating a cry and giving oxygen with a bag and mask. But most premature infants need help with breathing, as described later in this chapter.

Translating medical jargon in the delivery room

Labor and delivery rooms in large hospitals are frequently busy places. The normal activity can be intensified after a premature birth, and team members often use shorthand medical terms to communicate. Following are expressions you may hear, and their translations:

- "We pinked her up"—Babies are normally dusky blue until they are born. After birth, a baby may need assistance to ensure that the normal increase in oxygen takes place, changing the hue of lips and tongue from blue to pink.
- "He's pretty grunty"—Newborns, particularly premature babies, sometimes make a grunting sound when having difficulty breathing. Their vocal cords compress to help increase air pressure in their lungs. Sustained grunting means the baby needs help with breathing.
- "Bagging up" or "we bagged her"—An inflatable bag, operated by hand, is used to administer controlled breaths of an oxygen-air mixture to the baby.
- "Let's put him in a hood"—A "hood" is a see-through box that fits over the baby's head; it provides additional oxygen for a baby having breathing difficulty.
- "She'll need CPAP" (SEA-pap)—This is a two-pronged tube that fits in the baby's nose. It's attached to a device that provides continuous positive airway pressure (CPAP) to the lungs.
- "We gave her a dose of surfactant"—The baby received a medication to help his or her lungs work more effectively.
- "We'll place a U.A.C." (umbilical artery catheter)—This is a thin plastic tube that's inserted in an artery in the umbilicus to measure blood pressure, obtain blood samples and administer glucose or other medications.

That First Look

"David was born at 11:03 p.m. Several hours passed before Jack and I saw him in the intensive care unit. He was in a small bed that had clear plastic sides and a warming device above.

"He had on a tiny diaper. Tubes and patches and monitors seemed to be hooked up to every part of his body. He was tiny, less than 3 pounds, but he still looked like a baby."

If your baby is born prematurely and you and your partner are like most people faced with this experience, you'll be both amazed and perhaps a little shocked by that first close-up view of your baby in the NICU.

Parents are often amazed at the size of this tiny person and somewhat overwhelmed by the array of tubes, catheters and electrical leads typically attached to the baby's body. Premature babies can be so small that a man's wedding ring can serve as a loose-fitting bracelet.

Compared with full-term babies, premature babies have less body fat to help keep them warm. They are placed on a warmer (or in an isolette), where they will maintain a normal body temperature even though they lack body fat. They may remain unclothed and not wrapped in blankets so that the nursery staff can closely observe their breathing and general appearance.

Tubes and wires are often attached to a premature baby. As intimidating as these devices may be at first glance, they help keep the baby comfortable and the medical staff continually informed about the baby's health status.

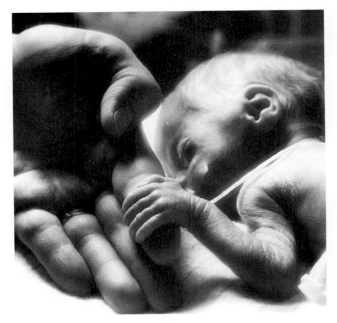

Size doesn't always indicate the amount of assistance a premature baby may need. Even though this little girl weighed a mere 1 pound 15 ounces, she needed only tube feedings and time to grow.

After a while, you'll get used to the NICU setting and to the small size of your baby. In fact, parents of premature babies sometimes come to view their small babies as normal-sized and full-term babies as huge.

Your premature baby may be covered with more of the fine body hair (lanugo) than is common in full-term babies. The skin of your baby looks wrinkled because he or she does not yet have the layer of fat that plumps out a full-term baby's skin.

Your baby's skin may look thin and fragile, especially in babies born earlier than the 28th week of pregnancy. Usually the skin begins to look like normal newborn skin a few days after delivery. The skin and cartilage that form your baby's outer ears will also be uniquely soft and pliable.

Watching your baby, attending to his or her needs and monitoring all the equipment is a specialized NICU staff typically comprised of the following people:

- Neonatal nurses—registered nurses with special training in caring for premature and high-risk newborns
- Neonatologists—pediatricians who specialize in the diagnosis and treatment of problems of the newborn
- Pediatric surgeons—surgeons trained in the diagnosis and treatment of newborn conditions that may require surgery
- Pediatricians—physicians who specialize in treating children

- Pediatric resident physicians—physicians receiving specialized training in treating children
- Neonatal respiratory therapists—staff trained to assess respiratory problems in newborns and adjust and monitor ventilators and other respirators

Other personnel may be present or available in the NICU, including pediatric nutrition specialists and X-ray technicians. Many hospitals have social workers who assist families in adjusting to the problems of caring for a premature baby.

Getting Acquainted

"The nurses encouraged us to hold David the day after he was born. I wanted to hold him, but I was afraid I'd hurt him or knock one of the wires loose. After the first few times, I gained more confidence. Almost from the beginning he seemed to respond to our touches."

You may be given a gown to wear in the NICU. If you have a cold you may be given a mask for your mouth and nose. Once appropriately gowned, you'll look like a member of the health care team. After a few visits to the NICU you may begin to feel like a team member too.

The sight of your premature baby hooked up to so much equipment can be intimidating and scary. Some of the tubes deliver fluids, nutrition and medication intravenously, and other equipment monitors the baby's blood pressure, heart rate, breathing and temperature. Here, an overhead warmer helps the baby maintain a normal temperature. The baby is deliberately left unclothed so the staff can watch breathing and skin color. A ventilator provides extra help with breathing. Eye patches shade the baby's eyes while under the bright bilirubin lights, used for treatment of jaundice.

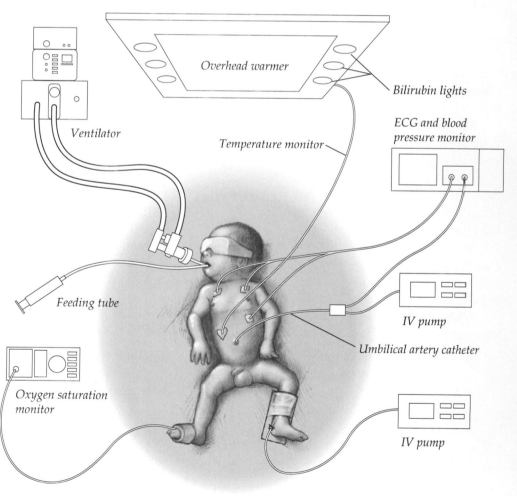

Overhead warmer

Bilirubin lights

ECG and blood pressure monitor

Ventilator

Temperature monitor

Feeding tube

IV pump

Umbilical artery catheter

Oxygen saturation monitor

IV pump

Your baby's caregivers will encourage you and your partner to become physically involved with your baby as early as possible. Until your baby is able to be held, you'll be encouraged to reach through the openings in the isolette to stroke your baby gently. As your baby's condition improves, you'll be able to hold and rock your baby. Help your newborn get to know you: Hum a lullaby, talk softly, stroke your baby gently or just spend time silently watching him or her.

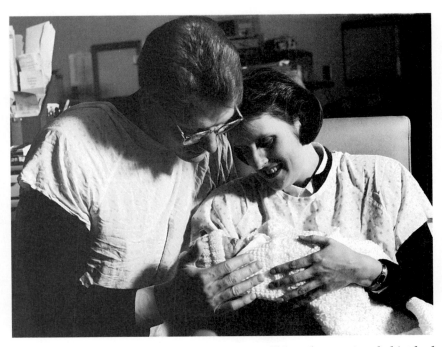

You may be surprised at how quickly this tiny person will come to recognize and respond to your voice and touch. The doctors and nurses can help you avoid or minimize difficulties with tubes, wires and monitors. Sometimes parents of premature babies can get involved with their baby's care a day or two after birth, but almost always within a few weeks. At some point, you will be encouraged to feed and bathe your baby.

Although premature babies look tiny and fragile and parents may hesitate to pick them up, parents' gentle contact helps premature babies thrive.

The time you invest in becoming well acquainted with your baby early on serves several purposes. Loving care is important to your baby's physical and psychological growth and development. Babies of all ages and levels of maturity need the attention and ready affection of their parents.

Your active involvement with your baby can also help overcome disappointments or fears you may otherwise harbor regarding your baby's health and the eventual outcome of his or her hospitalization in the NICU.

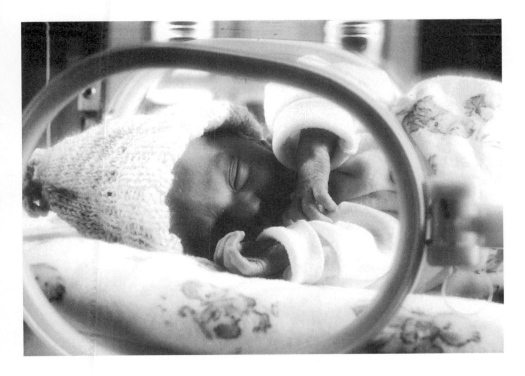

Premature babies need help maintaining their body temperatures because they have so little body fat. An isolette, an enclosed plastic box that is warmed, provides a comfortable environment. A stocking cap helps minimize heat loss.

Feeding Your Premature Baby

"Having a premature baby can make you feel so helpless. But breastfeeding was something I could do for David that no one else could do. I was amazed that eight weeks before I was due my body could produce breast milk. I was encouraged to pump breast milk, and after a few days we started giving him breast milk through a tube. At first, the idea of a tube down his throat bothered me, but it didn't seem to bother David. During the first week, he developed jaundice and we had to stop using breast milk temporarily to make the jaundice go away faster. But nine days after he was born, we gave him an opportunity to nurse. He seized the opportunity, and this was so satisfying."

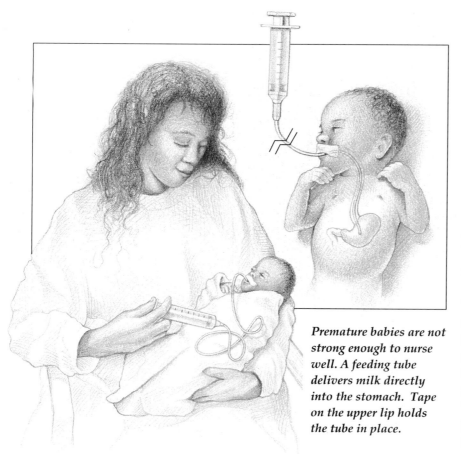

Premature babies are not strong enough to nurse well. A feeding tube delivers milk directly into the stomach. Tape on the upper lip holds the tube in place.

For the first few days or weeks after delivery, premature babies are usually fed intravenously. Their gastrointestinal systems are too immature to absorb nutrients safely. The components of the intravenous solution can include water, protein, fat, carbohydrates, electrolytes such as sodium, potassium and chloride, and minerals such as calcium. Because no two babies are exactly alike, the solution will be tailored to your baby's needs as determined by blood samples, and by the baby's health and rate of growth.

Within a few days, the intravenous feeding probably will end and a new form of feeding will start. Your baby will receive breast milk or formula through a tube that delivers the food directly to the stomach or upper intestine. This tube permits feeding to begin before your baby is mature enough to swallow reliably or even to suck. At first, only small amounts of nourishment will be administered through the tube. Once your baby's stomach and intestines demonstrate that they can absorb the nourishment, the amount will be increased. If all goes well, you'll be encouraged to attempt regular feeding without tubes.

There's no set timetable for breastfeeding or bottle feeding. The rate of advancement in feeding will hinge mainly on your baby's strength, which generally accompanies his or her growth and maturity. After your baby can nurse, supplemental tube feeding may be necessary for a while because your baby may tire too quickly when nursing and miss out on the nutrition he or she needs to

Tube feeding

Feeding tubes are used until a premature baby has gained enough strength to nurse. This type of tube feeding is often called gavage feeding. Staff in the NICU choose from an array of plastic feeding tubes designed to deliver food by various routes directly into the baby's stomach or upper intestine. Abbreviated names for the tubes reflect routes and destinations.

For example, you may hear the nurse ask for an OG tube, or just an OG. The "O" stands for oral (mouth), and the "G" for gastric (stomach). So the nurse's call for an OG feeding tube means your baby's meal is about to be delivered through a tube that goes through his or her mouth, down the esophagus and directly to the stomach.

An NG tube delivers food through the nose to the stomach, and an OD tube delivers food through the mouth to the duodenum (the portion of the small intestine into which your baby's stomach empties). An OJ transports food to his or her jejunum, just a bit further past the duodenum.

When first informed that their premature baby is to be fed by means of a tube, adults might envision skin incisions in their baby's throat, perhaps even permanent scars. Don't be alarmed; there are no incisions, only a simple plastic tube that might be taped on the baby's "mustache" area of the upper lip.

As unpleasant as it seems to most adults, premature babies generally don't seem to mind the tubes, which are soft and pliable and administered gently, by well-trained nurse specialists.

---

continue growing and gaining strength. Even though your baby is still in the NICU, you'll probably be urged to attempt breastfeeding because breast milk is generally preferred.

Even if your baby remains on tube feeding, he or she may be offered a miniature nipple or a tiny pacifier. A nipple or pacifier encourages the development of your baby's sucking and swallowing reflexes, and it can be soothing when your baby is fussy.

In the NICU, babies are often fed every one to three hours, so you'll need to provide a supply of your breast milk. Nurses in the NICU will show you how to pump your breast milk, which is refrigerated and stored for use as needed.

Premature babies grow at a rapid rate. It's a challenge to supply them with nutrients at a rate similar to what they would have received while still in the uterus. The composition of breast milk in a mother who gives birth prematurely is different from the milk in a woman who gives birth to a full-term baby. Therefore, your baby may receive your milk supplemented with extra protein, sodium, vitamins E, D and folate, calcium, phosphorus and iron. If your breast milk is unavailable, your baby will receive a formula specially designed for premature infants.

Complications of Prematurity

There's a reason babies generally remain in the uterus for almost 40 weeks before greeting the world: They need this time to grow. Premature birth can have serious health consequences. Babies born prematurely are at risk for several medical problems because their body systems are so immature. Some of these problems are apparent soon after birth; others may develop weeks to months later. The likelihood that a premature baby will develop these conditions, their severity and their seriousness are related to the degree of prematurity; the more premature babies will have the greatest problems. Some common medical problems for premature newborns are briefly described below.

Respiratory Distress Syndrome (RDS)

This is a breathing problem caused by immature lungs. The lungs lack a liquid substance called surfactant that gives normal, fully-developed lungs the elastic qualities required for easy breathing. In the 1960s this condition was called hyaline membrane disease; many babies died from it. Today, it is called respiratory distress syndrome (RDS). It can often be prevented or lessened in severity. Although the tiniest premature babies still are at greatest risk, today's survival rates and outcomes are excellent.

When labor begins prematurely, it's sometimes helpful to determine whether the baby's lungs would be mature if he or she were born immediately. In general, most babies would have immature lungs before about 36 weeks of gestational age, but there are exceptions. Some babies have surprisingly immature lungs, and others have amazingly mature lungs for their gestational age. It's sometimes possible to test amniotic fluid to assess the degree of lung maturity. Lab results that report a "high LS ratio" or "positive PG" are good news and generally indicate that the baby's lungs are mature. Sometimes medications, such as betamethasone or dexamethasone, are given to a mother in preterm labor to hasten the maturation of the baby's lungs. Even only one or two days of this treatment can sometimes make an important difference in the lung maturity for the newborn.

The diagnosis of RDS usually becomes evident within the first minutes to hours after birth and is based on the extent of breathing difficulty and on abnormalities seen on a chest X-ray.

Premature babies with RDS require various degrees of help with their breathing. Supplemental oxygen is usually required. The air we breathe contains 21 percent oxygen. Premature babies with RDS can receive various percentages of supplemental oxygen, up to 100 percent oxygen. Many babies with RDS may require supplemental breaths. A ventilator, sometimes called a respirator, gives carefully controlled breaths that can range from a few extra breaths per minute to entirely taking over the work of breathing. Some babies will benefit from respiratory assistance called CPAP (continuous positive airway pressure). A plastic tube that fits in the nostrils provides additional pressure in the air passages to keep the tiny air sacs in the lungs properly inflated.

Because RDS is due to an insufficiency of surfactant, babies with severe RDS are given doses of a surfactant preparation directly into the lungs. Other medications frequently used in babies with RDS include diuretics, medications to increase urine output and rid the body of extra water; dexamethasone, a cortisone-like medicine that reduces inflammation in the lungs; bronchodilators, agents that reduce wheezing; and theophylline or caffeine, agents that minimize pauses in breathing (apnea).

Babies who require assistance with their breathing or extra oxygen are monitored carefully to ensure they are receiving a proper amount of oxygen. A device called an oximeter or saturation monitor continually indicates the baby's blood level of oxygen. Blood samples from an artery are frequently measured to check levels of oxygen and carbon dioxide and the pH of the blood in order to judge how well the baby is breathing and make any necessary changes in the degree of help given to the baby.

Broncho-pulmonary Dysplasia (BPD)

The lung problems of premature babies generally improve within several days to several weeks. Babies who still require assistance with ventilation or supplemental oxygen a month after birth are often described as having bronchopulmonary dysplasia (BPD). Various medications can be used to help their breathing. Babies with BPD continue to need supplemental oxygen for an extended period. If they develop a bad cold or pneumonia, they may need assistance with their breathing, such as a ventilator. Some of these babies need supplemental oxygen after they go home from the hospital. As these babies grow, their need for supplemental oxygen lessens and their breathing becomes easier, although they are more likely than other children to have episodes of wheezing or asthma.

Apnea and Bradycardia

When watching your baby, you may be disturbed, even alarmed, by his or her irregular breathing patterns. Premature babies typically have an immature breathing rhythm, compared with the pattern of full-term babies. They tend to breathe in spurts: 10 to 15 seconds of deep breathing, followed by five- to 10-second pauses. This condition is called periodic breathing.

If the intervals of pauses in breathing last longer than 10 or 15 seconds, the baby is said to be having an apneic episode, or an A and B spell. "A" stands for apnea, a pause in breathing, and "B" stands for bradycardia, the medical term for a slow heartbeat. This reduction in breathing and heart rate will trigger alarms from your baby's monitoring device to alert the baby's caregivers.

A premature baby's reduced breathing and heart rate often spontaneously and promptly return to normal. If breathing and heart rate do not promptly return to normal, the nurse will gently stimulate your baby by rubbing the back or wiggling your baby awake. If your baby experiences frequent apneic spells, your doctor may prescribe a medication to help regulate breathing. Aminophylline, theophylline and caffeine are medications that can serve this purpose.

Patent Ductus Arteriosus

The route for blood circulation is different before birth than it is after delivery. Before birth, a baby's lungs aren't used and therefore they require minimal blood flow. Consequently, a blood vessel, called the ductus arteriosus, diverts blood away from the lungs.

The fetus makes a chemical compound called prostaglandin E. This circulates in the baby's blood, keeping the ductus arteriosus open. At birth, levels of prostaglandin E are supposed to fall sharply, causing the ductus arteriosus to close. Then the baby's lungs receive the blood they need to function properly.

Occasionally, especially in premature babies, prostaglandin E continues to flow at about the same level after birth as it did before. The open (or patent) ductus arteriosus can cause mild to severe breathing difficulties.

A patent ductus arteriosus is often treated with a medication that stops or slows the production of prostaglandin E. If this medication (indomethacin) is ineffective, an operation may be required. For more information on patent ductus arteriosus, see page 389.

Intracranial Hemorrhage

Premature babies who are born at less than 34 weeks of gestation are at risk for bleeding in their brains. This is called intracranial hemorrhage (ICH), or intraventricular hemorrhage (IVH). The earlier a baby is born, the higher the risk of this complication. If premature birth seems inevitable, certain medications given to the mother may help lessen the likelihood of a severe intracranial hemorrhage in the newborn.

Intracranial hemorrhages occur in approximately one-third of babies born at 24 to 26 weeks of gestational age. These very premature infants have delicate, immature blood vessels that may not tolerate the changes in circulation that take place after birth. Bleeding usually occurs within the first three days after birth. The condition shows up on an ultrasound exam of the baby's head. There is no risk from performing the exam—in fact, it is similar to the ultrasound exam you may have had during pregnancy.

The mildest degrees of intracranial hemorrhage require only observation. Various treatments may be required for more severe degrees of bleeding. Babies with severe intracranial hemorrhage are at risk for developmental problems such as cerebral palsy, spasticity and sometimes mental retardation.

Necrotizing Enterocolitis

For reasons that are not entirely clear, some premature babies in the first several weeks encounter a serious problem called necrotizing enterocolitis. A portion of the baby's intestine develops poor blood flow that can lead to infection in the bowel wall. Symptoms include a bloated abdomen, vomiting, breathing difficulty and bloody stools.

Treatment may include intravenous feedings and antibiotics. In severe cases, an operation may be needed to remove the affected portion of the intestine.

Retinopathy of Prematurity

In the 1950s, some very premature babies who survived were left with severe impairment of vision, sometimes even blindness. In those days, this complication was called retrolental fibroplasia. It was attributed to excessive use of oxygen. Eye complications still exist in premature babies, but the current understanding of these complications has prompted an entirely different name—retinopathy of prematurity (ROP).

ROP is most common in the most premature babies. In babies of 24 to 26 weeks of gestational age, most will have at least some temporary changes of ROP. It's uncommon for babies beyond about 33 or 34 weeks of gestational age to have ROP.

The retina develops from the back of the eye forward during fetal life, and this process is complete just about the time the baby is full-term. Therefore, if the baby is born prematurely, the retinal development is incomplete. Many factors can disturb the forward growth of the retina. ROP results from a disturbance in this delicate development of the retina. Vision problems related to prematurity are unlikely to be due simply to administration of oxygen.

If your baby is at risk for ROP, an eye specialist (ophthalmologist) will examine the eyes after 6 weeks of age. Fortunately, most of the changes of ROP are mild and will resolve without additional treatment. More severe degrees of retinopathy are often successfully treated with a technique called cryotherapy. Today, retinal detachment and blindness are uncommon and affect only the very smallest and most unstable premature babies.

Jaundice

Jaundice, a yellowing of the baby's skin, affects more than half of all newborns. It's caused by the buildup of a substance in the blood called bilirubin—the product of spent red blood cells. The problem is more common in premature babies because their livers are less mature than those of full-term newborns, and less able to process bilirubin effectively.

The doctor probably will place your premature baby under a bilirubin light to help rid your baby's body of excess bilirubin. This treatment, called phototherapy, may be given for a week or 10 days. (For more information on jaundice, see page 352.)

Going Home Before Your Baby Does

"I felt as if I were betraying my baby when I left the hospital without him. Intellectually I knew he couldn't come home with us, but emotionally I felt like I was letting my baby down. Somehow I felt I was giving him strength and that if I wasn't there, something bad might happen. David was a healthy 4-pound boy when we finally took him home, six weeks after he was born. Other parents, we discovered, must leave their babies for longer periods or return for medical treatments."

If your baby is born prematurely, you'll probably be discharged from the hospital before your baby is ready to leave. Even though you may understand why your baby must stay, dealing with your emotions is another thing entirely.

It may seem unfair that you get to leave but your baby doesn't. You understand clearly that once you depart you'll see your baby less frequently, and you may wonder how he or she can get along without you, especially if your home and the hospital are miles apart.

The doctors and nurses probably will be reluctant to speculate on the date of your baby's departure. So you may be left wondering just how long it will be before you can resume the role you've been planning for most of the preceding year—that of being a mother.

"Will anyone be there to hold him when he cries? Will he be fed promptly? Will his diapers be changed often enough? What if something goes wrong when I'm not there?"

These and other questions might be racing through your mind as you get ready to leave the hospital. But after you've visited a few times you'll find that your worries are unfounded and that you gradually adjust.

Don't hesitate to call the NICU during times you can't be there. Some parents avoid calling for fear of bothering the staff. Actually, interest and involvement from parents are encouraged.

Friends and relatives will probably ask you how big the baby needs to be before he or she can come home. In fact, most hospitals have no arbitrarily determined weight. Your baby is ready to come home when she or he:

- Has no medical problems requiring continuous hospital care
- Has a body temperature that is stable, and no longer needs the isolette
- Can nurse well enough to be able to gain weight, and very likely is also showing a good weight gain

---

Maternity leave for premature birth

Working mothers whose babies are born prematurely often face special problems. Neither they nor their employers were prepared for a sudden, unexpected absence or for the additional time off that care of a premature infant demands.

Mothers who plan to return to work often have a dilemma: do they take maternity leave to recuperate right after the baby is born, or do they save leave time to be used to care for the baby at home after they are discharged from the hospital?

If you return to work a week or two after your premature infant is born, you may encounter difficulty arranging for additional time off later, when your premature baby is ready to come home. To some employers, maternity leave is the equivalent of sick leave or recuperation after an accident; when you return to work, life is back to normal. If you return early, say before the end of a typical six-week maternity leave, your employer may interpret this as a signal that you're simply ready to return sooner than most new mothers and may feel no obligation to allow for additional time off for child care when your baby is released from the hospital.

Special problems created by premature birth are not always easily solved and, as health insurance becomes increasingly restrictive, may require negotiation with your employer.

Don't make assumptions about maternity leave policies. Before you make decisions regarding absences, discuss your needs with your physician and your employer. (See page 124 for more information about maternity leave planning.)

Often, discharge from the hospital takes place at or near the time that the birth would have occurred had the baby been full-term. However, if your baby is doing well and is ready, he or she may go home several weeks before your due date.

Many NICUs offer a rooming-in experience just before you take your baby home. Having the opportunity to take care of your baby yourself, yet having the comfort of knowing that nursing help is close by, can give you confidence before you go home. Your NICU nurses can help plan any special arrangements before the baby's discharge.

A premature baby might need treatment that can, or should, be scheduled for a later date. For example, the baby may need to return to the hospital later for additional treatment or surgery, such as the repair of an inguinal hernia. (For more information on inguinal hernia, see page 636.)

At Home
With Your Premature Baby

"We probably picked up a few habits from the hospital that are unusual for parents of full-term babies. We kept a log from the moment David came home of every time he ate, every medication he took, even every bowel movement. On the days when you're exhausted—and that's most days—it helped to know when you last gave medication, for example. I continued this practice with my child care provider. It gave me a sense of knowing how David's day went. Feeding him every three hours was the most difficult part. I put snacks and a pitcher of water by my bed to get me through the nighttime feedings. Another part I wasn't prepared for was the sense of isolation once we came home. During the weeks David was hospitalized, we were constantly busy going back and forth to the hospital. We had the support of all the nurses and doctors. Once we came home, it was an adjustment to have so little contact with anyone but David. I looked forward to doctor visits because that was about the only time we left the house."

Regardless of preparation, and even under the most desirable of circumstances, adjusting to the arrival of any baby is a challenge. Babies require lots of attention, especially during the first few weeks and months.

A premature baby poses a special challenge. Compared with a typical full-term baby, your premature baby may be more irritable and difficult to console. Premature babies generally need to eat every three hours, and sometimes more often. Because they tire easily when nursing, they usually take longer to feed.

Your emotional energy may be drained by worry, perhaps never before having had the responsibility for caring for a baby, let alone a premature baby. Despite instructions you may have received when leaving the hospital, you still can't know precisely what to expect. In a short time, you may feel mentally and physically exhausted, increasingly less effective as a parent and doubly burdened by the belief that your premature baby needs exceptionally attentive parenting.

There are no pat answers for these common difficulties. For the long term, you can take heart in knowing that most premature babies, once dismissed from the hospital, do well at home. With time, they mature—that is, they gain strength and require less of your time and energy. But faced with a premature baby newly arrived at home, you need short-term solutions.

Team parenting is the best approach to dealing with the homecoming of a premature baby. Simply put, your partner needs to share the responsibility fully. If your parents or in-laws offer their services, give this idea serious consideration too. Seek out and accept help from family, friends and neighbors. Trade off with your partner so each of you has a chance to get out of the house occasionally. These breaks can help protect you from exhaustion and isolation.

Common Questions

Is my baby eating properly? Getting enough sleep? Gaining enough weight? Should we send out birth announcements? Can I take my baby to the shopping mall? How old is my premature child? These are issues parents of premature babies often ponder as they anticipate release of their babies from the hospital and in the weeks that follow.

> *"We didn't send out birth announcements. It's something you feel unsure about when your baby is born early. It has taken us about two years to stop worrying about when David will "catch up" in his growth. We were lucky because he didn't seem to be delayed in developmental milestones. We kept expecting that his small size would be overcome. It takes a long time to feel content and confident that whatever size he is will be just fine. As time passes, size becomes less of an issue."*

Your baby's birthday, of course, is on the day he or she was born. But doctors usually apply a correction factor when they assess the development of a premature baby, counting age from the normal due date. Thus, from a developmental standpoint, your doctor will calculate age based on your due date. For example, no matter when a baby was born, he or she will be considered as a "1-month-old" developmentally at one month after the due date.

Avoid comparing the development of your baby with that of babies born full-term, and be cautious when interpreting developmental charts; sometimes they mislead parents of premature babies. Keep in mind that your baby's premature birth means that, for the first year or two, a more accurate comparison is to assess development based on the age your baby would be if birth had been at term.

Before your baby leaves the hospital, your doctor will answer your questions and provide you with guidelines on the care of your baby at home. These instructions are generally thorough and easy to understand. Still, don't hesitate to ask questions.

A follow-up visit will be scheduled for a few days to several weeks after dismissal from the hospital. Your doctor will want to examine your baby, visit with you about how things are going at home, answer any additional questions you may have and make plans for future checkups.

"Sometimes when I hold David now—a strong, wiggly toddler—I think back to when he first came home. He weighed less than our cat! When I'd hold him snuggled against me, he'd only stretch from under my chin to below my ribs. It's hard to believe the progress we've made. I'm sure all parents feel a sense of amazement and pride in the growth and development of their children. But when you start where we did, I think you're extra thankful."

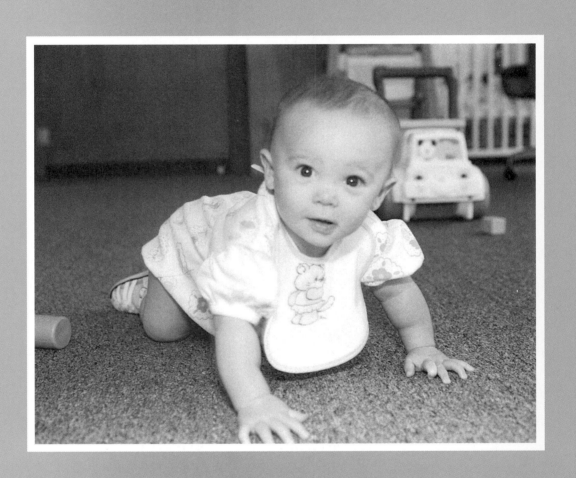

CHAPTER TWENTY-THREE

When a Baby Is Born With Problems

The vast majority of infants are born full-term, healthy and free of medical problems. Unfortunately, a few babies are born prematurely or with birth defects or medical complications. When lungs or other organs don't function properly, infants may require special care, often for weeks or months.

The birth of a seriously ill baby is heartbreaking, but today the outlook is far from hopeless. With good prenatal care, most difficulties that can arise are known ahead of time so that, before the infant's birth, arrangements can be made for prompt medical attention after the birth. The availability of specialized neonatal units for ill newborns has been a dramatic force in improving their chances of survival.

Where to find it

Parental Reactions

When a baby is born sick, parents are often overwhelmed by a barrage of hard-to-handle emotions.

Fear　The most difficult aspect is the "waiting," the "not knowing," the uncertainty of your child's future. You want to know everything, right now. Many parents are particularly concerned about brain damage, although they may not voice that specific worry. Getting a midnight phone call about a possible infection, or being told that a complication has occurred, can become a recurring nightmare.

> *"The baby was not breathing and had no heart rate when they got her out. They resuscitated her for six minutes. She had an Apgar score of zero. They hooked her up to a life support system and told us she was not going to make it, and just as the chaplain got there she turned pink. It was unreal. She just came back. Then four days later her kidneys failed, and they said she was definitely going to go. We went through this up-and-down, life-and-death thing time after time."*

If your baby's condition is unstable, you may wonder whether or not to send out birth announcements. One couple solved this dilemma by waiting until their daughter "graduated" from the neonatal intensive care unit. Then they sent cards that joyfully announced, "Fiona is home at last."

Inadequacy

Many women feel they have failed when they give birth to a child with problems. "I felt inadequate, a total failure," said one. "The most basic of biological functions, the one thing a woman is supposed to do, and I'd messed it up completely." Such feelings are normal, but there's probably nothing you did to cause your baby's problems.

Guilt

All the joyful expectations that you anticipated during your pregnancy come to a sudden halt when your baby is born with problems. You may needlessly blame yourself for everything, from taking your migraine medication when you had such a splitting headache, drinking wine on your anniversary, getting too little or too much exercise, to eating the wrong foods.

"I was convinced that it was my fault. I don't think any woman goes through nine months of pregnancy without 'breaking the rules' a time or two, and if something goes wrong with the baby, every single incident comes back to haunt you."

If you initially have negative feelings toward the baby, you might later feel guilty about that. All of these emotions are normal; many women experience them.

Grief

The joy of childbirth and the celebrations that go along with it are shrouded by grief, for this has indeed been a loss: you did not receive a perfect baby.

"We felt such sorrow for ourselves and sadness for the baby. We thought it was the end of the world, that he would have no future. We started grieving for him immediately. We didn't give him a chance. But now that he's been with us for three years, we appreciate what he's added to our lives. He's taken a lot out of us, but he would have anyway—most children sap you. If I had known in the beginning what I know now, it wouldn't have been so hard."

It's normal to go through stages of grief, those reactions that accompany bad news but that ultimately help you come to terms with it. See page 394 for more about the grief process.

Doubts

A hundred questions swirl through your mind. Will you be capable of caring for a child with this particular problem? Will you be able to bear up under the stress? What will be the quality of your child's life? How will you cope with your lifestyle changes? How will you manage financially? You can't resolve these all at once; you can only move forward one step at a time.

Isolation

You may feel very alone. This isn't what you had planned. You may even have trouble discussing the issue with your partner.

"Roger and I were not talking. He's not much of a talker anyway, but the pain was so great that we could not talk. He went to work and I drank a lot. At night we'd watch TV and go to bed. This went on for all the time the baby was in the hospital."

Family members and friends may not know what to say and as a result don't say anything. This reaction contributes to your feeling of isolation. Here's how one couple, who had a baby with Down syndrome, solved this dilemma.

"Brent and I discussed how we were going to handle this and decided we were going to be extremely open about it. We didn't want people to feel uncomfortable. We wanted them to ask questions, because they probably didn't know any more about it than we did. We made a point of telling everybody that he was a beautiful baby, so they wouldn't be afraid. That helped people a lot. There was non-stop traffic through this house. People weren't afraid to come."

Newborn Intensive Care Unit (NICU) and Specialists

By bringing together a group of highly trained personnel, the newborn intensive care unit (NICU) specializes in the care of babies who are born prematurely or who develop problems after birth. The doctors are neonatologists—pediatricians trained to deal with the unique medical problems of the newborn. Specially trained nurses help carry out the high level of demanding and exacting medical care that is needed. An NICU has the technology to diagnose and treat conditions that require immediate intervention. Pediatric radiologists, pediatric surgeons and other subspecialists staff an NICU.

The NICU has warmers, isolettes and bassinets available for babies. Most babies are monitored continuously for heart rate, blood pressure, breathing pattern and other vital signs. (See the illustration on page 360.)

The specialized equipment in the NICU can be intimidating. The ventilator sounds, IV pumps, tubing, electrical cables and technical terminology used by medical personnel are just a few of the new things you are exposed to. Monitor readings that fluctuate may frighten you because you don't know what is normal. Alarms can make you panic. Initially you may feel overwhelmed, so ask the staff to explain the condition of your baby and the purpose of each piece of equipment used for monitoring and treatment.

There are likely other babies in the same room as your baby, some probably sicker and others less sick than yours. It helps to stay focused on your own baby. It will be challenging enough to absorb the information about your baby, and confidentiality precludes the staff from discussing details of the other babies.

If your primary care doctor is unfamiliar with a rare condition, he or she may refer you to a specialist. Genetic specialists, in particular, are a good source for medical information and for putting you in touch with other families that have been through similar experiences. Pediatricians, neonatologists, nurses, social workers and clergy can be of tremendous help as well. They can give advice and connect you with support groups, advocacy groups, newsletters and national organizations that deal with a particular problem. Public health agencies also can help.

Welcome to Holland

I am often asked to describe the experience of raising a child with a disability—to try to help people who have not shared that unique experience to understand it, to imagine how it would feel. It's like this...

When you're going to have a baby, it's like planning a fabulous vacation trip—to Italy. You buy a bunch of guidebooks and make your wonderful plans. The Coliseum. The Michelangelo David. The gondolas in Venice. You may learn some handy phrases in Italian. It's all very exciting.

After months of eager anticipation, the day finally arrives. You pack your bags and off you go. Several hours later, the plane lands. The stewardess comes in and says, "Welcome to Holland."

"Holland?!?" you say. "What do you mean Holland?? I signed up for Italy! I'm supposed to be in Italy. All my life I've dreamed of going to Italy."

But there's been a change in the flight plan. They've landed in Holland and there you must stay.

The important thing is that they haven't taken you to a horrible, disgusting, filthy place, full of pestilence, famine and disease. It's just a different place.

So you must go out and buy new guidebooks. And you must learn a whole new language. And you will meet a whole new group of people you would never have met.

It's just a *different* place. It's slower-paced than Italy, less flashy than Italy. But after you've been there for a while and you catch your breath, you look around and you begin to notice that Holland has windmills... and Holland has tulips. Holland even has Rembrandts.

But everyone you know is busy coming and going from Italy...and they're all bragging about what a wonderful time they had there. And for the rest of your life, you will say, "Yes, that's where I was supposed to go. That's what I had planned."

And the pain of that will never, ever, ever, ever go away...because the loss of that dream is a very very significant loss.

But...if you spend your life mourning the fact that you didn't get to Italy, you may never be free to enjoy the very special, the very lovely things...about Holland."

—Emily Perl Kingsley, 1987

Medical Problems in Newborns

Blood Problems

Polycythemia. Newborn polycythemia occurs when an infant's red blood cell count (hematocrit) reaches a level so high that the blood is too thick to flow effectively through the body. Signs and symptoms include low blood sugar, seizures, lethargy, poor feeding, jitteriness, respiratory distress and possibly blood clots.

Babies with these signs and symptoms must receive prompt medical attention. If polycythemia is confirmed, treatment may include a partial exchange transfusion. For this procedure, some of the infant's blood is removed and replaced with albumin or other fluid. The effect is to "thin out" the baby's blood, bringing the red blood cell count into a normal range. After treatment, the outlook for infants with polycythemia is excellent.

Potential causes of polycythemia are intrauterine growth retardation (see page 382), diabetes in the mother, asphyxia, some maternal medications, maternal smoking and pregnancy at high altitude.

Anemia. Anemia occurs when the red blood cell count decreases to a low level. Newborn anemia can be caused in three ways:

- Blood loss may occur due to problems with the placenta.
- Blood cells can be destroyed inside the baby's body by infection, by a blood group difference between the mother and baby (see page 167 and page 223), by inherited diseases such as thalassemia (see page 62) or by red cell disorders.
- Decreased production of red blood cells can occur from congenital infections or bone marrow inactivity.

Because of the many potential causes of newborn anemia, its cause usually is investigated before any therapy is given. This investigation includes blood tests to examine the responsiveness of the bone marrow, a search for the presence of unusual antibodies and inspection of the appearance of the red blood cells. Only for circumstances in which anemia threatens the well-being of the baby will your doctor suggest a blood transfusion. Anemia can complicate other problems such as respiratory distress and infections. In these cases, the need for blood may be more crucial than it would be for an otherwise healthy child.

Breathing Problems

Respiratory distress is the most common problem in the newborn and often the first sign that the baby is ill. Fast breathing, labored breathing or periods of no breathing at all (apnea) can result from several medical difficulties.

Infants with respiratory distress need prompt medical attention. This can range from supplemental oxygen for mild cases to a ventilator for severe cases, in addition to intravenous fluids and medications. Babies remain in the hospital until they are able to breathe room air on their own, take oral feedings (by breast or bottle) and maintain their own body temperature.

Asphyxia. Asphyxia occurs when the amount of oxygen in the baby's circulation drops and stays low. In addition, there is a buildup of carbon dioxide and a decreased pH in the baby. The causes vary. In an unborn baby, the flow of blood through the umbilical cord may be reduced, for example, because of blood loss from the placenta (placental abruption), a knot in the umbilical cord or low maternal blood pressure. If the baby shows signs of asphyxia before birth, an emergency cesarean birth may be necessary.

A newborn can have asphyxia if breathing is difficult, due to causes such as respiratory distress syndrome, meconium aspiration or infection. The infant may need cardiopulmonary resuscitation (CPR) if asphyxia is particularly severe.

The term asphyxia is often loosely applied to any newborn with problems. Technically, however, it applies to cases in which an infant's problems are in response to a lack of oxygen, buildup of carbon dioxide and low pH, rather than being due to other identifiable problems such as infection or metabolic disease.

The level of oxygen in an unborn baby's bloodstream is normally quite low compared with that of a child or adult. As a result, babies are resilient to lower amounts of oxygen and tolerate the normal birth process well in the vast majority of cases. They often go through a period in which their oxygen content drops but no problems result. Also, individual babies have different tolerances for a decreased oxygen supply. For example, an anemic infant might not tolerate a period of a lowered amount of oxygen as long as an infant with a normal blood count. For these reasons, the diagnosis of asphyxia is difficult to pinpoint.

Women at increased risk for delivering babies with asphyxia are those with diabetes mellitus, anemia or hypertension; those who use drugs; or those who have a premature birth or a pregnancy that extends beyond 42 weeks.

Apgar scores (see page 349) are not a good measure of asphyxia, particularly at one and five minutes. An infant with an Apgar score of 5 or less at 10 to 15 minutes, however, is at greater risk of lasting problems occurring as a result of asphyxia. Also, seizure activity or an abnormal neurological exam in the first few days of life increases the likelihood of lasting neurological problems. Asphyxia can affect virtually all organ systems in the newborn baby's body and can result in severe developmental delay, mental retardation or damage to the brain or other organs.

Meconium aspiration. Meconium refers to the thick, dark bowel movements that a baby has in the first day or two of life. Occasionally, in response to stress, the baby has this bowel movement before birth and the meconium mixes with the amniotic fluid. This rarely occurs before 34 weeks of gestation, but it becomes increasingly common in a postmature baby. About 10 to 15 percent of all births show some evidence of meconium being present in the amniotic fluid. In most cases, this causes no problem, and the baby has an uneventful birth.

If the meconium gets into the baby's lungs, however, it can cause breathing problems. When the meconium is thick or full of particles, the infant is at risk for asphyxia. If meconium is present when the membranes rupture, it sometimes is possible to perform a procedure called amnioinfusion. A catheter is inserted through the cervix, and a saline solution is instilled into the uterus to dilute the concentration of meconium.

When thick meconium has been present in the amniotic fluid, the doctor makes an extra effort to suction the baby's mouth, nose and trachea at birth. Even so, some infants will have difficulty breathing. The presence of small particles of meconium in the airways and in the lungs prevents the normal exchange of oxygen and carbon dioxide. Sometimes, no matter how much suctioning is done, the meconium remains deep in the lungs. A ventilator might be required to get oxygen into the bloodstream.

Sometimes a newborn with meconium aspiration will develop an accumulation of air between the lung tissue and the chest wall. This is called a pneumothorax (see below).

There is no "cure" for meconium aspiration; rather, the baby's own healing processes have to clear the lungs. The goal of medical therapy is to support the baby with oxygen, fluids and medications until the lungs can breathe effectively on their own. An extended stay in the hospital is often required. A specialized type of heart-lung bypass called ECMO (extracorporeal membrane oxygenation) is available in some hospitals for severely affected infants who don't respond to more conventional methods of treatment.

Transient tachypnea. Infants born with this form of respiratory problem often have no symptoms other than rapid, shallow breathing. In some babies the skin may have a bluish tinge, which can be alleviated with small amounts of oxygen. The problem usually resolves within three days. Until it improves, the breathing difficulty may prevent the baby from feeding well and also from going home at the same time you do.

Respiratory distress syndrome (RDS). RDS is a specific diagnosis that refers to a lack of surfactant in the lungs of premature babies. (See page 364 for a complete description.)

Pneumothorax. One to 2 percent of newborns develop a pneumothorax, a rupture in the lung's tiny air sacs (alveoli). This allows air to collapse the lung and put pressure on the heart and major blood vessels. Initial treatment can range from simple observation to giving extra oxygen or removing the trapped air with a needle.

The severity of pneumothorax can range from mild to life-threatening. Usually it is not life-threatening, but it can require the placement of a chest tube (a plastic tube placed in the chest to drain away air) for several days.

Low Blood Sugar (Hypoglycemia)

Following birth, the baby no longer receives nutrition from the placenta, the major energy source throughout pregnancy. At that point, the baby's own ability to regulate blood sugar (glucose) becomes important. A newborn's blood sugar level is commonly measured in the nursery to be certain that it is in a normal range. If it is decreasing to low levels, feeding the baby breast milk or formula usually will cause the level to return to normal.

Occasionally an infant's blood sugar will test repeatedly low. Symptoms of hypoglycemia (jitteriness, poor feeding, rapid breathing, lethargy and seizures) might or might not be present. Prompt treatment is necessary. Often an IV is started to infuse glucose directly into the circulation while the potential causes for the hypoglycemia are investigated. These include prematurity, asphyxia, infection, a cold environment, congenital heart disease and being small for gestational age. Uncommon causes include metabolic disturbances that interfere with the normal production of glucose in the body.

Babies of diabetic mothers are at particularly high risk for hypoglycemia because they are born with increased levels of insulin in their bodies. After birth, this extra insulin causes their blood sugar level to decrease. These babies may need glucose infusions from an IV to achieve a normal blood sugar level. If you have diabetes, regular glucose monitoring throughout your pregnancy should prevent your baby from having serious difficulties. Even if the baby is born with hypoglycemia, prompt recognition and treatment provide an excellent outlook. (For more information about maternal diabetes, see page 231.)

Infections

Serious bacterial infections occur in about two or three of 1,000 newborns. Bacteria can infect the baby before, during or after birth. A baby with a bacterial infection may need hospitalization in a newborn intensive care unit. Depending on the type of bacteria and the type of infection, the baby may require anywhere from one to four weeks of treatment.

Bacterial infections are potentially serious because they can invade any organ or the blood, urine or spinal fluid. Prompt treatment with antibiotics is necessary, but even with early diagnosis and treatment, a newborn infection can be life-threatening. For this reason, doctors are cautious when dealing with a possible or suspected infection. Antibiotics often are given early, and their use is stopped only when it is proved that an infection does not exist. About 19 times out of 20, when antibiotics are given, the test results come back showing no evidence of infection. It is better to err on the side of safety by "overtreating" than risk not treating a baby with an infection soon enough.

Viruses can cause infections too. Some cause serious infection in the mother; others interfere with the growth and development of an unborn fetus. (See page 212 for a more detailed discussion of maternal infections that can affect pregnancy.)

Group B streptococcus (GBS). This bacterium is found in the reproductive tract of up to 30 percent of women. Fortunately, only a small percentage of babies born to women with GBS become infected. More and more commonly, doctors are screening for it and treating it with antibiotics before birth.

Women who have preterm labor, preterm ruptured membranes, a prolonged period of ruptured membranes (usually more than 24 hours), fever, a urinary tract infection or an undetermined infection are likely to be tested for GBS. If signs of infection in the uterus are present—maternal fever, foul-smelling amniotic fluid and elevated white blood cell count—antibiotics may be given as a precaution, even before test results are available.

If GBS infects a newborn, the illness takes one of two forms. In early-onset infection, the baby becomes sick within hours after birth. Symptoms might be breathing problems, gastrointestinal or kidney problems or heart and blood pressure instability. Even with immediate treatment, up to 20 percent of babies with early-onset GBS infection die.

In late-onset infection, which occurs a week or more after birth, meningitis— infection of the fluid in and around the brain—usually results. Although meningitis is serious, the death rate is not as high as in the early-onset form. Children who survive either type of infection can have neurological problems.

Problems of Metabolism and Growth

Metabolism involves the physical and chemical processes of the body. If a chemical or hormone is seriously out of balance, problems can result.

Congenital adrenal hyperplasia (CAH). Congenital adrenal hyperplasia occurs in one of approximately 5,000 newborns. One of several possible blockages in normal metabolism can result in a range of problems in the newborn. These can include vomiting, diarrhea, failure to gain weight after birth and ambiguous genitals (the genitals of a newborn girl may be formed such that she appears to be male). Additional problems might include severely low sodium and seriously high potassium levels in the blood.

A test done on a sample of blood taken in the first few days of life can identify many of these infants before serious symptoms develop. Treatment is very effective for these infants and usually consists of giving cortisone-type medications and sometimes surgery.

Congenital hypothyroidism. The thyroid gland produces hormones essential for mental and physical growth and development. For the one in 4,000 babies born with an underactive thyroid, prompt thyroid hormone supplementation allows for normal growth and intelligence.

Galactosemia. This disorder prevents metabolism of galactose, one of the sugars normally present in milk. It occurs in one of 40,000 newborns and, without treatment, results in cataract formation and brain, liver and kidney injury.

Babies with galactosemia cannot be fed breast milk or standard infant formula. Their dietary intake of galactose must be carefully regulated. With careful diet modification, medical problems can be avoided.

Phenylketonuria (PKU). PKU is an inherited enzyme deficiency that results in an abnormal accumulation of phenylalanine. Only one of 10,000 babies is born with the disorder, but if treatment is not begun promptly, mental retardation results. Treatment is dietary: at first a special formula, and later a restricted diet. Nutritional guidance from a registered dietitian is essential.

Intrauterine growth retardation (IUGR). An infant who is born extremely small for gestational age—usually below the 10th percentile—may be small because growth has been insufficient. This is termed intrauterine growth retardation (retardation refers to physical growth, not mental development).

IUGR occurs when the fetus does not get adequate nourishment through the mother's placenta. This deficiency results in too little body fat and decreased nutrition stores, and the newborn then has difficulty in maintaining a normal body temperature and blood sugar level. Many medical conditions and lifestyle characteristics can produce IUGR (see page 196), although some babies who initially are suspected to have IUGR are small simply because parents or other family members are small.

Many growth-retarded infants grow slowly throughout early childhood, then go through a "catch-up" phase in which they eat more and grow rapidly. In most cases, there are no long-term problems.

Birth Defects

According to the March of Dimes, about 3 to 5 percent of babies born in the United States have some type of birth defect. Although these numbers may sound scary, remember that many of the problems are relatively minor.

Most couples have a small risk of recurrence in a subsequent baby, but in some families the risk could be much higher. A geneticist can carefully analyze your family's history to assess the likelihood of a particular defect occurring again.

Central Nervous System Disorders

During the first four weeks after conception, the embryo develops a neural tube that eventually forms the brain and spinal cord and their surrounding tissues. Should something go wrong with this delicate system, during its formation or after, several parts of the body can be affected.

Spina bifida. About one of 500 babies is born with spina bifida, a condition in which the lower portion of the neural tube fails to close. The defect can occur anywhere on the back but usually is located in the lower part. The effect on the child depends on the severity of the defect.

In the mildest form, called spina bifida occulta, a small separation of the bones causes no problems and shows up only on an X-ray, with perhaps a small dimple or birthmark on the skin above. Most children with this form are unimpaired, although a few have spinal cord defects.

The more severe form of spina bifida, myelomeningocele, involves a lesion that can be as large as an orange, with nerves, muscles and spinal fluid exposed. The exposed nerve tissue is at high risk for infection and requires prompt surgical correction to place the exposed tissue inside the body and cover it with skin. Neurosurgeons are the specialists who perform this surgery, occasionally assisted by plastic surgeons. The degree of physical impairment depends on the degree of myelomeningocele. The child can have trouble with muscular control of the legs, with foot and knee function and with bladder and bowel control. Mental retardation and learning disabilities are other possible outcomes, and hydrocephalus is common (see below and page 67). Children with myelomeningocele need close and extensive follow-up care and observation. Coordination of medical care, along with physical therapy and developmental assessments, is necessary if these children are to achieve their full capabilities.

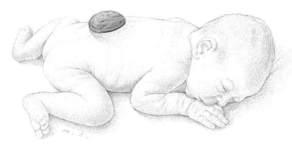

Myelomeningocele, a severe form of spina bifida, is an outpouching of tissue over the spine. Exposed nerves and muscles may become infected, so prompt surgery is needed after birth.

Myelomeningocele often can be diagnosed by ultrasound testing before the baby is born, allowing optimal plans for the birth. There is some evidence that cesarean birth produces a better neurological outcome than vaginal birth. (See page 67 for more information on myelomeningocele.)

Anencephaly. In the most severe form of neural tube defect, the upper end of the tube fails to close. The result is anencephaly, in which portions of the skull and brain never form at all. The condition is always fatal; if the baby is not stillborn, death occurs soon after birth.

Hydrocephalus. A child born with hydrocephalus has an imbalance between the brain's ability to produce cerebrospinal fluid and its ability to absorb it. The resulting accumulation of fluid in the skull produces an extremely large head. This birth defect occurs in about one of 1,000 newborns.

Medication is sometimes effective in treating the disorder, but the usual treatment is a neurosurgical procedure. An opening in the brain can be created or a plastic shunt inserted (ventriculoperitoneal, or VP) to drain the fluid to another part of the body.

A positive long-term outlook for babies with hydrocephalus depends on effective medical management and the absence of other central nervous system disorders.

Cerebral palsy. Cerebral palsy is an abnormality in areas of the brain controlling motor function. The cause can be abnormal development of the brain before birth, oxygen deprivation, infection, bleeding in the brain or physical damage that occurs during birth. It also can be caused by injury in early infancy. Often, however, there is no obvious explanation, although new studies are showing that a considerable number of children with otherwise unexplained cerebral palsy have an abnormality in brain development.

Physical symptoms of cerebral palsy range from weakness and floppiness of muscles to spasticity and rigidity. Convulsions or mental retardation might or might not be associated with the condition. There is no cure for cerebral palsy, but special education and physical therapy can help compensate for the motor deficit and any learning disabilities. Surgery is sometimes helpful in dealing with limb deformities and gait disturbances.

Cleft Lip and Cleft Palate

These conditions occur in one of 700 newborn infants and can have a definite recurrence risk in families. The defect can range from a small notch in the lip to a complete separation that extends into the nose. If the palate is also cleft, the roof of the baby's mouth has failed to close. Clefts in the lip or palate are separate birth defects that may or may not occur together.

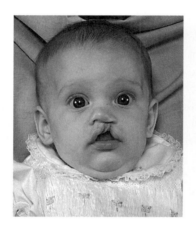 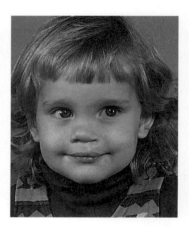

Cleft lip can be effectively repaired surgically, as evidenced by these unretouched before- and after-surgery photographs. The photo on the left was taken at age 3 months, and the photo on the right was taken at age 2½ years.

Depending on the position and extent of the cleft, surgical repair usually is performed within the first 12 months of life. Apart from difficulties with eating, the biggest concern for children with cleft palate is speech development. With satisfactory repair and follow-up, more than 85 percent of these children will be able to speak normally.

Gastrointestinal Tract

The gastrointestinal (GI) tract extends from the mouth through the esophagus, stomach, small and large intestines, rectum and anus. If at any point along this route a portion has not formed correctly, it interrupts the continuity of the entire system. Surgical correction is necessary for GI obstruction in newborns.

Prenatal ultrasound exams can't always identify birth defects of the GI tract. In some cases, however, an excess of amniotic fluid will accumulate, giving a clue to an obstruction of the baby's GI tract.

Usually, GI obstruction is evident within the first day or two of life. The baby will not feed properly, may spit up and vomit, might develop a distended abdomen and possibly will not have any bowel movements. The condition can quickly worsen, requiring referral to a newborn intensive care unit, where the condition usually can be diagnosed with the aid of X-ray studies and evaluation by a surgeon.

After surgery, the continuity of the GI tract must be reevaluated as feedings are introduced. The healing process may be complicated, and more operations may be necessary. The outlook for most children with GI obstruction, however, is favorable.

The causes of most newborn GI problems are unknown, and the problems usually do not recur in subsequent children.

Pyloric stenosis. Pyloric stenosis is a narrowing of the pylorus, the part of the stomach that empties into the small intestine. It affects approximately one of every 150 male babies and one of every 750 female babies. About 15 percent have a family history of the abnormality, but the precise cause is not known. Symptoms of persistent vomiting and weight loss usually don't appear until four to six weeks after birth. Surgery is required to correct pyloric stenosis; the prognosis is excellent.

Esophageal atresia. One of 3,000 to 4,500 infants is born with an esophagus that has not developed normally. The defect often occurs along with abnormalities of the trachea, heart, urinary tract or central nervous system. Symptoms are apparent soon after birth. The baby may have an abundance of secretions coming from the mouth, or may choke, cough or turn blue when feeding is attempted. An operation usually is needed promptly.

Intestinal atresia. Obstruction of the intestines occurs in about one of 1,500 births. It can occur anywhere in the intestines, such as the duodenum, jejunum, ileum or colon. Treatment for complete obstruction requires surgery; for partial obstruction, treatment depends on the severity. Most infants tolerate the operation well and recover completely.

Hirschsprung's disease. Hirschsprung's disease is the cause of one-third of all colon obstructions in full-term newborns. Characteristically, babies with Hirschsprung's disease have an abnormally large or dilated colon, causing symptoms of vomiting and poor growth. Treatment is usually done in two steps. First, the surgeon creates an opening on the outside of the abdomen (stoma) so that stool can pass into a disposable pouch. When the child is between 12 and 18 months old, the opening is closed, and the abnormal portion of colon is removed.

Imperforate anus. Congenital abnormalities of the anus and rectum are fairly common; minor abnormalities occur in one of 500 births, and more serious abnormalities occur in one of 5,000 births. If the anal opening is simply narrowed, it can be dilated with an instrument. Sometimes the anus lacks an opening (imperforate); an operation is required.

Diaphragmatic hernia. A diaphragmatic hernia occurs when an abnormal opening in the diaphragm enables part of the abdominal contents to push up into the chest cavity. In babies with large hernias, the stomach and a large part of the intestines displace the heart and lungs, and emergency surgery is necessary. About 50 percent of these babies die. Babies with less sizable hernias may not have problems, or the hernia may not be detected until they are a few months old.

Genetic Disorders

Chromosomes are the genetic material carrying the information that determines how our bodies develop and how they work. Chromosome material from both the father and the mother combine to provide this information. On occasion, these chromosomes may come together in such a way that there are too many, too few or perhaps incomplete chromosomes. Birth defects caused by abnormalities of the chromosomes occur in about one of 250 newborns.

If you have a baby with a genetic disorder, or if certain disorders tend to run in your family, you can receive genetic counseling to determine the cause of the problem and what the risk is for having more children with the same problem. This will give you the information you need to make decisions concerning future pregnancies.

An in-depth discussion of genetic disorders is beyond the scope of this book, but following is a brief summary of some of the common problems.

Trisomy 21 (Down syndrome). About one of 700 babies is born with Down syndrome, which is caused by the presence of an extra chromosome number 21. The child with Down syndrome has a small body stature and several facial features characteristic of the disorder. Developmental delays are always present, and heart and gastrointestinal problems are common.

The severity of developmental delay plays a major role in determining the quality of the child's life. Many persons with Down syndrome live with their families, go to school and enter the workforce under supervision or in sheltered workshops. Other children are profoundly delayed and require significant care.

Full genetic evaluation of the child and both parents is required for accurate determination of the origin of the extra chromosome and the risk for having another child with Down syndrome. The risk for Down syndrome increases with advancing maternal age, particularly after age 35, although it can occur in children born to younger mothers.

Trisomy 13 and trisomy 18. These chromosome abnormalities are less common but more serious than trisomy 21.

Trisomy 13 prevents normal development of the heart, eyes, brain and other organs. Most children with trisomy 13 die within the first year of life. Those who survive have profound developmental delays.

Children with trisomy 18 have small eyes, abnormally formed ears, feeding difficulties and heart problems and are small for gestational age. Many other malformations have been described. Children with trisomy 18 are severely mentally retarded. Half die within the first two months of life, and the rest seldom live past their first year.

Turner syndrome. About one of 3,000 baby girls has an abnormality of or is missing one of the sex chromosomes. This affects their growth and development. Most girls with Turner syndrome have normal intelligence but grow up small for their age unless they receive hormone supplements. They are at higher risk for certain heart and kidney problems. Puberty usually is delayed, and the vast majority of these girls are infertile, although advanced reproductive techniques have allowed some women with Turner syndrome to have children.

Sickle cell anemia. This hereditary condition is relatively common in blacks, occurring in about one of 600 black newborns. In sickle cell anemia, the red blood cells, rather than remaining flexible and round, become rigid and shaped like crescents or sickles when oxygen concentrations decrease in the blood. They are fragile and tend to break up much sooner than normal red blood cells.

Bacterial infections and blockage of blood vessels are the two most serious complications of sickle cell anemia, although various other problems may occur. Infants with this disease are often born preterm and may have intrauterine growth retardation.

Sickle cell anemia occurs when both parents are carriers. Then each child has a 25 percent chance of having sickle cell anemia, a 50 percent chance of being a carrier (sickle cell trait) and a 25 percent chance of inheriting two normal genes.

Cystic fibrosis. This condition affects the respiratory and digestive systems. It is the most common fatal hereditary disease in white children in the United States, affecting approximately one of every 2,000 infants. If both parents carry the altered gene, each child has a 25 percent chance of having cystic fibrosis, a 50 percent chance of being a carrier and a 25 percent chance of having normal genes.

Cystic fibrosis causes chronic respiratory disease, diarrhea, malnutrition and exercise limitation. The disorder is ultimately fatal, but recently developed treatments have enabled some persons to live beyond their thirties. Efforts are currently under way to develop gene therapy for this disorder. (For more on genetic disorders, see page 56.)

Genital Abnormalities

Undescended testicles. The testicles normally descend two months before birth from an area near the kidney, through a small opening in the abdominal muscles, into their normal position in the scrotum. In about one of 30 full-term baby boys, one or both of the testicles have not descended into the scrotum. The incidence is higher in premature infants. Sometimes hormone supplements can bring an undescended testicle into place. If it has not descended by 12 to 15 months of age, the condition should be treated surgically.

If the condition is left untreated, the child can grow up to be infertile, particularly when both testicles are involved. A boy born with an undescended testicle has a higher risk of testicular cancer, generally when he is in his twenties or thirties. Correction does not reduce the risk of cancer, but it does allow for better examination and earlier detection.

Hypospadias. In this condition, the urethral opening is located on the shaft or the base of the penis rather than at the tip. In its mildest form, the opening is just on the underside of the glans; in its most severe form, it may be located at the base of the penis, on the scrotum. Surgical correction provides a better cosmetic appearance and allows normal function of the penis. This type of operation is commonly done by a pediatric urologist.

Ambiguous genitals. Sometimes a female who has been exposed to an excess of male hormones in the womb is born with ovaries but male-like genitals (female pseudohermaphroditism). A male can be born with testicles but with ambiguous or completely female genitals (male pseudohermaphroditism). Rarely, newborns have both ovaries and testicles and ambiguous genitals (true hermaphroditism). The causes of ambiguous genitals include tumors, chromosome abnormalities and hormone excess or deficiencies. (For more information, also see "Congenital adrenal hyperplasia," page 381.)

When a newborn's gender is in question, an endocrine specialist should be consulted promptly. Only after thorough testing and evaluation can a correct diagnosis be established and the correct assignment of sex be made.

Hand and Foot Abnormalities

Some deformities result from the way the baby was positioned in the mother's uterus. These positional deformities usually resolve on their own. Other abnormalities are rare but complex, requiring surgery or other treatment.

Clubfoot. One of every 1,000 babies is born with a complex foot deformity known as clubfoot. Early treatment is essential and should be initiated soon after birth. This usually involves stretching, splinting or casting. Sometimes an operation is necessary, but about 50 percent of the time the problem can be corrected with casts and corrective shoes. Children with clubfoot are commonly treated by pediatric orthopedic surgeons.

Congenital absence of a part or all of the upper extremities. Rarely, a child may be born with only part of one finger missing, or an entire arm may be absent. Additional birth defects occur in some of these children.

Webbing (syndactyly) of fingers or toes. Webbing of the toes is rarely more than a cosmetic problem; because the feet usually function normally, surgery is unnecessary. In the case of the hands, however, the joints of the fused fingers do not line up, and the fingers are difficult to use if they are not separated surgically. Orthopedic surgeons who specialize in hand surgery treat these conditions.

Extra fingers or toes. Extra fingers or toes are usually surgically removed. The timing of the surgery depends on whether the extra digit consists of only skin and soft tissue or contains bone or cartilage. Extra toes should be removed before the child begins to walk and wear shoes.

Heart Problems

Approximately one in 125 babies is born with a heart defect. Some types of heart disease cause problems immediately after birth, whereas others may not become apparent for days to weeks to years. The survival of these babies has improved considerably during the past several years, thanks to improving methods of diagnosis before and after birth and to improvements in medical and surgical techniques.

Pediatric cardiologists specialize in diagnosis and medical management of heart problems in children. Pediatric cardiovascular surgeons specialize in operations to correct congenital heart defects.

The heart has four chambers and two major blood vessels. It pumps blood to the lungs, where the blood receives oxygen and returns to the heart. The heart then pumps this oxygenated blood out to the body. Any of the heart chambers or blood vessels can be affected during development. Birth defects involving the heart generally occur within the first six weeks of pregnancy.

A common sign of congenital heart disease is a heart murmur, heard when the flow of blood does not take its normal path through the heart. Most murmurs don't reflect a serious problem, but they may lead the doctor to investigate further. Other signs of cardiac problems include bluish skin (cyanosis), caused by blood going to the body without first being oxygenated in the lungs. Rapid, shallow breathing (tachypnea) and rapid heart rate (tachycardia) also occur in babies with certain congenital heart defects. These are ways in which a newborn baby tries to compensate for a heart problem. Signs and symptoms of some heart problems can include feeding difficulties, poor growth rates, recurrent respiratory infections and cardiac failure.

Specialized testing by electrocardiography (ECG), echocardiography (ultrasound test of the heart) and heart catheterization may be performed to better study the baby's heart. Some problems can be treated with medication. Others require surgical repair.

In most cases, the cause of a congenital heart problem is unknown. There are instances of heart problems recurring in families, but few cardiac diseases have a clear inheritance pattern.

Ventricular septal defect. This is the most common heart malformation, representing 25 percent of cases of congenital heart disease. An opening between the lower chambers (ventricles) of the heart increases blood flow, under high pressure, to the lungs. The size of the opening determines symptoms and treatment. Approximately 30 to 50 percent of small defects close spontaneously during the first year of life. Otherwise, surgery is usually done before the baby is 1 to 2 years old.

Patent ductus arteriosus. The ductus arteriosus is a vessel that leads from the aorta to the pulmonary artery. Normally, this closes immediately after birth. In premature babies, the ductus simply has not had time to close and often closes spontaneously within weeks or months. In full-term infants, failure to close is considered a congenital malformation. Surgery is necessary, usually between the first and second years of life.

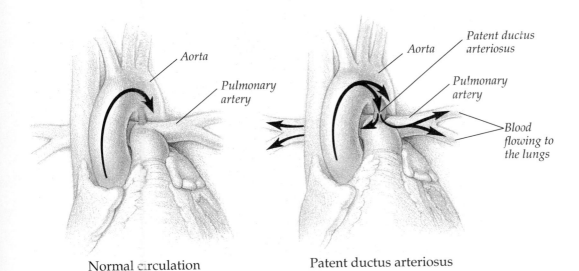

Normal circulation   Patent ductus arteriosus

Patent ductus arteriosus is a heart problem in which blood that should flow out the aorta to the body is misdirected to the lungs through an opening that normally closes after birth.

Pulmonary stenosis. An obstruction of the blood flow from the heart to the pulmonary artery is called pulmonary stenosis. Children with mild to moderate stenosis can lead a normal life but should be under the regular care of a physician. Those with more severe stenosis require surgery.

Atrial septal defect. An opening high in the heart, between the upper chambers (atria), produces abnormal blood flow. It is more common in girls than in boys and often occurs in children with Down syndrome. The condition often has no symptoms in early infancy. Surgical closure is the recommended treatment, usually between the ages of 3 and 6 years.

Coarctation of the aorta. Coarctation (constriction) of the aorta results in increased blood pressure above the obstruction. There are usually no symptoms, but heart failure may develop because of other associated heart abnormalities. Even in the absence of symptoms, a significant obstruction should be surgically repaired between the ages of 2 and 5 years; this treatment will help prevent future complications.

Tetralogy of Fallot. This consists of a large ventricular septal defect, obstruction of blood flow from the heart's right ventricle to the lung (pulmonary arteries) and a shift of the aorta toward the right side of the heart. The right ventricle also is enlarged. The result is decreased blood flow to the lungs. The main symptom of this disorder is cyanosis (bluish skin because the circulating blood doesn't contain enough oxygen). Cyanosis may not be present at birth but rather may develop slowly during the first year. Corrective surgery after infancy is the usual treatment, although it may have to be performed earlier.

Aortic stenosis. Aortic stenosis—a narrowing of the valve through which blood leaves the heart to enter the aorta—is more common in male infants. It is the cause of 5 percent of cardiac malformations. If severe, it usually is detected in early infancy. If mild, it might be heard as a heart murmur later in childhood. Severe stenosis requires surgery. Children with mild or moderate obstruction should remain under medical care because of the possibility of the obstruction increasing in severity.

Transposition of the great vessels. This is a complex defect in which the two arteries arising from the heart are reversed. Blood returning to the heart from the body is pumped back to the body without passage through the lungs. Infants with transposition are blue (cyanotic) and must have immediate surgery.

Orthopedic Conditions

Congenital hip dislocation or developmental dysplasia of the hip. When the upper leg bone (femur) is not in proper position at the hip socket, the development of this joint may be hampered. Congenital hip dislocation can sometimes be recognized in the first few days of life by examining the movement of the hip joint. Your doctor will examine the hips in the hospital as well as at follow-up visits for well-baby care. If present, congenital hip dislocation requires proper positioning of the joint, usually by means of a special brace. This treatment is often successful within six to eight weeks. Persistent problems, or those that develop later in infancy, occasionally require a cast or surgical treatment by a pediatric orthopedic surgeon.

The cause of the hip dislocation is unknown. It occurs 10 times more frequently in girls, and also more frequently in firstborns and babies who are born in the breech position. Furthermore, a family may have a history of developmental dysplasia of the hip. With early detection and prompt attention, the outcome is excellent.

Urinary Tract Problems

The kidneys filter impurities out of the blood and help maintain an appropriate chemical balance in the body. The ureters, bladder and urethra are conduits and reservoirs through which the urine formed in the kidneys passes. At any point along the urinary tract, an interruption or malformation can occur that might interfere with the normal functioning of the entire urinary system.

Some of these problems can be identified by ultrasound testing before birth. (It is important to note that not all unusual urinary tract findings on prenatal ultrasound tests indicate problems; some will revert to normal either before or after the child is born.)

Because much of the amniotic fluid volume is made up of fluid passed from the urinary tract of the developing fetus, decreased amounts of amniotic fluid can be another sign of urinary tract problems.

Urinary tract problems include the following:

- A malpositioning of one or both kidneys
- Hydronephrosis (kidney enlargement caused by obstruction to urine flow out of the kidney)
- Obstruction where the ureters join the kidneys
- Obstructions in the urethra (one type which is more common in boys is posterior urethral valves)
- The absence of one or both kidneys (if both are absent, the condition is fatal)

One kidney may be sufficient to clear the body of waste products even if the other has been severely affected by a medical condition. Some defects of the urinary tract never require surgery, even those caused by obstruction. Careful medical follow-up is important to determine whether complications are developing. Some complications might lead to a recommendation for corrective surgery by a pediatric urologist.

Deciding on Care for a Baby Who Is Dying

Loving care in medicine often means intervention with medications, machines and occasionally operations, but sometimes, instead, it means focusing on comfort care rather than painfully extending a life that is inevitably going to end.

Making decisions about a baby's care should be a team effort. The role of the doctors is to provide the parents with enough information to understand the medical implications of the available choices, of what *could* be done. Together, parents and doctors decide what *should* be done.

If a decision is made to discontinue medical support, ask whether you might be able to hold the baby, or perhaps even take the baby home for whatever time you can have together. Talk with your doctor and nurses about what you might anticipate when medical support is discontinued. Also, ask for recommendations about what arrangements are needed after the baby's death.

You also may want to discuss whether an autopsy should be done and whether organ donation is a possibility.

When a Baby Dies

Sometimes babies die. When a baby dies, the emotional trauma to the parents is profound. Death shatters the hopes and dreams that the pregnancy inspired; it seems as if the future has died along with the baby.

About 1 percent of babies die within 28 days after birth; this is termed neonatal death. Most of these deaths can be attributed to four causes: low birth weight, asphyxia, congenital defects and infections.

Another 1 percent of babies are born dead. The death of a baby after 20 weeks of gestation but before birth is called a stillbirth. Most of these deaths are due to genetic or congenital defects, umbilical cord or placenta problems or medical conditions of the mother.

Usually the mother is unaware of the death of a fetus. One day a woman might notice that she does not feel the baby move. Perhaps she calls her doctor, who asks her to come in, and when she does the doctor can't detect a heartbeat. The absent heartbeat in combination with other monitoring determines that the baby has died. This news is devastating.

There are two options for labor after a fetal death. Your doctor might recommend inducing labor. Or, if your cervix is not yet ripe, you might be asked to wait until labor begins naturally. Most often labor begins within two weeks after fetal death, although it can take longer in middle pregnancy. The wait can be excruciating. In this circumstance, many women prefer not to go out in public, where others might ask when the baby is due.

Decisions

A number of decisions must be made after a baby dies. No decision needs to be made immediately, and there is no one "right" way to do things. Get as much information and support as you can, and then let your heart be your guide. You are treading an unfamiliar path and will find your way more easily with help from others who know the way. Most hospitals have a chaplain, and an increasing number of hospitals have a perinatal loss support team. Or you might prefer to call your own minister, priest, rabbi or spiritual support person. You might want to wait until your family or friends arrive before making major decisions.

Baptism. Customs for baptism vary. Some religious groups baptize a baby who is not born alive and some don't. Others have rituals such as dedication or naming. The hospital chaplain, if requested, can perform a simple, informal service.

Organ donations. Because of their tiny size, newborns who die are often not candidates for organ donation. Your doctor may discuss this issue with you, though, so that you won't later wonder why you weren't offered the option. On occasion, a baby's death can give life or enhanced quality of life to another child. If organ donation is possible and is something you desire, your doctor will contact the appropriate organizations.

Autopsy. After a stillbirth or neonatal death, doctors might recommend having an autopsy done. The purpose of an autopsy is to answer questions about the baby's death or contribute to the understanding of the baby's medical condition. Finding out all you can about why your baby died might be helpful to you, particularly if you plan future pregnancies. This decision is yours, and you need to do what is comfortable and right for you. Your doctor can explain autopsy procedures and answer any questions you may have.

Funeral and burial arrangements. Planning a funeral can be overwhelming at any time, but it is particularly difficult when death supersedes what was supposed to be a new beginning. A young couple, especially, might have little experience in making these arrangements.

Most people who have had a baby die stress the importance of having a memorial service to recognize the baby by celebrating the birth and mourning the death. The sense of closure may help start you on your way toward acceptance and healing. In addition, it will allow others to better understand the depth of your loss.

Services can be held in many different locations: your hospital room, hospital chapel, funeral home, church or synagogue or graveside. The mother must not be excluded from attending the service, even if that means waiting until she is out of the hospital. If you're worried about the cost, babies' funerals are seldom as expensive as those for adults. Some funeral homes even provide them free, as a community service.

The baby's parents should participate in the planning. Delegate some of the details, if that will help, but make sure that your wishes are heeded. The choice of music and other personal touches might be important to you.

Announcements. You have several choices about how to tell people that your baby died. You can make phone calls or delegate someone else to make the calls. You can place an obituary in the newspaper. You can mail printed announcements or write personal notes.

> *"We lost the baby just before Christmas. Instead of sending Christmas cards, I handwrote notes to everyone. As painful as this was, in a way it helped me. By the time I had written 'Our baby died' a hundred times, I finally began to believe it."*

Creating Memories

When an older person dies you are left with years of memories. When a baby dies you have to make as many as you can in just hours or days—you have to "create" memories.

Parents used to be denied the right to see a baby who had died. It was thought they'd "forget" more easily if they didn't see their baby. But parents didn't forget; in fact, they had a harder time dealing with their grief when they hadn't had a chance to see their baby and to say good-bye. Now we know that the best way to begin accepting what has happened is to spend time with the baby.

Some parents might initially be hesitant to see their baby after she or he has died, but most professionals now agree that it is important to look at and hold your baby. Parents have their own perceptions of how their baby will look, particularly if there are birth defects. These perceptions almost always are worse than the baby's actual appearance. Parents are more likely to notice and remember features of their family that they see in their baby.

"Few babies are more malformed than our daughter was, but we were able to concentrate on the features that were properly made rather than on the imperfect ones. We accepted her as the child we had conceived in love, and as time passed, the physical image softened until she became, to us, the most beautiful child in the world."

Hold your baby. Explore the fingers and toes. Feel the hair. Make the most of this brief time together with your baby.

Others also might need to see the baby: grandparents, aunts and uncles. Some families gather in the room, holding the baby, perhaps even bathing or dressing the baby. If you have other children, it may help to let them see their sister or brother. They also have suffered a great loss and, depending on their age, may surprise you with their ability to accept death.

State law permitting, some people go a step further and take the baby home for a brief time. They place the baby in the cradle that was so lovingly prepared, in the room that was so painstakingly decorated. They accept the baby into their home to say their good-byes.

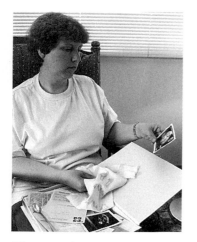

Photographs and other keepsakes can provide comfort and memories of a baby who died.

Naming the baby. If you had already chosen a name, it's probably best to use it for this baby and no other. Don't "save it for the next one." By naming the baby, you make him or her real. You may be surprised at how much it means when you and others can refer to the baby by name.

Photos. Taking photographs is now a common practice after a stillbirth or neonatal death. Instant photographs don't always last as well over time, so you might prefer to take conventional prints from negatives. If you initially feel that you don't want to save any pictures, keep them anyway. Many parents are grateful that they saved pictures that they could look at when they were ready.

Ideas for keepsakes. Save objects associated with your baby. Ask for the hospital ID bracelets, the crib card, the knit cap that newborns wear and perhaps ultrasound images that were taken. If you don't have a set of the baby's footprints, ask the nurses to help make a copy for you, or make tracings of a hand or foot. Snip a lock of hair to put in a locket. Keep the blanket the baby was wrapped in and any clothes or stuffed animals you brought with you to the hospital.

Later on you can create more keepsakes. Get a certificate of the baby's birth or death. Frame the baby's handprints or footprints.

Grieving

Grieving is the emotional and physical response to a loss, the process of coming to terms with it and letting go. Grieving takes a long time, and it is hard work. The death of a baby may be a young couple's first experience with grieving, and many are unprepared for its intensity.

Stages of grief. Grief is often divided into stages, but these have no set time-line or even sequence. You might skip a stage, remain for a while in one or experience several at once.

Denial and protest. For the first days or weeks, you may have trouble believing that the baby died or even was born. Your mind may seem fuzzy, and you may have trouble concentrating on much of anything; you may hear only half of what people say to you.

"Shortly after I got home from the hospital, I drove across town to my sister's house. It's a route I've taken a million times but I somehow missed a turn. I couldn't for the life of me find it, and nothing looked familiar. I pulled over and just went to pieces. Then I had to get out a map to figure out where I was. I was only a block from that darn turn, could even see it from where I had parked, but I just wasn't able to integrate the information."

Despair. The pain of new grief is so raw that you may feel it physically. You might have recurrent dreams about the baby, hear the baby cry or feel the baby kicking again.

Anger is common. You have every right to be furious at what life has dealt you. You might lash out at those around you. The medical staff is a common target: how they gave you the bad news, how they treated you or your perception that they rushed you into decisions. You might strike out at family and friends and those you most love and need, or even at yourself and at the world in general.

"I was angry at what had happened to my body. To be such a physical wreck with nothing to show for it was unbelievably unfair. And I was furious at all the other women who were mothers, when I couldn't be."

Express your anger rather than letting it turn inward. Talk it out with family and friends or, as soon as your body has recovered sufficiently, unleash it in physically constructive ways like exercise or gardening.

Grieving is also a time of searching for answers. Why me? Why this baby? You may become preoccupied with the details of your pregnancy, labor and birth. You might want to make a list of questions for your doctor. Why did the baby die? Was there anything I could have done differently? What are the chances of the same thing happening again? What can we do to minimize that possibility? If the problem was genetic, you might ask for referral to a geneticist, who can help answer your questions.

Depression. This longest of the grief phases might last for 18 to 24 months. You may have difficulty sleeping, or you might want to sleep all the time. You may lose the motivation to perform even ordinary daily activities at home, and doing anything outside your home can be nearly impossible.

Symptoms of grief

- Sleep disturbances ranging from insomnia to exhaustion and a desire to sleep all the time
- Weight loss or gain
- Inability to concentrate
- Disorientation
- Tightness or pain in chest and throat
- Headaches
- Aching arms
- Withdrawal from social activities
- Lack of interest in normal routines such as cooking, shopping or personal hygiene
- Sighing
- Anger, resentment, bitterness
- Irritability
- Sexual difficulties
- Mood swings

"When I moved into this stage it was almost a letdown. The rawest pain was gone, but the flatness that replaced it was not a welcome substitute. At the beginning I had no interest in anything, not even food, which was amazing; usually I head for the fridge at the slightest sign of stress. My husband cooked every night and practically had to spoonfeed me. On my own I probably would have starved."

It helps to frame your days with simple routines to keep some semblance of balance. Try to care for yourself in simple ways, like making the effort to look nice each day, eating healthful foods and getting some exercise even if all you do is take a walk around the block.

Social withdrawal is common during this time because you feel detached from the community. You might need to stay close to home and restrict your social life to people you feel emotionally safe with.

Resolution and acceptance. For a long time—maybe a year or two—you have been working through your grief, but it's still not over. The final stage is just beginning.

"It's not something I sit every day and try to work out, because I have to keep living, keep going for the people who depend on me. But every now and then when I have a little time to myself, all of a sudden it will hit me and I'll think, 'I'll deal with this little part of it right now.' Then I'll put that part away. Then something else will surface. It's an ongoing growth."

Slowly the sun begins to shine. Your energy level picks up, you feel more comfortable in social situations, you can talk about the baby without falling apart and you can enjoy yourself without feeling guilty. You will not forget, though. You will still have bad days, but you will rebound more quickly.

Resolution means accepting that you will live the rest of your life without this child. It means accepting the new person you have become through the growth of grieving. Resolution comes in its own time; it takes courage to go through the process and learn to live again.

Husbands or partners.

No two people grieve in the same manner. Each person finds his or her own way to make sense of the loss of a baby, and this difference can cause tremendous strain on a relationship. Some studies show that the divorce rate is higher among couples who have lost a child.

A mother—*"He just went back to work, as if nothing had happened. I was left in that screamingly silent apartment, with nothing to do but wallow in grief. The fact that he could even function made me resentful. He didn't cry all the time, like I did, which made me think he didn't care as much."*

A father—*"I'm a pretty private person. I hurt as much as she did, but I needed to deal with it by myself. She needed to talk about it all the time, to anyone who would listen. She even wrote articles about it. The fact that she made money writing about our private tragedy seemed like she was using our baby for personal gain. It wasn't until we had a blowup over it that I finally understood her need to pour it out in that way and to help others in similar situations."*

If you don't talk about misunderstandings, they can build to unmanageable proportions. This is the time to try harder than ever before to share your feelings.

If you can't talk things out, try writing letters to each other. If the strain is still too much to deal with, it's time to seek counseling. (For more information on professional help, see page 400.)

Children. Teaching children to grieve losses and to respect the grief process is an important gift. It might be tempting to shelter them from some of the pain you are feeling, but even very young children will sense that something terrible has happened. If they don't know exactly what it is, they'll be scared. They may be frightened by what is most likely their first experience with death and by the changes that have occurred in their parents. Home is no longer happy, and they have new worries. Might I die too? What if mom or dad dies? What if my bad thoughts about the new baby caused the death?

The best way to cope with your children's anxiety is by talking about it. Just as you need someone to listen to you, they need you to listen to them. When children grieve they feel the same gut-wrenching pain that you do. "My stomach hurts," they might say, and that's when you need to hold and cuddle them and reassure them of your love.

"I was so sad after our baby died. I simply couldn't find the energy to be a good parent to our 2-year-old, and I was thinking of sending him to my mom for a while. Then one day after I just about drove away from the gas station without paying, Matthew looked over at me from his car seat and said, "Our baby dead and we really sad, aren't we?" I hugged him and cried. After that day I knew he needed me and I needed him too."

Dealing with hurtful comments. Some people think you can't be hurt by losing a baby you never got to know. They expect you to "put the death behind you," to "forget about it." Their lack of sensitivity can cause them to make comments that hurt deeply. Others might mean well but are so uncomfortable with the situation that they blurt out things they wouldn't say if they just took a moment to think. Some of these remarks will stay with you for a long time and may be hard to forgive. Try to remember that most people are doing the best they can in a situation they haven't previously faced. Just as you are in unfamiliar territory, so are they.

Dealing with children's grief

Speak in clear terms. Children are concrete thinkers and take what you say literally. Terms such as "laid to rest" or "gone to sleep forever" may make them fearful of napping or going to bed. If you say the baby went up to heaven, the child may respond with, "Well, let's get in an airplane and go get him back!" "Mommy lost the baby" is similarly confusing to a young child.

Reassure them that the baby's death was not their fault. Young children are magical thinkers. They often think that their thoughts, words or actions had the power to cause the death. They need to know that the baby didn't die because they didn't want to share their room and toys, because they told mom she couldn't bring the baby home if she had a boy or because they bounced the ball on mommy's tummy. They also need to realize that their wishing can't bring the baby back to life.

Name your sadness. "The baby died, and you hurt deep inside. Even though you can't see the hurt or put a bandage on it, the pain is real bad. It's called grief."

Let your children share in the rituals of death. Even very young children can benefit if you have prepared them for what to expect and are open to their questions. Viewing the body—if they choose to—is less frightening than what their fantasies may be. Children are curious about "what dead looks like" and "what dead feels like." Explain everything in advance. However, be sensitive to a child who does not want to participate.

Ask your older child's health care provider if you're unsure about how to discuss death with a child of a particular age. Don't expect to have all the answers. There are no easy answers when talking about the death of a baby, not even for professionals. The most important thing for your family is being together, talking about the baby and how you feel. Although there are some things in life you have no control over, children will sense that the power of love within the family can help all of you cope with even the most difficult of times.

Express your love. Touch is healing, so hug and hold your children and tell them how much you love them.

Anniversaries and holidays. As the anniversaries of the child's due date, birth and death approach, you might temporarily go back to an earlier state of grief.

> *"My grandmother lost a baby, and each year when that anniversary rolled around she grieved. Even when she was in her nineties, the pain felt fresh. She's dead now, but it helps to know that she survived her loss and that she would be thinking of me on my baby's birthdays if she were still alive."*

Anniversary pain is intense, but its duration is short. Planning a celebration gives you a focal point. If you have other children, ask them how they'd like to remember their baby sister's or brother's birthday. They might want a little family party, complete with a birthday cake. One family makes a special dinner and sets a place for the baby, with a single white rose to decorate it. Another releases a balloon with a message inside to the baby.

Holidays such as Mother's Day, Father's Day, Christmas or Hanukkah also can be times of great sadness. Some families develop specific methods for expressing their love and feelings of loss for the baby. They might plant a bush, light a candle, hang a Christmas stocking or buy a tree ornament each year in memory of the baby. Rituals like these keep the baby's place in the family.

Multiple births—when one baby dies. When you lose a twin or triplet, your emotions swing from one extreme to the other. One minute you're cooing over the baby who lived, and the next you're mourning the one who died. And your loss is double: you have lost not only a baby but also the opportunity of raising multiple children. Each day that you watch the surviving baby or babies grow, you're reminded of the one who is not with you. Other people can be especially hurtful if they assume that because you have at least one live baby, your loss is somehow less.

Finding Support

When a baby dies, many parents feel isolated. Friends and family may not know what to say or might stay away. The sight of other parents holding and cuddling their children can further amplify that feeling of isolation.

> *"I have finally joined what I jokingly used to call the Mothers' Club. I have experienced pregnancy and birth, but I can't join in conversations about them without someone asking, 'And how old is yours?' The answer to that inevitably is the conversation-stopper of the week."*

Unfortunately, we live in a death-denying society that doesn't allow enough time and support for grieving, particularly for babies. We don't even have a name for the significant life passage of bearing a child who died. If a woman loses her husband, she becomes a widow. If a child loses his parents, he becomes an orphan. Yet when parents lose a child—what some would call the greatest tragedy of all—no word exists to describe the loss.

No one should grieve alone. More than at any other time of your life, you need to surround yourself with people who can listen to you, reflect with you, care for you, hold you, cry with you, remember with you.

Family and friends. When a death occurs in a family, every member is affected. Most families and friends draw together to share their grief and let their strong ties support them. Sometimes, though, even close family members

A message for friends and relatives and suggestions for talking with parents whose baby has died

Nothing you can say to parents will make the pain of their baby's death go away, so avoid statements that may cause anger and resentment. If you don't know what to say, say "I'm sorry" or say nothing; just offer your presence, your arms and your ears. Acknowledge, rather than minimize, the grieving parents' heartache. They do not want the memory of the baby forgotten.

Do not say:

- "You can always have another." Parents wanted this baby, and this baby is the baby they are grieving for. Nothing will replace this pregnancy or child.

- "At least you didn't have time to get attached to her." The parents loved this baby long before the birth. Their hopes and dreams were centered around a future that now has died along with the baby.

- "Think of the hard life he (or you) would have had if he'd lived." Whatever might have been wrong with the baby, the parents nevertheless loved and wanted him. The pain is not diminished just because the baby had birth defects or medical problems.

- "It was God's will." Many people find themselves in confusion about their religious beliefs. They can't understand how God would take the life of an innocent baby and cause them such pain.

- "At least you already have one (or more) at home." Other children don't make up for the child who has died.

It's helpful if you say:

- "I'm so sorry."

- "How can I help?"

- "We've been thinking of you so much."

- "Do you want to tell me about the baby's birth?"

- "I feel so sad for you."

- "I can't begin to imagine what you're going through, but I want you to know how much I care."

Also, refer to the baby by his or her name.

let you down. They might not have the capacity to understand the depth of your loss, might be afraid to let themselves try or might think they have to keep a brave front. Then you may need to turn elsewhere for support.

Support groups. Grief is a private journey and different for everyone, but you can be helped by being with others. Parents who have lost a child often feel that no one who hasn't been in the same situation can understand the depth of their loss. Many hospitals and communities offer organized support groups in which people can share their experiences, problems, feelings and fears. If you're not yet ready to be with people, support groups offer sympathetic voices on the phone. Their members are willing to listen to you long after others think you "should be over it."

Helping yourself. Finding support means reaching out to others. Much of your grief work, however, must be done alone, and tools are available to help you. Search the library for books and articles that deal with infant death. Such reading makes you aware that you are not alone; others have suffered the death of a child and have survived. Their words can help you move forward. You can try expressing your feelings in a diary or journal or by writing poems or stories. What's important is that you deal with your grief, not run from it.

Professional help. If you are having difficulty coping despite all your efforts, it may be time to consult a professional. Social workers, clergy, psychologists and psychiatrists are specially trained to help people work through grief. You can ask for recommendations from doctors, nurses, social workers, religious organizations, organized support groups or your funeral director.

Moving Forward

When you lose a baby, your life will never be the same because you will never be the same person. This is not to say that all the changes will be negative. True, you'll have lost your ability to take life for granted, but you'll grow and stretch in ways you never dreamed possible. Introspection, developing new coping styles, questioning values and lifestyle and the process of grieving all help you find inner strength and resiliency. You emerge a more caring and compassionate human being.

CHAPTER TWENTY-FOUR

Adoption

One way to build a family

Many situations and events in your life may have led you to consider adoption as a way to build your family. Most of what you need to know about caring for a baby is already in this book: all babies require love, nurturing, guidance and medical care. But because you may have no control over the prenatal and postnatal care of the child you adopt, you may have some unique concerns. This chapter offers basic advice on adoption and addresses medical and emotional issues that may be on your mind.

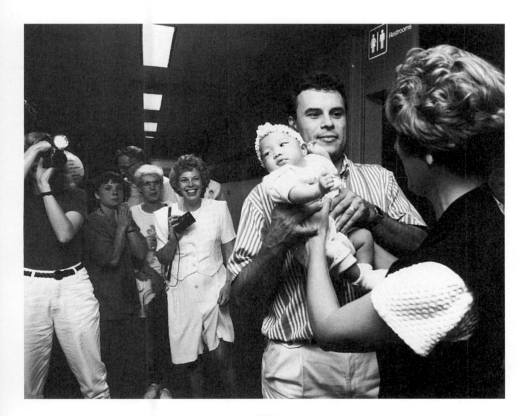

The waiting over, many families celebrate the arrival of an adoptive daughter or son with a festive gathering at the airport, including relatives, close friends and cameras to record the happy occasion.

Beginning the Adoption Process

Each year in the United States, there are about 50,000 domestic adoptions and thousands more international adoptions—each one of them as unique as the children themselves. Experienced parents say that the key to making an adoption proceed smoothly is to gather as much information as possible:

- Talk to friends who have adopted and seek their advice.

- Contact the adoption branch of your state's health or welfare department, your county social service agency and your public library for up-to-date information on public and private adoption agencies (religious or non-denominational). Call the agencies listed in the Yellow Pages under "Adoption."

- Ask agencies what types of children they place, what services they provide and their requirements. Many people are surprised to find that agencies differ greatly in the fees they charge, the waiting time for a placement and the age, health, fertility, marital status, income, education and religious affiliation required of applicants.

- Ask about independent adoption, in which you locate a birth mother or birth parents who agree to transfer their parental rights directly to you, using an attorney or agency as an intermediary. Some states permit only agency-assisted adoptions.

- Think carefully about the kind of child you can parent successfully. Would you prefer an infant or an older child? What sort of physical, medical or emotional problems are you willing to accept? Would it matter to you, your family or your community if the child is of a different race? The waiting time for healthy white babies in the United States is usually considerably longer than that for minority infants, older children, sibling groups or children with medical or emotional needs. Often, the waiting time is less for a child through international adoption.

- Investigate the reputation of each agency or attorney you consider.

- Familiarize yourself with the adoption laws in your state. If you pursue independent adoption, find an attorney who knows these laws well. It can help you avoid involvement in a situation with a tragic ending.

- Have your agency or lawyer spell out every step in the process so there won't be surprises along the way. Some people find it helpful to make a time line or flow chart and list all the variables: who does what and when, which forms are needed and how much each procedure costs.

Handling the Stress of Adoption

For most people, the adoption process can be stressful. In addition to the pressures felt by anyone anticipating a new baby, adoption involves forms to complete, personal questions to share with strangers, home studies to complete and agency fees to work into the budget, all of which can be overwhelming.

For others, adoption spells freedom from yet another miscarriage or infertility evaluation. As one mother put it, "After three years of trying to get pregnant, beginning adoption procedures felt like we were finally making progress."

Whether or not you find the process emotionally taxing, adoption groups can be invaluable sources of information and support. If you are already working with an agency, it might have its own support group or be able to refer you to a local one.

An organization called Adoptive Families of America (AFA) provides parents with important information about resources, agencies, international adoption and support groups, and it keeps members up to date on adoption issues through its bimonthly publication, *Adoptive Families*. For more information, contact the AFA, 3333 Hwy. 100 North, Minneapolis, MN 55422; telephone (612) 535-4829.

Couples who first need to come to terms with their infertility may benefit from RESOLVE, Inc., a national organization that offers information and support to infertile couples; it has many local chapters around the country. Contact RESOLVE, Inc., 1310 Broadway, Somerville, MA 02144-1731; telephone (617) 623-0744.

Inquire about "open adoption"

"Open adoption" implies an ongoing relationship between the birth parents and the adoptive parents, based on a shared love and concern for the welfare of the child, with full disclosure of identifying information. Both the birth parents and the adoptive parents are involved in making an adoption plan, and they agree to share information and maybe some contact (photos, reports or even visits) as the child grows up.

In the past, most agencies practiced "closed adoption"—the original birth certificate and adoption records were sealed to protect the confidentiality of the birth parents, adoptive parents and adoptees. However, for a growing number of American birth parents who place their babies for adoption, open adoption is gaining popularity because it offers them some control in choosing the adoptive parents and the option of continuing communication with the adoptive family after they have transferred their parental rights. Open adoption may offer adoptive families more direct access to the child's medical history.

Many agencies now offer a range of openness in their programs. Some even allow birth parents to select who will adopt their children from books of family profiles. Ask if contact with the birth parents is a possibility or a requirement at your agency.

Coping With the Wait

Unlike a nine-month pregnancy, adopting a child can take anywhere from several months to several years. Some applicants report nothing but smooth sailing, but others have trouble tracking down the multitude of documents required by the adoption agency, the state and federal government and, with intercountry adoptions, the foreign government. "The hardest part was not being able to hope too much," recalled a father who waited two years for a child. "Putting too much faith in any one date would only set us up for disappointment."

One mother coped with the long delay by writing a journal to her daughter, explaining in regular installments what the rest of the family was doing and feeling as the adoption procedure dragged on. Sharing this with her daughter as she grows up might help her daughter realize how much it meant to her parents when she joined the family.

Adoption support groups can be great sources of encouragement. It might help you to talk about your experience with others.

When a Placement Falls Through

Just as pregnancies are subject to miscarriage and stillbirth, adoptions can also fall through if either of the birth parents changes his or her mind before legal rights are terminated. Adoptive parents who find their hopes dashed in such a way need to give themselves permission to grieve for their loss, and they need the emotional support of those around them.

"You start accepting a child as your own as soon as you get any information about a specific child, such as a photograph," said one adoptive mother. "If the birth mother changes her mind, it feels similar to the death of a child. You go through the normal stages of grieving."

If this happens to you, take as long as you need before requesting another placement. Although the child will never be forgotten, time will lessen the pain. If you believe the problem was with the agency, seek a new agency. Adoption support groups can be valuable sources of leads on children available for adoption.

What is a home study?

A home study is a document required by all adoption agencies and other countries to ensure that prospective parents can provide a safe, loving home. It includes a physical description of the home, current health reports, income statements, criminal background checks, letters of reference and reports of interviews with agency or social service workers.

Prospective parents are usually asked to write autobiographies describing their own strengths and weaknesses, employment, lifestyle, relationship with their spouse, their childhoods and upbringing, and their anticipated parenting styles. They will be asked their reasons for adopting and the type of child they want to adopt. The home study also reflects the steps they have taken to educate themselves about adoption issues and the culture of the child they are adopting.

The final home study document prepared by an agency may be six to 10 pages long. It shows that a family has been carefully screened to increase the odds that the family is psychologically and physically capable of meeting the needs of a child. It also indicates the family has been informed about adoption issues and that the agency supports the adoption application.

Medical Issues in Adoption

Tracking Down the Medical History

Try to acquire any medical, genetic and social records of your child's history in writing from the birth parents or adoption agency. There might not be much information, but it will be easier to track down now rather than years later.

It is especially important to gain full disclosure from the agency before you adopt, so you have a more accurate representation of any medical conditions your child may have. But even if no prior medical history exists for your child, your health care provider will know what screening tests, immunizations and developmental tests are needed.

Choosing a Health Care Provider

The best time to choose a health care provider is before your child arrives. Unfortunately, not all providers have experience with adoption, and most have no special training in it. Talk to other parents who have adopted and ask for recommendations. Call a few of those health care providers to say you are planning to adopt, and ask if there is any specific medical information you should request from the agency concerning your child. If you will be adopting internationally, ask the health care providers if they have had experience with international adoptions. This information will provide insight into their attitudes about adoption and allow you to determine which personalities are best suited to you and your family.

Schedule a pre-adoption visit with the health care provider you prefer. If this visit does not go well, don't hesitate to schedule another one with a different provider. Most health care providers appreciate the opportunity to meet parents before the child arrives so they can discuss issues like sleeping, eating, making the house childproof and any pertinent medical concerns. They can also discuss with you general developmental expectations based on the age your child will be on arrival. Parents who will be traveling to another country to meet their child might have additional questions about what medicines to bring and health precautions to take

Some people confer with their health care provider to help them make sense of medical reports on children referred from their adoption agency. He or she can explain the implications of a medical condition, or perhaps alert prospective parents to what might be missing from the records.

Examinations and Immunizations

Most children adopted from within the United States do not need a medical examination right away, unless they have a known medical condition or arrive ill. If they appear healthy when they join your family, doctors recommend waiting a couple of weeks or even a month. This time gives the child a chance to adjust and the parents a chance to get to know the new arrival so they can better answer the doctor's questions about their child's "usual" behavior. However, first-time parents, especially if they did not have a pre-placement visit, may want to consult their health care provider sooner if they need information and support.

At the first appointment, your health care provider will review the child's immunizations and perform any age-appropriate screening tests, as well as any further tests indicated by the examination.

Some children have no official birth date. Determining their age can be difficult if their growth is delayed because of prematurity, problems at birth, malnutrition or neglect. Your doctor will try to make an educated guess based on a developmental examination, but when children are developmentally delayed, sometimes skeletal or dental X-rays will be suggested for a more accurate determination.

Some children who are behind in their gross motor skills are able to catch up eventually after being on an adequate diet, coupled with a stimulating, nurturing environment. One 11-month-old girl did not know how to crawl when she was adopted from abroad, because she had never had an opportunity. In her orphanage, children were kept three to a crib, day and night. She quickly learned to crawl when her adoptive mother placed her on a blanket with a toy slightly out of reach.

After your child's first medical examination, it is important to follow the schedule of examinations and immunizations recommended by your health care provider.

Medical Conditions in International Adoptions

Sometimes the agencies require an immediate medical examination for children adopted from another country, even though the children may be experiencing jet-lag and culture shock when they arrive. Certain countries have such high incidence rates of infectious diseases or parasites that prompt testing and treatment, if necessary, are recommended, both for the care of the child and for the protection of the rest of the family.

In addition to a complete physical examination, your health care provider might recommend some or all of the following screening tests:

- Hepatitis B profile, because hepatitis is common in some countries
- PPD (purified protein derivative, or Mantoux) test to test for tuberculosis, which is widespread in India, Korea and Central and South America
- Stool examination to test for intestinal parasites, with follow-up stool tests in a few months, or if diarrhea or other symptoms develop
- Blood test for syphilis
- Complete blood cell count to check for anemia and blood disorders
- Urinalysis and urine culture for cytomegalovirus (CMV), which is prevalent in India and other Asian countries
- Vision and hearing screening
- HIV screening to test for AIDS, which is becoming increasingly common around the world

Some authorities also suggest tests for thyroid hormone and certain enzyme deficiencies. Ask your health care provider for advice.

There is a higher incidence of lactose intolerance among Asians, blacks, American Indians and Hispanics, but it usually doesn't become a problem until children are 8 to 12 years old. If your child has persistent gastrointestinal symptoms such as vomiting or diarrhea, or fails to gain weight, ask your health care provider about the possibility of lactose intolerance or food allergies.

For more information about the international health concerns of your child, contact the International Adoption Clinic, Box 211 UMHC, 420 Delaware St. SE, Minneapolis, MN 55455; telephone (612) 626-2928.

Breastfeeding an Adopted Baby

Many adoptive mothers are surprised to learn that nursing their babies is an option for them. Because lactation, or the production of breast milk, can be induced by regular pumping or stimulation of the nipples, a woman might be able to breastfeed without ever having been pregnant.

Adoptive mothers who choose to nurse usually do so to enhance their relationships with their infants. Although most adoptive mothers can't produce all the milk their infants need, even limited nursing allows them the opportunity for physical and emotional attachment with their babies.

When the baby's arrival can be anticipated, some women try to establish a milk supply in advance by using an electric breast pump at regular intervals.

Others wait until the baby arrives, because the baby's sucking will stimulate lactation better than any pump on the market. These mothers use a supplemental nursing device that allows infants to receive formula through a soft tube inserted in their mouths while nursing. Even after their milk comes in, many mothers continue to use supplemental nursing devices if they need to increase the volume their infants receive at the breast.

Babies are usually more willing to nurse if they are younger than 8 weeks of age, but some adoptive mothers have reported success with older infants too.

If you think you might like to nurse your adopted baby, discuss the advantages, disadvantages and techniques with your doctor or a lactation consultant. There may be one on staff at your hospital, or you may contact the International Lactation Consultant Association, 201 Brown Ave., Evanston, IL 60202-3601; telephone (708) 260-8874. Information on adoptive nursing is also available from La Leche League International, P.O. Box 4079, Schaumburg, IL 60168-4079; telephone (800) 525-3243, or (800) La Leche.

Attachment

Before he adopted his 11-month-old son, one father worried, "Will he ever learn to trust us?" Because his son had spent six months with his birth mother and five months in foster care, the adoptive father was afraid the boy wouldn't be able to transfer his trust another time or, worse, that he might have never learned to form an attachment. As it turned out, their attachment experience began happily at the airport encounter, and the father reports a continuing joy from their deepening relationship.

Psychologists say that the optimal period for attachment is in the first six months of life, so parents who adopt children beyond that age are naturally concerned. Although older children may need more help in resolving loss, grief or fears related to the separation and change, studies have shown adoptive families form attachments as successfully as biological families.

The key is to realize that strong two-way attachment between any parent and child does not happen in one magic moment but develops gradually over time. Researchers Dorothy Smith and Laurie Nehls Sherwen divided the bonding behaviors of adoptive parents into specific time periods: pre-adoption, first encounter (entry), and after adoption.

I n the pre-adoption phase, attachment begins as parents fantasize about their child-to-be and resolve issues about their role as parents. Sometimes fantasizing is difficult for adoptive parents who may have no information about the child's age, date of arrival or what he or she might look like. Parents might wait for months with no information and suddenly get a call saying, "A baby boy is available. Can you pick him up tomorrow?"

Smith and Sherwen found that adoptive parents often lack the traditional support systems of family and friends to help prepare them for parenthood during this "pre-entry period." This situation develops partly because family attitudes about adoption may not be supportive and partly because prospective parents don't always share their adoption plans, fearing something could go awry.

"I found myself getting jealous of pregnant women," said one adoptive mother. "They got lots of attention because everyone could see they were expecting a child, but nobody knew my baby was due on a plane from Korea in two weeks."

The Pre-Adoption Phase

The First Encounter

At the first encounter, Smith and Sherwen found that attachment was facilitated if the child matched the parents' expectations. Although some parents experienced initial disappointment when their child arrived sick, dirty or not fitting the agency's description, true attachment did not depend on that moment. It was helpful, however, if the persons present with the adoptive parents at the first encounter were supportive and positive.

The After-Adoption Phase

Once the child joins the family, parents and children use verbal and nonverbal communication to work out what Smith and Sherwen call "a harmonious routine of interaction." The same activities can foster the attachment process for biological and adoptive parents: lots of touching, hugging, skin-to-skin contact and engaging baby with smiles, sounds and games like peekaboo. Here are some other tips.

Allow time for adjustment. Parents who adopt have sometimes waited so very long for a baby that they cannot wait to smother the child with love and attention. Remember that your child has just been separated from everything that was familiar and needs time to warm up to you and take in a new environment.

Holding children close helps them get accustomed to your scent, to hear your heartbeat and to feel your body warmth, but don't overdo it. Pay attention to their signals. If they look away from you, cry or stiffen, chances are that they have had enough attention and need some quiet time alone.

Talk, sing and read to your baby. These activities allow the child to get used to the sound of your voice. This is especially important for children who come from another country because it helps them get acquainted with the natural rhythms of a new language.

Respond to your baby's needs. Be quick to find out why he or she is crying, but also investigate if your child doesn't yet signal his or her discomfort.

> One father remembered, "It was almost scary at first, because our son never cried when he was wet or hungry. It made us wonder what his life had been like; perhaps crying didn't do him any good. Now he fusses like a regular kid."

Find out as much as you can about your baby. Inquire about the child's environment and routine before he or she entered your family, so you can help smooth the transition. For instance:

- A child who shared a crib in a crowded orphanage or slept on a mat with her entire foster family may be frightened at night in a room by herself. Place a stuffed animal in her crib for her to snuggle with, and put the crib in with you or a sibling until she is ready for her own space.

- A child who was carried everywhere on the back of his foster mother, as is the custom in Korea, may feel right at home if you put him in a back carrier. Even a child who isn't used to it may enjoy the security of being carried close to you in a front or back baby carrier.

- A baby who is used to falling asleep with the room light on may be extremely attached to that simple routine. Be sensitive to any behaviors that seem important to your child, and allow some time before gradually trying to change habits.

- A child who comes from poverty may experience sensory overload with a nursery full of toys, unable to decide what to play with first. Introduce one toy at a time, as the child is ready.

Be familiar with your baby's developmental age. On joining your family, your child's developmental age can affect how he or she interacts with you. For instance, in the first four months, babies cry mostly when they need something and will bond most easily with the person who responds immediately to their cries. After four months, they begin learning cause and effect and may cry just to see what happens. This behavior could frustrate parents meeting their child for the first time at this stage. At nine months, separation anxiety can be very intense for a child who has been attached to another caregiver.

Read the chapter in this book that corresponds with your child's developmental age. You will find that some of your child's behavior is indicative of the developmental age rather than of his or her personality.

If you are adopting a child who is 6 months or older, keep in mind that he or she may also have begun to learn certain cultural behaviors. For instance, a child from a country where passivity is encouraged may appear unresponsive.

If you are adopting a child of 12 months or older, it may take more time and understanding to get acquainted and develop mutual trust. You may find reassurance in reading about parenting and in doing what you can to help your child feel loved, secure and wanted.

Problems With Attachment

Sometimes parents do all they can to form an attachment and still are unhappy with the way things are going. If you are feeling discouraged, or if your child exhibits behavior problems or doesn't seem to be building a relationship with you, seek professional help. Your health care provider, adoption agency, a social worker or a therapist may be able to help you understand and solve behavior problems.

The Grieving Child

All children are individuals, with definite likes, dislikes and inborn personality traits. Some adjust quickly and respond with joy to their new families, but others might have a difficult adjustment period. Babies who have experienced maternal loss have been known to exhibit symptoms similar to grief: they may cry inconsolably or erratically, look sad, rock back and forth, eat less or not be interested in playing.

Telling Children They Are Adopted

Years ago, parents did not always tell their children they were adopted. The news might be revealed by a relative, or come as a surprise in childhood or adulthood, leaving the children feeling puzzled, angry or betrayed.

Today, parents are advised to be open about how adopted children joined the family. There is some disagreement about how early to tell, but most adoption experts feel that deceiving children for even a few years can jeopardize trust in their adoptive parents. Experts agree that if parents demonstrate they are comfortable talking about adoption as a positive, normal experience, their children will be much more likely to feel comfortable with it themselves. They will also be more willing to share their questions and concerns about adoption as issues arise.

Parents need to examine their feelings about their children knowing or having a relationship with their biological relatives. Resources are available to help make these contacts, even for international adoptions. Some children gain a sense of history by being able to find this information and meet their birth parents. Sometimes just knowing whom they resemble can be a comfort.

Whether to search for a child's birth parents should be the personal choice of the child. Some children are not interested in looking, just as not all birth parents want to be found. Helping your child understand this feeling is important too.

"You have to be honest with your child and face the questions you fear the most," advised the mother of one adopted and two biological children. "You need to be willing to grow with each other."

The Adoption Story

Some experts recommend that parents develop an "adoption story" and tell it to children from the very beginning. Children won't understand everything at first, but the words and phrases will become a natural part of their vocabulary, and they love hearing stories about themselves.

One mother tells her Korean daughter a story like this:

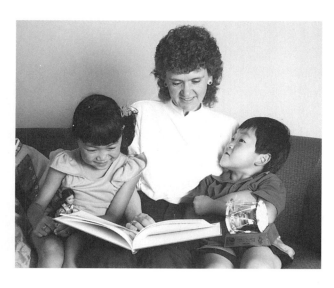

Children love to hear stories. Many experts recommend that adoptive parents develop an "adoption story" they can share with their children from the very beginning.

"Once upon a time, your daddy and I had no children. We were very, very sad. So we went to the (name of adoption agency). Meanwhile, in a country far, far away, a beautiful baby girl was born. Her birth parents were sad because they could not take care of any baby at that time in their lives, and they knew she needed to be cared for and loved. They were so happy when the adoption agency told them they had found nice parents like us to take care of their little girl. And we were so happy because the little girl was you, and we could be a family!"

This story introduces her birth parents in an understanding way, explains why her parents chose adoption to build their family and gives her a sense of personal history and belonging. Any details you can add to such a story about the joy of your first encounter will make it more delightful to your child.

Creating an adoption book for your child is another way to celebrate the unique way he or she joined your family. Save any mementos such as letters, toys, hospital name tags or documents that came with the child at the time of placement; they can serve as a source of "roots" later. Include photographs of the official adoption and "before and after" family pictures.

Attitudes Toward Adoption

Your Own

Let your language reflect your own positive attitudes about adoption. Grown-ups who were adopted as children advise that it is most important to say "my child," and not "my adopted child." Be open and honest about the adoption, but don't use it as a label.

Certain phrases are best avoided. For instance, "put up for adoption" refers to a 19th-century practice of literally "putting up" homeless children on platforms for better viewing by local citizens who might adopt them, often just for cheap labor. And "given up for adoption" leaves children feeling there was something wrong with them that made their parents give them away.

Instead, talk about the decision made by the birth parents (biological parents) to "make an adoption plan" or "arrange for an adoption." It is important for children to understand their birth parents could not take care of any baby at that point in their lives, and so they "transferred their parental rights" to the adoptive parents. The adoptive parents are their real parents, because they have made a lifelong, legally binding commitment to do the parenting.

Grandparents

Sometimes grandparents may have their own attitudes and expectations that they need to work through before they fully accept adoption as a way their son or daughter chooses to build a family. For instance, your mother may feel guilty that something she did during her pregnancy is the cause of your infertility.

"Talk to your family ahead of time," advised one adoptive mother. "Be open and honest, but expect to hit some roadblocks. Some people aren't going to approve right away."

If you are involved in an adoption support group, invite the grandparents along to a meeting. Share some of your books or magazines with them. Introduce them to friends who have adopted so they can see that adoptive families are the same as other families.

If you can find a way to involve grandparents in your preparations, like helping to decorate the nursery, your excitement and enthusiasm may be contagious.

"My husband came from a family of nine, and they'd never heard of infertility," recalled one mother. "They were initially unsupportive, but they came around as soon as they saw the baby."

Sometimes, however, certain family members never accept adoption. If this happens to you, it is important to think about how you are going to deal with the situation in order to lessen the impact on your children. Adoption support groups can prove invaluable in this process.

Dealing With Insensitivity

Adoptive parents and children may be faced with hurtful remarks at one time or another. It isn't always easy or appropriate to speak up when someone says something offensive, but it is important to keep your child's well-being in mind. Your response may be more for your child's benefit than to educate the naive person who may just be making conversation.

Here are some responses suggested by adoptive parents to frequently asked questions:

"Who are his real parents?" We are. We aren't imaginary. We are the ones who do the parenting. (Information about the birth parents is the child's to give.)

"Are they really brother and sister?" Yes, they are. They have the same parents. (Whether or not they are biologically related is also the child's information.)

"I don't know how any mother could give up her child." The decision to place a child for adoption is a painful, difficult decision for any woman, but it is always made in the child's best interests. It is not because a birth mother doesn't care, but because she and the birth father could not care for a child at that time in their lives.

"Too bad you couldn't experience pregnancy." You don't get to experience everything in life. I may never get to Africa either. But my adoption experience has been wonderful, and I wouldn't trade it for anything.

Parenting Is Parenting

Many families are built through adoption. What makes adoption unique is that it is an active process, often involving a great deal of paperwork, introspection and scrutiny by outsiders. In addition, because adopted children have experienced separation from their birth parents, their initial adjustment and attachment process with their new families can be affected. And in the future, it may result in questions about who their birth parents are and why they could not parent them.

Other than that, parenting is parenting.

"I feel exactly the same way about my adopted child as I do about my biological children," said one mother. "If anything, adoption has given me a real sense that each child is a special gift."

CHAPTER TWENTY-FIVE

Your Physical and Emotional Health

The first year after childbirth

Don't be surprised if the days, even months, after your baby's birth are characterized by one word: chaos! If it's any comfort, you have good reason to feel stressed. First, you may find that giving birth tests the upper range of your physical limits. Then, you're suddenly responsible for a tiny new person who, initially, may not communicate his or her needs well at all. You may need to redefine your identity both as an individual and as a partner, and you also need to adjust to becoming a parent and relating to others as a family. Stress also may affect other family members, including the baby's siblings and grandparents—or even your pets!

Everyone's attention, which was fixed on you during your pregnancy, may now seem focused on this newest member of your family. Most of the preparation throughout your pregnancy probably focused on childbirth, although some parents also use this time to learn about the care and development of their new baby. It was a time of anticipation and dreaming. Parents often expect the after-delivery (postpartum) time to flow as smoothly. For most women, it doesn't.

This chapter focuses mainly on you, the new mother. Although your partner will understand some of the feelings discussed here—and will benefit by reading this chapter to understand what you're experiencing—this chapter is all about you and the months after you've given birth. Every pregnancy is different, so even if you've had a baby before, you may learn something that you didn't experience the first time around.

Years ago, mothers stayed in bed, often in a hospital, for a week or more after their baby's birth. Now, one to two days in the hospital is typical. Traditionally, many doctors think of the postpartum time as six weeks, because this is usually the amount of time it takes your uterus to shrink back to approximately its pre-pregnancy size.

However, you may experience physical changes related to the birth for as long as a year. You may experience breast problems, discomfort, infections or nipple irritation. Women are often concerned about fatigue, hemorrhoids, poor appetite, constipation and acne and sometimes are concerned about increased sweating, hot flashes, and numbness and tingling in their hands. As a new mother, you are more likely to have respiratory ailments (including coughs, colds, sinus infections and bronchitis). You may be more susceptible to bacterial or viral infections that you're exposed to at work or that your baby contracts at the child care center.

In addition to physical changes, the vast majority of new mothers also struggle with emotional adjustments. In short, for most new mothers the postpartum time is stressful. Although some are energetic, ready to go and feeling great, others simply are too stressed or exhausted to immediately jump back into their earlier pace.

This chapter will help you understand and deal with the physical and emotional changes you're likely to experience as a new mother. Although it cannot replace the personal advice of your doctor, it may help you when you realize that other women have gone through many of the changes you're experiencing. And it should also help you know when you need to seek further professional advice.

Physical Changes

Did you believe the myth of "bouncing back" after your baby's birth? If so, you may be disappointed. In fact, you may wonder if your body will ever get back to normal. "Normal" postpartum physical changes can vary widely. If you are concerned that you may be outside that normal range, discuss your concerns with your doctor. Let's look at the common physical changes you can expect.

Breasts

Your breasts may remain enlarged for a while after your baby's birth. As women age, breasts will gradually droop from stretching of tissue within the breast. To prevent premature sagging, wear a bra at all times until your breasts return to their pre-pregnancy size.

If you're nursing, you will notice that you have colostrum for the first few days after your baby is born. You may think that your milk supply is inadequate, but it will become sufficient as your baby nurses. Breastfeeding can seem awkward at first. Try to maintain a positive attitude. If something isn't working, ask for help and try something else. You may avoid sore nipples if you alternate which breast you offer your baby first (but still offer both, to avoid engorgement). Varying your position while nursing may also help.

Engorgement. You may experience the discomfort of breast engorgement when your milk comes in. If you're not nursing your baby, your breasts may become engorged and hard until you are no longer producing milk. You can relieve engorgement pain by wearing a well-fitting bra. Cold washcloths or ice packs can reduce swelling. Engorgement usually lasts less than three days. Avoid pumping or massaging your breasts, because this encourages milk production.

Mastitis. Regardless of whether you breastfeed or bottle feed your baby, call your doctor if your temperature is more than 100.4 degrees Fahrenheit (38 degrees Centigrade) or if one area on your breast is reddened, sore, hard and hot. These are symptoms of mastitis, an infection that can occur when bacteria enter the breast, usually through a crack in the nipple. Acetaminophen will help bring the fever down, and your doctor will prescribe antibiotics for infectious mastitis.

If you are breastfeeding, continue nursing to empty your breasts. You may be more comfortable nursing the baby more often but for shorter periods. The antibiotics you are taking are not harmful to your baby, although you may notice a change in color of the baby's bowel movements. With treatment, mastitis usually clears up in a few days.

Breast self-examination. Monthly breast self-examination can be more difficult during pregnancy and breastfeeding. Because breast cancer may be curable if detected early, regular breast self-examination is important for all women. Women who practice regular breast self-examination are most likely to detect breast changes before a doctor will, because he or she checks your breasts only at periodic examinations. Mammograms can be safely done during pregnancy, but they are rarely needed. If there is a suspicious lump found during pregnancy, a biopsy is sometimes done to determine whether it is breast cancer.

Regular breast self-examination is easier if you find a convenient time and establish a routine. Examine your breasts one week after the start of your period, because your breasts usually are less tender then. Or, establish a routine; for example, do breast self-examination the same day your monthly phone bill arrives.

If you're breastfeeding, it's best to do breast self-examination right after you've fed your baby, when your breasts are emptier and any abnormalities will be more obvious.

There are three steps in breast self-examination. It's important to perform all three each time. For example, you may discover a breast change when lying down that you might not notice in the shower.

Step 1: Visual inspection in front of a mirror

- Disrobe to your waist and stand in front of a mirror with arms at your sides, inspecting both breasts for changes since your last breast self-examination. Turn from side to side to view the outer portions of your breasts, looking carefully for changes.

- Rest your palms on your hips. Press down firmly to flex chest muscles and firm your breasts, and again, turn from side to side looking for changes.

- Raise both arms above your head and press your palms together to flex chest muscles and firm your breasts. Again turn from side to side looking for changes.

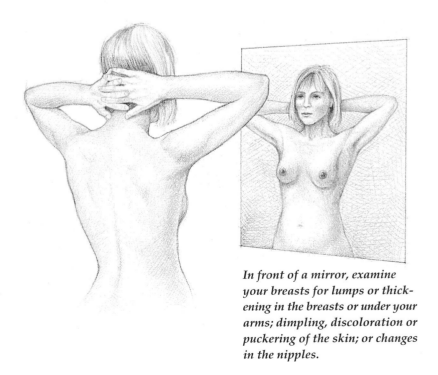

In front of a mirror, examine your breasts for lumps or thickening in the breasts or under your arms; dimpling, discoloration or puckering of the skin; or changes in the nipples.

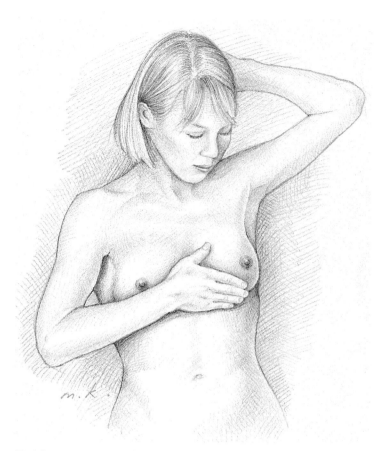

Raising one arm overhead allows your breast tissue to lie flat over the chest wall. Use the pads of your three middle fingers, not your fingertips, to examine your breasts.

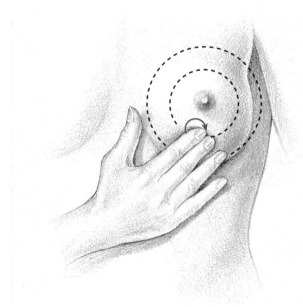

Make small circular motions with the pads of your fingers (as shown by the purple arrow), applying light, moderate and deeper pressure. Move your fingers from spot to spot, repeating the same circular motion to cover the entire breast (as shown by the dotted lines).

Step 2: In the shower or tub

- Lather your fingers and breasts with soap so your fingers can glide smoothly over wet skin.
- Use your right hand to examine your left breast. Raise your left arm overhead to allow the breast tissue to lie flat over the chest wall. If you have larger, more pendulous breasts, support your breast with the left hand.
- Use the "pads" of your three middle fingers to examine your breast. The pads are the inside tops of your fingers, not your fingertips.
- Imagine your breast to be the face of a clock. Find your collarbone. Place your fingertips approximately one-half inch below the collarbone at the 12 o'clock position.
- Making small circular motions with the pads of your fingers, apply light pressure, moderate pressure and deeper pressure. Slide your fingers to each hour on the imaginary clock, 12 o'clock to 1 o'clock to 2 o'clock...repeating the circular motion with light, moderate and deep pressure at each hour.
- Carefully examine your underarm area where lymph nodes are located. (Lymph nodes are bean-sized nodules that filter foreign material.) They lie under your arm, as well as near the collarbone and along the breastbone. Usually you can't feel your lymph nodes.
- After completing one circle around the outermost portion of your breast, move in toward the nipple about one-half inch and complete another circle. Continue using the same pattern until you examine every part of your breast, including the nipple.
- Cover the entire breast from collarbone to bra line, breastbone to underarm. A ridge of firm tissue in the lower curve of each breast is normal.
- Look for discharge by squeezing the nipple gently from top to bottom and side to side.
- After you have completely examined your left breast, examine your right breast using the same method.

Step 3: Lying down

Use the same procedure and pattern described above, plus these additional guidelines:

- To examine your right breast, place a folded towel under your right shoulder blade. Place your right hand behind your head to distribute the breast tissue more evenly on your chest.

- Repeat the exam on your left breast with the folded towel under your left shoulder blade and your left arm behind your head.
- You may want to use lotion or powder on your finger pads so your fingers can glide more smoothly.
- Reach deeply under your underarm where the lymph nodes lie.

Remember that there are various kinds of breast lumps, and the vast majority are not malignant. Breasts are normally lumpy. Some women have more lumps than others because of fibrocystic changes. If you have this condition, note how many lumps you have, where they are located and their approximate size. Check for changes each month. If you find breast changes that concern you, see your doctor.

Uterus

Your uterus shrinks immediately after your baby's birth, decreasing to normal size over six weeks. By two weeks after delivery, you may no longer feel your uterus when you press on your abdomen. Your uterus may be slightly larger if this is not your first pregnancy or if you have uterine fibroids. As your uterus shrinks, you may experience after pains or contractions for several days. After-pains may increase during nursing and are more common and more intense if you've had multiple pregnancies. Medications used to control hemorrhaging may increase the cramping. Your doctor may prescribe an analgesic to help ease the pain, but if pain persists for more than a week, or if you have a fever, you should see your doctor. These symptoms could indicate a uterine infection.

Vaginal Discharge

Vaginal discharge after birth varies widely in amount, appearance and duration. This temporary discharge (the medical term for it is "lochia") is initially bloody, then becomes paler after about four days and white or yellowish after about 10 days. Vaginal discharge may last from two to eight weeks; doctors aren't usually concerned about the duration, but about whether the amount of discharge diminishes. If your vaginal discharge has been otherwise normal, don't be alarmed if you pass occasional blood clots—even up to golf ball size.

Call your doctor or the labor and delivery nurses if:

- You're soaking a sanitary napkin every hour for four to five hours (sooner if you become dizzy or notice increasing blood loss)
- The discharge has a foul, fish-like odor
- Your abdomen feels tender or your bleeding increases and you're passing numerous clots

Episiotomy

If you had an episiotomy, it will heal and the stitches will dissolve in two to three weeks. It may be painful to walk or sit while your episiotomy is healing. Let the pain remind you that you need to rest and pamper your body. A small squirt bottle of water is handy for rinsing off your episiotomy after you use the toilet. Many women find that the pain they attribute to their episiotomy is actually from hemorrhoids. If you find that your episiotomy becomes hot, swollen and painful or produces a pus-like discharge (which could indicate an infection), call your doctor.

Gently cooling your episiotomy with ice can decrease swelling. Some women find that adding ice cubes to a bath of room temperature water provides good relief from the pain.

When you lower yourself to sit on a soft surface, squeeze your buttocks together. You may be more comfortable sitting on hard surfaces, because soft surfaces allow your bottom to stretch and pull on the stitches more. You'll do a real favor for your muscles if you do 30 to 50 Kegel exercises frequently, perhaps every time you feed your baby. (For more information on Kegel exercises, see page 180.)

Hemorrhoids

Women frequently develop hemorrhoids during pregnancy and the birth process. Your nurses or doctor may have discussed this possibility with you, or you may discover them yourself after you return home. If you notice pain during a bowel movement and feel a swollen mass near your anus, you probably have a hemorrhoid. If your hemorrhoid causes discomfort, it may be helpful to soak in the bathtub. You can also avoid some discomfort by keeping your stool soft. Eat a fiber-rich diet, including fruits, vegetables, whole wheat and bran. Avoid using laxatives, because they may aggravate the problem. A cotton pad soaked with cold witch hazel cream applied to the area of your hemorrhoids may help relieve discomfort. If you still have problems, talk with your doctor, who might suggest a prescription medicine.

Urinary Incontinence (Leakage of Urine)

Some new mothers may pass urine inadvertently, especially when coughing, straining or laughing. This is usually caused by stretching of the base of the bladder by pregnancy and birth; fortunately, it usually improves within three months. Do Kegel exercises to hasten urinary control, and wear protective undergarments or sanitary napkins in the meantime. (For more on Kegel exercises, see page 180.)

Fecal Incontinence (Inability to Control Bowel Movements)

Fecal incontinence is a somewhat common problem for new moms. It is associated with stretching and weakening of the pelvic-floor muscles, tearing of the perineum (the area between the vaginal opening and the anus) and nerve injury to sphincter muscles around the anus. You are more likely to experience fecal incontinence if your vaginal delivery followed an unusually prolonged labor. Fecal incontinence usually resolves after a couple of months. Talk with your doctor about exercises to restore the muscles. Sometimes persisting incontinence can be helped by surgical repair.

Other Physical Changes

Here are some additional physical changes you may notice.

- Abdomen. After your baby's birth, your abdomen will likely remain enlarged and the muscles quite lax. Abdominal muscle tone will return with exercise. Stretch marks will probably be permanent, but they may fade with time. If you developed a dark line on your abdomen (linea nigra), it will probably fade over the next several months. Be sure to call your doctor if you have continuing lower abdominal pain.

- Skin and hair. The texture of your skin and hair may change as a result of your pregnancy. In the months after birth, some women lose a lot of hair. (See page 16 for more information about hair loss.) Generally, these changes are temporary, and you'll find that by the time your baby is 6 months old, your body has returned to normal. You may have noticed small red spots on your face after baby's birth. They are a result of small blood vessels breaking during the pushing stage of labor. These spots will disappear in about a week. Usually, any skin that darkened during pregnancy, such as on your face (the mask of pregnancy, or chloasma), will eventually fade back to its normal color.

- Muscle pain. You may feel overuse muscle pain in your arms, neck or jaw from the exertion of labor. This will ease in a few days.

- Blood clots. During the first two weeks after delivery, your body's protective mechanisms to prevent bleeding may result in blood clotting and vein problems, especially in your legs. Try to avoid these problems by walking and delaying the use of birth control pills for the first two weeks after delivery. If a vein in your leg becomes sore and tender or if one leg swells, call your doctor. Also, be sure to contact your doctor immediately if you experience chills or shaking.

Recovering From a Cesarean Birth

A cesarean birth is a major operation. Your body will need extra time to mend, and your hospital stay will be longer than if you had given birth vaginally. If your cesarean birth was unexpected, you may have emotional as well as physical issues to deal with. Tips to help speed your recovery are discussed here.

In the Hospital

- Consider a private room. If you had an unexpected cesarean birth and you find yourself sharing a room with a new mother who delivered vaginally, consider a private room. You may want the privacy as you sort out your emotions, discuss your feelings with your partner and begin the recovery process.

- Accept pain medications. Don't hesitate to take a pain reliever, even if you plan to breastfeed. To be successful with nursing, it's important to be comfortable. Comfort is especially important during the first several days of your recovery, when your incision is beginning to heal. Take the pain medicine about a half-hour before you nurse. Very little of the medication will find its way into your breast milk.

    Even with pain medications, you may be uncomfortable after your cesarean delivery, especially for the first 24 hours. Keep in mind that the discomfort does diminish. Most women feel much better in a day or two.

- Don't be overly concerned about your incision. Your nurses and doctor will clean it daily for the first day or two and check to see that it's healing properly. The sutures or staples are strong, and you need not worry about pulling your incision apart as you move about in bed.

For the first two or three days, bathing will be by sponge bath, but soon you'll be allowed to shower, with assistance. As your incision begins to heal, it may itch. Resist the urge to scratch your incision. Lotion is a better alternative.

Most incisions heal without incident, but any incision can become infected. If the skin on the sides of your incision is reddened and swollen, and especially if pus is draining from your incision, it may be infected, and your physician may prescribe an antibiotic.

- Secure a helper. After a cesarean birth, you'll find it difficult to move about at first. Many hospitals, but not all of them, give priority to taking babies into the rooms of new mom. Your partner or another helper at your bedside, at least for portions of the day, can help bring the baby to you.

- Move about in bed. You can begin gentle exercises almost immediately. Ask your physician or a nurse about abdominal tightening exercises, foot and arm movements, bending and straightening your knees and a pelvic lift exercise.

- Take a walk. Be sure to have a supporting arm nearby for those first short walks, but get out of bed as soon as you can. Early walking is one of the best ways to speed recovery. You'll probably be anxious about standing and stepping away from your bed. Once you're under way, you'll discover that slow walking is not as difficult or painful as you thought it might be.

- Avoid flatulence (gas) and constipation. Flatulence is a common, major discomfort in women who've had a cesarean delivery. Suppositories can help, but walking is the best preventive measure.

  Limit your diet to clear liquids for the first several days. Your digestive system needs time to "wake up." If you eat solid foods too soon, you may have a problem with constipation.

  Exercise can help prevent constipation, as can a diet that includes fiber. If you breastfeed your baby, drink eight to 10 glasses of fluids daily. A loss of fluid from breastfeeding can lead to constipation.

- Expect a vaginal discharge. Shifts in hormones after delivery cause a vaginal discharge called lochia, regardless of whether you had a cesarean or vaginal birth. The brownish to clear discharge will last several weeks. Some hospitals provide pads held in place by a T-belt. Avoid them. These pads can irritate your incision and delay healing. Pads with adhesive strips work better.

At Home

- Avoid exhaustion. Excessive fatigue is a common problem for moms who've had a cesarean. Once you're home, you'll discover there's much to do, and although you may still be taking an oral pain reliever, you'll be feeling pretty well. There's a tendency to do too much! Remember that unlike mothers who delivered their babies vaginally, you're still recovering from an operation.

- Avoid stairs and lifting. Ask your doctor for recommendations about everyday activities such as walking up and down stairs or lifting anything heavier than your baby. Until your body has recovered from the operation you aren't able to move as quickly, and therefore you have a higher risk of stumbling or pulling sore muscles. Driving is also not recommended until you can make sudden movements of your legs or trunk without discomfort.

(For more information on the effects of cesarean birth on moms and babies, see page 327.)

Menstruation

The resumption of menstruation varies widely after pregnancy. If you're nursing your baby, you will probably begin menstruating again from one to three months after you wean your baby, although some women (usually those with high levels of estrogen) begin menses while they are still nursing. Nursing lowers the level of reproductive hormones and stimulates the production of prolactin (the hormone responsible for milk production). Consult your doctor if menstruation has not begun six months after you've weaned your breastfed baby. In this case, the first thing your doctor probably will do is administer a pregnancy test.

If you're not nursing, you'll probably begin menstruating again within four to 16 weeks. Because ovulation usually occurs about two weeks before menses, you may be fertile before your first period and should be sure to use some form of birth control if you resume sexual activity during this time and don't want to get pregnant right away. Your period may be further delayed if you take medications (some tranquilizers, antidepressants or sleeping pills), exercise excessively or have marked weight loss.

Weight Loss and Diet

You'll probably lose about 10 pounds during birth. This includes the weight of your baby, the placenta and amniotic fluid. Oxytocin, the hormone that stimulates labor, initially causes your body to retain fluid. So, during the first week after delivery, when that hormone is no longer released, you'll lose additional fluid weight.

Don't plan to lose all the weight you gained during pregnancy in a few weeks, but more realistically over three to six months. Remember, it took nine months to gain that weight, and it's going to take a while to lose it. Don't be surprised or embarrassed if you are still wearing maternity clothes at your next checkup—many mothers do.

Most women are concerned about their weight after having a baby. Be patient. The best weight loss plan allows for loss of about half a pound each week. Remember that good nutrition is important to your well-being—and your baby's, if you're nursing. At least 90 percent of people who go on fad diets to lose weight regain that weight within a year. It's much more important to change your lifestyle. Look for a gradual reduction in your weight if you maintain a healthful eating style, get a moderate amount of exercise and reduce your stress.

To calculate the approximate number of calories you need to have in a day, multiply your weight in pounds by 12. This is a rough guide to maintain your current weight. To lose half a pound a week, you need a deficit of about 250 calories a day. It's important for your long-term health that you lose weight

How much should you weigh?

Your weight is healthful if:

1. You have no medical problem that's caused or aggravated by your weight

2. Your family history doesn't increase your risk of a health condition related to weight

3. Your weight falls within the acceptable range for your height and age.

Within each age range in the chart below, the lower weights generally apply to women, and the higher weights generally apply to men, who tend to have more muscle and bone.

Height (without shoes)	Weight in pounds (without clothes)	
	Ages 19-34 years	Ages 35 years or older
5'0"	97-128	108-138
5'1"	101-132	111-143
5'2"	104-137	115-148
5'3"	107-141	119-152
5'4"	111-146	122-157
5'5"	114-150	126-162
5'6"	118-155	130-167
5'7"	121-160	134-172
5'8"	125-164	138-178
5'9"	129-169	142-183
5'10"	132-174	146-188
5'11"	136-179	151-194
6'0"	140-184	155-199
6'1"	144-189	159-205
6'2"	148-195	164-210
6'3"	152-200	168-216
6'4"	156-205	173-222
6'5"	160-211	177-228
6'6"	164-216	182-234

slowly. If you restrict your calories too severely, you risk a permanent drop in your metabolism, which will make losing weight even more difficult.

The most important dietary recommendation is to reduce fat to no more than 30 percent of your total calorie intake. In addition to adding weight, fat may increase your cholesterol level and your risks of developing some types of cancer, gallbladder disease and high blood pressure. Reduce your fat intake by limiting spreadable and pourable fats (oils, margarine, butter, salad dressings) and by sautéing foods in water rather than oil. Decrease your consumption of meat and cheese.

To lose and then control your weight:

- Don't skip meals
- Add fiber with whole grains and raw vegetables and fruit
- Avoid all fad diets
- Increase your exercise

If you need further help with weight loss or if you have specific concerns or questions about diet, ask your doctor to refer you to a registered dietitian.

Exercise

Regular daily exercise will help restore your strength and return your body to its pre-pregnancy state. It will increase your energy level and your sense of well-being while helping you fight fatigue. Exercise also helps your circulation, which will improve skin tone.

If you had a cesarean or complicated birth or complications after giving birth, you may need to go slowly. Talk with your doctor if you're uncertain.

If you exercised regularly before and during your pregnancy, you will probably be able to resume exercising as soon as you feel ready. But don't expect to return immediately to your pre-birth level of exercise. If you didn't exercise much during your pregnancy, you'll need to start more slowly and work gradually into more vigorous exercise. Walking and swimming are excellent exercises to help you get back into shape after your baby's birth. Here again, begin slowly, and pick up the pace and distance as you feel up to it. Some new moms enjoy exercise classes specially designed for women who have recently given birth.

During pregnancy, your body probably developed extra padding in the thighs and buttocks. This padding is often difficult for women to lose. When you are up to it, 20 to 30 minutes of non-stop aerobic exercise three times a week will help you control your weight. Combine that with toning exercises three times a week to give your muscles a sleeker definition.

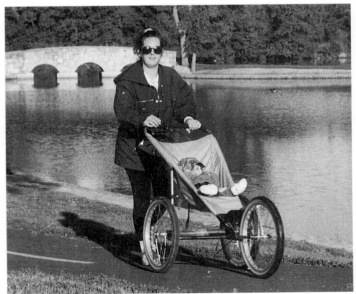

Brisk exercise along with some fresh air helps to revitalize your body and spirits.

Emotional Adjustments

We've known for a long time that giving birth often brings about emotional changes. We don't totally understand why these emotional changes are so strong after childbirth. These emotions are certainly not just from the fluctuation of hormone levels after birth, although this may be a contributing factor.

Changes in your daily routine can affect your emotional adjustment during this time. If you're used to feeling "in control" and organized, you may be disheartened when your fairly controllable lifestyle vanishes after you give birth. For a woman with a career, giving birth brings on an identity change, a shift from a capable worker to a novice caregiver. You may find it difficult to explain to your partner who has been away at work just what you've done all day that exhausts you. You may find it difficult to adjust to limited time spent with adults—combined with the 24-hour responsibility of caring for your baby. You probably feel a desire to talk about the experience of giving birth, but you may find that others around you easily tire of the topic.

Fatigue

It would be wonderful if a woman's body could store energy during the pregnancy for the fatigue she'll encounter during the baby's first year. Unfortunately, we're not made this way—fatigue will inevitably occur. When you are caring for an infant around the clock, your sleep is frequently interrupted. It's probably a major challenge just to find time for a shower or a few minutes alone. You may feel isolated when your partner goes to work. Exhaustion may make it difficult to separate physical from emotional problems.

Here are a few suggestions for dealing with fatigue:

- Arrange for help. If someone asks if you can use help, put their good intentions to work. Accepting help doesn't indicate a dependent personality or weakness; it is a good coping skill. Your mother, mother-in-law, sister or good friend might be pleased by an invitation to spend a few days with you. Most are glad to help out with some meals, the housework or errands—or watch your baby while you run the errands. It's usually best to establish the expectation that their role is to help you, rather than focusing on the baby.

  Many communities have services available for new mothers. To learn about services available in your area, talk with nurses at the hospital or call your local public health department. Some women even hire a woman experienced in helping new mothers and new babies. Look in the Yellow Pages or check local newspaper listings under maternity care or postpartum services.

- Spend time away from home. Take your baby out for a walk or find someone to watch the baby for a few hours while you get out. You'll be surprised at how much better a change of environment helps you feel. Consider seeking out other new moms and swapping child care for brief periods. There may be a child care cooperative in your area, through which parents trade time caring for each other's children.

- Take your phone off the hook. You don't have to answer phone calls if you don't feel up to it. If you have an answering machine, turn it on while you take some time off for yourself. If you don't have an answering machine, leave the receiver off the hook when you want to rest.

- Expect and accept a little clutter. This is especially important for those who take pride in having an organized, spotless household. Forget about having an immaculate house. You'll be a much better, happier mother if you care for your baby, not your home. Don't worry about cleaning before friends or relatives visit—they'll understand.

- Work with your partner to use the "divide and conquer" approach to housework. If sharing this work is something new for the two of you, be sure to offer plenty of compliments to the novice. Try to avoid being overly critical about how the work is done; just be grateful that it's done. Focus on the most important points; the dishes don't have to be put away, just put away the perishables.

- Simplify mealtimes. Before the birth of their babies, some women fantasize that when they are home with their babies they'll finally have a chance to indulge in preparing romantic, exotic dinners. In reality, you'll probably use shortcuts such as paper plates, frozen dinners or take-out foods. The romance isn't in the menu or even the setting; it's in the mealtime sharing and celebration of your experiences as a family.

- Are you over-committed? Don't feel guilty for saying "no" to requests for your volunteer time. Similarly, you may need to bow out of current commitments. These activities can come later. Don't be reluctant to say that the demands of new motherhood are taking a higher priority.

- Exercise can help. Start slowly and add a bit more exercise each day until you're back in shape. (Yes, that day will come, eventually!) Exercise will give you the strength to meet more of the day's challenges while it improves your self-esteem and body image. Use exercise tapes, TV workouts or a fitness club with baby-sitting services to get yourself moving.

- Make sure you're nourished spiritually. Give priority to refilling your spiritual well, from which you'll be drawing heavily during this time. Talk with people you find uplifting, and share your thoughts with them. Parenthood helps us appreciate the gift of life. We become more aware of how important others have been in our lives and how we contribute to the well-being of others. This awareness helps you keep in perspective that you're part of a bigger realm.

Financial concerns may also be adding to your or your partner's fatigue and stress. Many parents will tell you that no matter your income level, there's almost always a money shortage when you have children. Although many parents work extra hours successfully, it's important not to overdo it and add unmanageable stress to the family picture. It's also a good idea to postpone major financial and time commitments such as home improvement projects until things are more settled.

Depression

If you are fatigued and overwhelmed, it's natural to feel depressed. Many factors can contribute to this depression: the many bodily changes you are experiencing, illness, difficulties during your pregnancy, changes in your family's finances, unrealistic expectations of childbirth and parenting, perhaps unresolved issues from your own childhood, an unexpected pregnancy and insufficient social or emotional support. Some degree of depressed mood affects most new mothers.

There are three levels of postpartum depression, and these are discussed below.

"Baby blues." The "baby blues," a mild form of depression, affect more than 80 percent of new mothers. Contributing factors may include some or all of the following:

- Disappointment about not having the mythical "perfect birth," although virtually all births result in some unexpected outcome
- A response to postpartum pain or discomfort
- A letdown from an exciting event
- Concerns about dealing with your new baby or surprise about the amount of work involved in caring for the baby

Symptoms of baby blues include episodes of anxiety, sadness, crying, headaches, exhaustion, feeling unworthy and irritability. The blues can occur within a day or two after the birth, or they may not surface for several weeks. You'll get over baby blues more quickly if you get extra rest, good nourishment and medical care—and some help caring for yourself and your baby. You will probably get over baby blues in a few days or several weeks. Occasionally, baby blues turn into postpartum depression.

Postpartum depression (PPD). This affects between 10 and 20 percent of all women who have just given birth. It is more common among second-time moms than first-time moms. PPD is a treatable form of depression. This depression is different from the "blues" we all feel from time to time. Rather, it is a physical illness affecting the brain.

Just like other organs in your body—your heart, lungs and kidneys, for example—your brain also can become ill. When it's your appendix that's acting up, you feel physical pain, because the nerve fibers that come from your appendix send "pain" signals. When it's the area of the brain that generates emotions, you feel emotional changes, because the nerve fibers that come from your brain send "emotional" signals. You can't think your way into or out of these feelings any more than you can think yourself into or out of the pain of appendicitis.

You may be having PPD if you feel a sense of sadness that doesn't go away or frequent mood swings, anxiety or guilt. You can distinguish PPD from other depression by the fluctuations, a good day followed by several bad days and back to another good day.

PPD usually begins from two weeks to three months after your baby is born. Your most effective preventive tool is educating yourself about PPD. If you're struggling with PPD, seek out information and support to overcome the sense of isolation, depression, fear or even guilt. The sooner you realize you have PPD and do something about it, the better your chances for treating and curing the problem. Because PPD is a physical illness, doctors use medications to relieve its symptoms. Be sure to discuss your concerns with your doctor if you think you might have PPD.

Postpartum psychosis. Postpartum psychosis is a fairly rare and more severe form of depression. Some women who have postpartum psychosis have never had any prior psychiatric illness, and others have experienced depression previously. Some have experienced a recent significant loss, divorce or separation, abuse or a difficult birth. Others have a perfectionist personality.

Postpartum psychosis may begin within days or weeks after a baby's birth. The symptoms are the same as those of PPD, but more extreme. Women with postpartum psychosis are severely depressed and may be confused, paranoid and unable to function. Times when they can think clearly may be interspersed with periods when they can't. Postpartum psychosis can be life-threatening. Women with this condition may consider harming themselves, their baby or others. They might or might not realize that they are having problems, and they may be unable or unwilling to seek treatment.

It's important to recognize postpartum psychosis as early as possible. It's critically important to seek medical help if you suspect that you or someone you know may have this problem. Depression and confused thinking can be very frightening to experience or to observe in a friend. It's important to know that waiting and hoping for improvement are not enough and that medical treatment is likely to be very helpful.

It's helpful to know that the feelings of depression after birth are common, they aren't your fault and you can feel normal again. Explore and accept your feelings without judgment. Discuss whether your expectations are appropriate. Allow yourself to grieve over unfulfilled expectations, and try to let go of guilt you may feel. Take a look at the other stressors in your life; do what you can to relieve or postpone them until you're handling things well again. And recognize that you may need treatment or medication to help you function and relieve your symptoms.

Ask your doctor about support groups available in your area for new mothers. It can be helpful to talk with another new mother who has faced problems you're experiencing and can guide and reassure you. For additional information on "blues," depression and psychosis that can follow birth, contact:

Postpartum Support International
927 North Kellogg Avenue
Santa Barbara, California 93111
Telephone: 805-967-7636
(From 8 a.m. to 8 p.m., Pacific standard time)

Stress

You will likely have the opportunity throughout these early months to consider your techniques for dealing with stress. Remember that different things prove stressful for different people. One common characteristic of much of our stress is that it involves something over which we have no control. For new mothers, major stress points often include the following:

- Your baby's birth didn't go as you expected; perhaps you had a long labor or unexpected cesarean birth. It's not unusual for new moms to feel that they weren't adequately prepared for the pain and length of labor.

- You're finding the adjustment to caring for your baby at home difficult; you may not feel up to the task.

- You, or your partner, find it difficult to return at the end of a workday to a chaotic household, rather than the serene family many of us envision.

- You're finding it difficult to return to your job. Your employer expects you to perform a full day's work, you've had to deal with child care hassles (perhaps including leaving a crying baby) and you're feeling overwhelmed with caring for a child and maintaining your home while holding down a job. You may simply not be ready to return to work, yet feel compelled by family or personal needs to do so.

- You may find a significant change in your sexual activity. Most couples struggle with a temporarily less-satisfying marital relationship after the birth of a baby. Mothers often feel less interested in sexual activity for a while after they deliver a baby. This decreased interest may be due to fatigue, discomfort from the physical stress of delivering a baby, hormonal changes that women have as their bodies return to a pre-pregnancy state or dissatisfaction with body image.

Don't feel alone! During the postpartum period, most women are concerned about their ability to deal with new demands and responsibilities such as the possibility that you won't find any personal time, your ability to care for your baby properly and the difficulty of juggling all your other responsibilities while managing to maintain a good relationship with your partner. You can discuss your concerns with your doctor, obstetrics nurse, childbirth educator or social worker. They have helped others with similar concerns. The pediatrician, family doctor or nurse-practitioner you see for baby checkups is very interested in helping new parents.

Sexual Relations

Becoming new parents frequently affects a couple's sexual relations. Your partner may have a renewed interest in sexual activity, but you may experience a decrease in sexual activity in the first year after childbirth, for several reasons.

Literally, you may be too tired. You may find intercourse painful, or fear that it will be. Many women feel a decreased sense of attractiveness in the postpartum period, and some have difficulty achieving orgasm. Differences between you and your partner may add tension to your relationship.

Work with your partner to make room for each other's feelings, and share them openly. He needs to understand that even finding time to talk and laugh together takes more effort than either of you ever expected. Resuming sexual activity is even more challenging. Whether you've given birth vaginally or had a cesarean birth, your body will probably need several weeks to heal. During this time, aim to maintain emotional and sexual intimacy; lovemaking without intercourse can resume soon after birth if you wish.

Most women wait three to six weeks before resuming intercourse (less, if you didn't have an episiotomy). If you had a cesarean birth, your doctor will probably advise you to wait six weeks. A good indicator of the earliest you should consider resuming sexual intercourse is when you no longer feel pain when you press on your vaginal opening or episiotomy.

Breastfeeding may affect your and your partner's attitudes about sexual intimacy. You may think of the intimacy of nursing as a replacement for intimacy with your partner—or, you may become less receptive to your partner's overtures if you think of your breasts as simply nurturing rather than erotic. Some men find that they feel greater closeness with a nursing partner, whereas others become jealous of that mother-infant bond. You may experience some milk flow with breast stimulation. Some couples find this pleasurable, but others adjust their sexual practices to avoid stimulating milk flow.

The following suggestions may make resuming sexual activity more pleasurable for both of you:

- Rest before you attempt intercourse.

- Hormonal changes mean you may experience vaginal dryness and a thinning of the vaginal wall. When menstruation resumes and breast-feeding ends, these will improve. Meanwhile, lubricating creams or lotions may help.

- Use a position that allows you to control penetration. Usually this works best if the woman is on top, where you can determine the depth and pressure of the thrusting. It's important to find a way that intercourse is pain-free, or your body's muscles will tighten each time you anticipate that pain. Kegel exercises may help you learn to relax and tighten vaginal muscles.

- Talk with your partner about family planning and, unless you want to become pregnant again immediately, select the best birth control method for your needs.

Birth Control

Because some women who have unprotected intercourse before their first postpartum menstrual period become pregnant, it's important that you and your partner—with your doctor's help—discuss your birth control options and make a reasoned decision. What's best for you isn't necessarily the same method that's best for another couple. You doctor can help you medically evaluate your options. Here is a brief discussion of birth control options.

Birth Control Pills

This method uses synthetic hormones to prevent ovulation and impair fertilization. The pills are generally either a combination of estrogen and progestin or progestin only (the "mini pill"). The estrogen-progestin combination pills, used as directed, are the most effective reversible form of contraception available, but progestin pills are also highly effective. Because progestin-only pills do not affect breastfeeding noticeably, many physicians recommend this method as long as you breastfeed. Although the combination pills may reduce your milk supply slightly and cause slight amounts of hormones to be excreted in breast milk, combination-type oral contraceptives are considered safe to use when breastfeeding.

Your doctor will usually prescribe the pills within two to six weeks after birth. It takes about a week for the pills to become effective, so you should use another method of protection if you have intercourse during this time.

The safety of oral contraceptives for most women is well established. Birth control pills may help reduce the risk of endometrial and ovarian cancer and may help prevent osteoporosis.

If you take birth control pills, you will probably have regular menstrual periods with less flow. You do need to remember to take the pills daily, and you may notice some side effects, including nausea, breast tenderness, headaches and weight gain. A few women have problems from blood clots. Some women (for example, smokers older than 35) should probably not use the combination birth control pills, but often they can use the progestin-only pills successfully. Progestin-only pills should be taken at nearly the same time each day. They may cause irregular menstrual bleeding.

It is important that you and your doctor decide if birth control pills are the right choice for you. Your doctor can then prescribe a pill that is best for you, depending on your history and physical condition. Never use birth control pills that were prescribed for someone else. Fewer than 3 percent of women become pregnant while taking birth control pills.

Contraceptive Implants

These are similar to progestin-only birth control pills, in that they contain hormones that impair fertilization and prevent ovulation. Your doctor can implant these small, flexible, match-sized hormone sticks under the skin of your upper arm. They will last for five years, and there's no need to remember to do anything. Contraceptive implants may have the same side effects as oral contraceptives, except that they also may cause some irregularity in your menstrual cycle or spotting, and they may adversely affect glucose control in women with diabetes. This method is somewhat expensive initially. Fewer than 5 percent of women who use the implants will become pregnant.

Important: Recent reports have surfaced concerning difficulty in removing implants when desired. If you opt for implants, be careful to select a physician well trained and experienced in placing and removing implants.

Birth Control Shots

Similar to contraceptive implants, birth control shots contain progestin. You need to get a birth control shot in the arm or buttocks every two to three months to maintain protection. This method is safe immediately after childbirth and while you are breastfeeding. You may experience irregular monthly periods and spotting, and chances are good you may stop having periods entirely after a while. When you stop getting the shots, return to fertility may be delayed. This method is highly effective in preventing pregnancy. There is a slightly higher rate of pregnancy among women who weigh more than 160 pounds, and as such, your doctor may need to adjust the amount of medication you receive.

Diaphragm With Spermicidal Jelly or Foam

The diaphragm is a dome-shaped rubber cap that fits over the cervix. For effective birth control, it must be used with spermicidal foam or jelly applied around the rim and in the center. Diaphragms come in different sizes, and your doctor will determine which size you need. If you used a diaphragm before becoming pregnant, you should have your doctor check to see if you now need a different size.

Some women do not like the requirement that the diaphragm needs to be inserted less than two hours before intercourse and left in place for six to eight hours after intercourse. Doctors attribute the varying pregnancy rates of women using diaphragms and a spermicide—sometimes as high as 20 percent—to vary-

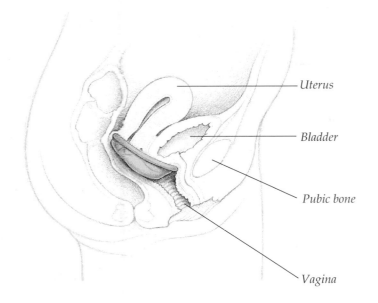

A diaphragm, a flexible disc, fits over the cervix to prevent sperm from entering the uterus.

Uterus

Bladder

Pubic bone

Vagina

ing levels of motivation and correct use. Diaphragms may also provide partial protection from some sexually transmitted diseases.

The cervical cap is similar to the diaphragm, but smaller. It must also be used with spermicidal jelly or cream. Failure rates are comparable to those of the diaphragm.

Male Condom

The condom, a thin rubber sheath worn by a man over his penis, is another barrier form of contraception. Condoms are effective in preventing pregnancy about 90 percent of the time. They are most effective when the woman also uses spermicidal foam or jelly. Condoms are inexpensive and don't require a doctor's prescription.

Condoms made of latex rubber are the only reasonably effective protection against sexually transmitted diseases; other methods may diminish the risk somewhat but not significantly.

Female Condom (Vaginal Pouch)

This new form of the condom, worn by the woman, comes in several forms. Many are made of thicker latex than typical male condoms. All extend to the outside of the vagina, and several have a diaphragm-like end that fits on the cervix. Insertion methods vary. Breakage rate is generally less than half that of male condoms. These devices have been approved only recently by the Food and Drug Administration.

Spermicidal Vaginal Sponges, Jellies, Suppositories, Creams and Foams

These methods rely on a substance that destroys sperm cells before they can fertilize an egg. They do provide a good backup to barrier techniques such as diaphragms or condoms. They are easy to obtain without prescription, but they require planning. Small plastic vaginal sponges contain spermicide and are inserted in the upper part of the vagina. The other spermicides are placed in the vagina near the cervix. Some people consider spermicidal jellies, creams and foams messy. About 20 percent of women who rely solely on these methods become pregnant in a year, although when used consistently and correctly, pregnancy rates tend to be only about half that high.

Intrauterine Device (IUD)

Your doctor inserts this small device into your uterus to prevent pregnancy. This device interferes with successful implantation of the fertilized egg. An IUD is not a good choice if you have ever had a sexually transmitted disease. Users appreciate that they don't have to remember to do anything for birth control. However, IUDs may cause increased cramping with menstruation, are sometimes expelled spontaneously or need to be removed, and they may increase your risk of acquiring sexually transmitted diseases. You should be in a monogamous relationship if you use this method. IUDs are generally a rather expensive option for birth control. About 5 percent of women who use this method will become pregnant in a year.

Rhythm Methods

With these techniques (also called natural family planning), you assess your fertile time and avoid intercourse during that time. They require no medication or devices, but your partner must cooperate, and you may find it difficult to judge your fertile time.

The calendar rhythm method estimates that ovulation occurs about 14 days before onset of a menstrual period. The temperature rhythm method, by which you detect ovulation when your basal body temperature is slightly elevated in the morning, directs users to avoid intercourse from the first day of a period through the third day after the temperature rise. The cervical mucus rhythm method relies on changes in the cervical mucus throughout the menstrual cycle.

Failure rates are as high as 40 percent a year for the various methods, largely due to inaccurate estimation of the time of ovulation.

Surgical Sterilization

Tubal ligation for women or a vasectomy for men is usually a permanent means of preventing pregnancy. Failure rates are less than 1 percent. Tubal ligation can be done any time after your baby is born. It involves cutting or closing off the fallopian tubes to block the sperm from reaching and fertilizing the egg.

If you decide to have a tubal ligation shortly after giving birth, the procedure involves making a small incision below your navel, tying off a small portion of both fallopian tubes and then cutting or sealing them off. When complete, it stops eggs from moving through the fallopian tubes, where they could be fertilized by sperm.

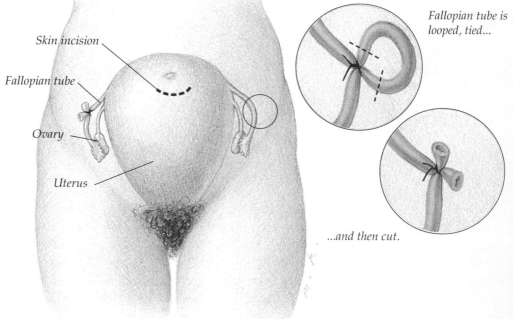

Skin incision

Fallopian tube

Ovary

Uterus

Fallopian tube is looped, tied...

...and then cut.

A vasectomy seals the passage out of the testis, the vas deferens, to prevent release of sperm. You need to be sure that you do not want to have another pregnancy before opting for these methods, because there is no guarantee that the procedure can be reversed. Surgical sterilization is usually rather expensive. Insurance companies often pay for surgical sterilization, but they will not pay for attempts to reverse the procedure.

Postpartum Checkup

Doctors generally want to examine mothers at four to six weeks after birth. The purpose of this exam is to determine if you are physically and emotionally returning to your pre-pregnancy state. You should expect to have a pelvic exam to examine your vagina and cervix and to assess the size and shape of your uterus. Your episiotomy or other incisions can be checked. Your doctor will also likely do a breast exam and check your weight and blood pressure.

This is a good opportunity to ask questions about nursing and discuss birth control. Don't hesitate to bring up other health concerns or how you are feeling emotionally.

The next scheduled medical visit after your postpartum checkup might be in six to 12 months, perhaps for renewal of your prescription for birth control pills or for a Pap smear and breast exam. If you want an earlier appointment, just ask. Remember, if you think you should see a doctor, make arrangements to do so.

Sometimes women who see an obstetrician may be reluctant to ask about non-pregnancy health concerns. Don't worry whether you should call your obstetrician or someone else; it's okay to check with an obstetrician who knows details of your health. Your obstetrician can either handle your concerns or assist you in deciding whom to see.

Celebrate Motherhood

The first year for a new mother is likely to prove more challenging than you thought, and also to become more joyful and energizing than you imagined. At a time when even a break to go to the bathroom can be the ultimate luxury, it's essential to maintain your sense of humor. Be good to yourself; take care of yourself. One mother of teenagers regretfully confesses that she really short-changed herself by not taking more time for herself when her children were small. There never seemed to be time to do that. She'd always figured that she'd have more time when the kids were older. Of course, that time never came. Give yourself some little gifts: a short trip to the store, a fragrant bubble bath, lunch with a friend.

Celebrate motherhood, take delight in the joy of caring for your baby. Build a store of the rich memories of this special time.

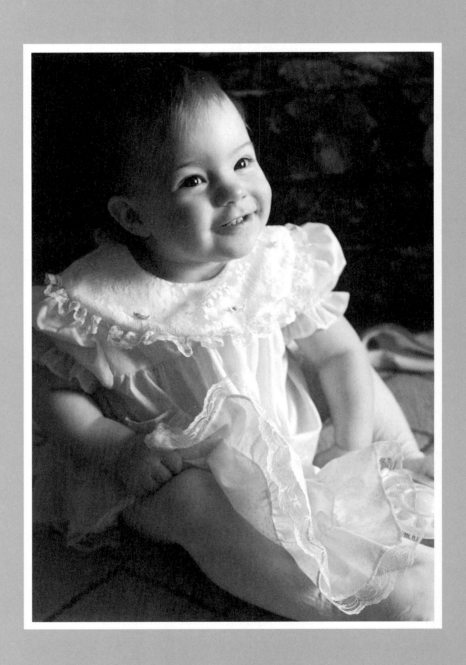

Part Three

Living With and Understanding Your Baby

CHAPTER TWENTY-SIX

Your Newborn Baby

Labor and birth are behind you. Now you can relax. Perhaps you're gently holding a warmly swaddled, completely content daughter or son. Cherish this time.

Look into your baby's eyes. He or she has felt your warmth and movement, heard your voice. Now your baby is seeing you for the first time.

Touch your baby's skin. Caress its smoothness. There's nothing quite as soft and supple as a newborn's skin. Listen to the baby's small, gentle breaths.

Put your finger into your baby's hand. Feel the grasp of the tiny fingers as they hold onto you.

Even though your baby will, in many ways, resemble you and your partner, this is a one-of-a-kind, new human being—a person with a unique appearance, temperament, personality and potential.

The individuality of your baby will shape your relationship with him or her. At the same time, this relationship will shape your baby's development. Your loving responsiveness is the most important foundation for your baby's intellectual, emotional and social development.

Every day, as you watch and listen to your baby, you become more of an expert on this new little person. You will come to trust your infant to express his or her needs, and to trust your common sense and growing expertise. The information in this chapter will help you gain familiarity with the way newborns look and act.

What's a Newborn Baby Like?

Your baby undergoes tremendous change during the birth process. It may take a while to settle into the new world, both physically and emotionally. Your baby will adapt and change rapidly in the first few hours and days after birth. As you well know, the experience of labor and childbirth had its impact on you. Your baby was affected too. For example, by now the puffiness that may have been apparent in your baby's face at birth is diminishing, but you both may still feel exhausted.

From the moment of birth, most parents focus on two features—eyes and hands. The eyes and hands convey what is most human about a newborn baby. Both are essential in the communication and feedback that help establish a strong bond between parents and child.

Eyes

It is normal for a newborn's eyelids to be puffy. The puffiness might be symmetrical or more to one side and will last only a day or two.

Developing in the uterus, infants have no need for vision. But once born, an infant experiences the world as a symphony of shapes and colors. Your baby's eyes can focus on and follow a slowly moving object. Newborns notice various patterns and shapes. Faces especially seem to catch their attention.

Immediately after birth, babies often keep their eyes closed because the room may be too bright. A newborn hasn't learned yet how to squint in bright light. Turn down the lighting in the room and your newborn will be more comfortable opening his or her eyes; now you can enjoy watching your baby look around. Don't be alarmed if your newborn looks cross-eyed at times. This appearance is normal in newborns; as your baby matures, it will likely disappear.

What color are your baby's eyes? You'll probably have to wait at least a few months to know for sure. At birth, most babies have dark bluish brown, blue-black, grayish blue or slate-colored eyes. By the time your baby is 2 to 4 months of age, you can usually distinguish blue from brown eyes, but it may take six to nine months or even a year to know your baby's permanent eye color.

Sometimes babies are born with red spots on the whites of their eyes. They are caused by the breakage of tiny blood vessels during the birth process. The spots are harmless; they will not interfere with your baby's sight and will probably disappear in about 10 days.

Hands

Babies have beautiful hands; premature babies have slender fingers, and full-term newborns have pudgy hands with dimpled knuckles. When sleeping, babies often hold their hands in peculiar poses. This tendency is unique to very young infants and is outgrown within a few months.

Your baby will grasp things with a mitten-like motion for the first six to nine months before learning to pick up small objects with the thumb and index finger.

Fingernails began to grow on your baby's tiny fingers many weeks before birth. Your baby's nails may need to be trimmed shortly after birth to prevent scratches.

Head

At birth, a baby's skull is not one smooth, hard bone, but consists of several sections of relatively soft bone that can withstand the pressures exerted on it during birth. If your baby was born vaginally, the head may be changed in shape (molded) during labor. At birth the head may appear flattened, crooked or elongated. Usually within 24 to 48 hours the head resumes a more rounded, normal appearance. Then, your newborn will look more like the baby you've envisioned.

As you gently stroke your baby's head you may feel two softer spots. One is toward the front of the scalp, the other further back, toward the crown. These spots are called fontanelles, where the skull bones do not yet join.

The fontanelle in front (anterior) is a diamond-shaped soft spot approximately the size of a quarter. Normally, the fontanelle is flat, but it bulges when your baby cries or strains when having a bowel movement. You might feel it pulsate.

For the first six months, as your baby's head grows, this fontanelle will grow slightly larger. Then, the covering over the fontanelle gradually hardens, and by nine to 18 months, it is completely filled in with hard bone.

The fontanelle at the back of the head (posterior) is the size of a dime and closes around six weeks after birth. Often it is barely noticeable at birth.

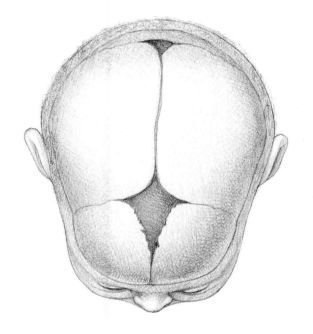

The soft spots on your newborn's head are called fontanelles (see shaded areas). During birth, the fontanelles enable the soft bone plates of your baby's skull to flex, allowing the head to pass unharmed through the birth canal. Before your baby's second birthday the plates will fill with bone and harden.

Hearing

Babies hear well. Your baby will respond to various noises, but especially to the sound of your voice. Loud noises may startle your baby. Quiet music may soothe your baby. An interesting noise, such as your voice, may prompt your baby to stop and listen; however, looking toward the source of sound won't come for several months.

Skin

Many parents expect their newborn's skin to be flawless. More commonly, you'll see some blotchiness, bruising from birth and skin blemishes unique to newborns. For example, most babies have milia, tiny white "pimples," on the nose and chin. It is common to see a red patch, called a salmon patch, over the nape of the neck, between the eyebrows or on the eyelids; these are sometimes called "stork bites" or "angel kisses." They disappear during the first several years.

Sometimes, small white or yellowish bumps surrounded by pink or reddish skin are present at birth or, more typically, show up a few days later. The condition is called erythema toxicum. It causes no discomfort and is not infectious. It requires no treatment and disappears in a few days.

Infantile, or newborn, acne may occur within the first six to eight weeks. In this condition, whiteheads appear on the face, neck, upper chest or back. Again, it disappears without treatment and does not predict future skin problems. (For more information on baby's skin, see page 499.)

Genitals

In boys, the testicles begin developing early in pregnancy, up inside the baby's abdomen. In the later stages of pregnancy they move down into the scrotum, the sac-like structure at the base of the penis. At birth, the scrotum is typically swollen. In most full-term boys, the testicles are in the scrotum. If the baby arrives early (premature birth), one or both testicles may remain higher in the groin or even up inside the abdomen. Often the testicles descend into the scrotum on their own over the next six to 12 months. Erections occur normally in infants, especially before urinating or when they may be slightly chilled, perhaps when having a bath.

In newborn girls, the labia are swollen. In dark-skinned infants, the labia are deeply pigmented at birth. You may notice a small amount of mucous discharge, which is perfectly normal. Don't be surprised if in the first few days you also notice a small bloodstain on your baby daughter's diaper. This is bleeding from her uterus, set in motion by the drop in maternal hormone levels that occurs with birth. It is common, normal and temporary.

Weight

Newborns typically lose several ounces after delivery—up to 10 percent of their birth weight. At birth, their bodies normally contain extra water. During the first few days of life, they lose the water through urination. This water loss typically accounts for the loss of several ounces in weight. By the fourth or fifth day after birth, babies begin to regain some of the lost weight. This weight gain now results from growth rather than water retention.

Temperature Regulation

Babies are born without much insulating tissue—that is, fat. After birth a baby is wet and may lose heat rapidly. That's one reason babies are dried with a towel or blanket and wrapped snugly in a blanket (swaddled) shortly after birth. Sometimes, when a baby is held by the parents immediately after birth, keeping the baby warm can be forgotten in all the excitement. Unless the room is rather warm, the newborn should either be wrapped in a blanket or be snuggled skin-to-skin on mother's chest and covered with a blanket.

Smaller babies sometimes have trouble maintaining body temperature and are kept under a warmer or in an incubator to keep them warm. In a few days they can generally maintain their own temperature. Most heat loss occurs from the baby's head; hats or stocking caps are sometimes used to help babies stabilize their temperatures.

Urination and Bowel Movements

Sometime during the first 12 to 24 hours, your baby will pass urine. It is normal for baby boys to have an erection just before urination. Pay attention to this to avoid getting sprinkled at diaper changing time!

Your baby's first soiled diaper—usually within 48 hours after birth—may present a surprise. During the first few days the stools are thick and sticky—a greenish black substance called meconium. Once the meconium is passed, the stools become greenish yellow. The color, frequency and consistency vary considerably, depending on how your baby is fed. In babies who breastfeed, stools are more frequent, generally soft, watery and golden yellow, resembling mustard with seed-like particles. Some breastfed babies may go several days without a bowel movement, and others stool every time they nurse. Yellow, watery stools in a breastfed baby are not a sign of diarrhea; they are normal. In bottle-fed babies, stools are less frequent, more formed and tan-colored.

Jitteriness

Babies are often jittery or easily startled during the first few days of life, especially when undressed. Usually, this jitteriness subsides when the baby is held or swaddled, or when the baby nurses. Jitteriness generally is a reflection of the normal immaturity of the newborn's nervous system.

Occasionally, jitteriness can be a sign that the baby's blood sugar or calcium level is low. If jitteriness is marked or persists, your doctor may order a blood test to check your baby's blood sugar and calcium levels. In babies born to mothers who take cocaine or other drugs, jitteriness can be a symptom of drug withdrawal.

Umbilical Cord

A newborn's navel (umbilicus) has a short, transparent cord. It may be colored dark blue by an antiseptic solution used by many hospitals to cleanse the umbilical cord. Over the next few days, the cord will dry up and turn black. Within two to three weeks, it will loosen and fall off. Occasionally, this event causes brief, mild bleeding.

When your baby cries, a bulge may appear beneath the navel. This is called an umbilical hernia. An umbilical hernia does not require treatment and will usually disappear on its own, by the time your child is 2 years of age.

Hiccups

Most babies have frequent bouts of hiccups. A hiccup is simply a twitch of the diaphragm, the muscular membrane separating the chest and abdominal cavities. It's unclear why babies have hiccups so frequently. Hiccups commonly occur after a feeding, and particularly after burping. Hiccups are not harmful to a baby but sometimes a baby with hiccups will fuss or cry. Unfortunately, there's no reliable way to stop hiccups.

Sneezing

Most babies have episodes of sneezing. Sneezing is a baby's way of clearing mucus from the nose—especially important because babies breathe primarily through their noses.

Babies also make other odd breathing noises. Their nasal passages are relatively small, creating "nose noise." Sneezing and noisy breathing don't necessarily mean your baby has a cold. If breathing and feeding don't seem difficult, then most likely there is nothing that needs to be done about the noisy breathing. As your baby gets bigger, the "nose noise" usually decreases. If your baby seems to have difficulty feeding because he or she can't breathe easily, call this to the attention of your baby's health care provider.

States of Attention

From the moment of birth, babies are able to notice and respond to their environments. This information is important to know because babies develop in response to their environments—and you are the most immediate and most important part of your baby's world, at least for the first few months.

Babies are born with a social orientation—the inborn ability to distinguish people from objects. Your baby will notice your voice or an interesting sound, such as a rattle. Your baby can focus on a nearby face or follow your movements. Babies have social skills for meeting the family, and you can best make use of them when your baby is alert.

The amount of time a newborn spends in a quiet, alert state is minimal, but it increases rapidly over the first year. You may notice that your baby is most alert and receptive when she or he focuses attention on something interesting. This alert state is the ideal time for playful stimulation of your baby. Your baby's alertness depends on whether your baby is hungry or has just been fed or is tired or rested, and also on how stimulating the surroundings are. Thrusting movements of arms and legs and brief fussy noises or cries are clues that she or he is trying to shut out the stimulation or may be hungry or tired. At first, you will be discovering the limits of your baby's capacity for alertness, but over time, you will be helping to expand this ability.

Reflexes

It takes time for your baby's nervous system to become fully developed. As a result, newborns often appear uncoordinated in their movements, and might even appear a little "jerky" at times. You are likely to see several reflexes, automatic muscle responses, in your new baby. They are normal and a sign that your baby's nervous system is functioning well.

Rooting reflex. The rooting reflex causes newborns to turn their heads toward something that touches their cheeks. This response helps an infant search for food. Stroking your baby's cheek with your finger or nipple will help him or her find the breast.

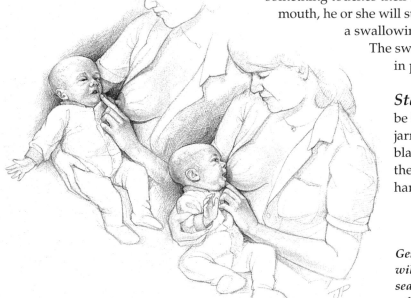

Sucking reflex. The sucking reflex causes newborns to suck when something touches their lips. If you slip a finger into your baby's mouth, he or she will suck on it. The sucking response then causes a swallowing reflex, which is essential for feeding. The swallowing reflex is initially less developed in premature infants.

Startle reflex. The startle (Moro) reflex can be triggered by sudden changes in position, a jarring of the crib, loud noise or jerking of the blanket or clothes. When babies are startled, they suddenly reach out their arms and hands, extend the neck, then bring the arms

Gently stroke your newborn's cheek and she or he will turn in the direction of your finger and begin searching (rooting) for the nipple. The rooting reflex generally stops after four months.

together and may even cry loudly. The reaction is normal, and it even occurs during sleep. This reflex gradually disappears after a few months.

Grasp reflex. The grasp reflex prompts newborns to grasp an object placed in their hands and cling to it briefly. As your baby grasps an extended finger, you may be able to carefully pull your baby into a sitting position. Although infants can't grasp objects with their feet, stroking the bottoms of their feet prompts their toes to turn downward as if trying to grasp.

Events Occurring in the Hospital

Newborns receive care after birth in various settings: the well-baby nursery for healthy newborns, the observation nursery for babies needing closer attention or the newborn intensive care unit, sometimes called the special care nursery, for babies born prematurely or with serious medical conditions.

The traditional well-baby nursery is usually located near the rooms where new mothers stay. It typically has big windows, so that your visitors can see your new baby. Your baby will be brought to you regularly for feedings.

Many hospitals now allow your baby to stay in your room, either around the clock or during the daytime, so that you can care for and feed your baby as you wish. This arrangement is called rooming-in. While the baby is with you in the room, visitors are usually limited to the immediate family. During visiting hours, when more family members or friends are around, babies are taken to the nursery. Rooming-in can help you build confidence in caring for your baby.

Increasingly, however, as hospital stays for childbirth are routinely shortened to one or two days, the location in which you and your baby stay is undergoing change too. Depending on your hospital's facilities, you may experience labor, give birth and stay with your baby in one room. With this arrangement, you are usually given the option of having your baby stay with you through the night or sending your baby to the well-baby nursery. Nurses help new moms get acquainted with their babies. In this arrangement, you can learn about your baby's needs and how to meet them while expert help is available. Some hospitals provide parent-education programs in these rooms around-the-clock on closed-circuit television. Others have VCRs available for parent education tapes.

Circumcision

If you choose to have your son circumcised and the procedure is to be done in a hospital, it is usually done early in the morning. The morning feeding is delayed until after the procedure, which usually takes less than 15 minutes.

Typically, the arms and legs are restrained on a tray designed just for this purpose. Since most newborns prefer to be snuggled in blankets, many babies cry when they are undressed. The penis and surrounding area are cleansed, and an anesthetic may be injected into the base of the penis. The injection stings but blocks further pain.

To remove the foreskin, doctors use a clamp designed for newborn circumcision or a specially designed plastic ring.

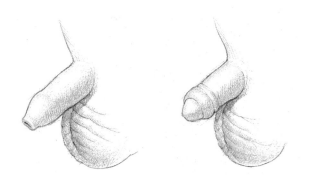

Before circumcision (left), the foreskin of the penis extends over the end of the penis (glans). After the brief operation, the glans is exposed (right).

After removal of the foreskin, the end of the penis (glans) appears red and sore. Usually an ointment, such as petroleum jelly, is applied. A strip of gauze is loosely wrapped around the glans to keep it from sticking to the diaper. If the plastic ring is used, it will remain on the end of the penis until the edge of the circumcision has healed, usually within a week. A small amount of bleeding is common on the first day or two. It's okay to wash the penis as it is healing. For a few days, apply petroleum jelly to prevent the penis from sticking to the diaper. (For information on the pros and cons of circumcision, see page 184.)

Screening Tests

Sometime within the first few days after birth, a small amount of blood is taken, often from the baby's heel, and sent to the state health department. There it will be analyzed to detect the presence of rare but very important medical conditions such as congenital hypothyroidism (see page 382), galactosemia (see page 382), phenylketonuria (see page 382), and sickle cell anemia (see page 387). These screening tests differ slightly from state to state. Early diagnosis and treatment of these conditions are extremely important. The results of the tests are sent to your baby's health care providers within a week or two.

Don't be alarmed if your baby needs to have the screening test repeated. To ensure that every newborn with one of these conditions is identified, even borderline results must be rechecked. Sometimes this rechecking is necessary to verify the accuracy of the lab testing. Retesting is especially common for premature babies. Your health care providers are very familiar with newborn screening and will be able to help answer any questions that arise about your baby.

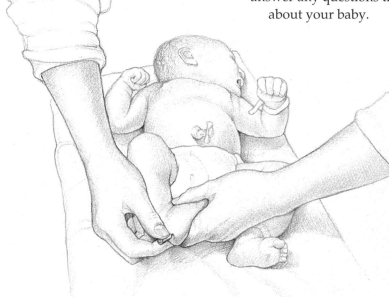

State laws require screening for certain rare medical conditions when your baby is a few days old. The tests involve sending a blood sample, usually obtained from your baby's heel, to a lab for analysis.

Hepatitis B Vaccination

Hepatitis B is a viral infection that affects the liver. It can cause illnesses such as cirrhosis, liver failure or the development of liver tumors. Hepatitis can be spread to a child during pregnancy and birth. Adults can contract hepatitis through sexual contact, shared needles or exposure to the blood of someone with hepatitis.

Babies should receive the hepatitis B vaccine to protect them from any possible contact with this virus. Your baby may be given this vaccine in the hospital, shortly after birth. Two additional hepatitis B vaccinations will be given in your baby's first year.

Jaundice

More than half of all newborn babies have jaundice, a yellowish discoloration of the skin and eyes, in the first few days of life. It is most apparent on the fourth or fifth day after birth and may last up to several weeks. Jaundice reflects the relative immaturity of the newborn's systems and is not a cause for alarm. It does not cause discomfort for your baby. Typically it disappears on its own, causing no lasting harm.

Babies are born with a generous supply of hemoglobin, the oxygen-carrying portion of blood cells. This supply decreases as red blood cells are broken down and recycled in the body. When the red blood cells break down, bilirubin is formed. This imparts a yellowish color to eyes and skin. Bilirubin is transported to the liver, where it is processed, sent to the intestine and eliminated in bowel movements.

Several conditions can make jaundice, or an elevated level of bilirubin, more likely to occur:

- A baby who has bruises as a result of birth may have a higher level of bilirubin because of the breakdown of more red blood cells.
- Sometimes when the mother has a different blood type than the baby, the baby may receive maternal antibodies that break down red blood cells faster. If so, a higher level of bilirubin may result.
- In premature babies the liver may not be mature enough to process the bilirubin as rapidly as in a full-term infant.
- Breast milk may increase the amount of bilirubin reabsorbed from the intestine, and thus the blood will have a higher level of bilirubin.

Jaundice in the newborn is usually not a major problem but can sometimes require a longer stay in the hospital. Blood tests can measure the level of bilirubin. If the level is elevated, treatment can lower it. Methods of treatment include:

- Feeding the baby more frequently, so that the baby takes in more fluid and has more bowel movements, which increase the amount of bilirubin passed with the stool
- Placing the baby under a bilirubin light, a special light that acts through the skin to change the bilirubin into a form that can be eliminated by the kidneys
- Rarely, if the bilirubin level becomes extremely high and approaches a level that might be harmful to the baby, giving the baby an "exchange" blood transfusion to reduce the level of bilirubin

The birth certificate

By law, the birth of every baby must be documented. However, state laws vary in regard to some of the details of the birth certificate. You'll be asked to fill out a birth certificate information form shortly after your baby's birth.

The birth certificate provides legal proof of age, parentage and citizenship, and it may be needed later for obtaining a driver's license, a Social Security number or a passport or for other purposes. Birth certificates are also used extensively by health researchers because they contain carefully selected questions about the health of the mother and baby and about the pregnancy. The medical information is maintained in a private file; it is not part of the public legal record.

In the hospital, parents are asked to provide the personal information that goes on the birth certificate—your ages, birthplaces and education; your marital status; and your baby's name. Other information will be added by your baby's doctor or a certified nurse-midwife, who must sign the birth certificate before it is filed by the hospital with the clerk of court, county recorder or auditor of your county.

The birth certificate must be filled out and filed within five days of your baby's birth, perhaps before you've decided on a name. You will be responsible for adding a name, or making any amendment or alteration. In choosing the name to put on your baby's birth certificate, remember that it is a legal record of your child's identity.

Many hospitals send parents home with souvenir birth certificates. These documents can't be used for legal purposes. You can get an official copy of your baby's birth certificate by writing to the vital records section of your state health department or the local filing agency of the county of birth. There is a fee for this record. If you call first you will probably be given complete instructions about how to obtain what you need.

Keep an official copy of your child's birth certificate in a secure place. Double-check the information for accuracy. Most information on the birth certificate can be amended. However, it takes legal action to change your child's last name.

Sometime before his or her first birthday, you'll need to obtain a Social Security number for your child. The easiest way is to check the box on the birth certificate. A number will be automatically assigned, and you will be notified within three or four months. If you do not check the box on the birth certificate, you'll be responsible for getting the application from the Social Security office and filling it out yourself.

Going Home

For the trip home from the hospital, most babies are dressed in a T-shirt and sleeper and wrapped in a baby blanket. A hat or bonnet is not necessary, but certainly is cute for pictures. In cold weather, a hat, snowsuit and extra blanket may be needed. There's a common tendency to dress babies too warmly. Ask your nurse if you're uncertain.

The most important piece of baby gear you'll need for the trip home is a car seat. Under most circumstances, what place could be more secure for a new baby than in a parent's arms? But in a moving vehicle, that is a hazardous place indeed. In the event of a crash, your body could crush your baby against the dashboard and windshield. Even if you are wearing a seatbelt, your baby would be torn from your arms by the force of a collision.

Because of this danger, car seats are required by law in every state. The proper use of car seats is one of the best ways parents can protect their children—and drivers can pay attention to the road. Start now with the rule that the car doesn't move until your baby is secured in a car seat.

There are two types of seats for babies. The first decision you'll make is whether to buy a seat designed specifically for infants (it will have to be replaced when your baby is older) or to buy a convertible seat that accommodates infants and older children. Your choice may depend on the type of vehicle you drive and on regulations where you live. Check on the regulations with your local hospital, discuss them in prenatal education classes or ask the baby's health care provider. Remember that many hospitals have rental programs for infant car seats.

Infant-only car seats fit newborns best and accommodate babies from birth to approximately 20 pounds. They are small and portable, holding the baby in a gently reclining position. These seats are installed so that the baby always faces the back of the vehicle. Such a seat allows you to carry your baby to and from your car while leaving him or her undisturbed in the seat.

The seat belts of your vehicle are used to anchor the car seat in place. Follow the car seat manufacturer's installation instructions carefully. Also check the owner's manual for your car for any special

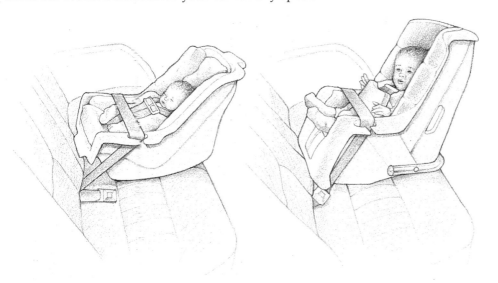

Securing your baby in an approved car seat is one of the most important safety precautions you can take. The infant-only seat (left) is small and portable. It faces the rear of the car. You can use this type until your baby weighs about 20 pounds. Or, you can choose a convertible safety seat (right). Your baby also faces backward in this type of seat until he or she weighs about 20 pounds. When your child weighs between 20 and 40 pounds, you can use the same seat, facing it forward in the car.

instructions about installing car seats in a car with air bags or shoulder restraints. The center of the back seat is the safest place for a car seat. With more than one adult in the car, one of you can sit next to the baby in the back seat. If you're driving alone with the baby, you may decide to put the car seat in the front seat. Make sure to follow instructions carefully for fastening the car seat in the front seat.

A harness on the car seat itself is strapped snugly between your baby's legs and over the torso. You'll need to dress your baby in clothes that leave the legs free so that harness straps can go between them. For your newborn, you might also need to tuck in rolled-up baby blankets on each side to support your baby's head and shoulders.

The alternative to an infant-only seat is a convertible safety seat. This type of seat, which can hold a child who weighs up to 40 pounds, is used in a rear-facing position until the baby weighs about 20 pounds, when the seat is turned to face forward. Such seats are bulky and less portable than infant-only seats. They also must be anchored by your vehicle's seat belts. A harness on the safety seat holds the child securely in place.

If your baby has a medical condition that prevents him or her from comfortably sitting up, your doctor may recommend that your baby be secured lying flat while riding in a car, at least for the first few months. In that case, you will need to invest in an infant car-safety bed. You can purchase car beds that convert into infant seats.

The bills for baby supplies can add up, and you may consider borrowing a seat that another child has outgrown. Besides making sure all parts are in working order and that fasteners operate easily enough to encourage regular use, check the date of manufacture. Seats manufactured before 1981 may not meet current federal safety standards.

A special baby?

Special safety restraints are available for babies born with exceptional needs. For information, write James Whitcomb Riley Hospital for Children, Automotive Safety for Children Program, 702 Barnhill Drive, #1601, Indianapolis, Indiana 46202.

CHAPTER TWENTY-SEVEN

The Basics of Baby Care

Visualize your baby's life before birth, nestled in your uterus—the ultimate in controlled environments. From the beginning, he or she has been constantly rocked and securely held. Before birth, your baby never had to feel the discomfort of cold, hunger or indigestion.

Even the gentlest of births can be a jolt for the typical newborn. No wonder that babies often quiver and startle so easily at first, or that bright lights and loud noises take some getting used to. It's not surprising that being unwrapped or put down is frightening. As you might expect, even learning to eat often requires extra effort, with mealtime frequently followed by hiccuping, spitting up and a bout of gas.

Of course, you can't protect your child from all the struggles that go into adjusting to life outside the uterus. But knowing about your baby from his or her perspective might help you appreciate all the changes this new person will experience. Usually, by the time your baby is approaching a week or two of age, the initial shock of birth, hospital activities, learning to eat and moving home is past. You're beginning to notice individual behavior patterns. And as with people in general, the range of "normal" infant behavior is broad.

Wouldn't it be wonderful if newborns could talk? You could avoid the guessing game you often play in the beginning—wondering if your baby is hungry, frightened, lonely, in pain or tired. As you become better acquainted with your baby, your guesses will become more educated.

Meanwhile, every new parent naturally looks for clues to the baby's needs. Body movement and posture, facial gestures, sucking motions and "states"— from drowsiness or asleep to alert, squirming or crying—all communicate your baby's basic needs for physical comfort, food, rest and feeling loved. These clues will help direct what you do for your baby: whether you should continue what you've been doing, try something different or simply step back and wait.

In this chapter we'll discuss many aspects of your baby's basic needs. And in Chapter 28 you'll read more about getting started with feeding your baby.

Supplies and Equipment

Friends and relatives will suggest that different items are "musts" for you to have on hand for the newest member of your family. Of course, family budgets vary greatly, as do personal circumstances and preferences. Families with limited storage space, for example, may want fewer items to fold, sort and store.

Make a list of items you need. Your list will probably not be identical to that of other parents, but it may be helpful to ask experienced parents what supplies and equipment were most useful to them.

In addition to buying new items, you may also want to explore garage sales or visit outlets for used baby clothes and equipment. A word of caution is necessary, however, about used cribs and car seats. In recent years, safety experts have made major strides in product design and regulations for manufacturing these items, so be aware that cribs and car seats manufactured a few years ago may not meet current safety requirements. (See page 447 for more details on car seats and page 453 for what safety features to look for in a crib.)

Suggestions for a layette list

Clothing

When you're buying clothes for your newborn, choose a three-month size or larger so your baby doesn't immediately outgrow them. Cotton fabric tends to retain odors less than other fabrics and is more comfortable for your baby's sensitive skin. Select sleepwear that is treated with flame-retardant chemicals, and make sure everything you buy is washable. Look for snaps or simple closures to make dressing easier, and avoid buttons, which are easily swallowed. Items to include:

- Four to six undershirts
- Four to six gowns or kimonos
- Four to six receiving blankets (knit blankets work well for swaddling)
- Three to six stretch coveralls (look for those with snaps on both legs for easy dressing and undressing)
- Cardigan sweater, jacket and bunting or snowsuit (depending on your climate)
- Dress-up outfit
- Hat, for warmth in cool weather and sun protection (depending on your climate and time of year)
- Booties and socks

Bath and toiletry articles
- Three or four baby towels (with hoods)
- Three or four washcloths
- Baby soap (mild, with no perfumes)
- Baby shampoo
- Brush and comb
- Bathing tub
- Baby nail clippers or scissors
- Rubbing alcohol (for care of umbilical cord)

Bedding
- Waterproof mattress
- Mattress pad
- Waterproof pad
- Four to six crib sheets
- Two crib blankets
- Crib bumpers

Diapers
- 80 to 100 disposable diapers per week
- 80 to 100 cloth diapers per week from a diaper service
- Three to six dozen 100 percent cotton diapers, if you plan to buy cloth diapers. The number you'll need is determined by how often you wash diapers. With three dozen, for example, you'll probably need to wash them every other day
- Diaper pins
- Diaper pail and deodorizer
- Diaper liners (can be used inside cloth or disposable diapers)
- Six diaper covers or plastic pants
- Diaper rash ointment
- Premoistened towelettes, alcohol- and fragrance-free

For outings
- Carriage or stroller
- Diaper bag
- Front carrier or backpack (also handy around the house)
- Car safety seat (required by law; check with your hospital for rental or purchase options)

Room furnishings
- Crib, optional cradle or bassinet for early weeks
- Changing table
- Chest of drawers
- Reclining infant seat
- Lamp
- Rocking chair
- Mobiles, cradle gym, rattles, crib mirror
- Swing
- Nursery intercom, for listening to baby from other parts of your home
- Tape player and "white noise" tapes (for example, the sounds of ocean waves)

Later additions
- High chair
- Playpen
- Open toy box or shelves

Diapers

You have several options when it comes to diapering your baby. You may choose to buy and wash cotton diapers. Some of the newer types have waterproof nylon shells with convenient Velcro-type closures. Or you may prefer to use cotton diapers provided by a diaper service. Perhaps you'll select disposable diapers or end up using a combination of types.

If you use disposable diapers, you'll find it helpful to have a dozen cloth diapers on hand to use if you run out of disposables or to drape over your shoulder or put on your lap while burping your baby. Some parents even introduce cloth diapers as their baby's "security blanket" instead of trying to keep track of a favorite blanket or stuffed animal.

Your specific needs and lifestyle will influence your choice of diapers. Factors to consider are discussed below.

Cost and time. Buying and washing cotton diapers yourself may be your least expensive option, but be sure to factor in the value of your time, the cost of water and detergent and wear and tear on your washer and dryer.

Using a diaper service or disposable diapers clearly will save you time and effort. It may be less expensive to use a diaper service than to buy disposable diapers, especially when you consider the price of the larger, more expensive disposable diapers your baby will need as he or she grows. If you have two or more children in diapers, a diaper service will probably be your most economical choice.

Environment. Disposable diapers consume about 2 percent of our landfill space. Each year, about 16 billion diapers are used, or 3.2 million tons of solid waste. But there is also continued controversy about whether the water, energy and other resources used to make, wash and dry cloth diapers make them a wise choice environmentally.

It's still unclear whether biodegradable diapers decompose any faster in landfills than regular disposables. It's also unclear whether there is a risk of infectious disease caused by diapers disposed of in landfills.

Diaper rash. Regardless of the type of diaper you use, it's important to change diapers frequently. You can reduce the frequency and severity of diaper rash by changing your baby's diaper and cleaning the skin well at least eight times a day. But don't wake your baby just to change a wet diaper.

Rules of child care centers. If your baby will be cared for outside your home, check to see if there are rules regarding the type of diapers used. Many child care centers do not allow cloth diapers because they are less convenient than disposables.

A Place to Sleep

In choosing a safe place for your baby to sleep, you have several options. In many non-Western cultures, it's common for infants to sleep with their parents. American practices range from welcoming the child into the "family bed" to providing a separate room and baby crib, but many families opt for something in between. Your choice will depend on personal preference and the needs of you and your baby.

Some breastfeeding mothers prefer to nurse while lying in their own beds. After feeding, they may choose to place their infants in a nearby bassinet, cradle or crib, or the baby may remain in mother's bed and nurse on demand throughout the night.

Regardless of your decision on sleeping arrangements, carefully consider your baby's safety. Prevent a harmful fall from the bed to the floor by staying one step ahead of your baby's considerable, and sometimes surprising, ability to roll and move about.

An important safety consideration in buying a cradle or bassinet is to check the base to be sure it will not tip easily or separate from the stand. And be sure to stop using it when your child exceeds the weight limit specified by the manufacturer. Before you invest in one of these options, however, be aware that babies outgrow them quickly, and in three to four months you'll need a safe, standard-sized crib for your baby.

Your child should be able to use a crib from birth until nearly 3 years of age. Whether you opt for a new or used crib, and additionally if there is a crib at your baby's child care facility, baby-sitter's or grandparent's home, be sure to look for the following safety features. These recommendations are based on studies of documented crib injuries.

- Look for side slats that are less than 2⅜ inches apart.

- Avoid cribs with additional openings (such as decorative cutouts).

- Make sure corner posts are less than ⅝ inch above the rails; cut down any that are higher (except for posts on a high canopy).

- With the mattress in the crib, the top edge of the raised crib sides should be at least 20 inches above the mattress surface. The lowered crib side should be at least 9 inches above the mattress. Boost sides, if necessary, with safety extenders (available at baby supply stores).

- Drop sides should be operated with a locking, hand-operated latch, secure from accidental release.

- Make sure the mattress fits snugly; you shouldn't be able to get more than two fingers between the mattress and the crib side.

- If you use bumper pads, place them around the entire crib and tie them into place in at least six places (trimming off excess length of ties after tying). Remove bumper pads when your baby learns to pull to a standing position.

- Never use any type of thin plastic as a mattress cover.

- Assume that any crib made before 1974 has lead-based paint (or check it with a commercially available lead testing product). Strip off lead-based paint carefully to avoid exposing yourself to lead. Make sure the surface is splinter-free, and repaint with high-quality, lead-free household enamel. Do not use old paint. Place plastic strips (available at most children's furniture stores) over the top of the side rails.

- Be sure that hardware fits properly and that all joints are tight.

- Never place the crib near a hanging window blind or drapery cords. In fact, it's a good idea to avoid placing a crib next to a window.

- If you choose a playpen or crib with mesh sides, keep all sides raised at all times.

Remove hanging crib toys and mobiles when your baby first begins to push up on hands and knees because he or she will soon be able to stand and reach for them. As your baby grows, adjust the crib accordingly, lowering the crib mattress before your baby can sit unassisted, so that it's at its lowest position before your baby pulls up to stand.

Changing Table

Some parents prefer a specially designed changing table, complete with storage for diapers and accessories. Others use an inexpensive dresser-top variation or place a pad on a table or countertop. Positioning the changing table near a wall reduces the chance for a fall. To completely eliminate falls you can even change your baby on the floor, taking care to cover the floor with a blanket, towel or changing pad.

Some parents prefer to change diapers near a toilet or in the baby's sleeping area. In any case, never leave your baby unattended, even if the changing area has a protective edge. Always keep one hand on your baby while reaching for diapering supplies. Before you start to change the baby, have all the necessary items within reach. Remember, turning to fetch a forgotten item or answer the phone, even for a moment, can result in a serious fall.

Laundering

Your newborn's skin is quite sensitive, and rashes are common. Rashes come from various sources and are not limited to the diaper area. Because the finishes on new garments and some detergents can be irritating to baby's tender skin, it's important to wash new clothes in a mild detergent before your baby wears them, taking care to rinse them well.

Washing cotton diapers. Right after you change your baby's cloth diaper, use a toilet to flush away solid stool. Keep used diapers in a diaper pail half-filled with water, to which you've added 1 teaspoon of bleach or ½ cup of vinegar to each 5 gallons of water.

Wash diapers separate from other clothing. First, select the spin cycle to rid diapers of presoak water. Then, wash them in hot water, using a mild detergent and 1 cup of bleach.

If the diapers seem to be irritating your baby's skin, run them through the rinse cycle twice to remove any remaining residue of detergent or bleach. Adding ½ cup of vinegar to the final rinse will help too. Then, line dry or use a dryer, as usual.

Safety Precautions

In the United States, babies are more likely to be hurt, become handicapped or die from accidents than from illness. Many parents are unaware of this sobering fact. You can prevent many accidents simply by knowing what your baby is able to do at each stage of development and making sure that the surroundings are safe.

Between birth and 4 months of age, babies eat, sleep, cry, play, smile and also wiggle a lot. They can easily roll off a flat surface and need to be protected at all times. You can decrease your baby's risk of accidental injury by taking simple precautions.

Bathing

Check the temperature of the bath water with your own hand before bathing your baby. Setting the thermostat on your water heater to below 120 degrees Fahrenheit can help prevent scalding. Always hold your baby with at least one hand during the bath, and if you are interrupted, take your baby with you. Never leave your baby alone in the bath!

When your baby is in the crib, be sure to keep the sides up. Never turn your back on your baby if he or she is on a table, bed or chair. If you're interrupted while you're with the baby, put your baby in a secure place, such as the crib, tucked under your arm or even safely on the floor. Do not leave a baby unattended in an infant seat that's placed on a table or countertop, because even very young infants have been able to flip out of them. Be aware, too, that infant seats are not stable on beds or other soft surfaces.

Falls

Place screens around hot radiators, furnaces, stoves or portable heaters. Don't smoke around your baby, and ask others who care for your baby to follow similar precautions. Drinking hot beverages while holding your baby or leaving a hot drink on a place mat or near the table edge can lead to a spill and a burn. Take special precautions if you heat baby food or formula in a microwave oven because the uneven heating can burn your baby's mouth. Most babies will take their food or formula unheated or slightly warmed. It's best to warm food and formula in hot water, making sure to test it on your wrist or taste it yourself before feeding your baby.

Burns

To prevent suffocation and choking, avoid using pillows in places where your baby sleeps and plays. Be sure to keep pins, buttons, coins, plants and plastic bags out of reach. Select crib and playpen toys that are too large to swallow, too tough to break and have no sharp edges or small parts.

Choking Hazards

When traveling in a car or other vehicle, always place your baby in an approved car safety seat in the position recommended by the seat manufacturer. Your baby is safest in the middle of the back seat of the car. Never allow someone to hold your baby in a moving vehicle—even if the person is buckled up. Your child can be easily thrown forward with a sudden stop.

Motor Vehicles

Never leave your baby alone with young children. Keep the phone numbers of your health care provider, rescue squad and poison control center near your phone, along with your address and directions to your home.

Supervision

Teach older children when and how to call the emergency 911 number. To avoid confusion, be sure to teach the number as "nine-one-one" instead of "nine-eleven." Install smoke detectors, and change batteries regularly. It may help to use a significant yearly date, such as your birthday, as a reminder to change them.

Household

Don't leave your baby unattended and within reach of pets. They could hurt or frighten a baby without intending to. Your baby may represent new and unwanted competition for your attention, and your pet may need time to adjust to the new arrival. Some parents feel more secure restraining pets on a leash or placing them in another room with the door closed. If you have questions or concerns about pets in your home, ask your health care provider for recommendations.

Pets

Miscellaneous   Never place a loop of ribbon or cord around your baby's neck to hold a pacifier or for any other reason. Use only pacifiers with a large ring attached and appropriate to baby's size. Do not put necklaces, rings, earrings or bracelets on babies. When your baby is unsupervised or sleeping, take all toys and small objects out of the crib.

As your baby grows, he or she will become more mobile and will do more exploring. Adapt your home environment to those changing safety needs.

Getting to Know Your Baby

By the end of your baby's first week home, you may start to notice specific behavior trends. Dr. T. Berry Brazelton, a well-known Harvard pediatrician who has written extensively about child development, identifies three types of infants: quiet, average and active. Although not all babies fall neatly into one of these three categories, a general description of the categories can help you understand your baby compared with other infants of the same age.

You may find that one behavior type more than another seems to apply to your baby. But keep in mind that one type is not better or worse than another, nor is it a permanent label for your child. The categories are simply descriptions of different activity levels in infants to help you relate to your baby and his or her needs and to show you the wide range of what's considered normal behavior.

Quiet   Quiet babies will often sleep at least 18 of 24 hours, and they fuss for less than one hour during the same period. They may seem uninterested in their surroundings initially, and they are not very sensitive to environmental stimuli or disturbances.

Quiet babies may communicate a need only by gentle squirming or quietly sucking their fists or fingers. Sometimes these babies need help moving to a more alert state once they're awake, and they may need encouragement in eating and socializing.

Average   Average newborns often sleep at least 15 of 24 hours, and they fuss for two or three hours throughout the day. They are moderately attentive to their surroundings and to environmental disturbances. These babies often are able, through sucking, looking, listening or changing body position, to calm themselves when mildly disturbed by a noise, by sudden movement nearby or by being transferred to a crib.

An average baby may appreciate some shielding from external disturbances, particularly when the day's routine has been disrupted or the baby is extremely tired.

Active   Active babies may sleep only 12 of 24 hours, and fussy spells may total from four to six hours a day. They are usually highly aware of their surroundings and are quite social, but they can also be highly sensitive to an environment that is too busy or noisy. Although active babies eat and grow well, they may be bothered by indigestion. You'll find that a quietly interesting and predictable environment is best for an active baby. Active babies need a lot of cuddling and reassurance at first, but they will gradually learn to relax and sleep more by about 3 months of age.

The intensity of an active infant could wear down even a Supermom. If you have an active baby, taking regular breaks is a must. A baby who is eating, growing and developing normally and has no signs of illness but who has extended fussy periods beginning at about 2 or 3 weeks of age and ending after about 3 months is often called "colicky." Neither specialists nor parents fully understand what causes or cures colic. (For more information about colic, see page 541.)

Regardless of behavior type, one thing is true of all children: As much as we try to figure them out, they are still individuals and often elude our analysis. So, don't be surprised if just when you think you have your child figured out, he or she throws you for a loop. It's just one of the challenges of parenthood.

Some of the ways that behavior type influences how your baby may respond to given situations are discussed below.

Responses to Disturbances

To find out how your baby responds to environmental disturbances, wait until your baby is asleep, then gently pick him or her up, lay the baby on his or her back covered loosely with a blanket, and slowly unwrap. Then observe what this tiny person does.

Quiet babies will typically squirm a bit and then fall back to sleep after a short while. Average babies will often squirm and fret a bit more, perhaps for several minutes, but will eventually return to sleep with minimal assistance. An active baby, however, may become distraught and find it impossible to fall back to sleep without being picked up, swaddled and rocked.

Another way to observe your baby's reaction is to gently pick him or her up, tummy-down on your forearm. Keep your body away from the baby's, holding the baby facedown. Hold your baby that way for a few moments and observe his or her reaction.

Quiet babies might have both arms and legs relaxed and hanging like a rag doll. An average baby may tuck in the arms and legs, startle and become a little fretful, but an active baby might actively wiggle arms and legs, rigidly arch the back and cry.

Cuddling

Is your baby a cuddler? Babies differ greatly in how they like to be held. How does your baby respond when held close? Does he or she seem to enjoy it? Do you sense resistance? Does your baby seem to want to stand up, facing outward, or prefer a tummy-down position instead of being held chest to chest? Not all babies are cuddlers.

Settling Down

How does your baby settle down after a minor disruption? Does your baby seem to be able to calm down without your help? In other words, does she or he have the ability to self-console? Do you find it necessary to settle your baby with rocking, cuddling or a pacifier? If you provide only the minimal necessary assistance in helping your baby settle, she or he will increasingly develop the ability to self-console.

Swaddling

Many babies settle down and drift off to sleep better in the first months if they are snugly wrapped in a blanket.

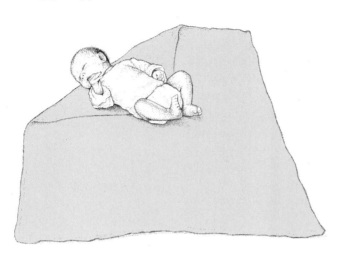

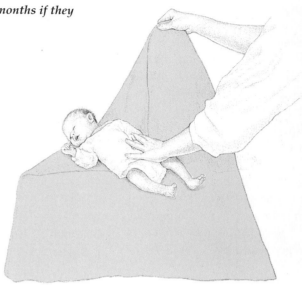

Step 1. Fold down one corner of a soft blanket and place your baby's head above the fold.

Step 2. Bring one corner of the blanket up and pull it taut. Bring the blanket across your baby's body with one arm tucked inside. Tuck the corner under your baby's bottom snugly.

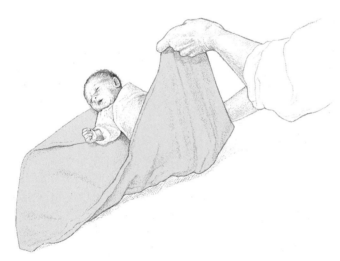

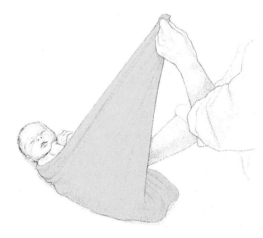

Step 3. Fold the bottom point up, leaving room for your baby's legs to move freely.

Step 4. Then bring up and pull the other corner taut and tuck it under your baby. Leave one hand and arm free.

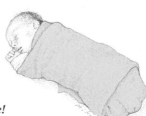

Step 5. Aah...a cozy bundle!

Sometimes your help may simply mean directing a flailing finger to your baby's mouth, and at other times it may mean wrapping your baby more snugly in a blanket (swaddling), massaging, patting, talking in a reassuring voice, rocking, cuddling or offering a pacifier. Quiet babies tend to require less help settling than active babies.

When you allow your baby to settle alone, helping only as needed, you're actually encouraging his or her efforts to self-console more than the parent who intervenes in every squirmy or fussy episode. Sometimes, of course, you will want to simply sit and rock your baby. This attention won't spoil a baby and is good for you also. And it will help establish the important priority of taking time for yourself and your baby. Remember, you have this opportunity for only a short while.

Settling down to sleep

Some babies settle down to sleep quickly. Others do not. Either way, there are steps you can take to encourage your drowsy, well-fed, comfortable baby to relax for sleep at bedtime.

Place your baby on his or her side or back in the crib, then expect some squirming and fussiness. If your baby doesn't settle independently within about 10 minutes:

- Present something interesting for your baby to look at, such as an unbreakable mirror.
- Introduce monotonous, continuous "white noise" such as a fan or a recording of ocean waves.
- Wrap your baby snugly in a blanket.
- Help your baby put a finger into his or her mouth.
- Pat or massage your baby while speaking softly or humming.
- Offer a pacifier.
- Pick up and rock or cuddle your baby.

Watching and Listening

Early on, your newborn will enjoy looking at you and listening to your voice. When your baby is comfortable and alert, your face and voice often can hold his or her attention longer than other surrounding sights and sounds. A newborn can best see objects or faces eight to 10 inches away.

Try holding your baby upright, about 8 inches from you. Talk to her or him, moving your face slowly from side to side. At first the baby's attention span will be short. Repeat your baby's name over and over. In time, your baby will turn toward your voice and learn to follow your face as it moves.

Elimination

A 4-year-old big sister, getting to know her new baby brother, packed a lot of wisdom in her comment that, "All Jason does is cry, eat, wet his pants and sleep!" So, it's no wonder that we spend some time on these "highlights" of your baby's life.

Babies vary a lot in their elimination habits, the primary factors being what your baby eats and how often he or she eats. Most babies urinate nearly every hour until they are 2 to 3 months old and every two to three hours for the rest of their first year. Notify your health care provider if you notice any of the following: fewer than three wet diapers in a 24-hour period, urinating more frequently than every half hour, changing color of urine, bloody urine or strained or painful urination.

The frequency of bowel movements varies widely. (See page 440 for a description of bowel movements.) Your baby may have as many as four to 10 a day, or as few as one every three to four days. After the first month, the number of bowel movements is usually less than three or four times a day, or even as seldom as once a week.

Babies may turn red in the face and cry during a bowel movement—or they may seem totally unaware of one. This whole range is normal. As long as the bowel movements are soft or runny, your baby is not constipated. If stools become hard, dry and difficult to pass, no matter how frequent, your baby may be constipated. Breastfed babies seldom have problems with constipation.

Babies with diarrhea have frequent, unusually loose or watery bowel movements that can come on suddenly. Dehydration, or the loss of essential body fluids, is the major concern if a baby has diarrhea.

Notify your health care provider if your baby has frequent large, watery bowel movements, if stools are watery and smelly, if stools are white (without color) or if you notice fresh blood on the diaper. He or she will also want to know if your baby is vomiting and not eating or if you have any other concerns about your baby's elimination habits.

Sleep

One major factor that will determine how readily your family adjusts to its newest member is your baby's sleep patterns. Sleep patterns change frequently during the first year, and although you have no control over how much your baby sleeps, there are things you can do to influence when sleep occurs.

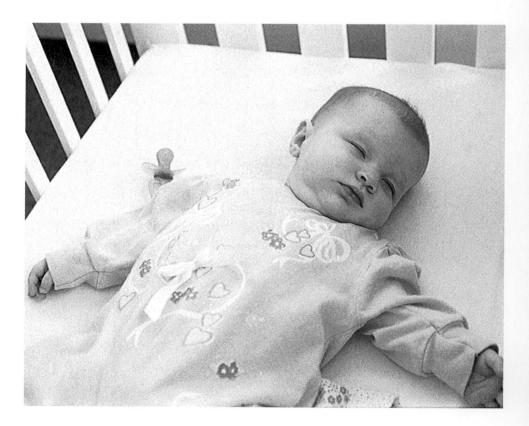

In the first few weeks, most babies spend at least half of their time sleeping. Place your baby on his or her back or side for sleeping, unless your health care provider recommends otherwise.

Typical Sleep Patterns

In the first few weeks of life, most babies sleep a great deal—12 to 20 hours during a 24-hour period, on average. As a baby's nervous system gradually matures, so do patterns of sleep and wakefulness. During the first month, babies usually sleep and wake around the clock, with relatively equal parts of sleep between feedings.

Because most of a newborn's energy is directed toward growing, many non-sleeping hours are spent eating. When you figure in the three or more hours it takes to feed, diaper, bathe and dress your baby each day, there is little time in that busy newborn's life for periods of "quiet alert."

A major change in a baby's sleep-wake patterns usually occurs between 6 weeks and 3 months of age. By 3 months, many babies shift more of their sleep to nighttime and can sustain wakefulness for up to two hours at a time. Most babies are awake for a longer time than usual during a certain time of day, often in late afternoon and early evening. By 6 months, the longest sleep usually follows the longest wakeful period, and a typical baby may be sleeping eight to 10 hours at night. Some infants, however, do not sleep through the night until 1 year or older.

Parental Influence

Numerous factors contribute to your baby's sleep-wake cycles, including your baby's maturity and inborn temperament. Breastfed babies frequently sleep for shorter periods between feedings in the first few months. There are ways you can influence your baby's sleep schedule. Chapters 29 through 34 each include a section about sleep habits of babies at different ages.

Sleep Positions

Place your newborn baby on his or her side or back to sleep. In the United States since the 1940s, it had been the custom for babies to sleep on their stomachs. Recent studies have shown that infants lying on their sides or backs have lower incidences of sudden infant death syndrome (SIDS).

SIDS, unexplained sudden death while an infant sleeps, occurs in about one or two in 1,000 newborns. It is not uncommon for parents to awaken their babies when they first sleep through the night because of worry about SIDS. This is a normal and understandable fear that will eventually subside. (For information on other risk factors associated with SIDS, see page 514. For information on sleep factors and the risk of SIDS, see page 528.)

A rolled-up blanket provides some support for keeping your baby on his or her side while sleeping.

Stirring Versus Waking Up

Drooping eyelids, rubbing the eyes and inconsolable fussiness are usual signs of fatigue in a baby. Many babies cry when they are put down for sleep, but if left alone, most will eventually quiet themselves. It often takes 20 minutes of restlessness for a baby to fall asleep.

If it's bedtime and your baby is not wet, hungry or ill, try to be patient with the crying and encourage self-settling. If you leave the room for a while, your baby will probably stop crying after a short time. If not, briefly try comforting him or her and allow the baby to try to settle again.

In the first few months, it's common for a pattern to evolve in which a baby is fed and falls asleep in a parent's arms. Many parents enjoy the closeness and snuggling of this time, but eventually this may be the only way the baby is able to fall asleep. To avoid this association between feeding and sleeping, try feeding your baby about a half hour before bedtime. Put your baby in bed while he or she is drowsy but still awake.

Babies who stir during the night are not necessarily distressed. When infants enter different sleep cycles (as discussed on page 538) and begin to move or cry, parents sometimes mistake these signs for waking up, and they begin a cycle of waking and feeding the child that often leads to exhaustion for both parents and baby.

Infants typically cry and move about while they pass through various sleep cycles. You might want to move your baby's crib to a location that enables you to hear cries of distress when true wakefulness occurs but promotes sleep when your baby is simply stirring.

Infant Crying and Fussiness

Babies cry somewhere between one and five hours out of 24. Crying usually peaks at about six weeks and then gradually decreases. It's your baby's first way of communicating and an important way to release tension.

It's difficult to listen to your baby cry, and you may find yourself wanting to comfort and quiet her or him. However, you will not always be able to calm your baby when fussing is simply to release tension. Babies do cry. It's part of being a baby. But if you feel the length or intensity of your baby's crying is unusual, trust your intuition and call your baby's health care provider.

It's normal to be frustrated by a crying baby. All parents have been in this situation. Consider arranging for needed breaks with understanding friends or a baby-sitter. Even an hour's break can renew your coping strength. If your baby's crying is causing you to feel emotionally out of control, contact your health care provider, your hospital emergency room, local crisis intervention service or mental health help line immediately.

Why Babies Cry

Although not all infant crying can be explained, there are universal reasons for crying. Because babies cannot talk, crying is their way to communicate their needs and desires. If you're puzzled by your baby's crying, consider the following possible reasons:

Hunger. Most babies eat six to 10 times in a 24-hour period, and for at least the first three months they will usually wake for night feedings. If hunger is the cause of your baby's crying, he or she will eagerly accept the feeding and stop crying.

Quiet babies may just squirm and root around or gently fuss when hungry. If they nap for more than three hours, watch closely for these subtle signs. Or, if they are partially awake, unwrapping and sitting them up may gently encourage them to eat.

Average babies will wake for feedings, eating well most of the time, but active babies may become frantic when hunger strikes. They may be so worked up by the time feeding begins that they gulp air with the milk and overeat, causing spitting up or indigestion.

You may avoid some of this frenzy if you try calming your active baby before feeding him or her, or try feeding before the fussing begins. Burp your active baby often, and stop feeding during the gulping episodes. This will give your baby an opportunity to catch his or her breath and calm down.

If your baby has six to eight wet diapers each 24 hours and is gaining 3 or more ounces each week, he or she is getting enough nourishment to discount hunger as an ongoing cause of prolonged fussiness.

Discomfort. The discomfort of gas or indigestion can cause your baby to cry, as can wet or soiled diapers and uncomfortable temperatures or positions. When babies are uncomfortable, they may try to relieve the discomfort by looking for something to suck on. Their sucking is often frantic, disorganized and chewy. Feeding will not stop the crying, and a pacifier may help only briefly. When the discomfort passes, your baby probably will settle down.

Quiet babies may only mildly fuss when they feel a burp, gas or a bowel movement, and they may not even mind wet diapers. If you can identify and relieve the discomfort, your baby will probably settle down.

Average babies may be fussy before passing gas or a bowel movement, and they usually burp easily. After you've burped your baby and changed wet or soiled diapers, he or she will usually settle down. If the fussing continues, try offering a pacifier or your finger to suck on as you rock or rhythmically walk your baby, periodically burping him or her.

Active babies often squirm and fuss after feedings, eventually winding themselves up to screaming before burping, passing gas or having a bowel movement. They may also become similarly agitated when they need a diaper change. Active babies tend to spit up more frequently than other babies.

When your active baby is fussy or agitated, try burping, checking the diaper, walking, rocking or letting the baby suck on a pacifier or your finger. Sometimes you can settle an active baby with a warm (but not too hot) water bottle on the stomach, accompanied by gentle patting or rubbing. Some babies may also feel secure and comfortable in a swaddle wrap. (The technique is described in the illustrations on page 458.)

Boredom, fear and loneliness. Sometimes a baby will cry because he or she is bored, frightened or lonely. The baby's arms and legs may flail a little, and the suck may be intermittent, chewy and lazy. If your baby is crying for one of these reasons, a feeding may not calm your baby, because this little person may be seeking old-fashioned TLC (tender loving care). A baby seeking TLC may calm down simply with the reassurance of seeing you, hearing your voice, feeling your touch, being with you, cuddling or being offered something for sucking.

Overtiredness or overstimulation. When it's clear your baby isn't hungry or in need of a diaper change, burping or TLC, he or she may simply be overtired or overstimulated, and crying is the baby's way to unwind and release tension. You may notice that your baby's fussy periods occur at predictable times during the day, and for average and active babies, they usually peak when the baby is around 6 weeks old.

If your baby cries from being overtired, reduce the noise, movement and visual stimulation in the area. "White noise," such as the continuous, monotonous sound of a vacuum cleaner or a recording of ocean waves, can often relax and lull your baby by blocking out other, extraneous sounds. Try placing your baby in the crib, closing the door and setting a kitchen timer for 15 or 20 minutes, letting your baby unwind until the timer goes off. If your baby still has not settled after this period, then it's time to check for other reasons for the crying.

Although many parents find it difficult to let their baby cry, think of it as giving your child an opportunity to unwind. Some babies continue this pattern of crying when overtired or overstimulated for about three months. Creating time for yourself and taking advantage of friends' and relatives' offers to assist can help you make it through this frustrating period.

Drying Those Tears

In assessing why your baby is crying, a checklist is helpful to assist you in figuring out the causes. The following suggestions might help you:

1. Check on your baby soon after you hear the crying.
2. Is the baby hungry?
3. Does the baby need a diaper change?
4. Does the baby need to be burped?
5. Is the baby too warm or too cold?
6. Does the baby need to be moved to a more comfortable position?
7. Does the baby just need to suck, whether on a finger or pacifier?
8. Does the baby need TLC: rocking, cuddling, stroking, gentle talking or singing? (You might try one of these for 15 to 20 minutes.)

If your baby continues to cry after you've exhausted the above suggestions, place him or her in the crib, and leave the baby alone for 15 to 20 minutes. Stay within earshot, however.

If, after going through the list, your baby still continues to cry, repeat the process. But if you feel your baby isn't acting "right," looks different or isn't eating as usual, trust your intuition and contact your baby's health care provider. At times, you may need the help of an expert to tell the difference between a well baby and a sick baby.

Don't take your baby's crying personally. She or he is not mad at or rejecting you. Remember, crying is a baby's way of communicating and letting off steam. Think of it as a first sign that your baby is developing independence. Meanwhile, as more than one mother will advise you, try to sleep whenever your baby does—even during the day. If you do, you'll have more energy for the late afternoon and evening, when your baby may be fussy and the demands of the rest of your family are greater.

Spoiling your baby. Don't worry about spoiling your baby during the early months of her or his life. The attention your infant gets from you and other care-givers during the first year helps build trust and security. You aren't spoiling your baby, you're responding to baby's needs with TLC. But it's also important to remember that sometimes it's okay and even necessary to let your baby have some crying time.

Early Physical Care

Now that we've spent some time addressing your baby's behavior tendencies and patterns, let's talk about some of the basics of taking care of this newest member of your family.

Holding Your Baby

Normal, careful handling won't hurt your baby, and with experience you'll feel more and more comfortable holding him or her. Increasingly you'll find yourself responding to your baby's moods by how you choose to play with and handle him or her.

During the first several months of life, babies differ in their ability to control their neck muscles and heads. Until you're certain your baby can hold his or her head up well, lift the baby slowly, always supporting his or her body and head.

If your baby is lying on his or her back, slide one hand under the lower back and bottom and the other under your baby's neck and head from the opposite side. Lift gently and slowly, so your baby's body is supported and the head doesn't flop back. Carefully transfer your baby's head to the crook of your elbow or onto your shoulder.

When your baby is on his or her side, slide one hand under the neck and head and the other under his or her bottom. Scoop your baby into your arms slowly and gently, making sure the head doesn't flop.

If you're picking your baby up from the tummy, slide one hand under the chest with your forearm supporting the chin, and slide the other hand under your baby's hips. Turn your baby toward you as you lift slowly, and slide the head-supporting arm forward until your baby is nestled in the crook of your elbow, while the other arm continues to support the baby's bottom and legs.

When putting your baby down, gently support the head and neck with one hand and the bottom with the other until he or she is on the surface.

As you become more comfortable holding your baby, you'll soon learn what positions he or she prefers. Experienced parents often identify a "best position" to calm their babies. Newborn babies usually feel secure and calm when they're cradled in the crook of an elbow, with head and limbs firmly supported. All babies have their own preferences.

If your baby is fussy and needs calming, you might try holding him or her along the length of your arm, facedown, with the baby's head at the bend of your elbow and the crotch at your hand (see page 542). Or hold your baby across your lap, with tummy pressing against your knees. Another comforting position is to lie on your back and place your baby facedown on your chest while gently rubbing his or her back.

Carrying Your Baby

Your baby will probably develop a preference for how he or she wants to be carried. Some enjoy being carried while they're facing outward, looking at the world, and others prefer the security of snuggling close to your body. Your baby may like being carried with arms and legs tucked in, or he or she may prefer a more relaxed position with just the body and head supported.

Infant carriers allow your baby to have direct contact with your body and body movements. They also enable you to have your hands free for other activities. Front or back carriers are especially good for the first three months, and the

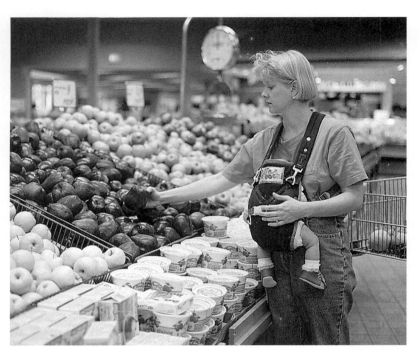

Some babies enjoy the closeness provided by a front carrier. It leaves your hands free for other activities.

earlier your baby becomes accustomed to being carried this way, the easier the adjustment for both of you. Some parents prefer front carriers, because it is easier to maintain close contact—including eye contact—with the baby. But remember, it's never safe to ride a bicycle or to drive or ride in a car with your baby carried in this way.

To use a front carrier:

- Buckle or tie the carrier belt around your waist before picking up your baby.

- Hold your baby against your shoulder, with your hand behind your baby's head.

- Sit down on a chair and lean back, so the weight of your baby's body is supported on your chest and stomach.

- Pull the pouch up and maneuver your baby's legs through the holes.

- Pull the shoulder straps up and over your shoulders, using one hand to support your baby as you adjust the straps comfortably. As you sit forward, the carrier will gradually take your baby's weight. Be sure to put your hand behind your baby's head to support it whenever you lean forward. To prevent backaches, adjust the carrier to a comfortable level.

Diapering Your Baby

On average, a child experiences 5,000 diaper changes before he or she is toilet-trained. Even though you are performing a necessary child care task, it also can provide a wonderful opportunity for closeness and communication with your baby. Your warm words, gentle touches and encouraging smiles can help make your baby feel loved and secure, and soon your baby will be responding to you with gurgles and coos.

Because newborns may urinate as many as 20 times a day, it's important to change your baby's diapers every two or three hours for the first few months. However, it's not necessary to awaken your baby to change a wet diaper. Urine doesn't usually irritate a baby's skin, but the acid content in a bowel movement can, so change a messy diaper as soon as possible after your baby is awake. Remember to clean your baby thoroughly at each changing.

If your baby is a boy, he may urinate as you remove his diaper. (This seems to be especially true at your baby's first checkup!) To avoid being sprayed, cover his penis loosely with a diaper or cloth while cleaning the rest of his diaper area.

Whether your baby is a boy or a girl, thorough cleansing is a must. Holding your baby's legs at the ankles works well during the cleaning. Use a cloth dampened with warm water or a premoistened baby wipe to wipe your baby's diaper area. Using alcohol-free and fragrance-free wipes may help avoid drying or irritating your baby's skin. When your baby has a bowel movement, use the

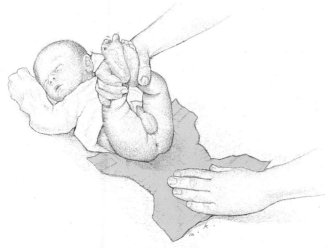

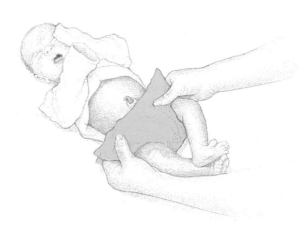

Changing a Disposable Diaper

Step 1. *When you open the diaper, make sure that the tapes, which are at the back of the diaper, are at the top, or away from you. Slide the diaper under your baby until the top edge (the edge with the tapes) lines up with your baby's waist.*

Step 2. *Then bring the front of the diaper up through the legs, without twisting it to one side.*

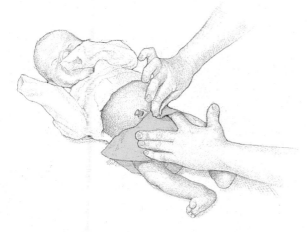

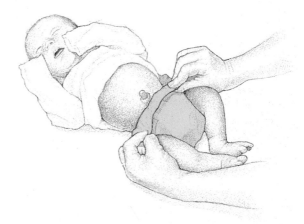

Step 3. *Hold one side in position while removing the tab from the tape, and pull the tape forward to stick to the diaper front. Repeat for the other side, making sure the diaper is snug around your baby's legs and not twisted to one side.*

Step 4. *For a newborn, fold down the top of the diaper so it won't rub against the healing umbilical cord. Disposable diapers should fit snugly around the waist, with room enough only for one finger.*

unsoiled front of the diaper to remove the bulk of the stool. Then gently finish cleaning with a cloth or wipe, using a mild soap as needed. You needn't apply lotion or powder, unless your baby tends to develop rashes easily.

Lift your baby's lower body by the ankles to slide the new diaper underneath. If you're using diaper pins, avoid accidentally poking the baby by always keeping the fingers of one hand between the diaper pin and your baby's body until the point of the pin is securely locked in the pin's hood. Cloth diapers should be worn snugly because they tend to loosen as your baby moves around. Tuck the edges of cloth into plastic pants to keep wetness inside.

If you use cloth diapers, you can fold them several ways. Experiment with different techniques for maximal absorbency and best fit. Fold the side edges in, making shallow folds for a large baby, deeper folds for a smaller baby. For boys, you may want to have extra padding in the front. Some people find that folding the front narrower than the back allows diaper pins to sit flatter on the tummy and brings the diaper around the legs more tightly.

When you use disposable diapers, be sure to buy the size corresponding to your baby's weight. Keep your hands grease-free and dry before trying to fasten the tape so the tape will stick.

Diaper rash

All babies get a red or sore bottom from time to time, even with frequent diaper changes and careful cleaning. Below are some of the common reasons for diaper rash:

- Irritation from a new product that has come into contact with your baby's skin. Possibilities include disposable wipes, a new brand of disposable diaper or a detergent, bleach or fabric softener used to launder diapers. If you suspect one of these culprits, change to a brand that has not bothered your baby before. Generally, you'll have better results if you use products that have few additives and little or no added scent.

- Chemicals used in manufacturing clothing. Wash all new clothing before your baby wears it for the first time.

- A bacterial or yeast infection. (For more information on bacterial and yeast infections that cause diaper rash, see page 627.)

- Sensitive skin. If this is the case, change diapers frequently, washing the area with clear water each time. Allow the baby's bottom to air dry. Use a soothing ointment, such as A & D ointment, Desitin or Constant Care ointment, any time pinkness appears in the diaper area.

To help prevent diaper rash, avoid using super-absorbent disposable diapers, because they tend to be changed less frequently. If your baby's bottom is sensitive, you may want to allow time each day for your baby to be without a diaper, exposed to the air. To control the spread of infection, make sure to wash your hands well with soap and water after changing your baby's diapers.

If you're using cloth diapers, be sure you wash and rinse them thoroughly, and select snap-on plastic pants, instead of those with elastic bindings, for better air circulation. In addition, try using absorbent liners with cloth diapers.

Call your health care provider if the diaper rash doesn't improve in a few days.

Bathing Your Baby

Your newborn baby doesn't need a complete bath every day and shouldn't be immersed in bath water until the area around the umbilical cord is healed. If your infant resists baths, give a sponge bath, cleaning the parts that really need attention (especially hands, head and face, neck and diaper area). Sponge baths are a good alternative to a bath for about the first six weeks. Some babies love baths from the beginning, but others take time to adjust to the experience.

Find a time for bathing your baby that is convenient for both of you. Some people bathe their babies before bedtime, as a relaxing, sleep-promoting ritual. Others prefer a time when their babies are fully awake and ready to enjoy the experience. You'll enjoy this time more if you are unrushed and unlikely to be interrupted.

Have all the bathing supplies ready (washcloth, cotton balls, a towel, diaper changing supplies and clothing) before you fill the tub and begin to undress your baby. Plain water baths are fine most times. When needed, use a mild shampoo and a mild soap that is free of fragrances and deodorant additives. Never leave your baby alone in the water!

Be sure the room where you bathe your baby is comfortably warm (about 75 degrees Fahrenheit) and free from chilly breezes. You may bathe your infant in a bathtub or sink, or you may prefer a plastic tub or dishpan placed on a table or countertop. In the beginning, especially until you are comfortable handling your slippery, wiggling, wet baby, use just a couple inches of warm water. You may want to lather your baby on a towel and use the tub only for rinsing.

Test the water temperature with your elbow or the inside of your wrist. Some people prefer washing face and hair before placing their babies in the water. Wash your baby's face with clear water. Use a damp cotton ball to wipe each eye, from the inside to the outside corner. Gently pat your baby's face dry.

When the bath is to begin, undress your baby, removing the diaper last. If the diaper is soiled, clean your baby's bottom before the bath. To protect yourself from being sprayed, drape a diaper or washcloth over your baby boy's penis. Some babies dislike being naked and fuss vigorously at this stage. If this is a problem, give your baby sponge baths and try again in a week or two.

It's important to support your baby's head and torso with your arm and hand, to provide your baby both safety and a sense of security. When shampooing, tip your baby's head back to avoid the irritation of shampoo running into the eyes. It's not necessary to shampoo your baby's hair every time you bathe your infant.

Bathe the cleanest parts of your baby first and the dirtiest parts last. Be sure to wash inside folds of skin and to rinse the genitals with water. If your baby is a girl, gently spread the labia to clean, and if your baby is a boy, lift the scrotum to clean underneath. Do not try to retract the foreskin of your baby boy's penis if he is uncircumcised. Let your baby lean forward on your arm while you clean his or her back and bottom, separating the buttocks to clean the anal area.

Be especially careful when your infant is slippery and wet. Immediately wrap him or her in a towel and pat dry. If you use a skin lotion, choose an unscented variety and warm it first by holding some in the palm of your hand.

Dressing Your Baby

It's not unusual for new parents to overdress their infants. A good rule of thumb is to dress your baby according to how you would dress to feel comfortable. Use the same number of layers you would use for yourself.

Your baby will enjoy being taken outside, if dressed appropriately. But remember, a baby's skin is more sensitive than the skin of adults or older children and it sunburns easily. If your baby will be outside for any length of time, protect the skin with clothing and a cap. It's also a good idea to place your baby in the shade to prevent overexposure to the sun. Babies don't sweat easily and can become overheated.

Nail Care

To prevent your baby from accidentally scratching his or her face, you may need to trim the fingernails shortly after birth. For the first few months, it's okay to tear the soft nails carefully with your own fingernails or to use a nail clipper or a small scissors for the task. Trim the nails straight across, and keep them short. This task may be easier to do while your baby is sleeping.

Toenails grow slowly, and they probably won't need much trimming for the first six months. Check for sharp edges, though, because catching them on clothing is painful. Be sure to mention any ingrown toenails to your health care provider.

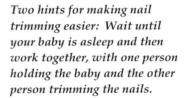

Two hints for making nail trimming easier: Wait until your baby is asleep and then work together, with one person holding the baby and the other person trimming the nails.

CHAPTER TWENTY-EIGHT

Feeding Your Baby

Getting started

Feeding your baby is about much more than nutrition. Your baby's first feelings of love, security, trust and comfort arise from your prompt and faithful response to your baby's hunger cry. Feeding is as much a social activity as a nutritional one, because your baby's growth and development are based, in part, on the powerful bond that forms at feeding times.

Of course, good nutrition is vitally important too. At no time in life does a person undergo such rapid growth as in the first year. You can expect your baby to double her or his birth weight by 6 months of age and triple it in a year. Your baby's brain will double in size during the first two years. The nutrients you feed your baby during these formative months lay the foundation for a lifetime.

Feeding can be a pleasant experience for you as well as your baby. It can be restful—a time to slow down and enjoy the simple pleasures of just being together.

Taking the time to give full attention to your baby is one of the most important things you can do. Let the bed go unmade. Let the phone ring (or use an answering machine). If you have help after you get home from the hospital, use it to insulate yourself from the rest of the world during feeding times. Give your full attention to your baby.

This chapter begins with an overview of topics about feeding that apply to all babies. If you plan to breastfeed, you'll find details and practical tips beginning on page 474. If you plan to bottle feed, recommendations begin on page 487.

The First Feeding

Many babies are surprisingly alert in the first several hours after birth. Newborns who are alert and healthy may be interested in nursing soon after birth.

Babies don't need to eat right away after birth, but they often like to suck. If you put your newborn to your breast, the sucking that may result will encourage your milk production even though your baby will receive only a small amount of your early breast milk, called colostrum.

Your baby may show an interest in nursing soon after birth, even while you're still in the birthing room or recovery area. If he or she is tightly wrapped in blankets, loosen or remove the wraps and snuggle your baby in the crook of your arm. Hold her or him against your body, skin to skin. The warmth of your body will help keep your baby warm.

Many women who have decided to breastfeed find it more convenient to room-in with their babies in the hospital rather than have the baby stay in the nursery. Frequent feedings on demand can help establish a plentiful milk supply.

To help your baby learn how to breastfeed, request that she or he not be given any supplementary bottles of water or formula, and preferably no pacifier, until breastfeeding is well established.

Most breastfed babies don't need water or formula. Some babies, those who have low blood sugar (hypoglycemia) in the first hours after birth, for example, may need an early boost of calories. In this instance, the required feeding is generally given by tube directly into the stomach, rather than by using a bottle. If the low blood sugar persists, a baby might need intravenous glucose. (For more information on hypoglycemia, see page 380.)

When to Feed

How often you feed your healthy full-term baby depends essentially on one thing—how often your baby is hungry. Most babies will let you know when they're hungry and will eat frequently and well enough to support their rapid growth.

If, however, your baby is very sleepy or was born prematurely, she or he may not always give clear signals, such as hunger crying. Many babies need encouragement with their first feedings. Most likely it won't be long until feedings begin to go smoothly in response to your baby's hunger cries. Letting your baby determine feeding times may make the first few weeks after birth seem unstructured and unpredictable, and they will be. But take heart, this situation won't last. In a short time you'll be better acquainted with each other, and feeding times probably will evolve into a natural rhythm.

Feeding your newborn on demand is suited to your baby's immaturity. This new person will have short periods of wakefulness, a nervous system that can't yet tell one sensation from another and a stomach with a small capacity. Allow your baby to set the pace, and your baby probably will eat better. Ultimately, your baby's healthy growth is evidence that he or she is feeding well.

Feeding your baby requires flexibility and alertness to your baby's cues. Being sensitive and responding to these cues form the foundation of a healthy and satisfying parent-child relationship. The relationship you foster during feeding is likely to carry over to all other aspects of parenthood and will benefit your child for a lifetime.

Generally speaking, your baby will let you know when she or he is hungry. Hunger produces discomfort that can make your baby cry. Your baby will learn to sort out different kinds of discomfort, and you'll learn to distinguish among cries for food, pain and tiredness.

Feed your baby promptly when she or he signals hunger. If you don't respond right away, your baby may become aroused by intense crying. Attempts to feed at this point may prove more frustrating than satisfying for both of you. Then the arousal and discomfort of hunger may combine to make your baby even more irritable. It can take considerable time, and patience on your part, for your highly upset baby to settle down enough to eat—and to learn to trust that future hunger will be promptly satisfied.

When your baby has had enough, you'll know. Generally, a baby will stop sucking and turn away from the nipple, or simply push the nipple out of her or his mouth with the tongue. If you try to continue the feeding, your baby may arch her or his back.

Your baby will determine how much and how fast to eat. It's normal for an infant to suck, pause, rest, socialize a bit and then return to feeding. If your baby is satisfied by feedings and is growing well, you can feel confident in knowing that you're doing great.

In the beginning, your baby will be feeding perhaps eight to 12 times daily. One feeding may seem to blur into another. Then gradually, feeding patterns and routines will begin to emerge after the first month or two.

Flexibility is important. Expect growth spurts, when your baby will need more milk and more frequent feedings. At other times, changing sleep/wake patterns may be reflected in changes in feeding demands.

Sleeping Through the Night

From birth through two to six months, expect your baby to routinely wake at night for feeding one or more times. The age at which babies sleep through the night without feeding varies tremendously. It depends on many factors, including your baby's temperament, maturation of the nervous system and feeding style. Some babies "snack" frequently. Others take larger amounts less often. Try not to compare your baby with anyone else's baby when it comes to sleeping through the night.

Growth

Generally, babies lose up to 10 percent of their birth weight in the first few days of life. This weight loss is mostly due to the normal decrease in body water, not loss of muscle or fat. By seven to 14 days, they regain the lost weight. Infants on formula may lose only 1 to 2 percent of their birth weight and regain it by the end of the first week. Both patterns are normal.

Feeding guidelines

Whether you breastfeed or bottle feed your baby, the best measure of your success is your baby's general pattern of health and growth. Here are tips to keep in mind:

- Follow your baby's cues about when to feed.
- Feed promptly in response to your baby's cues.
- Hold your baby securely but not restrictively.
- Stimulate the rooting reflex by gently stroking your baby's cheek (see page 442).
- Let your baby decide the pace and amount of feedings.
- Allow for natural pauses during feedings.
- Don't rush your baby; babies, like most adults, prefer to eat in a relaxed manner.
- Talk to and smile at your baby, but don't overwhelm your baby with attention during feedings.

Whether breastfed or bottle-fed, infants do not grow at a steady pace. They grow in sporadic bursts. There may be times when your baby will seem to grow overnight, and the days may seem to turn into feeding frenzies; your baby may appear insatiable. Feed your baby more frequently for the time being. Things will quiet down in a day or two.

The Sucking Reflex

During the first several months of life, your baby's sucking reflex will be strong. There will be times when he or she will want to suck without needing to be fed. Babies use sucking to calm themselves, and they often will suck on anything available.

As a new parent, you'll learn to distinguish the times when your baby is sucking because of hunger and when she or he is sucking to satisfy the need for sucking. You can assume that if it's two to three hours since the last feeding and your baby is putting fist to mouth, your baby is probably hungry.

Breastfeeding

Breastfeeding is wonderfully adapted to fulfill your baby's need for food and fluid. As your baby grows, the nutrient balance in breast milk shifts to supply what your baby needs.

Breast milk is the ideal food for a baby. Health professionals who provide care to mothers and babies have long recommended breastfeeding as the preferred method of infant nutrition. There are advantages to breastfeeding exclusively for the first five or six months of life and then adding supplements of solid foods until the baby is at least a year old. Even if you breastfeed for a short time, your baby benefits. In fact, there are advantages for both you and your baby. (For more information on these benefits, see page 182.)

Early in your pregnancy, your milk-producing (mammary) glands will prepare for nursing. By the fifth or sixth month of pregnancy, your breasts are ready to produce milk. In some women, tiny droplets of watery or yellowish fluid may appear on the nipples at this time. This fluid is called colostrum ("early milk") and will be the "milk" your baby gets for the first few days after birth. Colostrum is the ideal food for your baby's first few days. It's loaded with active, infection-fighting antibodies from your body.

The delivery of the placenta signals your body to start milk production. It prompts a hormone called prolactin to activate the milk-producing glands. The activation of milk production happens regardless of your plans to breastfeed or bottle feed your baby. The milk volume gradually increases and is often referred to as "coming in" between the third and fifth day after birth. Your breasts may feel full, hard or lumpy as glands fill with milk. The milk production and increased blood supply to your breasts might make them feel warmer and slightly tender.

Continuing milk production is based simply on the rule of supply and demand. The signal for continuing production of milk comes from the frequent and regular stimulation of the breasts by sucking and by regular release of the milk already produced. The more frequently your baby nurses and is allowed to remove milk from each breast, the more milk you will produce.

Dealing with engorgement. If your milk "comes in" rapidly, your breasts may quickly become so full, firm and tender that your baby won't be able to grasp your nipple. This swelling, called engorgement, also causes congestion within your breasts, which makes your milk flow slower. So even if your baby can latch on, she or he may be less than satisfied with the results.

If this occurs, don't be discouraged. You can release (express) milk manually. Support the breast you intend to express in one hand. With your other hand, gently stroke your breast inward toward your areola. Then place your thumb and forefinger at the top and bottom of the breast just behind the areola. As you gently compress the breast between your fingers, milk should squirt out the nipple. You can also use a breast pump to express your milk (for more information, see page 484).

As you release your milk, you'll begin to feel your areola and nipple soften. Once enough milk is released, your baby can comfortably latch on and nurse. As you nurse your baby, gently massage your breast to further relieve the fullness and promote the flow of milk. Wearing a nursing bra both day and night will help support your breasts and make them more comfortable.

Frequent, lengthy nursing sessions are the best means to avoid breast engorgement. Nurse your baby every two to three hours, night and day, even though it means waking your baby for feedings. Nurse your baby on each breast for at least 10 to 20 minutes. Once you settle into a pattern of breastfeeding, don't miss a feeding.

If your breasts are sore after nursing, apply an ice pack to reduce swelling. Crushed ice in a plastic bag will do, or cold packs are available at most pharmacies. If you continue to have trouble breastfeeding, contact your medical caregiver or a lactation consultant.

How Breastfeeding Works

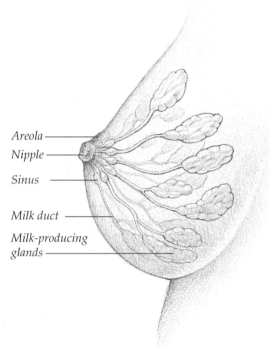

Areola —
Nipple —
Sinus —
Milk duct —
Milk-producing glands —

As your baby nurses, milk is released from the tiny sacs of the milk-producing glands and propelled forward through ducts into holding areas (sinuses) located just behind the areola. During nursing, your baby compresses the areola, forcing milk out through tiny openings in the nipple.

The let-down reflex. Your baby's sucking stimulates nerve endings in your areola and nipple, which signal the pituitary gland at the base of your brain to release a hormone called oxytocin. Oxytocin acts on the mammary glands in your breasts, causing the release of milk to your nursing baby.

This release is called the let-down reflex. Initially you may feel nothing at all. But within the first few weeks you may begin to feel a tingling sensation in your breasts when milk is released. Use the let-down reflex as your cue to sit back, relax and enjoy these precious moments with your baby.

Although your baby's sucking is the primary stimulus for milk let-down, other stimuli may have the same effect. For example, your baby's cry—or even thoughts of your baby, or the sounds of rippling water—may set things in motion. Gently massaging the nipples can also stimulate let-down.

Although the stimulation of frequent nursing builds up your milk supply, the let-down reflex is what makes your milk available to your baby. Because let-down may occur several times during the course of a typical feeding, be careful not to rush things. Your baby needs plenty of time at each breast.

Different techniques

Breastfeeding and bottle feeding require totally different sucking techniques for babies. Specifically, your baby's tongue plays a different role in the two types of feeding.

If you breastfeed, your baby will literally strip milk from your nipple with her or his tongue. With a bottle, a baby's tongue serves to limit the flow of milk from the nipple.

Because of the action of the tongue, the use of facial muscles and the pattern of sucking, many dentists believe that breastfeeding paves the way for proper development of mouth structure and positioning of the teeth without crowding; it also promotes healthy development of a wide dental arch.

Breast milk: how it's unique. Breast milk is uniquely designed to meet the complete nutritional needs of your baby in the early days and into the later months. It contains all the nutrients your baby requires for growth. It is easily digested.

Although formula and breast milk both contain proteins, fat and carbohydrates, the composition of human milk differs significantly from that of formula. In fact, as the composition of human milk is studied and important components are identified, formula manufacturers are continually challenged to alter their products to imitate mother's milk as much as possible.

No formula can exactly duplicate breast milk. The composition of your breast milk changes to meet the specific growth needs of your developing baby. In fact, the composition of your breast milk changes during a single feeding. The milk that comes first, the foremilk, is richest in protein for growth. The longer your baby sucks, the more she or he gets the hindmilk, which is richest in fat for energy needs, and probably the most satisfying.

Because breast milk is extremely well-absorbed, utilized and digested, breastfed babies probably will want to eat every two to three hours at first. Your baby's need for frequent feeding is not a sign that your baby isn't getting enough; it reflects the easy digestibility of breast milk.

Appearances. Many mothers take one look at breast milk and wonder, "How can it possibly be rich enough for my baby to grow on for four to six months, without any other nutrients, when it looks so watery?" Breast milk not only looks watery but also has a blue cast, making it look somewhat like skim milk.

Don't let looks deceive you. Breast milk is not skim milk. It's rich in exactly what your baby needs for growth. Breast milk provides about 20 to 22 calories an ounce. The nutrients and sodium content of breast milk are ideally matched to what your infant's still-immature intestines and kidneys can handle.

Babies and moms usually need help in initiating breastfeeding. Take advantage of the opportunity to ask questions while you're still in the hospital. Because of shorter hospital stays, however, breastfeeding may not be well established by the time you go home. Check back with your health care provider, a lactation consultant, the county health department or a La Leche League volunteer if you need extra support and suggestions.

Some babies have no trouble in figuring out what they're supposed to be doing at the breast. Simply bringing your baby up to the nipple and allowing him or her to nuzzle into the nipple may be sufficient, especially after your baby has had some practice. Others need prodding or encouragement.

Breastfeeding a sleepy baby. During the first few weeks you may pick up your crying baby and prepare to breastfeed only to discover you have a sleepy little person in your arms. To encourage breastfeeding under these circumstances, try gently tickling the crown of your baby's scalp. Softly talking to your sleepy baby may capture her or his attention, or gently rub the sole of your baby's foot with your fingers—but don't overdo it. Removing a few layers of blanket or clothing may also stimulate the baby to be interested in breastfeeding.

Newborn babies are normally sleepy for a few days. After all, the journey down the birth canal is difficult. Your baby may take only a few sucks and then stop. If she or he does not seem to be nursing well, ask your nurse or doctor for assistance.

Experimenting with positions. If your baby attaches and sucks correctly, even if the arrangement feels awkward at first, the position is correct. It won't be long before you'll be maneuvering easily and confidently.

Most moms try a sitting position first, probably because it offers maximal maneuverability. Others prefer to lie down. Whether you lie or sit, your baby's mouth must be comfortably near your nipple. Inexperienced mothers sometimes bend over to link baby with breast. Don't make this mistake. It's an uncomfortable posture that can lead to back pain. The important thing to remember is to get comfortable. Relax. Enjoy. You and your baby will find the way.

Here's a sampling of breastfeeding positions to try:

The cradle hold. Whether in your hospital bed or a chair, sit up straight. Put a pillow behind the small of your back for support. If you opt for a chair, choose one with low armrests.

Cradle your baby in an arm, with your baby's head resting comfortably in the crook of your elbow. Your forearm will support your baby's back. Your open hand supports your baby's bottom.

Next, move your baby across your body, tummy to tummy, so that she or he faces your breast, with mouth near your nipple. A pillow on your lap can provide support for the arm that's holding your baby. Your baby's arms should be on either side of the nursing breast.

Bring your free hand up under your breast to support it for breastfeeding. Place the palm of that hand under your breast with thumb on top of the breast, behind the areola. All fingers should be well behind the areola. Support the weight of your breast in your hand while squeezing lightly to point the nipple straight forward.

Getting Started

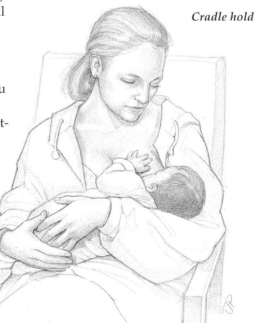

Cradle hold

If the little mouth doesn't open to accept your nipple, touch the nipple to your baby's mouth or cheek. If your baby is hungry and interested in nursing, her or his mouth should open. Move your baby's mouth immediately onto your breast so that your baby receives as much nipple and areola as possible.

As your baby starts sucking and your nipple is being stretched in your baby's mouth, you may feel some discomfort. After a few sucks the discomfort should disappear. If it does not, gently remove your baby from your breast, taking care to release the suction first, and reposition her or him. Repeat this procedure until your baby latches on correctly. Adjust your baby's position so that your baby's nose and chin touch your breast.

Once nursing begins you can relax the supporting arm and pull your baby's lower body closer to you. If your baby can comfortably remain attached, you may be able to stop supporting your breast with the other hand.

The cross-cradle hold. This position is similar to the cradle hold, with your baby across the front of your body, tummy to tummy, but instead you hold your baby with the opposite arm and support the back of his or her head with your open hand. This hold allows you especially good control as you position your baby to latch on.

What does it feel like?

What's it really like to breastfeed? Is breastfeeding painful?

Most new moms approach breastfeeding with mild anxiety. They've heard from other mothers that the experience can be somewhat painful, especially when a hungry newborn latches on firmly to the nipple of an inexperienced mother.

Experienced moms describe the sensation as an "ooh-ah," or even a flat-out "ouch," feeling. It's nothing you can't handle. But your baby is stretching your nipple for the first time, and you're not yet accustomed to the sensation.

This tenderness may last about a minute and may persist for the first several weeks of breastfeeding, after which your body will adjust and the discomfort will disappear.

You want your baby to latch on well and create a firm bond of suction. If your baby's cheeks remain smooth as she or he sucks, rest assured there's a good connection. If dimples appear on the baby's cheeks, she or he has not yet latched on properly. Gently remove your baby from your breast and reposition her or him for a better connection.

When your baby correctly attaches, a strong suction seal is formed between your baby's mouth and your breast. Between sucks, the suction pressure holds your baby's mouth to your breast. Even if your baby is not actively sucking, the hold is still powerful.

When it's time to switch from one breast to the other or to end a feeding, break the suction first unless, of course, your baby has already opened her or his mouth and released your nipple.

To break the suction, gently insert the tip of your finger into the corner of your baby's mouth. Push your finger slowly between your baby's gums until you feel the release.

The football hold. In this position you hold your baby in much the same way a running back tucks a football under the arm.

Hold your baby at your side on one arm, with your elbow bent and your open hand firmly supporting your baby's head face up at the level of your breast. Your baby's torso will rest on your forearm. Put a pillow at your side to support your arm. A chair with broad, low arms works best.

With your free hand gently squeezing your breast to align your nipple horizontally, move your baby to your breast until nipple meets lips. When your baby's mouth opens, pull her or him in close to latch on snugly.

Because the baby is not positioned near the abdomen, the football hold is popular among mothers who are recovering from cesarean births. It is also a frequent choice of women who have large breasts, who are nursing premature or small babies and whose babies tend to not take enough of the nipple and areola into their mouths.

For mothers of twins, it is virtually the only way to nurse two at a time.

Football hold

Lying down to breastfeed. Although most new mothers learn to breastfeed in a sitting position, there are times when you may prefer to nurse while lying down. For example, lying down might be the best position if your baby prefers to snack and doze at your breast. A lying position may help you in getting your baby correctly connected in the early days of breastfeeding, or when you both may simply be tired. If you're recuperating from a cesarean birth, reclining may be your only option for the first few days.

Lie on your side and place your baby on her or his side facing you, with mouth close to the nipple of your lower breast. Use the hand of your lower arm to help keep your baby's head positioned at your breast.

With your upper arm and hand, reach across your body and grasp your breast, touching your nipple to your baby's lips. After your baby latches on firmly, you can use your lower arm to support your own head and your upper hand and arm to help support your baby.

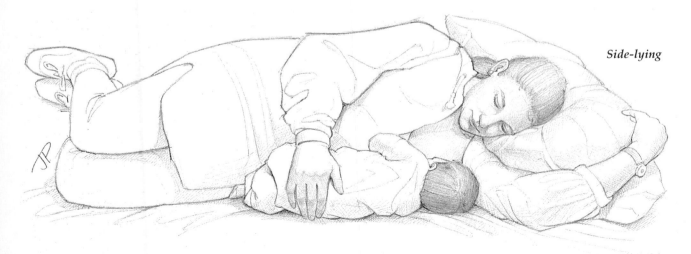

Side-lying

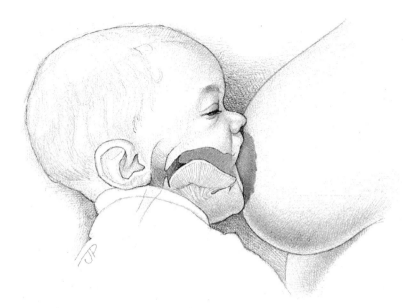

When your baby latches on properly, the nipple is stretched into your baby's mouth and milk is ejected toward the back of the baby's mouth.

Latching on properly. If your baby's gums cover your areola, your baby is in the correct position to nurse. When your baby sucks, he or she will compress the areola and underlying cavities (sinuses) in which milk has collected, forcing stored milk out through the nipple.

If your baby latches on to the nipple only, it may become sore and even bruised, the sinuses will not be sufficiently compressed and your baby will fail to get enough milk. You will both be left feeling frustrated and unhappy.

Alternate breasts. Offer both breasts at each feeding. Allow your baby to end the feeding on the first side, then, after burping your baby, offer the other side. Alternate starting sides to equalize the stimulation each breast receives.

Nipple care. After you finish nursing, leave your breasts uncovered (nursing bra flaps down) to air dry your nipples. Don't wash your nipples after nursing your baby. There are built-in lubricants around the areola that provide a natural salve. Soap removes these protective substances and promotes dryness, which may cause or aggravate sore nipples. (See page 507 for information about sore nipples.)

When you bathe, splash your breasts with water. Avoid soap. And again, allow your nipples to air dry. Don't towel dry your nipples.

Your Baby's Feeding Style

Every baby is different. Some are speedy, efficient eaters, consistently whizzing through feedings in minutes on each breast. Other babies are grazers, preferring snack-size feedings at frequent intervals. Still others, especially newborns, are snoozers. These babies may take a few vigorous sucks and blissfully doze off, then wake, feed and doze again intermittently throughout a typical nursing session. Sometimes a baby will be slow to wake and therefore reluctant to accept mom's breast. Babies often suck a few times, pause, then return to feeding.

Babies arrive in the world with different temperaments. Not surprisingly, their temperaments affect their feeding styles. To be successful with breastfeeding, your approach must be tailored to your baby's unique needs and preferences.

Most babies fall into one of three basic temperament types, all of them quite normal, according to Dr. T. Berry Brazelton, a pediatrician from Harvard. These temperaments, as they pertain to issues other than feeding, are also discussed on page 456.

The Quiet Baby	Suggestions
May shortchange himself or herself when feeding, ending the session before getting enough milk. May not awaken for daytime feedings in the first weeks. May need more frequent weight checks to be sure the baby is growing well.	Your baby may need special encouragement. Wake your baby for feedings at three- or four-hour intervals during daytime hours. Sit him or her up. Remove some clothing or blankets. Change diapers. Pay special attention to cues such as stirring during light sleep; this may be a good time to feed. In three to six weeks your baby probably will be more predictably hungry and may awaken regularly for feedings.

The Average Baby	Suggestions
Awakens for feedings and feeds well most of the time. May fall asleep during some feedings and, because of hunger, awaken early for the next feeding. May accept schedule changes. You may sometimes find it difficult to determine whether your baby is crying because of hunger or for some other reason, such as general discomfort.	Initially, feed your baby on demand; that's generally six to 10 feedings each 24-hour period. Gradually move to a modified demand schedule, waking your baby, if necessary, for feedings every two or three hours during the day while letting your baby "sleep through" at night. Offer to nurse if your baby cries. Once you begin nursing, if he or she falls asleep quickly, your baby was probably not hungry.

The Active Baby	Suggestions
Active babies may pose a special challenge. Expect piercing wails when your baby is hungry. May seem frantic to feed, and once nursing begins may be a greedy eater who gulps air as well as milk. May overeat, then spit up. May be frequently irritable, so don't make the mistake of viewing irritability as a feeding problem.	Nurse your baby frequently. If your baby is exceptionally upset, he or she may have difficulty latching on properly. Try to calm your baby before you attempt to breastfeed. Give your baby an incentive to breastfeed by expressing a little milk or colostrum onto your baby's lips. Gently remove your baby from your breast if he or she embarks on a gulping episode. After a brief "breather," offer the nipple again. Burp your baby frequently.

Going Home

The need for support when you breastfeed doesn't end when you leave the hospital. In fact, it may intensify once you're on your own. At this point your continued success may hinge on having an informed, supportive partner or another person, such as a family member, around to help at home.

Feeding frequency. Newborns need to eat frequently. Feedings satisfy their need to suck as well as their need for nourishment. Frequent feedings also will bolster your milk supply.

The idea that young infants are ideally fed every three to four hours can be misleading because it sets up the wrong expectations. If your baby wants to be fed more frequently, you may think there's something wrong with you, your milk supply or your baby.

Newborns vary greatly in the amount of time they spend nursing and the length of time between feedings. The best approach is to breastfeed as often as your baby is hungry. To establish your milk supply, feed by breast exclusively at first, without using bottle supplements. Let your baby set the pace; don't hurry her or him. Don't be surprised if your newborn baby requires a dozen feedings in a 24-hour period at first.

Remember that most nutritional needs will be met in the first five minutes your baby nurses on each breast, during which he or she will receive 70 to 80 percent of the total feeding.

Bunch feedings. All babies seem to need close-together feedings from time to time. Health care providers refer to these sessions as "bunch feedings." Most often, bunch feedings occur in the early evening, when a baby is most likely to feel cranky and irritable.

For example, you might find yourself feeding your baby three separate times between 6 and 9 p.m., after which your baby sleeps solidly for four or five hours. Then your baby may bunch another two or three feedings before he or she has another extended period of sleep—perhaps until morning.

Growth spurts. Intermittently through-out the first year, babies experience growth spurts. When your baby has a growth spurt, she or he will want to feed more frequently than usual. Some babies go through periods in which they just can't seem to get enough milk.

Putting your baby to your breast more often is the simple solution. Usually this lasts only a day or two.

Is my baby getting enough to eat?

Mothers who breastfeed often wonder if their babies are getting enough to eat. Although you can't precisely measure the amount of milk your baby's getting, there are clear signs that reveal how your baby is breastfeeding and whether she or he is getting sufficient nourishment.

For example, you'll know if your breasts are firm and full before feedings and softer and emptier after nursing. You'll hear and see your baby swallow milk, and you'll see your baby turn away from your breast when she or he has had enough.

Weight gain is perhaps the most reliable sign that your baby is getting enough to eat. Most babies lose a few ounces immediately after birth, then regain the weight—and then some—by two weeks. If you are unsure about whether your baby is gaining or losing weight, have the weight checked by your baby's health care provider. With shorter hospital stays that allow little time for establishing breastfeeding, your baby's health care provider may encourage a return visit within a few days after birth, or you can initiate the visit. Trust your instinct if you believe your baby isn't eating well. A baby who is excessively sleepy or irritable may need some help with feeding.

Another trustworthy sign of normal growth and development is your baby's pattern of stooling and urinating. Babies usually have six to eight wet diapers and two or more stools a day in the first few weeks. At first, they may pass some stool every time they eat. Contact your baby's health care provider if your baby is urinating or stooling less than these guidelines.

If you're like most mothers, your attention will be focused rather intensely on the needs and interests of your baby during the first several weeks and months of your baby's life. Although this commitment is completely reasonable, don't forget about your personal needs too. If your baby is to thrive, she or he needs a healthy mom.

Nutrition. The precise amounts of foods, fluids and calories you need to support breastfeeding are not universally agreed on, but you may need fewer calories to maintain your milk supply than was previously thought.

The best approach to your personal nutrition while breastfeeding is not unlike the best approach at other times in your life: Eat foods at regular intervals from various food groups—a balanced diet. And drink six to eight cups of fluids each day.

Rest. As difficult as it may be, work at getting enough rest. You'll feel more energetic, you'll eat better and you'll enjoy your new baby best when you're rested. Rest promotes the production of breast milk by enhancing the production of milk-producing hormones.

The tranquilizing effect of nursing can make you feel sleepy. Don't be afraid to nurse your baby lying down or even to take your baby to bed with you. Nursing's soothing effect may make you both sleepy, and lying down may be just what you need.

A nursing bra. Nursing bras provide important support for milk-laden breasts. They can help prevent backaches. They also help reduce leakage of milk. Many women find nursing bras to be comfortable and convenient to use.

You can buy nursing bras that fasten in front or in back. What distinguishes them from regular bras is that both cups open, usually with a simple maneuver that can be managed unobtrusively while you hold your baby. A common style has a slide hook that fastens the cup flap.

The cups of nursing bras are generally made of cotton fabric for comfort and are usually machine-washable—an important feature, because there will be times when your breasts leak milk, which can stain the cups.

Many small-breasted women wear no bra at all. Some get the support and convenience they need from a stretchy sports bra. But be careful to select a cotton bra; synthetics hold in heat, can create conditions that foster infections and can be irritating. Women who opt for a sports bra simply lift the bra over one breast at a time for feeding, and tuck themselves back in after a feeding.

Nursing pads. You may not be able to avoid excess milk from your breasts, but you can avoid leakage onto your bra and clothing. This is where nursing pads come in handy.

Absorbent and disposable, these slim pads can be slipped between breast and bra. Constructed much like an ultra-thin disposable diaper—some women make their own by cutting diapers into small squares—these pads soak up milk leakage while allowing air to circulate to the skin. Some models have an outer, leak-proof layer.

Nursing pads can be worn all the time or can be reserved for special occasions, to protect dress clothes, for example. Some women don't bother with pads at all.

Nursing pads are generally available in stores that sell nursing bras or in stores that sell disposable diapers.

Introducing a Bottle

Once your milk supply is well established, when you feel comfortable breast-feeding and you're confident that your baby is doing well, the occasional use of a bottle will not interfere with your milk supply. Babies drink differently from a bottle than from the breast. Don't let that difference undermine your success in breastfeeding.

When a baby drinks from a bottle, the suck does not need to be as vigorous as it does at the breast. Using a bottle could make your baby a bit lazy when returning to your breast.

Babies know when they are hungry and when they are full. If your baby acts satisfied—closes her or his mouth, stops sucking for a while, or turns away—you can assume your baby is satisfied, unless she or he needs to burp or is in the middle of a bowel movement. Then you can offer the bottle again, provided you heed baby's signals of fullness.

When you give your baby a supplementary bottle, follow your baby's cues as to the amount to give. There's no set amount that's right: your baby's behavior is the key to the correct amount.

If your baby is satisfied at 4 ounces, you should be too, even if milk remains. Eight ounces is probably plenty for a single feeding for older infants.

Breast Pumps

If you plan to skip an occasional feeding, you can leave baby a meal of breast milk by manually expressing milk ahead of time (see instructions on page 475 of this chapter). For women who need to express breast milk more than occasionally, breast pumps can be an important convenience.

You can purchase or rent breast pumps. Some are small manual pumps convenient for travel. There are also electric breast pumps that efficiently empty one or both breasts at one time. (See the illustration on page 593.)

Should you buy a pump or rent one? Even if you can afford to buy a pump, it may be better to rent one. An inexpensive electric pump may be far less efficient than an electric double-breast pump you can rent from a hospital or pharmacy. In the end, efficiency will serve you and your baby best by making it easy for you to continue breastfeeding.

Whatever the equipment, breast pumps are a special boon to mothers who want to breastfeed but must be separated from their babies for any reason, whether because they must return to work or because mother or baby must be hospitalized.

Breast pumps are especially helpful to mothers of premature infants who must be fed by tube in the hospital. Because of their immaturity and susceptibility to infection, mother's milk can be particularly important for such babies, and breast pumping makes it possible.

Milk can be pumped, collected and stored for a later feeding. If for some reason there is a period of time your baby cannot be breastfed, you can pump your breasts to maintain your milk supply. You can either discard the milk that you pump or save it. Breast milk may be used after it has been stored:

- For no more than six hours at room temperature
- In the refrigerator for up to five days
- Frozen in the freezer compartment of a refrigerator for up to two weeks
- In a separate or side-by-side freezer for up to six months

The same rules apply to breast pumping that apply to direct feeding—the more frequently you empty your breasts, the greater your milk supply will be.

Count on pumping your breasts every three hours for a newborn. If your baby is older, pump your breasts at the times you would be nursing.

Breast pumping is usually regarded as a substitute for breastfeeding, but for some women it can make it possible to breastfeed. The suction created by the machine can make an otherwise flat nipple stand out enough for baby to latch onto. For such women, having a breast pump on hand is helpful until baby learns to suck effectively.

Collecting and storing breast milk. Breast milk, like any other fresh food, is perishable. Follow these guidelines to maintain quality and preserve the nutrients in breast milk:

- Before pumping, wash your hands thoroughly with soap and water.
- It is not necessary to wash your breasts before pumping. Avoid nipple lubricants or creams.
- Pump directly into the bottles supplied in the kit. Most standard-sized bottles also will fit on the pump apparatus. Place a cap on each bottle.
- Label each bottle with the date and time of the pumping.
- You can combine the milk from each breast into one bottle. But don't "layer" milk, that is, don't combine milk from different pumping sessions in one bottle.
- After each use, wash the pieces in hot soapy water, rinse thoroughly and allow to air dry. You can use a dishwasher.
- Fresh breast milk can be stored at room temperature for six hours. However, it's safest to refrigerate it immediately.
- Freeze milk that will not be used completely by 48 hours after pumping.
- Full-term babies can be given breast milk that has been frozen up to six months. For premature babies, discard frozen breast milk that is older than three months.

Breastfeeding Myths

It's embarrassing. Most new mothers prefer privacy when breastfeeding. Experienced moms do too, but as they gain experience and confidence, they feel more comfortable nursing in the presence of others.

It takes little effort to maintain complete modesty when breastfeeding in public places. Wear clothing that lets you nurse freely without uncovering yourself or calling attention to what you're doing.

Many moms prefer loose, button-front tops that can be partially unbuttoned for feeding; opening from the bottom allows for greater modesty. The most discreet way to nurse is under the complete coverage of a very loose, oversized pullover top, such as a T-shirt. When you are ready to breastfeed, you simply slip your baby up under the garment. Most people won't even notice you're breastfeeding. You can also use a receiving blanket to cover your shoulder and baby.

I can't breastfeed because I'm going back to work. Some women choose not to breastfeed because they'll be returning to work and they can't imagine how breastfeeding can be compatible with employment. There are many ways to creatively combine work and breastfeeding. Moms these days are increasingly learning to do both, and employers are becoming more cooperative (see page 592).

I won't have enough milk. Many women quit breastfeeding after a few short weeks because of concerns about the adequacy of their milk supply. Some believe they run out of milk when in fact they run out of confidence.

What they need is guidance, knowledge about the breastfeeding process and support during the learning phase. New mothers need to know that the best way to increase the supply of milk any time is to feed the baby more often. If you have been nursing every four hours, try it every two hours or even once every hour during the day for a few days.

When your baby goes through a growth spurt, she or he will naturally want to nurse more often. If you are having a problem with your supply, regard it as a signal to increase the frequency of nursing. The more frequent and lengthy the feedings, especially in the early days, the smoother and faster you will establish an enduring milk supply.

Breastfeeding will ruin my figure. Some of the weight that you gain during pregnancy is intended as caloric reserve for nursing. Many lactating women experience a gradual weight loss—without dieting. However, a small number of women gain weight after childbirth—whether or not they breastfeed. Whether or not breastfeeding leads to weight loss, it helps your body return to its pre-pregnancy shape by stimulating contraction and shrinkage of your uterus. What's more, the milk supports the fatty tissue that makes up most of your breast. Women who develop sagging breasts after childbearing often blame breastfeeding, when the true cause is aging and the effect of gravity on the body.

My breasts aren't big enough for breastfeeding. The ability to breast-feed has nothing to do with the size of your breasts. Women's breasts normally differ in size and shape, but every woman's breasts are designed for their unique purpose—to nurture babies. Breast size is largely due to fat tissue, which is laid down at the time of puberty under the guidance of hormones. The size of the mammary glands inside the breast is what counts for producing milk, and mammary glands are the same regardless of breast size. Women with small or medium-sized breasts generally experience an enlargement of the breasts during pregnancy and the early months of nursing. After several months of nursing, the breasts usually reduce in size. In large-breasted women, breast size usually stays the same during nursing as during the last months of pregnancy.

Breastfeeding will restrict my lifestyle. Having a baby and caring for him or her will certainly change your lifestyle, but breastfeeding may be the least restrictive option. You never have to carry equipment. You never run short. And you never have to heat anything; milk is always at the ready. You can go virtually anywhere you can carry a baby. Even if you decide to travel to remote or foreign areas, your baby is well protected against gastrointestinal infection or other sources of contamination adults are often susceptible to. Many new parents, especially active ones, are surprised at the degree of freedom they experience to travel and engage in other activities during baby's first year. Because of the natural portability of baby's food supply, this freedom is greatest if you are breastfeeding. What's more, breastfeeding can allow you some freedom to be apart from your baby too. With a bit of advance planning, you can pump your breasts beforehand and leave milk for your baby for feeding times you plan to miss.

There's nothing I need to learn—breastfeeding is natural and easy.
Although breastfeeding is natural, it is a learned skill. Most women in America today grow up without the opportunity to observe other women breastfeeding. In other cultures, such an opportunity serves as a way of absorbing fundamental knowledge about breastfeeding and observing how new mothers handle the common problems that can be expected to crop up. Even for them, what appears natural has been learned over a long period.

The isolation that many new mothers experience after leaving the hospital compounds their lack of knowledge. It cuts off women from possible sources of support and information when they need it most. Many women today learn about breastfeeding by themselves and by trial and error, which can be frustrating.

Finding Assistance With Breastfeeding

There are many resources available to help with breastfeeding: lactation consultants, your health care provider, the baby's doctor or nurse, childbirth educators and the La Leche League. Help is usually only a phone call away.

Lactation consultants are not physicians. Most often they are registered nurses who specialize in helping moms and babies master breastfeeding. They are trained in, and knowledgeable about, various breastfeeding issues and are experienced in teaching breastfeeding. Nurses in the newborn nursery are also helpful in getting mothers started at breastfeeding.

There are existing networks of women all over the country who are happy to share practical information on breastfeeding. The best known is the La Leche League, an organization that for many years has helped thousands of women in countries throughout the world. Your local telephone directory probably has a listing for a La Leche League representative in your area. Or your hospital or childbirth preparation class may have established a network of women who have experienced the doubts and difficulties you're encountering.

Bottle Feeding

There's a long history of efforts to feed infants successfully when mother's milk is unavailable. In the past, these alternatives have not always been healthful or practical. The study of infant growth and nutrition and improvements in infant formula now provide safe and practical alternatives to breast milk.

Kinds of Formulas

Most infant formula comes from cow's milk; it is extensively altered so that it closely mimics breast milk, with the right amount of carbohydrates and the right percentages of protein and fat. The U.S. Food and Drug Administration monitors the safety of commercially prepared formula. Each manufacturer must test each batch of formula to make sure it has the required nutrients. It is also tested to guard against inadvertent contamination, such as with lead or pesticides.

Infants have very high energy requirements. Infant formula, like breast milk, is designed to be an energy-dense food—more than half its calories are from fat. Many different types of fatty acids make up fat; those that go into infant formula are specifically selected because they are similar to those found in breast milk. These fatty acids help in the development of the brain and nervous system as well as in meeting your baby's general energy needs. The butterfat naturally found in cow's milk is replaced with certain vegetable oils to provide essential fats.

The most common sources of protein in infant formulas are either cow's milk or soybeans. For healthy full-term infants, formula based on cow's milk is generally regarded as the first choice. About 90 percent of infants in the U.S. who are fed formula will do best on this type of formula.

> ### Common brands and types of formula
>
> **Cow's milk-based**
>
> Enfamil
> Gerber Baby Formula
> Good Start
> Similac
> SMA
>
> **Soy protein-based**
>
> Isomil
> Nursoy
> ProSobee
> Soyalac
>
> **Protein hydrolysate formulas**
>
> Alimentum
> Nutramigen
> Pregestimil
>
> **Formulas for premature babies**
>
> Enfamil Premature
> Similac Special Care
>
> **Special formulas**
>
> Lactofree
> Similac PM 60/40

Soy formula is an alternative for babies with lactose intolerance. Lactose is a sugar naturally present in milk. The ability to digest lactose depends on the presence of an enzyme called lactase. A small percentage of infants—about 1 to 3 percent of all babies—are born without the ability to digest lactose. They develop abdominal cramps, bloating, watery diarrhea and excessive gas if they drink more than a small amount of milk. For these babies, soy formula, or a cow's milk formula with the lactose removed, is the food of choice.

Parents sometimes consider switching to soy formula when a baby has colic, spits up or is fussy. It is best to check first with your baby's health care provider. Some fussiness and irritability are normal for newborns.

If you choose to give your baby a soy product, an important distinction is in order. Be sure to choose a soy infant formula, not soy milk. Soy milk is not nutritionally adequate for infants.

For some infants who come from families with a strong history of milk allergy, an alternative to standard formulas is a special cow's milk formula known as protein hydrolysate formula. Although more expensive, it is less likely to cause allergic reactions because the proteins in it have been broken down in a process that mimics digestion. Soy formula is generally not recommended for infants who are allergic to cow's milk formula, because a large number of infants allergic to cow's milk are also allergic to soy proteins.

There are several other types of formulas for special needs. For example, there are formulas specifically designed for premature infants, containing more vitamins, minerals, protein and calories. There are also specialized formulas for babies born with specific disorders, such as PKU (phenylketonuria).

Standard cow's milk formulas contain many vitamins, but most are relatively low in iron. Iron deficiency is generally not a risk in the first few months, but it can occur later in the first year. Many health care providers recommend starting formula-fed infants right off with iron-fortified formula; others prefer to begin iron supplementation after a few months. Infant formulas are available with and without supplementary iron. Check with your baby's health care provider in deciding on which is best for your baby.

Formulas come in three preparations: powdered, concentrated liquid and ready-to-feed liquid. Both the powdered and concentrated liquid formulas must be reconstituted with a specified amount of water.

Ready-to-feed formula is the most convenient. It is also the most expensive, especially when purchased in disposable bottles; you pay a price for convenience. Although it may be too expensive for general use, there are times, especially in the early months, when prepared formula in prepared bottles is very handy. You may want to keep a package on hand for quick use, perhaps by the baby-sitter. The ready-to-feed form is also handy for traveling.

There are many bottles and nipples on the market. It makes little difference which nipples you use, provided you do not select the overly soft nipples, designed for use by a premature baby, for a full-term baby. Some babies will prove to be a bit picky. It may be the way they suck, the size of their mouths or the shape of the roofs of their mouths, but they will make a fuss until you discover the right size nipple for them. Consistency is important; don't keep switching types of nipples. Remember, too, that old nipples can become hard and stiff; if so, it is time to buy new ones.

Regardless which nipple you choose, it is important to control the speed with which milk flows from the nipple. Milk flow that is either too slow or too fast can cause your baby to take in too much air, leading to stomach discomfort and the need for frequent burping. You can test the flow by turning a partly filled bottle upside down and timing the drops. About one a second is about right for the average baby. If the flow is too fast, you need a new nipple. If it is too slow, you can enlarge the nipple. Force a round wooden toothpick into the opening and, with the toothpick in place, boil the nipple for five minutes. Allow it to cool completely before testing it again.

There are several types of bottles. Lightweight plastic bottles have replaced the traditional glass bottles. Some bottles are shaped to better fit a baby's hands. It makes little difference to your baby which you choose. There are, however, two aspects of bottles that require special attention.

First, bottles come in two sizes, 4 ounces and 8 ounces. Remember, they are not an indication of how much your baby needs to drink in a feeding. Your baby may need less, or more, for any given feeding.

Second, in bottles that use disposable bags inside, the ounce markers on the side of the holder can be inaccurate indicators of how much the bottle contains. As a result, it is important not to mix formula powder or concentrate directly in the disposable bags. Use an accurate measuring container or cup for mixing formula to the correct concentration. Measure the water, then add the appropriate amount of powder or concentrate.

Types of Bottles and Nipples

Equipment needs

- Four 4-ounce bottles (optional, but useful in the beginning)
- Eight 8-ounce bottles
- Ten nipples
- Eight nipple rings
- Eight nipple covers
- One bottle brush
- One nipple brush

Preparation

Whatever type and form of formula you choose, proper preparation and refrigeration are essential, both to ensure the appropriate amount of nutrition and to safeguard the health of your baby.

New babies have few defenses against germs, even the common germs in our everyday environment; it takes a while for your baby to build up immunity. Even though it is no longer deemed necessary to sterilize formula at home, you still need to take some precautions to protect your baby. It is important to minimize the danger of bacterial contamination of your baby's formula by preparing and storing formula safely.

Wash your hands before handling formula or the equipment you use to prepare it. This is especially important if you have pets and handle them or their food.

Before every use, wash, rinse and dry all the equipment you use to measure, mix and store formula. If you use formula that comes in cans, it's advisable to keep a separate can opener just for the purpose. Be sure to wipe the top of the can carefully with a clean towel or napkin before you puncture the top.

After you open the container of powdered or liquid formula from which you will prepare your baby's bottles, close it promptly. Keep it tightly covered. Liquid formula can be kept in the can, but it must be covered and then refrigerated once it is opened. You can safely store opened cans this way for 24 hours; throw away any formula left in the can after that time, even if it has been refrigerated all that time.

Always mix powdered formula or concentrated formula with the exact amount of water the manufacturer specifies on the label. Using too much or too little water can be dangerous for your baby. If the formula is too diluted, your baby does not get enough nutrition for growth needs or to satisfy hunger. Your baby could also receive an excessive amount of water. Formula that is too concentrated can be even more dangerous. It puts a serious strain on a baby's digestive system and kidneys and can lead to dehydration.

Do not take shortcuts in measuring the ingredients. If you are using powdered formula, fill the scoop provided and shave off any excess with the flat of a knife; don't use a spoon or any other curved surface. Do not pack the powder. When using liquid concentrate, you can pour directly into the bottle to the exact measurement or into a measuring cup. Always hold the bottle or cup to eye level to check the amount; make sure that the quantity is exactly level with the correct measurement mark.

If you prepare and fill several bottles at one time, place any that are not for immediate use in the refrigerator. Keep bottles refrigerated until your baby is ready to feed, but empty any filled bottles remaining unused after 24 hours, even if refrigerated.

Once you warm a bottle, never put it back in the refrigerator, even if your baby goes back to sleep before you are able to give the bottle. If your baby leaves milk in a bottle after a feeding, even if most of it, do not put the milk back in the refrigerator. Throw out leftover milk once it's been warmed.

Cleaning Bottles

The days of sterilizing bottles are over. Unless your water supply has bacterial contamination, you do not need to sterilize bottles. It is sufficient to wash the bottles in a dishwasher or to hand wash them carefully with hot, soapy water. Use a bottle brush to clean hard-to-reach surfaces of the bottles. Pay special attention to the threads of the screw top, where formula tends to collect. Then put the nipple assembly on the bottle and squeeze the soapy water through the nipple to clean it. Rinse both the nipple assembly and the bottle well. Be sure to also wash the nipple covers. Rinsing and cleaning each bottle shortly after use prevents the buildup of dried milk and makes the cleaning process easier.

Is Your Water Safe?

If you are planning to use either powdered formula or liquid concentrate, both of which must be mixed with water, then the water you use in preparing your baby's milk is an important part of the formula. You need to make sure that the water contains no hidden contaminants.

If the water you drink comes from the municipal water supply of a large city, be confident that your water is safe. Regulations require that your water go through several steps of purification before it reaches your faucet. Smaller communities may find compliance difficult because of limited financial resources. If in doubt, check with your local water utility. Use cold, unsoftened tap water for preparing your baby's formula.

Well water sometimes poses a problem. If your house is supplied by well water, have your water supply checked. You need to be sure it does not contain trace levels of contaminants or heavy metals, such as lead. Well water sometimes contains such substances in amounts adults can tolerate but that pose a danger to babies. Bacterial contamination and nitrate content, for example, are potential problems. Bacteria can seep into ground water deposits from animal or human wastes, and nitrates are a result of fertilizer use. Large amounts of nitrates in well water used to prepare formula may lead to an illness known as methemoglobinemia, which can occur in adults but occurs more frequently in infants 3 to 12 months old.

If you are unsure of the water supply, use bottled water to prepare formula. Contact your county or state health department if you have questions about your well water supply or to arrange for testing.

Water caution

No matter the source of your water, it is advisable to take some simple precautions when preparing your baby's bottles.

- Whether cleaning the bottles or mixing the formula, let the water run for two minutes before using it. This precaution can help flush out impurities that may collect inside water pipes. It will also help guard against lead contamination. Older homes—those built before 1930—often have water pipes that contain lead. Even if the interior pipes have been replaced since then, the main line, bringing water into your home, may contain lead. Lead can get into the water from gradual corrosion of old pipes.

- Always use cold water for mixing formula. Hot water draws more lead out of pipes and so may have a higher lead level.

- Do not boil water intended for your baby's formula. "Sterilizing" the water by boiling it should not be necessary. Bottled water would be the preferred substitute if there is concern about contamination of water supplies, such as on a farm or after a flood. Boiling water concentrates minerals naturally found in water and can concentrate impurities as well.

Heating Formula

Warming a bottle of formula before giving it to your infant is not necessary. Usually, formula is served at room temperature. If it is served cold, a young baby may refuse it. Older babies may readily drink a cold bottle.

The best way to warm formula is to place the filled bottle in a bowl or pan of hot water and let it stand for a few minutes. If you hear your baby starting to stir, you can take a prepared bottle out of the refrigerator and start to warm it. Then, by the time you are ready to feed your baby, the milk is ready.

Always test the temperature before giving your baby a warmed bottle. You want to make sure it is not too hot or too cold. Shake the bottle after warming it, to distribute the warmed milk evenly. Then turn it upside down and allow a drop or two of the formula to fall on your hand. It should feel comfortable, barely warm.

Microwave alert

It is safest not to use a microwave oven for heating infant formula in bottles. Although microwave ovens are popular and convenient, bottles of formula heated by microwave can pose a serious danger of scald injury to your baby. This is especially true for bottles with disposable liners. Microwave ovens heat liquids unevenly. There may be hot spots of formula that burn your baby's mouth. This can happen even when a bottle's surface feels comfortable to the touch.

You can heat water more safely than formula. A bowl of water can be heated in the microwave. This hot water can then be used to warm the bottle. Alternatively, a measured amount of water can be heated in the bottle by microwave. Powder or concentrate is then added to the warm water and mixed thoroughly.

If you find yourself wanting to directly heat a bottle of formula in a microwave, you can do so provided you observe the following precautions:

- Use the microwave oven for heating formula only when amounts are 4 ounces or more.

- The bottle must stand up in the oven; do not use a small-capacity microwave oven that would require laying a capped bottle on its side.

- Keep the bottle uncovered (no nipple) during heating; this is essential to allow excess heat to escape.

- For 4-ounce bottles, heat at maximal setting for no more than 30 seconds.

- For 8-ounce bottles, heat at maximal setting for no more than 45 seconds.

- Replace the nipple assembly after heating.

- Turn the bottle upside down 10 times (you don't need to shake it vigorously); this is essential to eliminate the difference in temperature between the top and the bottom of the bottle and to eliminate hot spots.

- Always test the formula by placing several drops on your hand.

- Formula should feel cool to barely warm to the touch.

How to Bottle Feed Your Baby

Feeding is a very important experience for your baby. Every time you respond to your baby's cries of hunger in a timely way, you are teaching your baby to trust that the world is a safe place where important needs are met. It is also important to make sure feeding times are comfortable and enjoyable for you, so that you can provide the caring environment that will help your baby develop.

Holding your baby. The first step to rewarding feeding times is to make yourself comfortable. Cradle your baby in one arm, hold the bottle with the other and settle into a comfortable chair, preferably one with broad, low armrests. You may find yourself experimenting in the early days to find just the right combination of chair and position you and your baby like.

Support your arm by resting it on the broad arm of a chair, or by putting a pillow on your lap under your baby.

Pull your baby in toward you snugly but not too tightly, cradled in your arm with her or his head raised slightly and resting in the bend of your elbow. The semi-upright position makes swallowing much easier.

Now that you are ready to start the feeding, help your baby get ready. Using the nipple of the bottle or a finger of the hand holding it, gently stroke your baby's cheek lightly, near the mouth, on the side nearest you. The touch will cause your baby to turn toward you, often with an opened mouth.

Then touch the nipple to your baby's lips or the corner of the mouth. Your baby will open her or his mouth and gradually begin sucking.

Holding your baby during feedings can be soothing and rewarding. Sometimes busy parents are tempted to put their babies to bed alone, with a bottle propped up to maintain a steady flow. There are many reasons why you should avoid putting your baby to bed with a bottle. Here are a few:

- Your baby could choke. Your baby is not able to push the propped bottle away from her or his mouth.

- Just as much as your baby needs formula to grow, your baby thrives on human contact. The feeding experience is nature's way of ensuring that your baby gets plenty of close contact that is positive and rewarding.

- Putting your baby to bed with a bottle of formula promotes tooth decay. When a baby snoozes with a bottle in the mouth, there is prolonged contact between the baby's gums and teeth and the sugars in milk. Baby-bottle tooth decay can destroy your baby's teeth as they are developing.

Feeding time should be comfortable for both of you. Hold your baby securely, but not too tight, and position the bottle at an angle that keeps the nipple filled with milk.

Positioning the bottle. For your baby to suck properly, and to be rewarded with milk instead of air, you have to hold your baby's bottle in the right position. The bottle should be tilted so that the nipple fits back in your baby's mouth and the nipple is always full of milk. The bottle should be pointed down at an angle of about 45 degrees. The bulbous tip of the nipple should lie well back in your baby's mouth.

Holding the bottle at a 45-degree angle keeps the nipple full of milk. If the bottle is held too flat, the nipple fills with air as well as milk; your baby will swallow more air, which can lead to discomfort. Sometimes the nipple will flatten and your baby will not be able to get anything out of it at all. If this happens, gently pull the bottle against your baby's suction until it releases from your baby's mouth. Air will then bubble back into the bottle. You can resume feeding, holding the bottle so the bottom is tilted well upward.

In addition to holding the bottle at the proper angle, you need to hold it steady. If you hold the bottle too loosely, your baby will have trouble applying suction against it; the bottle will slip around in her or his mouth.

Amounts and schedules. Feed your baby on demand. Over time, your baby will come to trust that when hungry, she or he will be fed and will not need to fret with anxiety or signal you by prolonged crying.

Newborns have small stomachs and prefer small but frequent feedings. Your baby will take in as much milk as she or he needs, and no more. You can expect to feed your newborn at least six to eight times a day. There is a great deal of variability from infant to infant—in the way they eat, how much they eat, how often they eat—and babies change from day to day and feeding to feeding. Your baby may prefer a larger feeding at one time of day and a smaller feeding at another. Don't worry: You and your baby will figure it out together.

You can start with feedings of 2 to 3 ounces. It is not necessary to use a small bottle—just fill a regular 8-ounce bottle only partially. A small bottle, however, can help you maintain a realistic picture of your baby's needs and minimize pressures to overfeed your baby. As your baby gets older, she or he will probably want fewer but larger feedings.

As with breastfed babies, if your baby is producing six to eight wet diapers a day and seems satisfied after eating, you can rest assured that your baby is getting enough nourishment.

The following is a guide to how much and how often you can expect to feed a young infant. These amounts are approximations. They are based on the needs of an average-sized baby. If your baby is smaller, she or he will need slightly less and, if larger, possibly a bit more.

Your baby's age	An average feeding in ounces	Feedings in a typical day	Average total ounces daily
First 2 weeks	2-3	6-8	22
2-8 weeks	3-5	5-6	28
2 months	4-6	4-5	30

Resist the temptation to expect your baby to finish a bottle. That's the way eating problems start. Your baby is the best judge of when she or he is full. Watch for cues—turning the head away, arching the back or pushing the nipple out of the mouth with the tongue.

Burping Your Baby

When babies suck at the breast or at the bottle, they swallow a certain amount of air. Eventually, it gathers into a bubble in a baby's stomach, exerting pressure that can make a baby quite uncomfortable. Burping is the release of the swallowed air. Some babies are better than others at burping. Often, a baby needs to be helped with the process.

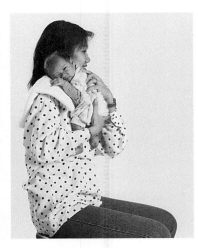

Hold your baby facing toward you against your chest and shoulder so that your baby's head is slightly above your shoulder and supported by it.

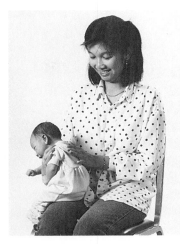

Sit your baby on your lap, facing sideways and leaning slightly forward. Support your baby's chest and head with one hand.

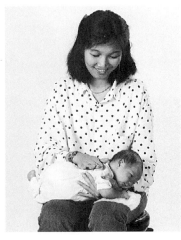

Lay your baby stomach-down across your lap.

In general, breastfed babies need less burping than bottle-fed babies. They probably take in less air because mouth-to-breast creates a more efficient suction than mouth-to-bottle. If you are breastfeeding your baby, it is not necessary to interrupt feedings to burp your baby. Generally, burping your baby twice during a feeding is sufficient—once after nursing from each breast.

Bottle-fed newborns need more frequent burping. You might try burping your bottle-fed baby after every 2 ounces. Or, following your baby's cues, take a burping break when your baby indicates lack of interest by turning away, refusing to open her or his mouth or arching the back.

Here are some tips to keep in mind:

- Remember to protect your clothing by putting a towel or cloth diaper on your shoulder or your lap. You can help your baby get the bubble up by gently patting the back or alternating gentle back patting with a rubbing motion.
- Newborns do not need to burp with every feeding.
- Don't spend more than a minute or two trying to burp your baby. If your baby doesn't burp in that time, she or he probably doesn't need to release air.

After a big burp, your baby may feel hungry again. Give your baby a little more time to suck. But be sure to remove the nipple from your baby's mouth as soon as she or he has finished drinking. Sucking on an empty nipple puts more air in your baby's tummy, making her or him uncomfortable.

Spitting Up

Spitting up is normal in all babies and is especially common in newborns. Babies may even vomit what seems like an entire feeding. Of course, vomiting can be a sign of illness, so if your baby is acting sick in other ways, or if vomiting persists, call your baby's health care provider.

Some babies are born spitters. Theirs is a case of physical immaturity; the muscles between the esophagus and stomach (the esophageal sphincter muscles) are not well coordinated yet. As the baby matures, often by two months, such nuisance spitting up is less of a problem.

Other babies spit up more because of the way they eat. Babies who gulp when they eat may be more likely to swallow a lot of air. When the air comes up, so does some of their latest meal.

Why Not Cow's Milk?

During the first year, don't be confused about what type of "milk" is appropriate for your baby—you have two choices, either breast milk or formula. Cow's milk—the kind that comes in a jug or carton at your local market—is a fine food for children, but not before your baby is a year old.

- Cow's milk is not suited for the intestines and kidneys of infants. Although it has about the same number of calories as breast milk, it has about three times as much sodium and three times as much protein. The protein produces large, indigestible curds in a baby's stomach. The protein puts a larger load on the baby's kidneys and increases the risk of dehydration.

  Because of the action of the protein in cow's milk (lactalbumin) on the intestine, cow's milk causes a microscopic blood loss in babies. This blood loss is not so obvious that a parent can notice it in the stool, but it can lead to anemia through iron loss.

- It can cause allergic responses. Cow's milk protein is also a foreign protein that can cross through the immature, highly permeable intestine into a baby's circulation and lead to allergic conditions.

- It may not contain sufficient fat. Infants have a need for fat; it is especially important for the developing brain and is an important source of calories. At least 50 percent of the calories in breast milk and formulas come from fat. Young children should not be fed skim milk, which has no fat, or low-fat milk, such as 1- or 2-percent milk.

CHAPTER TWENTY-NINE

Your Baby's First Two Weeks

You're finally home. When you left home to go to the hospital, you left your personal place of retreat, your haven. Now that you've returned, you may see it differently. Now it's your baby's home too—this little person's place of comfort and security.

For months, you've dreamed of bringing a baby into your home. You've probably wondered how life would change with the addition of your baby. Whatever is ahead, you know that you and baby have many adjustments to make as you become a family.

A bicycle built for two—if you've ever ridden one, you may be reminded of that experience often during the first two weeks after birth. Tandem bicycles are wonderful. They build relationships and promote teamwork. At least one person always gets to enjoy the scenery. But tandem bikes are like parenting an infant in two important ways.

First, beginning attempts can be tough. Synchronizing efforts is difficult. When one person is ready to go full steam, the other may want to coast. You can't get up to speed at first, so sometimes you wobble. In the beginning, you often stop and start over again. And sometimes you may even fall.

Second, people watching from the sidelines tend to believe it's easier than it looks.

In these first two weeks you may feel as though you and your baby are learning to ride a tandem bike. You may wobble a bit. You may not seem to cover much ground. You may have trouble working as a team. You may even seem to be going in different directions. And you'll hear lots of comments from the sidelines.

Although being a parent is a personal journey, many others have been down the same path before and succeeded. You will too. The minor troubles and fumbles of beginning parenting will not harm your baby. Here's one doctor's story:

"I was examining the 2-week-old baby of a new mother. She had had a great pregnancy. I thought she was doing a wonderful job as a mom.

"As I examined the child and was commenting on how good things were, she burst into tears. I wondered what terrible thing was going on. Through the

tears, she said, 'I just can't believe it; the baby is growing up well in spite of me.'

   "I remembered my own children and realized she was speaking for all good parents."

This mother was voicing the uncertainty and strong sense of responsibility that parents feel. Even when being a parent is difficult, try to relax and enjoy it. Don't try to be perfect. Your baby is a resilient little person.

During the first few days at home, your baby's reactions may surprise you. Still adjusting to the change from the womb to the nursery, your baby may take some time to process the new environment. New sounds, sights and touches may overwhelm your baby, who may retreat into sleep.

But your baby, when awake, is ready to take on this new world. Babies can see our faces and objects near them; they enjoy listening to human voices— especially their mothers'—as well as new sounds.

Each baby is different. Your baby's appearance, rate of growth, range of abilities and displays of personality will all be unique. As you embark on this journey with your child, take your eyes off the mile markers and take time to enjoy the companionship and scenery.

Growth and Physical Changes

During the first two weeks of your baby's life, you may not see dramatic growth. But this tiny body is going through many changes in the adjustment from life in the uterus. Through these first days of discovery, as you get to know this indi- vidual you brought home, you may notice these changes:

- The puffy, swollen eyelids of a newborn will subside in the first few days after birth. The fluid that causes this swelling is necessary to tide your baby over until feeding is established.

- Newborns, even male newborns, have swollen breasts in the first days after birth. This is normal and is a result of the mother's hormones passed to the baby in the uterus. During the first few days after birth, small amounts of fluid may be discharged from the baby's breasts.

- The feet and legs of newborns commonly look bowed or bent. Because their bones are pliable, they bend to fit snugly in the uterus. Their legs and feet gradually straighten; corrective measures are rarely needed.

- You may notice fine hair, "peach fuzz," covering your baby. This is called lanugo and gradually disappears over the first few months.

- Some blueness of the hands and feet is normal and may continue for a few weeks. However, a blue color of the lips and tongue may indicate heart or lung problems and should be reported to the baby's health care provider.

- Jaundice, indicated by a yellow tint of a baby's skin and the white of the eyes, may show up on the second or third day of life. Jaundice is caused by the inability of the baby's liver to deal efficiently with excess red blood cells that were needed in the uterus. As the liver catches up, the yellow tint will disappear, usually during the second week, although it may last longer in breastfed infants.

- Most young infants have dry, peeling skin—especially on their hands and feet—for the first few weeks. Rashes and birthmarks are also common.

Your baby's skin

The blemish-free babies in magazine ads may make you envious in the early weeks as you realize your baby's skin is less than flawless. Most babies—even those who later are in magazine ads—have rashes or blemishes in the early weeks. Most of the time, your baby's skin conditions are treated easily.

Common, temporary skin conditions

- Cradle cap—crusty, scaly skin on the baby's scalp. Periodic shampooing should help. If cradle cap persists, your baby's health care provider may suggest a medicated lotion or other treatment.

- Erythema toxicum—blotchy red rash, sometimes with yellowish centers. Most newborns have this rash. It most often appears on the face and torso. It generally disappears without treatment.

- Heat rash—fine red spots usually under the chin or on upper chest or arms. This rash may develop as a result of your baby being wrapped too warmly; it will probably disappear without treatment.

- Milia—tiny (pinpoint) white spots on the nose and cheeks. More than half of newborns have these cute little newborn spots. Milia eventually disappear and do not require treatment.

- Neonatal pimples—about 20 percent of babies have pimples at birth or in the first one or two months after birth. Periodic cleaning with mild soap and water is usually adequate. Neonatal pimples do not indicate that your child will have skin blemishes such as acne later in life.

- Peeling, dry skin—dry skin on the feet and hands is common in the first two weeks and will respond to over-the-counter lotions such as Eucerin, Vanicream, Nivea or Lubriderm.

- Diaper rash—redness caused by moisture, chafing of diapers or the acid in urine or stool. Frequent diaper changes may prevent the rash, but most newborns have diaper rash periodically because their skin is tender. To treat the rash, change the diapers frequently, and use a protective cream or ointment. Check with your baby's doctor or nurse-practitioner if the rash isn't improving.

- Yeast infection—a persistent, bright red rash in the diaper region that usually follows a diaper rash. Yeast infections are caused by a microorganism (*Candida albicans*) that flourishes in a warm, moist environment. If your baby has a yeast infection, an antifungal cream will help. In addition, frequent diaper changes will help promote dryness.

An important note: Although rashes are common and most often treatable at home, have your baby examined if you notice a rash that's purple, crusty or weepy or has blisters.

Birthmarks

- Salmon patches—Sometimes affectionately called "stork bites" or "angel kisses," these reddish or pink patches often occur above the hairline at the back of the neck, on the eyelids or between the baby's eyes. These marks are caused by collections of capillary blood vessels close to the skin. They fade within a child's first two years.

- Mongolian spot—This is the traditional term, but you may hear it called blue-gray macule of infancy. These large, blue-gray birthmarks sometimes resemble bruises. They are more common in dark-skinned babies, appearing on the lower back, less commonly on the buttocks and legs. They usually disappear later in childhood.

- Café-au-lait spots—As the name implies, these permanent birthmarks are light and coffee-colored, occurring most commonly on the baby's torso, arms and legs.

Weight Gain

In the first days after birth, all babies lose weight. Your baby will start to regain weight after four or five days, at the rate of about ½ to 1 ounce each day. This increase is difficult to monitor on a day-to-day basis, but by the two-week medical checkup, your baby will have regained birth weight and may have gained as much as a pound more.

Length

Generally, babies grow about 1 inch a month during their first year. By your baby's two-week medical checkup, you can expect a maximal increase of a little less than 1 inch.

Stools

The range of "normal" for a newborn baby's bowel movements is broad. Babies usually have wet diapers with every feeding, but they may have stools as frequently as after every feeding, as infrequently as once every week or, most often, in no consistent pattern.

You may notice your baby's stools differ in color. The different colors may indicate how fast the stools moved through the intestinal tract. In the upper part of the tract, stools take on a green color. As they move through the tract, they become yellow, orange, then brown. All of these colors are normal and are not indicative of diarrhea. A baby has diarrhea when the stools are watery, mixed with mucus and frequent. Mild diarrhea is common in newborns. If the diarrhea persists, call your baby's doctor or nurse-practitioner.

Constipation is not usually a problem for young infants, especially breastfed babies. Babies may strain, grunt and turn red-faced during a bowel movement, but these signs do not mean they are constipated. A baby is constipated when bowel movements are hard and infrequently passed.

Social Development: Your Baby's World

You've waited nine months to meet your baby and get acquainted. You've worked to prepare a place for this child in your home and family. You've anticipated quiet times of talking to your baby, studying the tiny features and sharing some of your dreams for this new life. But now that you're finally face to face, it may seem all your son or daughter wants to do is sleep and eat! When will you have the chance to get to know your baby better?

Remember, your baby is expending a lot of energy to make major adjustments from life inside the womb to a new, stimulating world. Restoring that energy requires lots of rest and nutrition. Feeding times can be times of cuddling, talking to and enjoying your new baby.

There will be periods when your baby seems especially ready to get to know you. Watch for times when your baby is calm and attentive, with eyes open. Newborns spend about 10 percent of their time in this state, often called "quiet alert." These times are especially enjoyable for getting to know your baby.

Your baby's alertness is governed by an effective on-off control. When stimuli are overwhelming, your newborn can simply tune out. For example, you will notice the baby startle at a loud noise, such as the vacuum cleaner or the pounding of a hammer. However, when the loud noise persists, the baby will no longer react to it. Even very young infants seem to know how much stimulation they can take.

Your baby will use this same on-off system when dealing with you and others. Don't be offended. It's just your baby's way of saying, "I've had enough. This is all the information I can handle right now. Give me a while; I'll get back to you."

E ven as a newborn, each baby has a distinct personality. And you may be surprised at how your baby—who for months was a part of you—now seems so different from you. Each day, you'll notice more individual traits that are distinctly your baby's. What personality traits can you see at this age? Cuddly? Assertive? Calm? Inquisitive? Easygoing? Intense? Independent?

When your baby is quietly alert, take advantage of this time to get acquainted. And let your baby get to know you. Explore these methods of socializing:

How Your Baby Relates to You

- Babies prefer the human face over other patterns or colors. Move within your baby's best vision range (about 12 to 18 inches) and allow your baby to study your features.

- Give your baby an opportunity to imitate you. Choose a simple facial movement such as opening your mouth or sticking out your tongue. Slowly repeat the gesture a few times, then wait. See if your baby will make attempts to mimic your gesture. Don't be discouraged if your baby isn't interested in this game, or tires quickly.

- Sing, hum or talk softly. Watch for your baby's reaction. Although he or she may not turn toward the sound, you will notice that your voice can cause your baby to settle down or become quiet. You can try various sounds to see whether your baby shows preferences for some sounds over others.

- Take advantage of times to cuddle and touch your baby. Newborns are very sensitive to changes in pressure and temperature. Babies love to be held, rocked, caressed, snuggled, kissed, patted, stroked, massaged and carried.

The quiet alert time generally lasts a few minutes. If your baby seems to spend even less time in this stage, perhaps the baby is receiving too much stimulation. Try to reduce your play activities to include only one stimulus at a time. For example, instead of moving into your baby's range of vision and singing softly, sing from farther away.

Your baby may give you very direct signals when playtime is over. Watch for these clues to let you know the baby is tired and needs a break:

- Closing eyes
- Turning away or dropping arm and shoulders away from you
- Stiffening or clenching fists
- Irritability
- Beginning deep, rhythmic breathing
- Tensing up, arching back
- Avoiding your gaze

How Your
Baby Relates
to Others

In the first few days of life, your baby will probably have many visitors and lots of attention.

If you have friends or family coming in to help during the first days at home, be specific about the kind of help you need. Accept their offers of help with housekeeping, meal preparation or errands. Most helpers will want some one-on-one time with the new baby. Don't be afraid to be the gatekeeper, letting others know when your baby needs a break from the action. Watch your baby for clues of tiredness or overstimulation and help others see them too.

Language Development: Early Communication

When you talk to your baby, remember that high-pitched voices are most appealing to babies. Encourage the baby's father and male friends to talk, sing or hum to the baby. Let them know that "baby talk" isn't as silly as it seems; babies actually prefer soft, rhythmic sounds.

By two weeks, your baby will begin to make sounds other than crying. But during the first few days at home, most of the sounds coming from the crib may seem to be cries.

Crying

Crying is a newborn's only verbal form of communication. Cries varying in pitch and intensity may be your baby's way of communicating different messages, but it may take a while to distinguish the unique cries of your baby.

"Her crying just broke my heart," one new mother said. "I couldn't tell what she needed and I was taking it personally. But by three weeks I was starting to tell the cries apart and by six weeks I was an expert."

When your baby's crying seems incessant, run down a simple list to determine what might be needed: Does she need a clean diaper? Is he hungry? Does she need to be burped? Is he bored? Would a different person's touch help? Is something pinching, sticking or binding him? Is she too hot or too cold? Does he just need to cry awhile? Has there been too much excitement or stimulation?

Young babies cry an average of three or four hours a day. If you've done all you can do, but your baby is still crying, it may be best to make sure the baby's dry, full, comfortable and wrapped snugly and then take a break. The baby may need a 10- or 15-minute period alone, even if crying. Check on the baby every few minutes from a distance.

If your baby has a prolonged, inconsolable cry, contact your baby's health care provider.

Calming a crying baby

If your baby has been fed and diapered and is well rested but is still crying, try one of the following actions:

- Gently talk to your baby face to face.
- Hold or swaddle your baby's arms close to your body.
- Use gentle motion, such as carrying your baby in a front carrier, walking, swinging or rocking.
- Hold the baby tummy-down on your lap.
- Gently rub or pat your baby's back.
- Hold the baby in an upright position on your shoulder or against your chest.
- Put the baby in a car seat and go for a drive.

Sensory Development: Exploring a New World

Evaluating your newborn baby's senses can be difficult. Even though your baby cannot indicate a degree of interest, you will notice when an object, sound or smell is engaging. Watch for your baby to "settle down" or become quiet when something new is introduced.

Your baby is nearsighted and sees objects best within 12 to 18 inches. This is about the distance between your baby's face and yours during nursing. Provide objects for your baby to look at during alert times. In addition to the human face, babies are interested in simple, high-contrast objects. Many toy stores sell black-and-white toys, mobiles and nursery decorations. Brightly colored decorations are also interesting.

When your baby is quiet and alert, hold a simple object within sight distance. Slowly move the object to the baby's right or left. From birth, most babies—if not too tired—will briefly follow moving objects with their eyes. Some babies will also move their heads to follow moving objects, but don't be surprised if your baby chooses not to play this game yet.

At times, your baby may appear to be cross-eyed. Because their ability to control eye movement is still immature, many babies are cross-eyed at times.

Vision

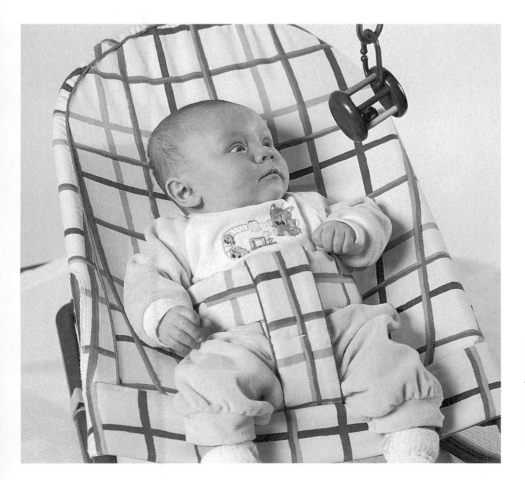

Your baby may enjoy studying a simple, bright-colored object for short times. However, most babies at this young age will quickly tire of this game, and they may not move their heads to follow a moving object.

Hearing New sounds will capture your baby's attention. However, because babies can so easily adapt to and "tune out" noises, your baby may react to a sound only once or twice. However, you may notice other subtle indications that your baby hears. In response to sounds, young babies may pause in sucking, widen their eyes or pause in their fussing.

Touch Young babies respond quickly to changes in temperature. They may startle when their skin is exposed to cold air and quiet again when they are wrapped warmly. Babies can detect differences in texture, pressure and moisture. These responses can work to your benefit when trying to calm your baby or rouse a sleepy baby for feeding.

You might notice your baby was born with several reflexes (automatic movements) related to touch:

- If you lightly touch one cheek, your baby will turn toward that cheek and open wide, ready to eat. This rooting reflex may be helpful in the early days of feeding.

- If you hold your baby's foot and press your thumb into the sole at the base of the toes, the toes will "grasp" at your thumb.

- When you press your thumb into a baby's palm, the baby will grasp tightly and the baby's mouth will often open. The baby may bring a hand to the mouth.

You may see some or all of these reflexes in your newborn baby. Soon your baby will outgrow them.

Smell Young infants have a keenly developed sense of smell. As young as 6 days old, they can distinguish their mothers by scent. Their interest in new, different smells can be noted by a change in movement and activity. However, similar to their sense of hearing, they easily become familiar with a new smell and no longer react to it.

Motor Development

Newborns are just learning to enjoy the freedom of unlimited movement. In their first few days, they may seem a bit reluctant to experiment with their mobility, preferring instead to be wrapped and held snugly. In time, however, babies learn to explore the range and limits of movement available to them.

From the day of birth, babies begin using their head and neck muscles. They can lift their heads up very briefly to look around. Babies may be able to briefly follow slowly moving objects or voices with their heads and their eyes by the second week.

When supported in a sitting position, babies will try to straighten their heads, but their neck muscles are still not strong enough to support their heads, which will drop forward. It will be several months before babies develop good head control.

A baby is born with a complete repertoire of reflexes. Many of them—like turning the head to avoid suffocation—are protective responses. Others, such as the rooting reflex, are transitional reflexes; they are present at birth but disappear when they no longer serve a purpose. Some additional reflexes you may observe include the following:

- Sucking—The sucking reflex is more than a mechanism for eating. Babies also suck to calm themselves. Ultrasound pictures show fetuses sucking their hands and fingers.

- Hand to mouth—Babies will try to find their mouths with their hands. This reflex may be why many babies bring their hands to the breast or bottle.

- Stepping—When firmly supported above a solid surface, with one foot on the surface, babies may step forward with the opposite foot and begin "walking" across the surface.

- Startle (Moro reflex)—When startled by a noise or a sudden movement, your baby may throw both arms outward and cry.

- "Fencing" (tonic neck reflex)—The classic fencing pose, one arm crooked and raised behind the head and the other extended away from the body, is common for babies. A baby lying faceup will often bow the body the opposite direction the head is turned and strike this pose. Sometimes, a little fist finds a clump of baby hair and can't let go.

- Smiling—In the first few days of life, most of your baby's smiles are involuntary. It won't be long, though, before you notice your baby smiling in reaction to a person or situation.

As you have opportunity—and your baby has energy—watch for some of these reflexes. But don't be discouraged if your baby isn't interested in showing off. These reflexes, present at birth, will diminish over the next few weeks, then disappear entirely as they are replaced by new, learned skills.

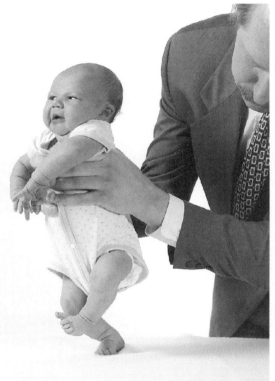

Of course, newborns can't walk, but when you hold them under the arms and let the soles of their feet touch the ground, they will place one foot in front of the other as if they are walking. This is called the stepping reflex. It disappears at about 2 months of age. Actually learning to walk and support their weight doesn't occur until nearly a year later.

Feeding and Nutrition

It may seem that most of your time in the first two weeks after birth is spent feeding your baby. Look at these feeding times as opportunities to be close to your baby, providing companionship, love and nurturing as well as nourishment. Keep in mind the importance of one-on-one, face-to-face contact between you and the baby during feeding times.

Feeding times are times of adjustment as you and your baby learn to work as a team. You will be surprised at how your baby displays his or her unique personality. The key at this point is learning to conform to your baby's temperament and schedule. "Giving in" to what the baby wants at this point will not encourage feeding or discipline problems in the future.

Pacifiers

Babies often suck as a means of calming themselves. Often, they need sucking beyond what is necessary for feeding. It's best to avoid using pacifiers until after nursing is well established.

It may be difficult to predict whether your baby will need a pacifier. Some parents who wanted their baby to take a pacifier have been disappointed when their baby preferred to suck on fingers or a thumb. Other parents who confidently predicted that their baby would never use a pacifier have been surprised when they realized that their baby needs one for the time being. To ease your baby's reliance on a pacifier later, use these techniques now:

- Encourage your baby to go to sleep without the pacifier.
- Find other methods for calming your crying baby other than the pacifier alone.

Water

Your newborn baby does not need any additional fluids beyond what is available through feedings. If you are taking your baby on an outing and begin to feel hot and thirsty, you should assume your baby is feeling the same way. At this age, babies may not sweat when hot, so watch for other clues of overheating, such as panting, crankiness or tiredness. An extra feeding may be needed to help baby quench a summer day's thirst. (For more information about protecting your baby from the sun, see page 633.)

Vitamin Supplements

Breast milk or infant formula provides all your baby needs for the first six months of life; additional vitamins generally are not needed.

During the last month of gestation, full-term babies "stock up" on iron. For premature infants, your baby's health care provider may prescribe iron or vitamin supplements.

Feeding Schedules

Although you're probably longing for some semblance of routine, your baby's feeding schedule is not going to provide that routine immediately. Although you can roughly estimate the amount of time between feedings, your baby's schedule will be erratic. During growth spurts, feedings will be more frequent for a day or two before settling back into a routine.

Bottle Feeding

During the first several weeks, most babies will be hungry six to eight times during a 24-hour period. However, there is tremendous variation among infants in how often and how much they eat. At first, your baby may be drinking about 2 or 3 ounces of formula at a time. Babies will generally give you signs that they are full—pushing the nipple out of their mouths, turning their heads away when you offer the bottle. (For more information on bottle feeding, see page 487.)

Breastfeeding

The key to success in the first days of breastfeeding is feeding your baby on demand, at the first indications of hunger. Because breastfeeding is a supply-and-demand operation, your baby's prompt and efficient eating will stimulate production of enough milk to meet the hunger. Also, prompt feeding will prevent common feeding problems such as an overly hungry baby who sucks too vigorously, an overly fussy baby too worked up to settle down and eat or breasts so engorged that the baby has difficulty latching on to them.

The synchronization of your baby's hunger and your body's milk production may take some practice. In the learning stage, breastfeeding may seem troublesome, discouraging and even painful. However, the best remedy for early breastfeeding problems is persistence. Within a few days, most breastfeeding problems will work themselves out.

When beginning breastfeeding, think in terms of prevention. Frequent nursing early on will prevent most breastfeeding problems from occurring. Your baby generally should be eating every one and one-half to three hours for a total of eight to 10 feedings a day, and the baby may spend 10 minutes on each breast.

As you begin breastfeeding, you may have several questions or concerns you'd like to discuss with an expert. Keep the phone numbers of your baby's health care provider, lactation consultant, peer support groups or other nursing mothers handy.

Mother's diet. Many women will tell about giving up various foods—such as onions, broccoli, garlic, beans and asparagus—while breastfeeding. Although it's true that some foods can noticeably alter the taste of breast milk, true allergic reactions in nursing babies are rare. If you believe a certain food causes a difference in your baby's disposition or stool patterns, it's unlikely that you need to eliminate it from your diet. Sometimes coincidental situations may cause you to suspect a food reaction, when in reality your baby is just having a tough day.

Many moms, even those who worked to avoid caffeine completely during pregnancy, may now want to have a cup of coffee or a caffeinated soda. If you drink large amounts of caffeine, you may notice irritability in your baby. However, one or two servings of caffeinated soda, coffee or tea each day should not cause a problem.

Alcohol can be passed on to your baby through breast milk. Your nursing baby is still in critical areas of development that can be hampered by the ingestion of alcohol. It's best to abstain from drinking alcohol while breastfeeding.

In families with a history of allergy to milk, a mother's ingestion of cow's milk can cause colic in her baby.

If you believe any food or drink you eat is causing a problem for your baby, make a note of your baby's reaction and discuss it with your baby's doctor or nurse-practitioner.

Sore nipples. Many nursing mothers have sore nipples when starting nursing. As with many breastfeeding problems, the best way to prevent sore nipples is to begin breastfeeding early with a frequent on-demand feeding schedule. However, if sore nipples do occur, these remedies may provide relief:

- Check the baby's position while feeding. The nipple should be toward the back of the baby's mouth; your baby should not be sucking directly on the nipple. (Proper latching on is reviewed on page 480.)
- Change the baby's nursing position.
- Allow nipples to air dry after nursing.
- Avoid nursing pads with plastic linings.
- Allow a drop of breast milk to air dry on the nipples between feedings.
- If using a lotion, make sure the nipple is dry before applying lotion.
- Apply ice on the sore nipple briefly before nursing.

Milk supply. The most common reason given by mothers who discontinue breastfeeding is that they believed their babies weren't getting enough milk. Unlike bottle feeding, when you're breastfeeding there is no easy way to measure how much milk your baby is getting. However, the supply-and-demand system of breastfeeding is designed to provide your baby with just the right amount of milk. It is rare that a mother cannot provide enough nourishment for her baby.

Watch for signals from your baby that will reassure you that he or she is getting enough milk. Do you hear your baby gulping when starting nursing? Does the baby seem satisfied after nursing? Do your breasts feel different, perhaps softer, after nursing?

Measurable clues of your baby's intake include wet diapers, number of stools and weight gain. However, these will differ greatly from baby to baby. Comparing your baby with another will not indicate whether yours is getting more or less nutrition.

On some days you may barely finish feeding your baby before cries of hunger start again. This crying is not necessarily a sign that the last feeding was inadequate. Perhaps your baby is ready to nurse again. When this happens, your baby is probably going through a growth spurt and for a day or two may require more frequent feedings before settling back into a new pattern.

Problems with let-down. The let-down of milk (see page 476) is called a "reflex," meaning it's an automatic response when baby begins to suckle. Rarely does anything interfere with this smooth process. When difficulties occur, they are most often related to psychological factors. Let-down may be inhibited by any of the following:

- Distractions
- A lack of needed privacy
- Embarrassment or anxiety about nursing
- Fatigue
- Pain

Most problems with milk let-down can be easily remedied by rest, change of atmosphere and support from family members and friends. Allow visiting "helpers" to relieve some anxieties by helping with household chores or older children.

Nipple confusion. If your baby has become experienced using an artificial nipple—a pacifier or bottle—before breastfeeding is firmly established, the result may be nipple confusion. Because different techniques of sucking are needed for bottle feeding than for breastfeeding, your baby may be confused when offered the breast again after using an artificial nipple and may not nurse effectively.

Babies who have trouble sucking. Babies are not always effective nursers. You may have an overly excited (and hungry) baby who cannot latch on well and so grasps and then loses the nipple. Or your baby may nurse just long enough to get a taste of milk and then pause before getting down to the business of feeding. The initial nursing may cause let-down, in which case the breast may become engorged. The baby may then have difficulty latching on well when he or she decides to really nurse.

Still other babies may nurse awhile, then rest before nursing again. Within a few days you should be able to determine when your baby is finished eating or is simply pausing to rest for a bit.

What your newborn needs most from you during feeding times is attention and social interaction. Make feeding time a time to develop trust and security. Hold your baby so eye contact is possible.

Sleeping Patterns and Habits

It's hard to estimate how much time your baby will spend sleeping during the first two weeks. Although it may seem like your baby never gives you any rest, you can expect your baby to sleep at least 12 hours a day, probably longer. Newborns may sleep for up to four and a half hours at a time, staying awake long enough to feed or for up to two hours before falling asleep again. But by the time your baby is 2 weeks old you will notice that the periods of sleeping and being awake are lengthening.

Babies have two stages of sleep, quiet sleep and active sleep. These stages alternate about every 30 minutes and will continue as long as the baby is sleeping. In quiet sleep, babies' faces and bodies are relaxed, with very little movement. You may notice a few startles or tiny movements of the mouth. The eyelids are still and breathing is regular. In active sleep, babies are more animated, moving their arms and legs or even their whole bodies and often making faces while they sleep. They breathe faster and their breathing patterns may not be regular. You can see eye movement under their eyelids, and their eyes may occasionally open. Like adults, they engage in rapid eye movement (REM) sleep and may even be dreaming during this stage.

Feeding sleepyhead

Undoubtedly there will be times when your baby rouses to eat, only to doze again when you begin feeding. Try one of these tips to feed your sleepy baby:

- Watch for and take advantage of your baby's alert stages. Feed during these times to prevent feeding a sleepy baby later.

- Partially undress your baby. Remember that your baby's skin is sensitive to changes in temperature. The coolness may rouse your baby long enough to eat.

- Rock your baby up into a sitting position. Just like the eyes of the "sleeping" dolls you may have had as a child, your baby's eyes often open when your baby is positioned upright.

- Give your baby a massage by walking your fingers up his or her spine.

- Stroke a circle around your baby's lips with a fingertip—clockwise and counterclockwise—a few times.

Baby's First Checkup

The baby's first medical checkup will probably be a low-key, relaxing appointment. The doctor or nurse-practitioner and the office staff will spend a little time getting to know you and your baby. They'll rely on you to provide answers to their questions, such as the following:

- How are you doing as new parents?
- How well is your baby eating?
- What has the baby's sleeping schedule been like?

- Does the baby seem to see and hear normally?
- What's your baby like? How active is your baby? Does your baby settle down easily after crying?

Your Baby's Growth

At the beginning of the visit, your baby's measurements will be taken—head size, length and weight. Head size is measured with a cloth or paper tape wrapped around the largest part of the head. Length is measured by stretching the baby out flat. Weight is measured on an accurate scale designed for weighing babies.

These measurements might be recorded in centimeters and kilograms. You might ask that they be written down for you in inches and pounds.

Your baby's measurements will be plotted onto a growth chart, which shows how your baby's height, weight and head size compare with those of other infants. But the most important information is how well your baby has grown since birth.

Although these charts help compare your baby with others, remember that the trend of your baby's growth won't follow along the exact line of the chart. Heredity, size at birth, growth spurts, illness and whether your baby was full-term at delivery all factor into your baby's growth patterns.

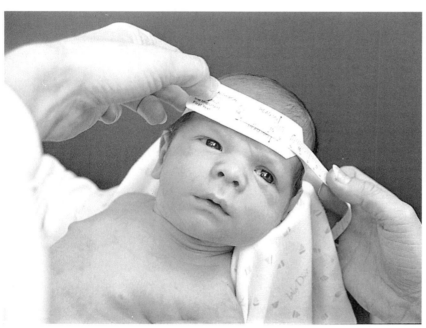

Measuring head circumference (the largest distance around the baby's head) is one way for your baby's health care provider to track growth.

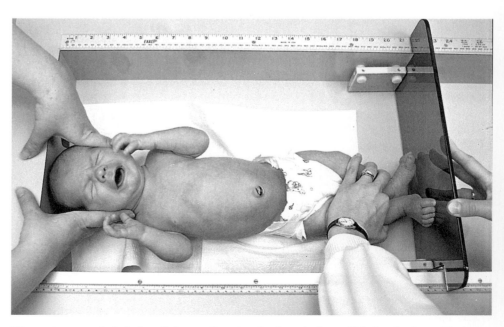

Measuring your baby's length is another standard part of a well-baby checkup. The procedure takes only a minute or two and is painless.

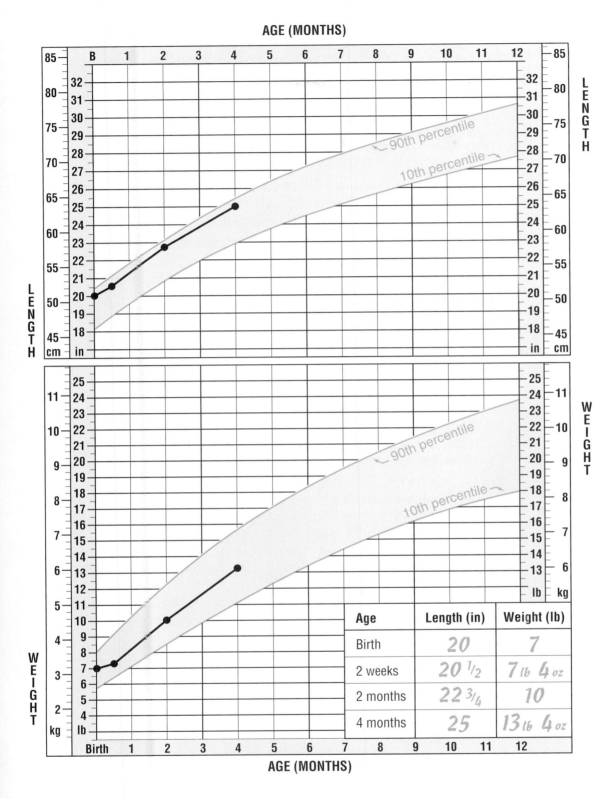

Age	Length (in)	Weight (lb)
Birth	20	7
2 weeks	20 ½	7 lb 4 oz
2 months	22 ¾	10
4 months	25	13 lb 4 oz

Throughout your baby's first year, your health care provider may record your baby's growth (length, weight, and head circumference) on charts similar to this one. In this simplified example, the baby has grown at a steady rate, as shown in the upward-sloping curves. Comparing the baby's length and weight indicates that the baby is well proportioned (length and weight are increasing at about the same rate). This baby's growth is in the average range. Babies whose height or weight is above the 90 percent mark on the chart are considered large, and those below the 10 percent mark are considered small.

How Are Things Going?

When the doctor or nurse-practitioner enters the room, he or she will probably ask you a few general questions about your baby, including, "How are things going?" This is your opportunity to bring up any concerns, frustrations or questions you have. Don't hesitate to write them down and bring the list with you. Sometimes you may feel that a question is personal and isn't directly related to the baby's health. However, your anxieties and concerns do affect your baby, so don't be afraid to ask any question you may have.

The Examination

The sequence and detail of your baby's examination will vary depending on your baby's mood, the questions you've asked, any noteworthy findings during the exam and how soon the baby will be examined again. Some common parts of the exam and their explanations follow:

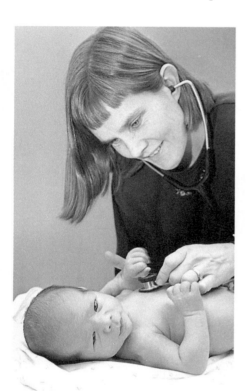

The first checkup is a time for the care-giver to evaluate your baby's health and to get better acquainted with your baby. It's also an opportunity for you to ask questions.

- Observing the overall responsiveness of the baby to the exam; does your baby act like a normal baby acts?
- Feeling the fontanelles (see the illustration on page 439), checking their size and softness
- Observing the baby's chest for signs of breathing difficulties
- Observing how the baby moves the arms and legs and whether muscle tone and strength seem to be normal
- Testing the baby's hips for smoothness of movement and proper placement of the hips within the hip sockets
- Feeling the abdomen for tenderness or masses
- Examining the genitals, including looking for an inguinal hernia
- Evaluating healing of a baby boy's circumcision
- Checking the navel; does it seem to be healing properly?
- Looking over the baby's skin for jaundice, rashes or birthmarks
- Listening to the baby's lungs (this is easy to do, even if the baby is crying); are the breath sounds normal?
- Listening to the baby's heart (this can be hard to do if the baby is crying). Is a murmur heard? If so, does it sound normal or worrisome?
- Peeking at the baby's eyes with an ophthalmoscope; do the eyes appear normal?
- Looking in the ears and mouth

Before the examination is completed, you will probably be asked again if you have any questions. If you want an explanation about any part of the exam, or have additional questions, now is the time to ask. Even if the office seems busy and there might not be time to discuss something today, you can always request another appointment or ask for recommendations on whom you could contact for more information.

When You Have Questions

There is nothing magical about the two-week time span before your baby's first medical checkup. You may have questions and concerns before this time. When calling with questions, the health care provider will need the following information to be the most helpful:

- Why are you calling? What are your concerns?
- What specific behaviors are causing your concern?
- Have you taken the baby's temperature? Does the baby have a fever?
- Is the baby eating and drinking? What? How much?
- Are you giving any medication? What? What dosage?
- Has the baby been exposed to illness? Is anyone else in the house sick?
- What have you tried to soothe or relieve the baby?

What Parents Worry About

Fussiness or Colic?

Many fussy babies are called "colicky," especially by concerned grandparents. Colic affects 10 to 20 percent of babies and is defined by these symptoms:

- Frequent fussy episodes, beginning about the second week of life
- Increased fussiness in the evening
- Prolonged, inconsolable crying for three or more hours

Colic typically peaks at about six weeks and then usually improves by three months, but parents of colicky babies can attest that those three months can seem unbearably long. If you have a colicky baby and find yourself frustrated, irritable and fatigued, you are not alone.

Experiment with various methods to calm your baby, but don't be discouraged if many of your efforts seem futile. Rocking and cuddling may help; try "white noise," such as the sound of a fan, humidifier or clothes dryer.

Be aware that your own anxiety and frustration over failed attempts to calm your baby may only increase the baby's frustration. Take a break and allow others to watch the baby so you can have some relaxation. If you're having trouble dealing with your crying baby, call your doctor or nurse-practitioner.

(For more information on colic, see page 541.)

Call for medical advice if your baby...

- Has a fever
- Is persistently irritable and inconsolable
- Shows no interest in eating or is feeding poorly
- Is vomiting forcefully
- Is lethargic, unusually difficult to arouse
- Has frequent diarrhea
- Has pale, light-colored, almost white stools
- Has a deepening yellow skin color
- Has a dusky, purplish hue to the lips and tongue
- Seems to sweat excessively when eating or crying
- Seems to have difficulty breathing

Umbilical Cord Care

The navel will heal best if the area around the umbilical cord is kept clean and dry. At least once a day, use a cotton swab to apply alcohol to the base of the umbilical cord. Once the alcohol has evaporated, dab the remaining moisture. Make sure the diaper is folded down, away from the umbilical cord, to prevent irritation.

It is not uncommon to see a dab of blood around the umbilical cord. A small amount of discharge does not indicate that the navel is infected. However, redness of the surrounding skin or a foul-smelling discharge may indicate infection and should be reported to the baby's health care provider.

The umbilical cord usually falls off by three weeks. Once the cord has fallen off, stop applying alcohol. The navel may "ooze" for a couple days after the umbilical cord falls off. Your baby can graduate to tub baths after the umbilical cord falls off.

Circumcision Care

Clean the diaper area gently and apply a dab of petroleum jelly to the end of the penis at each diaper change. This will keep the diaper from sticking while the penis heals.

In the first week, you may notice a yellowish mucus on the healing skin. This is a normal part of the healing and doesn't require cleaning.

Risk of SIDS

The term "SIDS" (sudden infant death syndrome), also referred to as "crib death," is used when an infant dies suddenly and unexpectedly during sleep.

Some conditions associated with a higher risk of SIDS (such as premature birth) are beyond your control. SIDS can't be predicted or prevented, but the following advice may help reduce the risk of SIDS:

- Sleep position—It's probably safest for young infants to sleep resting on their side or back, not on their stomach (see page 528).

- Diet—Breastfeeding may reduce the risk of SIDS.

- Secondhand smoke—Provide a smoke-free environment for your baby. This measure is as important during the baby's first year of life as it was during pregnancy.

- Room temperature—Your baby doesn't need a warmer environment than you do. If the temperature in the house is comfortable for you, it should be comfortable for your baby.

- Bedding—Babies should sleep on a firm mattress, not a beanbag or water bed. Avoid thick, fluffy padding under the baby, such as lambskin.

(More information on SIDS can be found on page 528.)

CHAPTER THIRTY

Baby From Two Weeks to Two Months

"What have we done?"

If you're asking that question, you're not alone. Most new parents reach a point at which expectations of pregnancy meet the reality of life with a new baby. Often, they're hit with doubts, questions and guilt.

"For the first month, I felt guilty because I wasn't enjoying motherhood as much as I thought I should," one new mom said. "I was worried people would think I was strange if I said anything."

It's perfectly normal to need time to adjust to the many changes that come with a new baby. You may wonder how your baby is fitting into the family, whether you're doing a "good job" as a parent and whether you'll ever have time for yourself again.

As you're going through these adjustments, your baby is making major adjustments, too. That tiny newborn you brought home is developing into a more predictable infant. And while you're thinking through the changes in your personal and social life, your baby is beginning to make social overtures. Just when you're asking, "What have we done?" your baby's first coos and smiles will begin to melt your doubts.

Social Development

At 2 months, most of your baby's social interactions are subtle. However, there are specific developments that point to your baby's continuing interest in building relationships.

From birth your baby is fascinated with faces. This fascination helps the baby learn language and sensory and social skills during the following months.

During the first two months of life, your baby will learn to smile. Although the first smiles are almost always due to gas, soon your baby will begin to smile in response to your talking, smiling and singing. During the second month, most babies begin communicating their moods and preferences with smiles.

515

By 2 months, more than half of all babies can recognize their parents. Babies show this recognition by reacting differently to their parents than to others and by more easily and quickly smiling for their parents than for strangers. They also begin to recognize objects by sight, before they have a chance to touch or taste them. A common example is when babies open their mouths for feeding after seeing their bottles.

Your baby is truly learning to recognize clues from others. Closely watching you and your responses and interactions will guide your child through continued social development.

Language Development

Early Communication

It's a treat when your baby first begins vocalizing. During the first two months of life, most babies begin to coo and make soft vowel sounds resembling "ooh" and "aah." A few babies may also begin early squeals and laughter. Most babies will continue to make sucking noises that soothe and calm them.

Talking to Your Baby

All of your baby's attempts at communication are unrefined at this stage. However, it's interesting to see the small developmental steps as the baby progresses. For example, watch your baby for subtle movements, expressions and gestures combined with vocalizations. Learning and interpreting this early body language will help you understand what your baby is communicating to you.

Although your baby will not understand your words at this age, talk to your baby in a pleasant voice. At 2 months, your baby may initiate a cooing game. If you respond to the cooing, your baby may "talk back" to you in a game of mimicry. Even if your baby doesn't respond by vocalizing, you may notice changes in the baby's movement when you speak. About half of all 2-month-old babies show specific responses to familiar sounds such as a parent's voice and will move their eyes or heads toward the sound of their mothers' voices, even when they can't see them.

When you take time out to talk face-to-face, give your baby a chance to "talk" to you in return, whether through vocalizations or body language. When you don't have time to talk one-on-one, your baby will still enjoy hearing your voice from across the room.

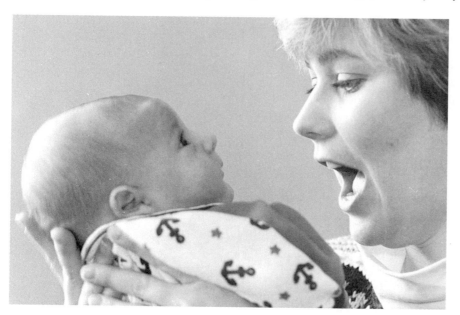

Talk to your baby, and give your baby an opportunity to "talk back." You'll both enjoy the experience, and your baby's response might surprise you.

Your newborn baby's crying patterns were no doubt confusing and frustrating to you. During the first two months, your child's different cries may become distinguishable to you, allowing you to respond more readily to your baby's specific need.

By the two-month mark, the crying's not over, but most babies are beginning to cry less often. Cumulative crying hours peak at 6 weeks, when babies generally cry about three hours each day. By 8 weeks, the average drops to two hours. (For more information on crying, see page 462.)

Crying Patterns

Sensory Development

As in many stages of the early years, the most important thing you can do for your baby's sensory development is allow the baby to be a part of your world. Your baby's sight, hearing and touch will develop when you expose your child to everyday activities. For example, watching you fold laundry gives your baby a chance to see color and movement, listen to your voice if you talk and even feel the textures of different fabrics if you brush them against your baby's cheek. At this age, your baby will be fascinated with the world of sound and activity within your home.

One of the most important tasks your baby has in the first days and weeks of life is learning to focus vision. At this age, babies are trying to focus both eyes together to see a single object. Because the tonic or "fencing" reflex (see page 505) in your baby is still strong, the baby has the advantage of always having an arm and fist to practice focusing on. And that extended fist is at the perfect distance for your nearsighted baby. At first, you may observe your baby staring at the extended arm and fist as if they had just appeared from nowhere.

Sight

Besides fists and faces, newborns and very young infants are fascinated by simple, high-contrast objects such as black-and-white checkerboard patterns and faces drawn with simple features. By 2 months, babies are beginning to prefer more complex designs, colors and various sizes and shapes. Having conquered focused vision, they are also learning to follow, or track, moving objects.

Providing visual stimulation for your baby is simple. Your everyday activity is fascinating to an infant. Just watching you cook, garden or exercise gives your baby a chance to observe movement and color. Other sights that might interest your baby include leaves, birds and cars outside the window; children playing; your mouth and expressions as you talk; ceiling fans; and mirrors. Your baby can watch any of these sights from the comfort of a carrier or a blanket on the floor.

You can use your baby's interest in bright toys and shiny objects to observe his or her ability to follow moving objects. Use shiny foil or a colorful toy, such as a hand puppet. Move the object side to side in front of the baby, then up and down. Objects moved up and down beside your baby's head will attract attention, but your baby probably won't be able to track vertical motion smoothly until about 3 months of age.

When providing toys and objects for your baby to look at, take into consideration the baby's motor development (see page 578).

Hearing

Babies as young as 1 month will respond to loud noises. Their responses include blinking their eyes, startling, frowning and waking from light sleep. Soft noises will also draw a response such as an increase in movement or a change in sucking movements. However, babies easily become used to noises and will tune them out if they're repeated.

You will soon be able to discern your baby's positive and negative responses to certain noises. Probably the sound that will most often elicit a positive response is the human voice. Your baby will love to hear you talk or sing. By 2 months, more than half of all babies recognize their parents' voices and respond with changes in movement or expression. They will also search for their mothers when spoken to, moving their eyes or heads to find the source of that familiar voice.

You can test your baby's interest in different sounds by holding a noisemaker (such as a bell or rattle) above your baby's forehead, out of sight. Lightly rattle the noisemaker and see whether your baby looks toward it. Then hold the noisemaker to the side of the baby's face and rattle it again. Keep in mind babies' ability to adjust to new noises. When babies hear the same noise several times, they no longer respond to that sound. So don't be surprised if your baby quickly tunes out this game.

Touch

Human touch is vital for every child. Your baby needs plenty of one-on-one contact (strokes, hugs, kisses and lots of affection) with mom and dad to learn security, trust and love. No one can teach your child these concepts better than you and your partner.

Changes in texture and environment are stimulating experiences for your baby. Babies enjoy fuzzy blankets, satin blanket edges, warm breezes, warm clothes from the dryer and stuffed toys.

Your baby will delight in gentle play and interaction.

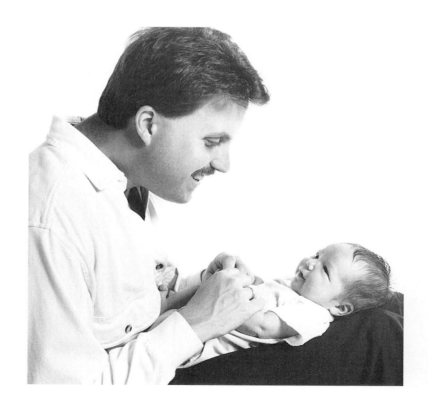

Motor Development

During the first two months, your baby is working hard on motor development—the baby's increasing ability to coordinate large and small movements. Motor skills include such activities as stretching, rolling, crawling and walking movements as well as grasping, reaching and pointing.

Jerky, abrupt reflexes from birth—such as the startle, crawling, grasping and tonic neck reflexes—are still present. But your baby has been practicing—stretching, moving, watching—and you can see the baby's movements becoming smoother and more controlled.

During the first two months, your baby is already learning how to get around. Don't leave your baby unattended on a changing table or any elevated surface. Babies at this age can't be trusted to stay in one place. They can use their feet to push off surfaces and scoot around. And even though they're just learning controlled rolling maneuvers, they can unexpectedly flip themselves over by their jerky, startled movements.

Hand coordination. As the startle reflex diminishes and your baby's movements become more steady, you will notice the baby making more deliberate hand movements. Some mothers note that their babies "discover" their own hands, bringing their hands in front of them and occasionally moving their hands toward their mouths. This type of play is a baby's early attempt at fine motor skills and hand-eye coordination; but most babies won't make any real strides in this refinement until 2 or 3 months of age.

Although hand coordination is still poor at this age, young babies will make attempts to grasp objects. A rattle or finger placed in the baby's hand will stimulate the baby's grasp reflex. Many times the baby cannot voluntarily let go of the object. The grasp used by babies of this age is called the palmar or "mitten" grasp because the four fingers work together as one unit opposing the thumb.

Head and neck. Each day, your baby's neck muscles are growing stronger. By 2 months, many babies can hold their heads at midline (facing straight ahead) while lying on their backs. On their stomachs, they can lift their heads about 45 degrees.

Although your baby's neck muscles are much stronger, they can't support the head completely. If you take your baby's hands and gently pull him or her up into a sitting position, you will notice the baby's head still drops back. You still need to provide head support when lifting or carrying your baby.

Knowing and understanding your baby's motor development will help you choose play activities appropriate to your baby's skills. Throughout the first six months, your baby will be interested in play that involves looking, listening, sucking or touching. And during these first two months, your baby will be most captivated by interesting sights and sounds.

Watching faces. Observing faces will continue to be one of your baby's favorite activities. At 1 month, most babies begin to enjoy face-to-face contact with others. Talking to your baby in this position allows your baby to see the many faces you make while talking: surprised, silly, happy, calm.

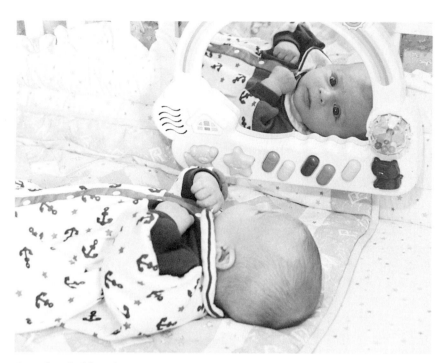

An unbreakable mirror is a wonderful companion, because babies are attracted to faces.

If possible, provide chances for your baby to watch his or her own reflection. Use a small, unbreakable mirror or one that's firmly mounted to the wall. Give your baby the chance to spend entertaining moments watching his or her own face in a mirror next to the crib or near a blanket on the floor. You'll want to supervise this play time if the mirror can be toppled, but take advantage of your baby's preoccupation by taking a moment to finish a task, make a phone call or simply relax and watch your baby play.

Even though human faces may be the most interesting to your baby, non-human faces can also be captivating. A doll, teddy bear or stuffed animal can provide additional face-to-face contact. Be careful, however, not to leave toys in the baby's crib. A fluffy animal near a baby's face can keep the baby from breathing easily.

Mobiles and crib toys. As you observe your baby's head and neck control, you will be able to make wise choices about mobiles and crib toys. In the early days and weeks of your baby's life, before the baby can support a midline head position, mobiles and objects hung across the crib are not practical. Instead, place pictures, mirrors or toys around the outside of the crib, just above mattress level.

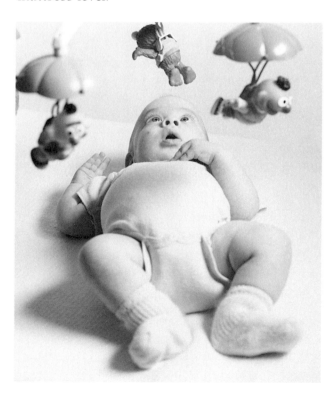

As your baby gains greater head and neck control, a mobile or other moving object becomes fascinating.

As the baby's head and neck control increase and the baby can face straight ahead while lying, mobiles are ideal toys. When purchasing a mobile, look at the mobile from the baby's perspective. Remember your baby's preference for simple shapes, high contrast and bright objects.

A homemade mobile can be just as entertaining as a purchased one. Simple faces cut out of paper plates, small, brightly colored toys or rattles and short strips of crepe paper or ribbons that flutter are all items suitable for a homemade mobile.

Make sure all items are secured completely and placed out of the baby's reach. When your baby is old enough to reach for tempting objects, remove the mobile.

Other toys. At this age, your baby is probably not interested in complicated toys. Most of the time your baby will prefer games that include watching and listening. Some squeaky toys and rattles will be appealing, but you will have to be the noisemaker. It will be several weeks before your baby can shake or squeeze these toys.

Movement games. Give your baby plenty of chances to experiment with movement. Put a blanket on the floor and let your baby kick and wiggle. Remember that your baby is stimulated by changes in texture and temperature. Use blankets made of different fabrics—fuzzy velour, bumpy knits, smooth flannel. In warm weather, take your blanket into the yard or to the park. In cooler weather, choose a sunny, carpeted spot for the baby's blanket.

When your baby is tummy-down on the blanket, put a bright object, noise-maker or mirror above the baby's head. Let your baby work on lifting up from the blanket to see the object. (This is tiring, so don't play the game too long.)

Playing on your baby's terms. Let your baby guide playtime. Watch for clues that the baby is tired or overstimulated. Some of the common clues are discussed on page 501.

Keep in mind your baby's physical limitations. During physical play, be gentle and careful not to shake your baby or toss the baby in the air. These activities can cause severe injury to your baby's eyes, neck and brain.

Feeding and Nutrition

The most important factor in your baby's feeding times is personal interaction. This is more than a time to be fed; it's also a chance for the baby to learn about you, how the two of you relate and the security and love you provide.

In the early days after birth, when you seem to be feeding the baby around the clock, it's hard to think about meeting your baby's social needs at each feeding. However, this doesn't require any effort beyond just being there and being attentive to your baby.

Babies should never be left unattended with a bottle. Besides robbing your baby of one-on-one interaction, propped bottles can cause choking if the baby cannot move the bottle to take a break from drinking. When a bedtime bottle is given, formula pools in the baby's mouth. This practice can lead to tooth decay.

How Your Baby Eats

Your baby's reflexes, motor development and eating skills are all interdependent. The tongue thrust, rooting and sucking reflexes are still very strong. These reflexes are the perfect skills needed to get nourishment from the breast or bottle. Cereals, fruits and solid foods require more advanced motor skills than your infant can master right now.

At the end of the second month, you will notice your baby is beginning to create more saliva. Saliva production is necessary for digestion, but the accompanying drooling and bubbles at this age are clues that the baby's ability to swallow is not developed enough to handle solid foods.

Diet   Breast milk or formula is still the only food your baby needs. Supplementing with water is unnecessary, but small amounts won't harm your baby. However, introducing other liquids such as juices, which your baby's gastrointestinal system is not yet mature enough to digest, could lead to allergies or cause diarrhea.

Cow's milk should never be given to young infants as a substitute for breast milk or formula. The effect of cow's milk on a baby's immature digestive system is discussed on page 496.

Sensitivity to formula. Except for specialized formulas designed for babies with specific nutritional needs or allergies, all infant formulas are very similar. Usually there is little to be gained by switching your baby's formula. Periods of fussiness, episodes of crying and spitting up are not indications of a baby's intolerance to formula and will not be solved by changing formulas.

If you wonder whether your baby's fussiness is connected to feedings, use the following checklist before talking to your doctor about switching formulas:

- Burp your baby often, after every 2 ounces of formula.
- Allow your baby to sit in a semireclined position for a couple of minutes before burping. This will help gravity take the formula to the bottom of your baby's stomach, and gas bubbles to the top.
- During feeding, place your baby in a reclining position. Never lay a baby flat on his or her back for feeding.
- Check the bottle's nipple for flow; sometimes changing nipples helps a baby feed more easily.

In a few babies, a true sensitivity to formula will develop. Look for these symptoms and report them immediately to your baby's doctor:

- Diarrhea—frequent, loose bowel movements mixed with mucus
- Persistent or increasing forceful vomiting
- The development of a rash

Feeding Schedule   Your baby is slowly becoming a more efficient eater. During this time, your baby's nursing schedule will become more predictable. Your baby will gradually need fewer daily feedings, will eat more at each feeding and will take less time to eat the same amount. At 2 weeks, babies usually nurse eight to 10 times each day. By 1 month, nursing might decrease to six to eight feedings (2 to 5 ounces each). By 2 months of age your baby may need only five to seven feedings each day (3 to 6 ounces each).

Although the numbers above are helpful as a point of reference, remember that each baby is a unique individual with unique calorie requirements. The number of feedings and amounts differ from baby to baby. Use the numbers above as a general guideline, but watch for your baby's hunger clues, as well as clues that tell you your baby is full.

Many factors will influence your baby's eating patterns. During a growth spurt, your baby may eat more at each feeding or require more frequent nursing. After a couple of days, the baby will settle back into a more predictable pattern. If your baby is sleeping longer through the night and skipping a night feeding, expect a morning "catch-up" feeding.

Because of the variations in feeding between babies, and each baby's individual nutrition needs and growth patterns, it's important to watch your own baby to know the schedule, feeding duration and amounts needed. Learn the communication clues that tell you when your baby is hungry and when the baby is full. Concentrate on your baby's desires and demands rather than on the amount your baby eats. If your baby seems to eat large amounts, but you are following your baby's communication clues, don't be concerned that your infant is overeating. The amount your baby eats at this age is not a sign of a future weight problem.

Sleeping Patterns and Habits

Newborns sleep off and on all day. Throughout the first two months of life, babies start "bunching" their sleeping time, staying awake longer during the day and sleeping longer at night. They still take frequent catnaps during the day, but are alert for longer periods. By 2 months, some babies can sleep six to eight hours at a time. Your goal is to make those hours nighttime hours.

Sleeping Through the Night

Experts give a wide range of ages that are "normal" for sleeping through the night. Although a few babies may be sleeping through the night occasionally at 2 months, many babies won't be developmentally prepared to sleep through the night until they're 6 months old.

The phrase "sleeping through the night" can be confusing. All babies—and adults, too—waken periodically through the night. Whether your baby will waken you depends on many factors, including the length of time the baby can go between feedings and the baby's ability to fall back to sleep without your help.

At 2 months, you'll probably begin subtle efforts to encourage your baby to sleep through the night. Any of the following steps will help:

- Put your baby to bed drowsy but awake. A baby who falls asleep in someone's arms may wake up in the night and not be able to fall asleep without being held.
- When your baby needs care or feeding in the night, use a soft voice and subtle body language to let the baby know it's nighttime, not playtime. Be business-like and boring. Let your baby know this is not the time for fun activities such as walking, rocking and playing.
- Think about your own sleeping habits. When you awaken in the night, it takes a couple of minutes to find a comfortable position, settle in and fall back asleep. The same is true of your baby. Unlike you, however, one of the only comforting mechanisms your baby has is crying. Expect some crying as the baby tries to fall back to sleep.
- Make sure your baby is comfortable and safe. If you've made sure the crib and area around it are safe, you won't immediately become concerned about the baby's safety if you hear cries.

- Establish a bedtime routine, a winding down of the day's activities. Perhaps you will want to turn off the TV and have a quiet time 30 minutes before you put the baby to bed.
- Try feeding the baby at least 30 to 60 minutes before bedtime. Babies who fall asleep on a full stomach may not sleep as well as those who fall asleep later after a feeding.

A goal, not a mandate. Don't feel pressured or rushed to have your baby sleeping through the night. Understanding your baby's schedule and communication clues takes time. Sleeping through the night should be a parenting goal you're working toward, not an issue that creates unnecessary guilt.

Sleeping and feeding issues. As you talk to others about how your baby sleeps, you will undoubtedly hear that your baby will sleep better if given solid foods. Unfortunately, this is not usually helpful. For the first three or four months, your baby's calorie requirements, small stomach capacity and rapid growth demand frequent feedings. Breast milk or formula is still the best source of the nutrition your baby needs.

Sleeping and personality. During the baby's first two months, you most likely will know whether you have a "night owl" or an "early bird." This is another area in which your baby will assert his or her unique personality. Even if you and your baby are opposites, create routines and schedules that respect your baby's preferences.

The Two-Month Checkup

The second medical visit will follow the same format as the two-week visit. Your baby will be weighed and measured. The numbers will be plotted on a growth chart, which will allow evaluation of your baby's rate of growth. Even though it's tempting to rate your baby's "success" by noting how the baby's numbers compare with the percentages on the chart, remember that it is more important to see steady growth since the last visit, regardless of how your baby's size compares with that of others.

Most of your baby's exam will consist of conversation between you and your baby's doctor or nurse practitioner. Most will follow the parent's lead, looking for clues that point to areas of concern or difficulty. Don't be afraid to direct the discussion toward specific topics or ask for information or assistance. Expect discussion about sleeping, feeding, schedules, development, immunizations, safety and your baby's personality.

Common portions of the exam, and their explanations, include:

- Check your baby's head, feeling the fontanelles (soft spots) to determine that the front fontanelle is still open, soft and flat
- Look over the baby's skin for signs of cradle cap, rashes or birthmarks; talk about bathing and skin care
- Evaluate the baby's sucking reflex; ask whether you have noticed the baby making more saliva

- Look in the baby's eyes; check for blocked tear ducts or discharge; watch the baby's ability to track objects
- Examine the baby's ears; talk about removing ear wax, if needed
- Ask about sneezing and congestion; give suggestions for using a bulb syringe, if needed
- Listen to the baby's heart and lungs
- Check healing of the baby's umbilicus (belly button)
- Feel the abdomen, checking for tenderness or enlarged organs
- Examine the genitalia; in boys, the doctor will check whether the testes are descended into the scrotum, and in circumcised boys, the penis will be examined to make sure it's healed properly
- Observe the baby's movements, commenting on the continued presence of reflexes
- Check hip movement

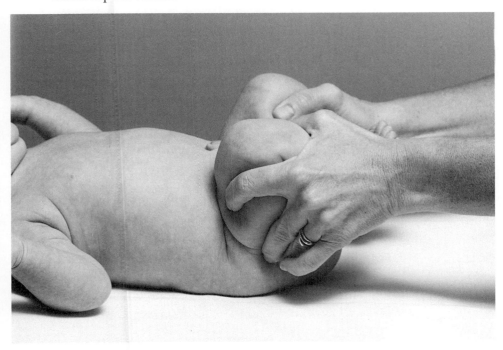

Your baby's caregiver will periodically check your baby's hips for dislocation or other problems with the hip joints.

Early immunizations are often just as hard for parents as for babies. It's tough to watch your baby deal with this brief pain; but it's harder still to nurse a child through a serious childhood illness. Keep in mind that your anticipation of the shots may be worse than the shots themselves. The person administering the shots knows the value of speed and can often be finishing a second shot before the baby reacts to the first one.

Immunizations are usually given at the end of the examination.

Immunizations

Diphtheria, tetanus and pertussis (DTP). Diphtheria is a serious disease that can cause paralysis, heart failure and breathing difficulties.

Tetanus is caused by bacteria growing in a wound. It affects the central nervous system and can cause pain, headaches, spasms and rigidity.

Pertussis, sometimes called whooping cough, is a bacterial disease that ranges from mild to severe. It is especially dangerous to babies. Under the age of 1, half of all babies with pertussis need hospitalization. One in 200 babies who have this illness die.

The DTP vaccine gives the immune system an opportunity to develop antibodies that protect against these illnesses.

Reactions to the DTP vaccine

It's common for babies to have mild reactions to the DTP immunization given at the two-month visit. Severe reactions, however, are rare. A severe reaction develops in less than 1 percent of babies. But contact your doctor if your baby has any of the following signs or symptoms:

- A fever of more than 102 degrees Fahrenheit
- Limpness
- Excessive drowsiness; difficulty awakening
- Convulsion
- Inconsolable crying
- Severe redness or swelling where the shot was given

Acetaminophen dosages

Weight (lb)	Weight (kg)	Drops (ml)	Elixir (teaspoon)
6-11	2.7-5.0	0.4	1/4
12-17	5.5-7.7	0.8	1/2
18-23	8.2-10.5	1.2	3/4

Note: Acetaminophen drops and elixir (such as Tylenol, Tempra) are two very different strengths. Follow the measurements specifically given for each type of acetaminophen.

The risks of the DTP vaccine are extremely low. Less than 1 percent of all babies have severe reactions to this vaccine.

The DTP vaccine, combined with the HIB vaccine described below, is often administered as a single shot in the thigh muscle. Common reactions to the DTP shot include a low-grade fever (less than 102 degrees Fahrenheit), fussiness and temporary feeding disturbances. The thigh area might appear red and sensitive. These symptoms may last up to two days. Your baby's doctor may recommend giving the baby acetaminophen.

A DTP vaccination may be postponed or canceled under some conditions. Talk with your doctor if your child is scheduled to receive a DTP vaccine and has, or has had, any of the following:

- A reaction to a previous immunization
- An infection or fever (a common cold should not prevent a vaccination)
- Convulsions (or if central nervous system disease is suspected)

Hemophilus influenza, type B (HIB). The common illness we refer to as "flu" is a viral illness. Hemophilus influenza, however, is a bacterial infection that causes ear and airway infections and is the leading cause of meningitis for children under age 2. Sometimes this illness acts quickly and responds poorly to medication. Therefore, an immunization is your child's best protection.

Hepatitis B. Three hepatitis vaccinations are given. Your baby may have had the first vaccination soon after birth. At this visit, your baby will receive a second vaccination. (The hepatitis B vaccination is described on page 445.)

Polio. Polio is a serious viral infection. It appears in mild and severe forms; severe forms of polio may result in crippling, paralysis and death. Your baby's grandparents may remember years past when polio was a common and dreaded summer disease. Because of vaccinations, polio has been virtually eliminated in the United States, but it is still present in other countries.

The polio vaccine is a live vaccine, made of weakened polio viruses. This is the only vaccine your baby might enjoy. It is administered orally in a fruity-tasting liquid.

Polio vaccine will be present in your baby's stools and mucus from a runny nose for a while—perhaps for as long as a month. People who handle the baby often will be exposed to these weakened viruses and may become re-immunized through the exposure.

If you or another caretaker has not been immunized against polio, tell the baby's doctor. The doctor should also be informed if someone in your family has a weakened immune system (is immunocompromised); such people include those who've had an organ transplantation and those with cancer. In such a situation, the baby could be given a vaccine prepared from killed viruses.

What Parents Worry About

Constipation

Your baby is constipated if you notice hard, formed bowel movements that are difficult to pass. Constipation is not defined by frequency of bowel movements. Some babies have a bowel movement every day; others may not have a bowel movement for five to seven days.

All babies turn red, make grunting noises and draw up their legs when having bowel movements. These signs do not necessarily mean they are constipated.

Pacifiers

A baby's sucking reflex is very strong. Young babies sometimes need to suck even after they're full. This non-nutritive sucking can be calming for your baby. Some babies choose to suck on their fingers or fists, but many babies prefer a pacifier. Using a pacifier is not harmful to a baby.

When choosing and using a pacifier, keep these tips in mind:

- Look for a one-piece pacifier. Pacifiers made of several small pieces may come apart and pose a choking hazard.
- Shop for dishwasher-safe pacifiers. In the early months of your baby's life, keeping the pacifier clean will help reduce the risk of infection.
- Watch your baby's pacifier for signs of deterioration. Replace a pacifier when the nipple starts to look worn; a worn nipple can tear off and choke a baby.
- Some days it will seem that your baby's pacifier spends as much time on the floor as in the baby's mouth. Many stores sell short straps that clip to your child's clothing and keep the pacifier within reach. However, never use a string or strap long enough to get caught around the baby's neck.
- Avoid a bedtime pacifier, which can be a nuisance because your baby loses it and wakes up.
- Many parents worry about starving their babies by unknowingly offering them pacifiers when they are really crying to be fed. Don't waste energy on this worry. If your child is hungry, the pacifier will be quickly rejected.

Sleep Positions

Recent studies have shown that babies who sleep on their stomachs have an increased risk of sudden infant death syndrome (SIDS). Experts are recommending that babies be put to bed on their backs or sides during the first six months of life. The back is the best position. (When putting your baby down on his or her side, pull the lower arm forward so your baby is not likely to roll forward.)

Sleeping on the stomach has not been shown to be a cause of SIDS, only an increased risk. The following sleep factors may also increase the risk of SIDS:

- A natural-fiber, too-soft mattress—Choose a firm mattress. A softer mattress may cause the baby to sink in and have difficulty breathing. Other soft surfaces such as water beds, beanbag chairs, sheepskins and thick quilts should not be used as sleeping surfaces.
- Improper bedding—Use lightweight blankets that will allow your baby to move about in the crib. If your baby is sweating around the face or neck, the baby is overheated and needs fewer covers. (If your baby is ill or has a fever, even fewer coverings are needed.) To keep your baby from becoming entangled in blankets, tuck the bedding in securely at the foot of the crib. Place the baby near the foot of the crib and allow the blankets to reach up only to the baby's shoulders. This positioning will reduce the risk of your baby sliding down under the blankets.

At the age when babies begin to move around the crib while they sleep, parents become concerned about maintaining a back- or side-sleeping position. However, when a baby has learned to roll over—both from back to front and from front to back—many of these risks decrease.

Some babies have medical conditions that require sleeping on their stomachs. If your baby's doctor has recommended this position, it is probably best to follow that advice. Remember that sleeping tummy-down has not been shown to cause SIDS; it is only one of the factors that may increase the risk of SIDS.

CHAPTER THIRTY-ONE

Baby From Two to Four Months

During these two months, your baby is changing from a passive infant to an active member of your family.

You may feel that most of your time with your 2-month-old baby is spent in basic caregiving. But you can see your baby's personality emerging. You can even understand the way your baby communicates with you subtly, with eye contact and cooing, and boldly, by crying.

By 4 months, your baby is even more communicative and is learning his or her place in your family. Just when you've started to believe parenting is little more than changing diapers, feeding and staying up all night, your baby will begin to show you how rewarding parenting really can be. Your 4-month-old baby really knows how to turn on the charm. When you're weary from the daily routine of caring for your baby, she or he will find new ways to thrill you—smiling, cooing, kicking, laughing and squealing.

"I wish he could stay this age forever," one mother said. "He adores me. Almost anything I do excites him and makes him happy."

In four short months, your baby has determined that this new family holds the most important people in the world.

Growth

Every baby is different. Although it's easy to make generalizations, it's difficult to predict your baby's exact growth during this time. Generally, babies grow 1½ inches and gain 2 or 3 pounds between their second and fourth months. Some smaller babies may have doubled their birth weights; other babies won't double their birth weights until around age 6 months.

Be cautious about relying on numbers or percentages to evaluate your baby's growth. Your baby is unique and will grow according to a personal schedule and timetable. Numbers and percentages should not be used to compare your baby with others, but to document steady, healthy growth in your own child.

It may be difficult to see your baby's growth until the baby is weighed and measured at the doctor's office. However, during these two months you will probably notice your baby filling out. By four months, babies may begin to look like those round-faced, smiling babies in magazines.

Social Development

At 2 months, your baby needs a lot of care and attention but may not interact with you as much as you had expected. Many parents find caring for their babies at this age especially challenging. Those who've struggled with doubts about their decision to become parents may even feel discouraged.

"The first couple of months of my baby's life were really a challenge," one mother confessed. "But I soon realized that each stage of her life was fleeting, both the difficult and the enjoyable ones, and I learned to take time to enjoy each one."

The stage at which your baby seems to require all care and to give little in response goes by quickly. Your baby is changing into a delightful, interactive little person. Getting to know your baby's subtle ways of interacting and communicating is part of the challenge and discovery of parenting. By 4 months, your baby will be actively responding to you and even initiating social interaction.

How Your Baby Relates to You

Parents and family are the most important people in a baby's life. Your baby is involved in your everyday lives, watching, listening and picking up clues on how humans interact. And your family will be the first persons with whom your baby interacts.

At about 3 months, your baby will begin to identify the behaviors that get your attention. A smile, for example, is one effective way. By the time your baby is 4 months old, the reaction to your presence will be even more vigorous. Your baby may respond to your presence, your voice and even your facial expressions with his or her whole body, kicking and waving arms. Your baby recognizes family members and will probably let you and the rest of the family know you're special people in his or her life.

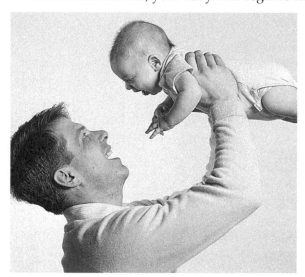

Your baby wants and needs your attention, and a smile is a wonderfully effective way to get it.

Getting to know brothers and sisters. If your baby has an older brother or sister, that child may be the baby's most popular playtime friend. Children can easily make a baby laugh and smile.

For siblings, this is a "honeymoon" time. At 4 months, the baby is old enough to thrill an older brother or sister with smiles and giggles but still too young to be "trouble," getting into toys and interrupting playtimes.

The daily grind. Your family is probably beginning to settle back into the schedules and routines you kept before the baby arrived. Car pools, a parent returning to work and routine errands all sap your time and energy. And when the family regroups at the end of the day, everyone is ready to relax, share stories of their day and tell one another about their stresses. Your baby can sense this change and may also need time to adjust, regardless of whether he or she has been home all day or in child care. You may notice your baby becoming fussier, as if to communicate, "I've been trying to be really good today, but now that we're all together, I'd like to tell you how tough my day has been."

Fussiness is common and variable in all babies. An increased fussiness at the end of the workday is normal and does not reflect on your success as a parent. All of us save some of our daily frustrations to share later with those we trust most.

When coping with this time of day, follow the baby's lead. What does the baby seem to need? Time alone? Someone to play with? Experiment with adjusting your evening routine to accommodate your baby's personality. Perhaps you can postpone your dinner hour or switch duties so each parent has a chance to spend time with the baby.

As you readjust your family's evening schedule, don't feel guilty about setting aside some much-needed time for yourself or for you and your spouse. Remember that taking time for personal relaxation and rejuvenation will benefit your baby too.

How Your Baby Relates to Others

At 2 months, your baby is pretty tolerant of other people and is probably willing to be held and cuddled by almost anyone. Usually, proud grandparents, relatives and friends are more than happy to oblige.

During these two months, your baby is growing into a real charmer. When others coo and smile, your baby is likely to respond. Share the joy of your baby with others, but watch for the clues that the baby is overstimulated. See page 501 for the signs that your baby needs a break from interaction.

Your baby's growing recognition of family members goes hand in hand with a realization that some people are strangers. At 4 months, many babies become picky about the company they keep. In a group or with an unfamiliar person, your baby may withdraw. Anticipate a transition time around strangers or when leaving your baby with someone else.

Language Development

Early Communication

Between 2 and 4 months of age, babies perfect the art of cooing. By 4 months, nearly all babies coo, both for their own pleasure and to initiate conversation with, or respond to, others.

Even though a coo is endearing, a baby soon learns that a laugh is irresistible. By 4 months, your baby probably laughs out loud frequently. The laugh may be intended to get your attention or just for the experience of making noise. About half of babies this age are beginning to make bubbling noises with their lips and tongues. Your baby may practice these sounds for hours.

Using real words and associating those words with objects is still beyond your baby's abilities, but by 4 months your baby recognizes all the sounds that make up human speech. Your baby will probably begin to experiment with these sounds. By 4 months, your baby may find one sound—such as mah or bah—and repeat it over and over, then a few days later discover a new sound and practice it repeatedly. Babies seem to enjoy playing with a new sound as much as they delight in playing with a favorite toy.

Talking to and With Your Baby

Your baby is building language skills by listening. It's important to talk to your baby. Don't be embarrassed to use a high-pitched voice. No matter what other people think, your baby actually likes it. Singing and reading to your baby also help your baby develop language skills.

Although words are still a jumble, your baby is picking up many communication clues by your tone of voice and inflection. Your baby begins to comprehend your daily routine and what's coming next—such as a diaper change or feeding time—by the way you talk.

When your baby's willing, play mimicking games. Respond to the baby's cooing or babbling with similar sounds. At 4 months, your baby may participate in a back-and-forth imitation game.

Crying Patterns

The total number of hours your baby cries each day is on the decline. At 2 months, most babies cry more than two hours each day. Between 3 and 4 months, most babies cry about one hour each day. Your baby may cry more or less than average. It may seem like more because your baby cries off and on throughout the day, not all at once. If your baby seems to cry excessively, try some of the tips for calming a crying or colicky baby discussed on page 541.

Sensory Development

The development of your baby's senses is not as easy to observe as the development of motor skills and coordination. Usually, parents notice sensory development when it affects motor development. For example, as a baby's sight improves, the baby notices more objects and may work harder to bat at or move toward them. Even though your baby can't tell you what he or she is experiencing, watching and playing with your baby will help you know how well the baby sees and hears.

At 2 or 3 months, your baby should be able to maintain eye contact with you. Although you may see the baby's eyes cross occasionally, the baby should grow out of constant eye crossing by 4 months.

Your baby's sight is maturing rapidly. In the next few months, your baby will begin to view the world in much the same way you do. Right now, your baby is learning that objects are three-dimensional. As the baby's eyes outgrow the cross-eyed stage and become better aligned, the baby develops depth perception.

At 2 months, your baby is still interested in large, brightly colored objects. But by 4 months, you may discover your baby testing a newfound, clearer vision by focusing on small objects such as prints on fabrics or wallpaper. An item as small as a raisin may catch the baby's attention, although items this small are a choking hazard and should not be left within the baby's reach. At this point, a baby's fine motor development lags behind sight development. The baby still grasps things with a mitten-like (palmar) grasp and will have difficulty picking up those fascinating small objects until he or she learns to use a finger-and-thumb grasp later.

Head and neck development work together with sight development to help babies at this age track moving objects. By 4 months, your baby will probably watch a brightly colored object as you move it slowly in an arc above the baby's head.

From birth, babies see color, but they have difficulty distinguishing similar tones or colors such as red and green. So they often prefer black and white or high-contrast colors. Between your baby's second and fourth months, color differences are becoming clearer, and the baby is starting to distinguish similar colors. Your baby may now prefer bright, primary colors.

Hearing

The sound your baby most wants to hear is the human voice. Singing and talking face-to-face or as you move around the room will delight your baby. At the beginning of this two-month period, the baby may quiet when hearing your voice. By the fourth month, your baby will respond more directly, even turning eyes or head toward you, searching for the sound of your voice.

Motor Development

How Your Baby Is Changing

Between the second and fourth months, most babies are beginning to move around to explore the world. Some of their newborn reflexes, such as the tonic neck reflex and Moro reflex, are disappearing. Babies are learning to use purposeful coordination of their large muscle groups to move around.

By 4 months, most babies are exercising their arm muscles by pushing up with their elbows or hands when on their tummies. Some may even use this newfound arm power to scoot around in a circle or even move a few inches forward or backward.

About half of 4-month-old babies can roll over. The first time your baby rolls over may come as a surprise to you—and to your baby. Unfortunately, many parents discover their baby's ability to roll when a baby placed on a couch or bed ends up on the floor. Take precautions not to leave your baby unprotected on elevated surfaces.

Babies don't need any coaching to learn to roll; it just happens. Usually, a baby first learns to roll over from front to back. All you need to provide is the opportunity and a little floor space.

Some babies make a nearly full-time game of rolling. Others are content to roll over only occasionally.

Don't be concerned if your baby isn't rolling over by 4 months. You will probably notice some rolling attempts in the near future. Remember, only half of babies are already able to roll over completely at 4 months.

As your baby's mobility increases, pay close attention to situations that could result in falls. At this age, your baby could easily roll off a changing table, bed or couch or out of an infant seat if not secured. An active baby can jiggle and wiggle enough to topple an infant seat off a counter; so stay close by, or don't use an infant seat.

Head and neck. Your baby's neck muscles are growing stronger. By 4 months, when you place your baby facedown, the baby can most likely lift his or her head and look straight forward. When held in a sitting position, the baby can sit with the head steady.

A 4-month-old, when lying on his or her back, may try to "help" when picked up. At this age, about half of all babies can be pulled up from this position by their hands, while their heads stay in line with their bodies.

Hands and arms. Your baby's hands may become preferred play-things during these months. Watching them, bringing them together at eye level and exploring them by mouth might be some of your baby's favorite pastimes.

During these two months, your baby mostly plays with toys by batting at them. But your baby's fine motor skills are improving. By 4 months, your baby can probably grasp a rattle or other small toy and may be learning to transfer objects from one hand to the other. Early in life, grasping is a reflex, and babies will grab onto anything that touches their palms. Now, your baby grasps objects by choice and holds them purposefully.

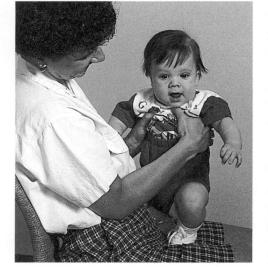

You may begin to feel like a human trampoline as your baby uses your lap for experiments with newfound strength in his or her leg muscles.

Legs. Between 2 and 4 months, babies seem to discover the strength of their legs. By 4 months, most babies can, with a little help, bear their own weight on their legs.

It may seem that every time you sit down with your baby on your lap, your baby is determined to stand. You may begin to feel that your lap is an infant trampoline as your baby learns to bounce vigorously in this position. Standing and bouncing while well supported won't hurt your baby's legs or hips. However, watch for situations in which the baby's bouncing could jostle a piece of furniture or a cup of hot liquid and cause an injury.

Playing With Your Baby

Your baby will continue to find new ways to explore the world. Each new development in coordination and mobility brings new adventures. These adventures require you to pay closer attention to safety issues, and they also provide you more opportunities for interactive play with your baby. In fact, as your baby approaches 4 months, you may notice that interacting with people, especially other children, becomes the baby's favorite pastime.

Toys. Throughout these months and until your baby's sixth month, your baby will do a lot of exploring by touching, holding, batting, turning and shaking objects. At 4 months, your baby may be especially interested in different textures. Shiny plastic wrap will be just as interesting as soft fabrics and fuzzy toys, but it is also more dangerous because it would likely end up in your baby's mouth. To help you identify objects that could be dangerous, see "Keeping playtime safe," page 536.

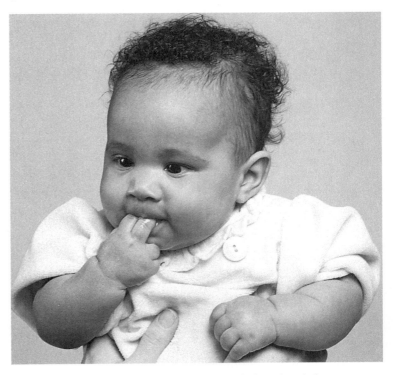

When choosing handheld toys for your baby, select toys that are lightweight and soft, easy to grasp and too big to swallow. Squeaking toys and rattles are appropriate for babies at this age.

Four months is also a good time to introduce your baby to soft, plastic baby books. An early introduction will allow your baby to see books as an everyday part of life, even if your baby prefers chewing the book over listening to you read it.

As your baby becomes more interested in toys, having toys handy will keep the baby from boredom in adult settings. Pack some of your baby's favorite toys or tie them to the stroller to provide entertainment as you run errands, work in the yard or visit with other adults.

Your baby's hands become fascinating playthings at this age. And most playthings, hands, feet and toys included, probably will end up in your baby's mouth.

Floor play. As your baby's head and neck strength increase, playing on the floor becomes more fun and allows your baby to work on motor skills.

You can share in floor-time fun by lying on the floor with your baby. Position the baby tummy-down on the floor and lie down on the floor facing the baby. Your baby will work neck and arm muscles to lift up and be face-to-face with you.

You can also encourage your baby to work those arm and neck muscles by putting toys just within the baby's reach.

At this age, your baby will also be interested in floor gyms. These toys usually have various brightly colored objects of different shapes. The baby will probably use both hands and feet to bat at and kick objects on the gym.

Bathtub play. As it becomes easier for babies to sit when supported, parents often turn bath time into playtime, sometimes even getting into the tub with their babies. Baths can be fun for both parent and baby. However, remember that bubble bath and soap can be irritating to a baby's eyes, skin and genitals. And keep a close eye and good grip on your baby. The water makes your wiggly, active baby extra slippery.

Keeping playtime safe

Your baby isn't crawling yet. Still, this is a good time to get into the habit of doing a "baby-level" safety check each time you put your baby down to play on a floor. Get down on your hands and knees, at your baby's level, and look for these items:

- Small objects your baby could accidentally swallow, such as coins, paper clips or small pieces of food or candy
- Toys with small parts
- Uncovered electrical outlets
- Pulls for window blinds, in which your baby could become entangled
- Electrical cords to irons, lamps or other appliances that could fall if the baby tugs on the cord
- Plastic bags or wrappings that could suffocate your baby
- Newspapers and magazines
- A pet's toys or treats
- Houseplants

Let older siblings become involved in the baby's care by helping with the safety search. Talk to them about the things that can be harmful to the baby. Communication and understanding can increase their awareness about the hazards of leaving toys and objects around the baby's play area.

Swings, jumpers and walkers. These devices were all designed to give a baby increased mobility while freeing the parent to tend to other tasks. However, they don't live up to their original intention. All of these "toys" need direct and attentive supervision because they can be dangerous.

By 4 months, your baby is probably outgrowing an infant swing. A baby who can wiggle, scoot and shift can possibly topple out of a swing.

Jumpers that hang on a doorway should always be positioned so the baby's toes barely touch the floor. The baby's heels should not touch the floor. A baby in a jumper should always be supervised. Injuries can occur if the jumper falls or the baby pinches fingers between the jumper and door frame.

Walkers have caused countless injuries and should not be used. Although parents often believe that using a walker will speed a baby's walking abilities, this simply isn't true. In fact, the use of a walker often robs the baby of time to crawl and walk alone. Walker injuries include pinches and falls. And walkers are especially dangerous because their use can result in a severe accident, such as a fall down a flight of stairs. Although many parents use child gates to help prevent such falls, gates can unintentionally be left unlatched in the midst of a busy day. A walker is one piece of baby gear you don't need.

Feeding and Nutrition

Your baby is changing, filling out and growing quickly. The amount your baby eats and feeding times may vary and be unpredictable as your baby grows. You are not alone if you're anxious about whether your baby is getting proper nutrition.

Diet

Breast milk or formula is still the best food for your baby. Its liquid form perfectly matches your baby's eating skills, habits and digestive abilities. And it provides all the calories and nutrition your baby needs for growth and development. Your baby doesn't need any other foods or vitamins.

Your baby's development and dietary needs are related. Watching the following areas of development will help you make wise choices about your baby's diet:

- The suck and swallow reflex. Your baby still manages milk or formula by moving it from the front to the back of the mouth by sucking, then swallowing. This sucking reflex is aided by the tongue-protrusion reflex, in which the tongue pushes forward to help the baby suck. This reflex is still strong, which means that it is difficult for a baby to manage solid foods. Babies at this age tend to push out cereals or solid foods rather than swallow them.

- Bringing hands to mouth. By 4 months, your baby is just beginning to bring one or both hands to the mouth. This is an early motor skill and shows that your baby is developing normally, but it does not indicate that your baby is ready to eat solid foods. The role physical development plays in readiness for solid food is discussed on page 553.

- Saliva production and drooling. From 2 to 4 months, your baby's saliva production increases. Drooling increases too. This drooling is further evidence that the baby's swallowing skills need to improve before the baby will be capable of handling new foods.

Your baby's excessive drooling might trick you into thinking the baby is teething, but the average age for a first tooth is 5 to 7 months, and many babies don't start teething until much later than that.

At 2 months, feeding times are times of concentrated, one-on-one interaction between you and your baby. As your baby nears 4 months, feeding times become less frequent, and the baby's attention is drawn to other people and activities during feeding. The baby may move around or stop feeding to play or "talk" to you. This distraction is not a sign that your baby is rejecting breast-feeding or is bored with formula. An easily distracted baby is normal as the baby discovers and explores the world. Your baby may discover that feeding time can be more than a time to eat; it's also a time to socialize, experiment and assert a little independence.

Distractions

As much as you want your child to learn through exploration and interaction, it can be frustrating to try to feed a distracted baby. Try to provide your baby with a quiet, uninterrupted feeding place, but acknowledge that everything is new and worthy of exploration to your baby. You may find that your baby's early morning feeding—when your baby is still sleepy and the room is dark—may be the best feeding of the day.

At 2 months, most babies need somewhere between five and seven feedings a day. By 4 months, the number of feedings decreases to four or five. It may still seem that your baby is eating often and large quantities. This impression is partly due to the baby's ability to sleep longer stretches at night. As nighttime feedings are eliminated, all the baby's feedings are compacted into the daytime hours. Those feedings should become more predictable.

Schedule

Just as your baby's feeding schedule becomes familiar, your baby may experience a growth spurt that disrupts the schedule. When your baby is growing quickly, he or she may eat more at a feeding or need more frequent feedings. Disregard timetables and absolute volumes. Instead, follow your baby's clues to know when the baby is hungry or full. After a growth spurt, your baby will probably settle into a new feeding routine.

Sleeping Patterns and Habits

Although every baby is different, by 4 months your baby may be sleeping well at night. These two months, then, are a time to help your baby continue building the skills needed to sleep through the night. In addition to creating a bedtime ritual that helps your baby anticipate sleeping, you may want to continue incorporating some of the tips on page 523 for helping your baby sleep through the night.

You may discover that your baby's idea of sleeping through the night differs from yours. Although your baby may sleep anywhere from six to 10 hours a night, those hours may not coincide with your personal sleeping hours. Perhaps your baby sleeps from midnight to 7 a.m. or from 9 p.m. to 3 a.m. At 2 months, your baby will probably awaken twice during the night, and by 4 months, he or she may awaken only once.

By 4 months, in addition to a predictable nighttime sleep, you can expect your baby to begin taking naps at regular intervals. These naps will probably last one to two hours, perhaps long enough for the baby's caregiver to accomplish some tasks or enjoy a good book. However, some babies just aren't "nappers" and may nap for just a few minutes at a time. Even though this schedule can be frustrating to parents, babies are experts at knowing how much sleep they need.

Your baby may fall into a pattern of a morning and an afternoon nap, a schedule that will probably continue for many months. If your baby is active, expect more frequent naps as the baby "recharges."

Fitting Into Family Routines

As your baby grows and develops more routine sleep habits, you'll probably get ample advice about your baby's sleeping schedule and patterns. While picking and choosing the tidbits that fit your baby's personality and situation, keep in mind that the most important consideration is how your baby's sleep schedule and habits interact with your family's lifestyle. Every family will discover different effective bedtime rituals and routines.

Where Your Baby Sleeps

Some young babies sleep in their parents' bed, others sleep in a crib in the parents' room and some sleep in their own room. As babies near the age of 4 months, they become very active sleepers, making noise, scooting around and often waking their parents. If your baby has been sharing your bed or room, this may be a time to reevaluate the benefit of this practice to the baby and to you.

Sleeping and Feeding Solid Foods

As eager as you are to have your baby sleep through the night, altering your baby's diet will not accomplish that goal. Adding cereal or other solid foods will not reliably help the baby sleep longer. Although your baby may be ready for solid foods in a few weeks or months, the decision to start giving solid foods should be based on your baby's daytime behavior and eating habits, not on sleeping issues.

Don't use a bottle of milk to help your baby drift off to sleep. A habit of falling asleep with a bottle increases the possibility of tooth decay, ear infections and inability to fall back asleep on waking in the night.

Your baby is changing quickly and becoming more mobile. New developments are exciting to both you and your baby. For your baby, each new skill affects every area of life, including sleep. At this age, your baby's ability to roll over may disrupt sleep. Until your baby learns to roll both ways, the baby may awaken after rolling out of a favored sleeping position and not be able to roll back. For a short time, your intervention may be needed to help your baby back into a comfortable sleeping position, but this problem will resolve after the baby learns to roll both ways.

How Development Affects Sleeping

Your baby's sleep cycles

Understanding how your baby sleeps will help you cope with sleep problems and night awakenings. Sleep is divided into two basic stages: REM and non-REM. REM stands for rapid eye movement, a primary trait of deep sleep.

REM sleep, often called active sleep, is characterized by:

- Eyes moving under eyelids
- Irregular breathing and heart rate
- Brain activity
- Dreaming
- Relaxed muscles
- Small twitches of face, hands and legs

Non-REM sleep, often called quiet sleep, is characterized by:

- A regular heart rate and breathing pattern
- Stillness
- Less mental activity
- Very little, if any, dreaming

Non-REM sleep is divided into four stages, beginning with drowsiness and progressing into deeper sleep. In the first stages of non-REM sleep, a person can be easily awakened. In later stages, breathing and heart rate start to become more regular, and the person is difficult to wake.

Dr. Richard Ferber, the Director for Pediatric Sleep Disorders at Children's Hospital in Boston, has defined the development of children's sleep habits and problems. According to Dr. Ferber, babies spend about half of their sleeping time in the REM state. Usually, a baby will fall asleep and go through a phase of non-REM sleep and a phase of REM sleep, then awaken. A baby may do this several times a night. The time spent awake may last just a few seconds or a few minutes. During this time, the baby may move around, fuss or cry. Whether the baby can fall asleep again may depend on the conditions the baby associates with falling asleep.

The sleeping patterns your baby is establishing will remain throughout her or his life. Everyone, even adults, goes through minor awakenings at night, although most people don't remember these awakenings in the morning. Viewing these awakenings as normal will help you teach your child to fall back asleep.

The Four-Month Checkup

By now, the routine of the baby's medical visit is probably becoming familiar to you. This examination will follow the same pattern as the previous well-baby exam.

Your baby will be measured and weighed, and the statistics will be noted on the baby's growth chart. The doctor will use these numbers to evaluate the baby's continued growth. Although percentages are available, the doctor will be most interested in how the baby's height and weight compare with those at the last visit.

Remember that all areas of development affect your baby's health and well-being. Don't hesitate to discuss sleeping patterns or problems, feeding, the baby's increasing mobility or safety issues. Bring a list of any questions you might have about your baby's development or care.

During the physical examination, the health care provider may do the following:

- Check the baby's head, feeling the fontanelles (soft spots) to see that they are open, soft and flat; look for signs of cradle cap (see page 627) or other skin irritations. As a baby's saliva increases, drool can collect in the folds of the neck and cause a rash.

- Examine the baby's eyes. By 4 months, a baby's crossed eyes generally will have corrected naturally.

- Look in the baby's nose. At this age, the baby doesn't rely on the nose as much for breathing. As a very young infant, your baby was primarily a nasal breather, which was necessary during feedings. Now, however, the baby will also breathe through the mouth.

- Check the baby's mouth and ask if you've noticed much drooling or chewing motions; feel the baby's gums for any signs of incoming teeth, although teeth usually don't appear until later.

- Listen to the baby's heart and lungs.

- Feel the baby's abdomen, checking for enlargement of the liver or kidneys or the possible presence of an umbilical hernia. (See page 543 for more information on umbilical hernias.)

- Examine the baby's hands and feet and check the movement of the baby's legs and hips.

- Assess muscle tone and strength.

- Look over the baby's skin, talking about any rashes or birthmarks.

- Examine the baby's genitalia and groin area, checking for rashes or a possible inguinal hernia. (See page 543 for more information on inguinal hernias.) For girls, the doctor might ask about any vaginal discharge. For boys, the doctor will check for hydrocele, a sac of fluid buildup within the scrotum. This condition is common, is usually present at birth and will resolve naturally as the baby's body matures during the first year.

At this visit, your baby will receive a second dose of immunizations given at previous visits: DTP, HIB and oral polio. Your baby's health care provider may give the DTP and HIB vaccinations in a single, combined shot.

Your 4-month-old may have a sore leg for a day or two after these immunizations. At a time when your baby tends to want to stand in your lap, bounce vigorously and generally view the world from an upright position, your baby may be temporarily subdued because of leg pain from the shots. To ease your baby's discomfort, follow the acetaminophen dosages listed on page 526. (For more information on vaccinations, their purposes and side effects, see page 525.)

Immunizations

What Parents Worry About

Colic is a frustrating and largely unexplainable condition. One of the only things experts know for sure about colic is that it doesn't last forever. In most cases, colic peaks at six weeks and disappears in the baby's third or fourth month.

Colic

Colic is a difficult experience for everyone. One doctor describes colic as "when the baby's crying—and so is Mom."

Doctors call colic a "diagnosis of exclusion," which means other possible problems are ruled out before determining the baby has colic. The parent of a colicky infant, therefore, can be assured that the crying is probably not a sign of a serious medical problem.

Studies on colic have focused on several possible causes: allergies, an immature digestive system, gas, hormones, mother's anxieties and handling. Still, it is unclear why some babies have colic and others don't.

Although the term "colic" is used widely for any fussy baby, true colic is determined by the following:

- Predictable crying episodes. A colicky baby cries at about the same time each day, usually in the evening. Colic episodes may last minutes or two or more hours.

- Activity. Many colicky babies pull their legs to their chests or thrash around during crying episodes as if they are in pain.

- Intense or inconsolable crying. Colicky babies cry more than usual and are extremely difficult—if not impossible—to comfort.

Generations of families have dealt with colicky infants. Many of them found consoling techniques that worked for their babies. Others simply had to endure their babies' weeks of colic. One of the suggestions listed may be the answer to comforting your colicky baby:

- Rock your baby gently. Avoid fast, jiggling movements.

- Lay your baby tummy-down on your knees and sway your knees smoothly and slowly, or cradle your baby tummy-down in your arms and rock gently.

- Cuddle your baby.

- Walk with your baby.

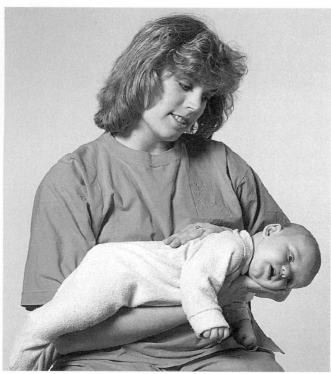

To comfort a colicky baby, lay him or her tummy-down and gently rock your baby on your arm or lap. But don't expect immediate success. There's no sure cure for colic.

- Use a front carrier, allowing your baby to be close to you while freeing your hands to do other tasks.

- Play a "white noise" cassette tape or create your own white noise with an appliance such as a vacuum or clothes dryer that makes a steady, uninterrupted noise.

- Give your baby a pacifier.

- Swaddle your baby.

- Put your baby in an infant swing.

- Buckle your baby securely in a car seat and set it on the floor near a running clothes dryer. (Don't place your baby on the dryer because vibrations of the dryer could cause the seat to move and fall off the dryer.)

- Provide a change of scenery.

- Lay your baby tummy-down on a warm water bottle.

- Give your baby a warm bath.

- Try singing or humming while walking with or rocking the baby. A soothing song can have a quieting effect on both parent and baby.

If none of these suggestions work and you can't end the crying, you'll need to shift your tactics and concentrate on finding ways to survive the colicky weeks:

- Put your baby in the stroller or front carrier and go for a brisk walk.

- Take your baby for a car ride.

- Leave your baby with someone else for 10 minutes and walk alone. You may be able to "trade" personal time with another parent or family member, to give each family member a short break.

- Put the baby down and do some on-the-spot vigorous exercises to re-energize yourself.

- If you are worried that your baby is sick or if you or others caring for the baby are becoming frustrated or angry because of the crying, call your doctor or bring the baby to the office or emergency department.

Remember that colicky babies are healthy babies. Colic isn't caused by anything you do, and it doesn't interrupt your baby's growth or development. Talk to your baby's health care provider for advice and support. And remember that your baby will soon outgrow colic.

Spitting Up

Spitting up is an everyday occurrence for babies. As your baby develops more saliva and drools more, you may notice an increase in spitting up. Spitting up causes the baby no discomfort. In fact, it may seem your baby isn't even aware of spitting up. Although spitting up is nothing to be worried about, you may be able to decrease the amount your baby spits up by trying these approaches:

- Feeding your baby smaller amounts at a time
- Feeding him or her slowly
- Limiting active and rough play after feedings
- Trying different positions during and after feedings
- Burping your baby frequently

Vomiting, however, is forceful and is obviously disturbing to the baby. A baby who vomits occasionally and is still gaining weight is normal. However, if your baby is vomiting persistently, contact the baby's doctor.

Pyloric Stenosis

In a few babies, a condition called pyloric stenosis develops; this is caused when a muscle between the stomach and small intestine (the pyloric muscle) becomes enlarged, narrowing the stomach outlet. Pyloric stenosis usually occurs between 2 weeks and 4 months of age and causes forceful—often projectile—vomiting and dehydration. It is corrected by surgery.

Hernias

An inguinal hernia can occur in either boys or girls, but it is more common in boys and premature infants. Caused by a weakness in the abdominal wall that allows the intestines to bulge outward, this hernia appears as a swelling in the lower abdomen or groin and is painless. Most of the time, inguinal hernias do not require immediate medical attention unless the swollen area seems tender. Let your baby's health care provider know if you suspect a hernia. An inguinal hernia requires an operation; it will not go away by itself.

Umbilical hernias occur around the baby's belly button. You might notice an umbilical hernia if your baby's belly button bulges when the baby cries. An umbilical hernia is caused by a small area of separation in the abdominal wall. It usually corrects during the baby's first two years without treatment.

Undescended Testicles

Before birth, a male infant's testicles descend from the abdomen into the scrotum via the inguinal canal. In some cases, this descent is not complete. One or both testicles may be undescended, causing the scrotum to seem small or unevenly developed. Undescended testicles are more common in premature infants or those with a low birth weight. The condition might be accompanied by an inguinal hernia.

In many cases of undescended testicles, the testicles will descend within the baby's first year. After a year, less than 1 percent of boys have undescended testicles.

Undescended testicles not corrected by operation or medical treatment within the first year or two of a boy's life may increase the risk of infertility or occurrence of testicular tumors as an adult.

If you suspect that your son has undescended testicles, bring your concern to the attention of the baby's doctor. Another condition, retractile testicles, can be easily confused with undescended testicles. Retractile testicles are those that retract close to the baby's abdomen or groin, often when he is excited or cold. The doctor should be able to feel these testicles and even get them to descend into the scrotum when the baby is relaxed and warm. A parent may notice descended testicles during the baby's warm bath but be concerned when the testicles seem to "disappear" later. Retractile testicles usually permanently correct during puberty and do not have the same risks as undescended testicles.

Feet   Your baby's stiff-legged stance and vigorous bouncing are not harmful to normal development. You will notice your baby usually stands with feet turned out, a position that gives more control and stability. Also, your baby's feet appear thick and flat. This appearance is normal. Your baby is unlikely to need special shoes or exercises.

CHAPTER THIRTY-TWO

Baby From Four to Six Months

From the beginning, parenthood is an adventure. During these two months, your baby is learning that all of life is an adventure and everything seems worthy of exploration. Life is not simply having someone care for your basic needs; life is full of toes and fingers and toys and colors and all sorts of things that need to be examined, touched and tasted.

Right now, your baby's exploration is limited to things within sight and reach, but your baby is working on expanding the horizons. Each physical development—reaching, grasping, rolling and sitting—is helping prepare your baby for adventures still down the road, like walking, crawling and climbing. Your baby is exploring people and relationships too. From four to six months, your baby is really learning how to interact with others.

Social Development

If you've ever wondered if your baby needed you for anything besides providing the necessities of feeding and changing, you're probably discovering now that the answer is an unwavering yes. Your baby not only is responsive to your actions but also will probably often demand interaction by squealing, dropping toys or repeating any action that has been proved to catch your attention.

For your baby, playing and socializing are serious activities. Your baby uses these seemingly casual situations to experiment with new discoveries. At this age, babies are learning about cause and effect and watching how people and objects respond to their actions. Your baby is learning that a good belly laugh gets a similar response from you. Pulling hair gets your attention. A funny face tempts you to respond with one of your own.

How Your Baby Relates to You

545

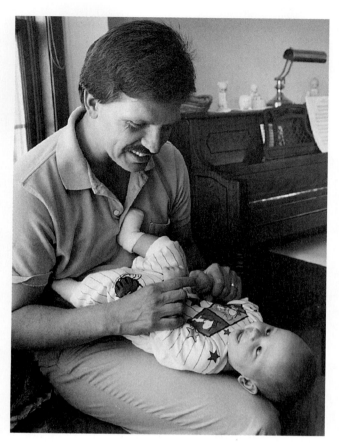

Give your baby a smile and you'll get one in return.

Like a scientist, your baby may test different actions over and over to see if they always get the same effect. And, like a successful scientist, your baby will be proud every time the response is the one expected. You can see your baby's smiles of accomplishment and self-confidence.

This is a fun age to socialize and play with your baby. Adults have the remarkable ability to express almost any emotion through facial expression, and babies love to watch and try to imitate these expressions. Your baby will probably enjoy this type of quiet play as well as more active physical play and will respond to the different play styles of parents and caregivers.

Don't be discouraged if playing with your baby seems uncomfortable at first. Remember, it's been a few years since you spent your evenings on the floor with a box of blocks and rattles. Give yourself time. And watch the "expert," looking at which toys your baby is drawn to and what the baby does with them. Then join in. Soon you'll know what games and toys make playtime fun for your baby. Your baby will give you the kind of immediate response—giggles, turn-taking, smiles—that make playtime rewarding for both of you. And your baby will let you know if playtime is too intense or has gone on too long. Watch for clues that your baby is overstimulated, such as turning away or becoming grouchy or tense.

Your baby needs a great deal of attention now. Left alone in a playpen, crib or infant seat, your baby will become bored. The stimulation of your company is necessary, but life doesn't have to be all games and playtime. You can meet many of your baby's social needs by including him or her in your daily tasks and errands.

Playing with siblings

An older brother or sister can get a lot of enjoyment out of a 4- to 6-month-old baby. At four months, a sibling is thrilled just to make the baby smile. By six months, the baby has moved beyond face-to-face interaction and may even play with toys offered by an older child. Your baby can probably entice a bigger brother or sister into picking up dropped toys or playing passing games.

At this age, it's important that your baby have personal toys separate from an older sibling's toys. Illnesses can be easily spread from one child to another through shared toys. Keep the baby's toys clean. Plastic toys should be washed often, and fuzzy toys that aren't as easily washed should be reserved just for the baby's play.

Babies love older kids mostly because they're fun to watch. Although babies will play some turn-taking games, they delight in being an audience and responding to what older children do. For safety reasons, play between your baby and an older child should be supervised closely.

Not only does your baby tolerate attention from others but also the baby may even initiate it. Most 6-month-old babies will work hard for attention, trying to get eye contact by wriggling or making noises and responding with grins if someone merely raises an eyebrow or smiles.

Because your baby most likely isn't afraid of strangers yet, he or she will probably interact with anyone who pays a little attention. This is a comfortable time for most parents. The baby is big enough that you're not overly concerned about safe handling, and you know the baby is comfortable with someone else. At this age, you can easily share the fun of your baby with others.

How Your Baby Relates to Others

Language Development

By four months, your baby understands all the basic sounds that make up his or her native language. Between four and six months, your baby discovers the ability to make some vocal sounds. Your baby will experiment with sounds during these two months, but still doesn't understand how these sounds work together to communicate. For example, you may hear your baby make a ma-ma or da-da noise, but the baby does not yet associate that sound with a parent, although it's tempting to imagine a connection.

Babbling usually begins with babies experimenting with vowel sounds. Later, consonants are added. By six months, about half of all babies babble by repeating one syllable over and over. A few babies have started adding more than one syllable to their babbling. You may hear your baby practice one sound, then move on to something else and not repeat the sound for several days.

Much of your baby's "talking" may seem more like sound effects than babbling. Squeals, sliding pitches and bubbling sounds are all common for babies at this age. Giggles and laughter are favorite sounds for both babies and parents. A gentle tickling game or blowing on your baby's tummy to hear laughter is a rewarding form of communication.

Your young infant was content to communicate with you through eye contact. Now, your baby is interested in watching everything else that's going on in the world. When your baby looks away from you and you follow the gaze, you and your baby are communicating. Perhaps your baby realizes that you're willing to help make the rest of the world accessible.

You can talk to your baby about events and people in your family. Although your baby won't understand your words, your tone of voice—whether soothed or rushed—communicates feelings and activities.

Turn-taking games are popular with your baby at this age. Allow your baby to be the leader and mimic vocalizations.

Talking to and With Your Baby

Sensory Development

Your baby's senses are now almost as fully developed as an adult's. Your baby sees and hears the world almost as clearly as you do, and this ability allows you two to understand and share many of the same experiences.

Sight By six months, your baby has more clearly focused vision and can smoothly track a moving object. Throughout these two months, your baby will be attracted to and can focus on small objects. Your baby's vision is maturing rapidly. During the next six months, your baby's vision will become adult-like, although it won't be fully developed for three or more years.

Your baby's depth perception has matured to the point that your baby understands that something out of sight may be just behind or under something else. This new awareness is called "object permanence."

Earlier, your baby was learning to distinguish similar bold colors. From four to six months, your baby learns to sort out subtle differences in pastel colors.

Hearing As a young infant, your baby would quiet and listen to a new sound. Now, your baby quickly realizes where sounds are coming from and will turn quickly in the direction of the sound. Your baby still has the ability to "tune out" a sound that's repeated over and over.

Motor Development

How Your Baby Is Changing At four months, your baby is probably fascinated by his or her own fingers. You might notice that your baby is content to lie faceup, intently inspecting her or his fingers. Many babies spend enough time in this position to wear a temporary "bald spot" on the backs of their heads. When your baby is lying faceup, you will also notice that your baby is beginning to look more "relaxed," arms and legs extended rather than pulled in toward the body.

One day, when fingers have lost a little of their appeal, your baby will discover toes. At first, your baby may explore those little toes just by grabbing them and feeling them. But by six months, many babies have learned to explore with their mouths and will suck on their toes.

"Let's see now...how many toes are there supposed to be on this foot?" Your baby is discovering that toes are wonderfully wiggly and well worth a careful examination.

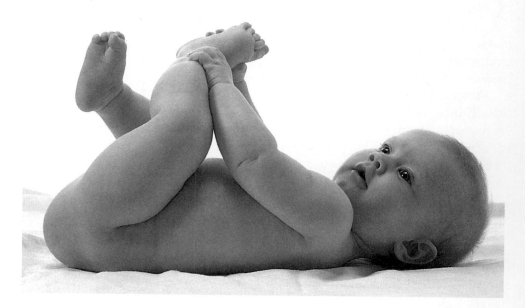

In fact, by six months, that little person in the nursery is no longer a baby, but a world-class explorer. Anything your baby can take hold of will be turned over, examined and most likely tasted. At six months, everything goes into a baby's mouth. This sucking, gumming and hand-to-mouth play is not necessarily a sign of teething; your baby is just discovering a new method of exploring. Keep items your baby might choke on out of reach. (For more information on choking hazards, see page 583.)

Each aspect of your baby's motor development gives your baby new tools to explore the world.

Picking up and letting go. At four months, your baby's hand control is still very basic. Because of the grasp reflex, your baby can grab a toy placed in her or his palm and can even hold that toy for a long time. But if your baby accidentally drops the toy or you take it away, your baby can't pick it up again. Your baby still manipulates objects by batting at them.

By five or six months, your baby's hand control is good enough that the baby can reach for a desired object using a rake-like motion and grasp it. This change from grasping as a reflex to reaching for things voluntarily is gradual. You may notice that sometimes your baby intentionally looks at and reaches for an object. Other times, your baby's hand may touch something and instinctively grab it, and your baby may seem surprised or intrigued by what has unexpectedly appeared in his or her hand.

After learning to grab a toy, your baby will practice moving things from hand to mouth, using both touching and tasting to explore the toy. You may even see your baby repeating the hand to mouth to hand movement, taking the object out of his or her mouth with alternating hands. Later, your baby will learn to move something directly from one hand to the other.

Your baby will soon discover that letting go of something is as much fun as picking it up. At first, letting go is almost accidental. The grasp reflex makes the baby hold onto something. When your baby learns how to let go of a toy purposefully, the baby's world becomes much more interesting—and messy. You may notice your baby beginning to organize things crudely, deliberately setting things down or piling objects together.

At this age, babies still use their whole hands (the "mitten" grasp) to pick things up. When babies are relaxed, their hands are open; by now they've outgrown the closed-fist pose of younger babies. You can see the slow progression from that tight-fisted infant to a more mobile and coordinated baby. Right now, your baby is just beginning to use hands and fingers for small tasks. And it's hard work! Watching your baby, you can probably see the amount of effort that goes into this kind of "play." When your baby reaches for an object, the baby's other hand may mirror the movement of the reaching hand. Both hands may close as one hand reaches for and grasps a toy.

It's too early to tell whether your baby is left-handed or right-handed. At this age, babies may seem to favor one hand for a while, then switch and use the other hand more often. True handedness is not usually determined until a child is about 3 years old.

Rolling over. At five or six months, most babies have learned to roll both ways. Keep a hand on the baby when changing diapers, and never leave the baby alone on a bed, counter, couch or any other elevated surface.

Sitting. Your little explorer will probably want to spend most of the day upright and will no longer be content to lie either faceup or facedown. When in your lap, your baby will probably want to sit or even "stand" on your legs. Your baby may also like sitting alone supported by pillows.

During these two months, your baby is working toward sitting up without help. A key development that makes sitting up possible is head control. By six months, your baby should be able to keep a steady neck and head position when pulled to a sitting position. Your baby's head shouldn't drop back and may even come forward as if "leading" the baby into a sitting position. Playing facedown on the floor and lifting the head and chest to see toys are good exercises to help your baby strengthen neck muscles and develop the head control necessary for sitting up.

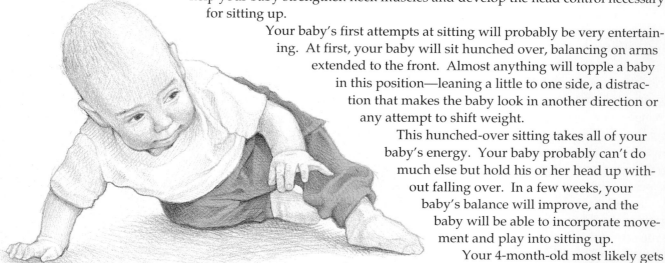

Your baby's first attempts at sitting will probably be very entertaining. At first, your baby will sit hunched over, balancing on arms extended to the front. Almost anything will topple a baby in this position—leaning a little to one side, a distraction that makes the baby look in another direction or any attempt to shift weight.

This hunched-over sitting takes all of your baby's energy. Your baby probably can't do much else but hold his or her head up without falling over. In a few weeks, your baby's balance will improve, and the baby will be able to incorporate movement and play into sitting up.

Your 4-month-old most likely gets great joy out of being upright and "standing" on your lap, and perhaps bouncing. All the bouncing your baby does is a part of normal development and is not harmful to the baby's hips, legs or feet. By about five months, you will notice your baby can probably bear full body weight on his or her legs without standing up on tiptoes. Standing alone and walking are still a long way off, but you can see how the small stages of development are preparing your baby for greater mobility.

Sitting is a skill your baby wants, and will work hard, to master.

Playing With Your Baby

As your baby becomes more of an explorer, playtime becomes more enjoyable for you and more intense for your baby. For your baby, every game is a learning experience. You might see outward signs of your baby's deep concentration, such as moving the mouth or tongue while playing. Your baby can't keep up that level of intensity and energy for very long, so keep playtimes short.

Give your baby plenty of opportunities to practice new developments. You can encourage reaching skills by putting your baby facedown on the floor with a few toys just out of reach.

One of the main concepts your baby is exploring at this age is cause and effect. Your baby is beginning to understand the results of simple actions. For example, squeezing or shaking certain toys makes noise. Hitting a toy against a table makes another noise. Your baby may repeat these actions, hoping for a response—a look, a smile, laughter—from you. This is an excellent age to start playing peekaboo.

Your baby will probably delight in play that involves taking turns. By six months, a favorite game for your baby is dropping things. Dropping a toy prompts mom or dad to pick it up. Most of the time, this game isn't nearly as much fun for the parent. Try variations that allow your baby to enjoy this game without wearing you out. Some possibilities might be:

- Tie the toys on short strings so you don't have to get on the floor to pick them up when your baby drops them.
- Find a big box and encourage your baby to drop the toys in the box. Turn the box over and empty it after the baby has dropped several toys.
- Try to get your baby interested in passing the toys directly to you rather than dropping them and waiting for you to pick them up.

Toys. Through their sixth month, babies are still interested in very simple objects and toys. By now, your baby will probably play purposefully with rattles and toys that squeak or make noise. Blocks and stacking toys are fun for banging and dropping. Teething rings and any other toys designed especially for gumming and chewing are also good, but remember that all toys will eventually end up in your baby's mouth. Keep toys that may be choking hazards out of your baby's reach.

Mobiles and toys to watch are still enjoyable for your baby. Keep an eye on these toys, and remove them from your baby's crib or play area when the baby is big enough to grab them or can sit up and reach them.

Playtime is intense for your baby, so be careful not to overstimulate the baby with too much activity or too many toys. Give your baby just a few toys at a time.

Safety

Each new stage of development requires increased attention to your baby's safety. During these two months, the two areas of development that cause new safety concerns are hand-to-mouth play and learning to sit up.

Infant seats. When your baby starts learning to sit up, chairs and toys that used to restrain your baby no longer will. Your baby can easily topple an infant seat left on a counter. An infant swing is no longer safe when your child is big enough to sit up and topple out of it. Use all safety straps provided, but don't leave your baby unattended in any infant seat or "sitting" toy. Avoid using jumpers and walkers. (The safety of jumpers and walkers is discussed on page 536.)

Bathtub seats. By six months, your baby may be big enough to use an infant seat made especially for the bathtub. These convenient seats have suction cups to hold the seat securely in the tub, but they should be used only as a toy that makes bath time more fun and convenient, not as a reliable support for your baby. Your baby is still unstable, wiggly and slippery and should not be left unattended in the tub even for a moment. Babies can drown very quickly in very little water. If something calls you away from the bathroom, take your baby with you.

Car seats. If your baby is still content to sit in a car seat facing backward, it's safest to keep the baby in this position. Some experts recommend turning the baby around when the baby reaches 20 pounds or six months of age. It's best to go by your own baby's development. When your baby can sit up without support, it's safe to turn the car seat around to face forward.

Choking. By six months, anything and everything makes its way into your baby's mouth. If your baby is eating anything besides breast milk or formula or is moving around more, the risks of choking increase. Remember that your baby's vision is improving, and the baby is learning to focus on smaller objects. Make sure these fascinating objects are not within your baby's reach.

Review the lists of choking hazards on pages 455, 583, and 648. Remind older children which of their toys they must keep away from the baby.

This is a good time to review infant cardiopulmonary resuscitation (CPR), explained on page 649.

Feeding and Nutrition

Many parents find feeding their babies between four and six months frustrating and confusing. They hear lots of opinions about what and how their babies should be eating.

There are no absolute timetables or specific rules about feeding your growing baby. Knowing when and how to start feeding solid foods and how to incorporate your baby's feeding time into the family's schedule are decisions you and your baby have to make together. But measurable developments in your baby's life and simple guidelines about dietary needs and nutrition can help you make a choice that's comfortable for your family.

Your Baby's Diet

Through most—if not all—of this two-month period, breast milk or formula is the best food for your baby. Breast milk and formula are easiest for your baby to eat and digest. They provide all the calories and nutrition your baby needs. Cereal is not nutritionally necessary during your baby's first six months.

The possibilities of food allergies are greatest during infancy. Maintaining a diet of breast milk or formula as long as possible reduces the risk of introducing allergens to your baby. As your baby's digestive system develops, the baby is better able to handle different foods without an allergic reaction. Also, waiting until your baby is developmentally ready for solid foods will shorten the transition time between your starting to feed solid foods and your baby participating in the feeding process.

If your baby seems to be increasingly hungry, it's best to increase the frequency of the breast or bottle feedings. However, you are probably beginning to think ahead to the time your baby will be eating solid foods. Deciding when to start giving your baby solids is a decision that should be made with a complete understanding of your baby's development and nutritional needs. Your baby's health care provider can give you information and support as you and your baby make this decision.

The iron your baby needs

By the time your baby's birth weight doubles, the baby has likely used up the iron stored during pregnancy. A dietary source of iron now becomes important to minimize the risk of anemia developing in your baby by the end of the first year. If your baby is breastfed and takes no formula feedings, talk about your baby's iron needs with the baby's health care provider. If your baby is receiving a low-iron formula, switch to a formula that is iron-fortified when the baby reaches this milestone.

When your baby begins eating cereal, choose a cereal with iron. When cereal is added to your baby's diet, it reduces the absorption of iron from breast milk or formula.

Solid Foods

Throughout our culture, opinions about when babies should start to eat solid foods have changed many times. In this century, popular opinion has recommended feeding solids as early as a few weeks old and as late as 1 year old. However, nutrition experts have maintained that solid food should rarely be started before the fourth month. Many suggest waiting until your baby is at least 6 months old.

Popular wisdom has a life of its own, and mothers have not always followed these recommendations. Many of today's mothers and fathers were raised by parents who started giving them solids early. Consequently, the issue of when your baby should be given solids may cause friction between you and the generation before you.

When to start giving your baby solids. You should introduce solids when your baby is ready to use new skills and is ready to build on those skills to learn more advanced ones. Introducing solids also should be coordinated with your baby's increasing nutritional needs. A lot of knowing when to start giving your baby solid foods is learning to read your baby's developmental cues.

Mouth. Your baby is interested in putting things in his or her mouth and exploring different tastes and textures. You may notice your baby making "chewing" motions, although they are usually up-and-down motions and don't incorporate the rotating, grinding motions needed for real chewing. Most of this mouthing is just play and experimentation. These are the preliminary steps toward readiness for solid foods, but they do not necessarily mean that the time has arrived for introducing solids.

Sitting up and head control. It's important for your baby to be stable and in control of body movements before starting solids. Watch to see if your baby can sit well when supported, can lead with his or her head when being pulled into a sitting position and can lift up from a tummy-down position and look around or play while holding his or her head up. It's important that your baby be able to maintain a stable upright position in order to eat solids off a spoon.

Tongue protrusion. From birth, your baby uses an outward push of the tongue to get milk from the bottle or breast, then sucks and swallows. This tongue protrusion reflex, which gradually diminishes during the baby's first six months, makes eating solid foods inefficient.

Swallowing. Being able to move food to the back of the mouth and swallow is a necessary skill for eating solids. As your baby learns to swallow efficiently, you will probably notice a decrease in the amount of drooling. The diminishing of the tongue protrusion reflex and your baby's ability to swallow without sucking go hand in hand.

Digestion. Although you can't outwardly measure how well your baby's digestive system is developing, the efficiency of your baby's intestinal absorption is increasing between the fourth and sixth months. By six months, your baby is much more efficient at processing food. Most babies can eat cereal at this age.

Hunger. Your baby's hunger cues are probably very familiar to you by now. If your baby seems increasingly hungry, add more frequent breast or bottle feedings.

Growth. Your baby's size may give you an indication as to when he or she is ready for solid foods. Most babies are able to eat solids after they've doubled their birth weights, which may be before or after their sixth month.

Sleep. Your baby's ability to sleep through the night is not connected with readiness for solid foods.

What to feed your baby.

Start your baby on the type of food that will be easiest to digest and have the least possibility of causing an allergic reaction in your baby's immature digestive system.

As your baby gets closer to 6 months old and is showing developmental cues indicating readiness for solid foods, you can introduce an iron-fortified cereal in your baby's diet. Baby cereals contain the type of easily absorbed iron your baby needs. Rice cereal is a good first food because it is easily digested and has little allergy potential. Buy cereals specially formulated for infants; they have the perfect balance of fat, protein and carbohydrate as well as iron amounts appropriate for babies. Commercial adult cereals contain iron, but not the type of iron babies easily digest.

Remember that, nutritionally, your baby still gets all the necessary vitamins and minerals through breast milk or formula with iron and doesn't need cereal or other solid foods in the first six months to meet nutritional needs. Therefore, when you start solid food, it should not take the place of breast milk or formula. Decreasing milk intake decreases the vital protein your baby needs. At this stage, breast milk or formula is more important to your baby's diet than cereal.

When your baby is used to cereal and is eating two cereal feedings a day, you may be ready to start introducing other solid foods. (Juice, fruits and vegetables are discussed on pages 566 and 567. Meats are discussed on page 583.)

How to feed your baby cereal. Cereal is a good food choice for your baby because it is soft and easy to manipulate. Mix your baby's cereal with liquid so the mixture is watery. Cereal can be mixed with your baby's regular diet of breast milk, formula or water.

When you're ready to start giving your baby solids, you should begin the feeding by giving your baby breast milk or formula. Remember that cereal is not intended to take the place of your baby's regular feedings, but to supplement them. Offer your baby cereal after he or she has had a regular feeding.

Place your baby in an upright position to eat cereal. At this age, you can put the baby in your lap or in an infant seat. After your baby has learned to sit without support, you can put the baby in a high chair. As your baby is learning to sit up, he or she will need close supervision while eating in an infant seat.

Feed your baby cereal with a spoon. Your baby needs to eat off a spoon to learn how to swallow without sucking. Putting cereal in an infant feeder or a bottle with a widened nipple may encourage your baby to overeat, which could lead to problems with obesity later in life.

Expect your baby to react to this new experience by pushing the food back out, making faces or even looking confused. When your baby gets used to the new taste and texture, he or she will probably open wide in anticipation of the food and swallow actively.

If your baby just doesn't seem to like the cereal, consider the possibility that it's not time for solid foods yet, or your baby isn't in the mood to put in the effort needed to learn something new.

Amounts and schedules. At first, your baby will seem to eat very little cereal. Start with about 1 tablespoon of rice cereal mixture once a day. This feeding does not have to be a morning feeding. Find a time of day that's convenient for you and the baby, keeping in mind that feedings will take longer as your baby is learning new eating skills.

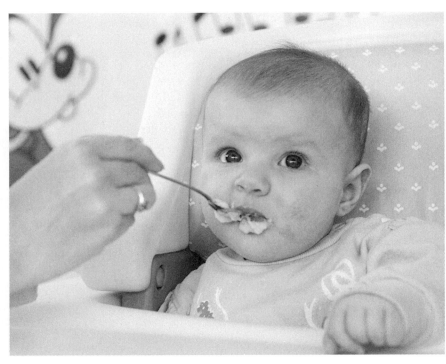

"This doesn't taste like milk at all." Your baby will learn to enjoy the texture and taste of solids; but don't expect immediate success with spoon feeding.

When your baby is eating 2 to 3 tablespoons of cereal once a day, add another cereal feeding. Your baby should be up to a total of about a half cup of cereal a day before you need to add any other solid foods. (You can read about adding new solid foods on page 566.)

The amount your baby eats may vary from feeding to feeding, so it's important to watch for cues that your baby is full. A baby who refuses to open up for the next bite, turns away or starts to play with the food is probably full.

Sleeping Patterns and Habits

You may feel that your baby expresses likes, dislikes and personality most strongly over the issue of sleep.

Remember that your 6-month-old is an explorer and is probably very reluctant to give up the day's adventures by going to sleep. Respect your baby's adventuresome spirit and provide plenty of time and a quiet atmosphere for winding down from the day's activities. Reading to your baby, playing music, giving your baby a bath and just cuddling are all activities that will signal your baby that bedtime is coming.

Babies are all different and operate on unique timetables. Your family's activities and schedules will also affect your baby's sleep schedule. Finding a sleep schedule that works for your baby and your family may take time. You may feel that your baby's schedule differs from day to day. Generally, your baby should be sleeping well at night by six months, perhaps as long as seven to 12 hours. In addition, your baby may take a couple of daytime naps, lasting anywhere from a few minutes to two hours. As in all aspects of development, each baby's patterns and needs vary.

Your baby's sleep schedule is probably becoming more predictable. It's reasonable to expect your baby to learn to fall asleep alone by this age. Reassure yourself that this goal is possible by remembering:

- Your baby is physically mature enough to go without a feeding in the night. If your baby cries in the night, it's most likely not because of hunger.
- Almost all babies cry almost every time they're put down to sleep alone. Your baby's bedtime crying is normal.
- Waking periodically throughout the night is part of everyone's normal sleeping patterns.
- Babies are very good at determining the amount of sleep they need. One way or another, your baby will get enough sleep.

Even after a calming bedtime routine, your baby may begin crying when put down to sleep. If you want your baby to fall asleep without your direct help, you may be able to help the baby fall asleep by allowing the baby to cry for a short time, then going in to comfort your baby, letting your baby know you haven't abandoned him or her. Be neutral and matter-of-fact, not playful or entertaining. Talk to your baby calmly and pat the baby's back, but resist the urge to pick your baby up. Leave the room and wait outside the door for a few minutes. If your baby doesn't fall asleep, repeat the calming sequence. Repeat this until your baby falls asleep. Each night, you may want to lengthen the amount of time between trips into the room to calm your baby.

How to deal with bedtime crying is a personal decision. If you choose not to leave your baby to fall asleep alone, you may choose to comfort your baby by rocking, reading or staying in the room.

Remember that your baby's sleep schedule is unique and personal. Even though you may talk to many parents whose babies seem to be sleeping perfectly, remember that it's normal and common to struggle with sleep issues at this age. As you get to know your baby's personality and sleep needs, you will be able to create a sleep schedule that works for your baby and your family.

The Six-Month Checkup

The six-month checkup should seem more familiar. You are probably comfortable with the office routine and can easily predict how your baby is going to react. Your baby's health care provider is becoming familiar to you, and you may be more comfortable talking about any questions or concerns you have.

Examination

Your baby will be weighed and measured. These measurements will be compared with those from the last checkup so you can see your baby's steady rate of growth. By six months, most babies have doubled their birth weight.

This physical exam may focus less on growth and physical changes; instead, the baby's health care provider may ask questions and evaluate your baby's activities, abilities and motor development. You can expect the exam to include:

- Listening to your baby's heart and lungs.
- Looking over the baby's skin for rashes.

- Feeling your baby's head and fontanelles (soft spots).
- Feeling for any incoming teeth.
- Checking head control.
- Testing your baby's ability to sit and stand with help; examining the baby's legs, feet and hips.
- Checking genitals.
- Assessing muscle tone and strength.
- Watching for and asking about your baby's reaching skills.
- Evaluating your baby's ability to grasp and let go.
- Examining the ability of your baby's eyes to focus straight ahead.
- Asking about your baby's sight and hearing. Although your baby's health care provider will try to evaluate these at the checkup, you can probably better tell how your baby sees and hears from the baby's day-to-day reactions and activities.
- Talking about sleeping and feeding issues.
- Discussing safety.

Immunizations

At this visit, the DTP and HIB vaccines are given, perhaps in a combined shot called DTP-H. These are immunizations your baby has received at previous visits. (These vaccinations, their purposes and any side effects are discussed on page 525.)

The oral polio vaccine is optional at this visit. Although your baby will have a third oral polio vaccine, it may be given anytime between 6 and 18 months of age. Your baby's doctor may give this vaccine now if you live in an area where polio may be an active concern.

Your baby may again experience discomfort from the shots given at this visit. Follow the acetaminophen dosages on page 526 to relieve your baby's pain. Any redness or swelling of the area around the injection site may be eased with a tepid bath.

Health Awareness

During these two months, the immunity your baby received while in the womb is waning, and the baby's own immune response is getting stronger. Your baby may experience an unpleasant "first"—an upper respiratory tract infection or other virus.

What Parents Worry About

Developmental Accomplishments

Most developmental timetables you read will show specific milestones most babies can reach during these two months: rolling over, reaching for toys, sitting up, bringing hands and toys to their mouths. If your child can't accomplish all the tasks, you may wonder, "Is my child normal?"

Developmental timetables are based on the average ages at which a study group of children accomplished certain tasks. The range of ages at which babies learn any new skill is wide. For example, one baby might roll over at 2 months of age and another may not roll over until 5 months. Both babies are perfectly normal, although neither is average.

If your baby is showing steady progress in learning new skills, don't be concerned about meeting specific dates on a timetable. Your baby may just be concentrating energy on another area of development.

If you are concerned that your baby is a little slower than average in learning new motor skills, talk to the baby's health care provider.

Daily Schedules

At the beginning of these two months, your baby's schedule probably seems erratic and unpredictable. In fact, your baby may seem to have several schedules, one for eating, another for sleeping and napping and still another for playing and socializing. You have a schedule too. Or at least you used to before the baby came, and you'd probably like to get back to it.

Many parents worry about forcing their babies into uncomfortable and unnatural schedules for the sake of creating a workable family schedule. You may worry that you're depriving your child of needed sleep, food or play in order to keep your own life in order.

This is not just a problem for families with babies. All families must learn to integrate the activities of all family members into one schedule. However, it may seem like a bigger problem now because you think your baby can't communicate personal wants and desires.

The truth is that your baby has a distinct personality and specific likes and dislikes. Babies know how to get their parents' attention when they aren't getting something they need or want. They also know how to regulate their own sleep and play to meet their needs. If you're watching your baby's cues, you should be able to make it through until the baby's schedule of eating and sleeping more closely matches your own.

CHAPTER THIRTY-THREE

Baby From Six to Nine Months

The period between six and nine months is a time of growing independence, which can be both exhilarating and frightening for an infant. You find your baby vigorously venturing into new things, but afraid to be too far away from the security of what he or she already knows—you.

Social Development

Your baby's wants, desires and distinct personality are probably clear to you by now. Between six and nine months, your baby will develop a personal and unique way to let you know what he or she thinks and wants.

Your 6- to 9-month-old baby craves your attention. She or he learns what behaviors—both good and bad—engage you. It takes some practice to conceal your reactions to your baby's mischievous antics and to lavish attention when you catch your baby being good.

During this time, your baby is torn between two desires: to be with you and to begin to learn independence. This struggle may surface in many situations as your baby searches for both predictability and adventure. Living with this new assertiveness may be tough for you as well as for your baby.

Your baby may seem most assertive when you make any attempt to separate from the baby—for a few hours or a few minutes. She or he may become more clingy—not wanting to let you out of sight—and may grasp or cry if you manage to break away. Your baby may even begin to strongly prefer the parent he or she spends the most time with. Both parents should understand that this situation is normal and will diminish with time.

How Your Baby Relates to You

Every baby goes through a stage of "separation anxiety," which may begin now or several months from now. Some babies pass through this phase quickly, but others struggle for a few months.

Part of your baby's frustration stems from not having the motor skills to follow you or keep up with you. And by nine months, your baby now understands the concept of "object permanence," the idea that something still exists even if it's out of sight. It's likely your baby knows you're just beyond sight range, but he or she can't get to you.

The positive side of this phase is that it shows a strong attachment between you and your baby. It may help to think of your baby's desperate cries at your separation as a compliment, although many parents have said, "I wish my baby didn't love me quite so much."

How Your Baby Relates to Others

Your baby's extreme attachment to you can result in a seeming dislike for everyone else. This can be crushing to caregivers, grandparents and friends who feel close to the baby. You can ease their feelings of rejection by explaining separation anxiety and helping to create a time of adjustment and transition.

If someone approaches your baby quickly, eagerly trying to engage the baby, the baby will probably cling to you even more tightly. Encourage others to spend some time just talking with you while you let your baby watch and listen. Your baby may eventually open up and jabber or want to play.

Peekaboo can be an icebreaker at this age because this game is so tempting for most babies. But don't be surprised if your baby will play this game only when you're close by. Assure others that your baby will outgrow this shyness.

Baby-sitters. Because babies react so strongly to separation from their parents, parents often are reluctant to leave their babies with sitters. You may wonder whether an evening out is worth the agony your baby seems to go through when left with a baby-sitter. You can help yourself and your baby through this stage by:

- Telling your baby when you are going to leave and providing reassurance that you will return. It's tempting to just sneak out when the baby is pre-occupied, but this approach won't help your baby overcome this anxiety. Instead, your baby could become more clingy, never knowing if you're going to leave.

- Encouraging your baby to adopt a transitional object—a toy, stuffed animal or blanket—something your child is attached to that will give a sense of security. During the next year or so, this special object can help your child move from dependence to independence.

- Assessing the quality of care your baby is getting when you're apart. If you are comfortable with your sitter and feel assured your baby is getting loving, qualified and competent care, you will be less bothered by your baby's crying when you leave.

- Remembering that your baby will only learn that you can be trusted to return if given the chance to be apart from you. Your baby will develop this kind of trust through experience.

Siblings. For a lot of big brothers and sisters, the honeymoon is over. That little baby loses some of the enchantment when the baby can scoot around and get into a sibling's toys.

For your baby—who has the increasing mobility to get around and explore—it's difficult to understand what's off limits. Encourage a spirit of cooperation with an older child. You may even want to create "my," "baby's" and "family" play areas.

Language Development

Your baby's understanding of words is far ahead of the ability to use them. At this age, she or he understands by listening to your tone of voice. Even the word "no" is understood by inflection and tone and not necessarily by the word itself.

The more you talk to your baby—whether it's while driving, dressing, feeding or cooking—the more your baby learns about communication.

By nine months, your baby knows his or her own name and is learning the meaning of many words that are associated with familiar people or objects, such as "doggy," "car" or the name of a brother or sister. At this age, some babies can follow simple one- or two-word commands even without being cued by hand gestures.

Continue to expose your baby to language. Give the baby books, even if your baby holds them upside down or just looks at the pictures. Point to the pictures and tell short, sentence-length stories. Follow your baby's lead, keeping in mind that most babies at this age have an attention span of just two or three minutes.

Your Baby's Speech

Your baby's babbling is probably starting to sound more like real words. At six months, your baby may make sounds like "dadadada" and "mamamama," but these are sounds only and probably aren't used to name people yet.

By nine months, almost all babies can babble by repeating one sound over and over as well as creating a string of alternating sounds. Some babies may have learned to name something or somebody, such as "mama." A few may even know another word by now, such as "baba" for bottle. However, most babies are still just experimenting with sound, imitating speech.

Sensory Development

Observing your baby's day-to-day activities is the best way to "test" your baby's sight and hearing.

Sight

Your baby's vision is almost adult-like in clarity and depth perception. By eight months, most babies' vision is 20/40. Although your baby still sees things close up better than far away, your baby's vision should be clear enough to recognize people and objects across the room.

Hearing

By six or seven months, your baby's hearing is almost fully matured. A baby at this age can quickly and accurately locate the source of a sound. Watch to see if your baby turns toward a sound, even if the sound comes from outside the baby's line of vision.

Be aware of noise overload. The constant drone of a TV or radio can make it difficult for your baby to sort out human voices.

Motor Development

How Your Baby Is Changing

Your baby's quick development during these months can be astonishing. In just a few weeks, your baby may go from barely sitting up without your help to bustling around the room by scooting, crawling and cruising.

No matter how fast your baby learns, there will probably be frustrating days when the baby wants to do more than he or she is able to.

Hand and finger coordination. At six months, babies have very clumsy hand movements and pick up objects by using a palmar grasp, with all their fingers pressing against their thumbs, as if wearing mittens. Between the sixth and ninth month, most babies will learn to use a "pincer" grasp, using the thumb and pointer finger to pick up small objects.

The graduation from a mitten grasp to a pincer grasp is gradual. First, you may notice your child using an "assisted" pincer grasp, resting the arm and hand on a surface to steady the hand and pick up a small object. Once that object is in hand, your baby may practice moving it back and forth from one hand to the other.

With the pincer grasp, your baby can—and probably will—pick up objects as small as a piece of lint. Because almost everything your baby touches goes directly into the mouth for further exploration, examine the baby's play area carefully and remove things that could cause choking.

Your baby is learning to use purposeful movements to control and move larger objects too. By seven months, your baby may use both hands to grab a toy. At nine months, your baby might pick up a different toy in each hand and practice banging them together.

Sitting up. By six months, your baby probably sits up with help or sits alone by leaning forward, hands to the floor. By seven months, your baby may be sitting alone with no support, even working to put arms to the side to keep from toppling over sideways. At eight months, your baby is even steadier and may be able to sit up for as long as five minutes without falling.

Your baby will learn to sit up before learning how to get from any other position into a sitting position. At nine months, about half of all babies can maneuver themselves into the sitting position.

Crawling. After your baby learns to sit up without much effort, you'll notice other movements that are predecessors to crawling—rolling, twisting, crouching and rocking back and forth on knees.

Your baby's desire and ability to crawl may differ greatly from another baby's. Crawling isn't even listed on many developmental charts. In fact, some babies aren't even interested in crawling, or may crawl just a few days before moving on to something else. Other babies seem to think crawling is the best and fastest way to get from one place to another.

Crawling uses the complex give-and-take movements of all four limbs that are necessary for walking later. It takes some time to understand how to make those little arms and legs work together. At first, a baby's arms are stronger than the legs, which makes for some funny crawling variations. Many babies begin crawling by using just their arms, scooting across the floor like a soldier in training. Others may find themselves up on their knees, give their arms a good push and begin moving backward.

Eventually, most babies will become experts at using their legs and arms simultaneously when they crawl. This is when parents look away for a minute, then look back and wonder, "Where did the baby go?"

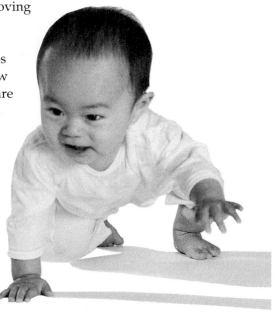

Standing. At eight or nine months, if you stand your baby up next to the sofa, the baby will probably be able to stand there, using the furniture for support. When your baby realizes how much fun standing is, he or she will probably start figuring out how to pull up to a standing position without your help.

By eight months, most babies can stand up with support. At nine months, more than half of all babies can pull themselves into a standing position, and some are beginning to "cruise" around the room, holding onto furniture for support. Some know how to lower themselves from a standing position instead of falling.

Learning to stand helps your baby develop the muscle control and strength needed for walking. However, most babies don't need help learning how to walk. Your baby will learn to walk when he or she is ready, as long as you provide opportunities for exercising and strengthening muscles.

Crawling can be the fastest and best way to get from one place to another. But getting those little arms and legs to work together smoothly does take practice.

Safe cruising

Get down to your baby's level and look around the room. What might your baby grab on to when standing, cruising or exploring? Watch out for:

- Dangling electrical cords
- Tablecloths
- Pull cords for window blinds
- Unsteady bookcases and other furniture
- Recliners with footrests left in upright position
- Floor lamps
- Garbage pails
- Pot handles
- Houseplants

This is a good time to review home safety (see page 454). Removing treasured or breakable items and making your home childproof will give your baby the freedom and confidence to explore and learn.

Playing With Your Baby

At this age, babies like predictability and will play the same game over and over. For example, many babies will engage in a back-and-forth game. At nine months, about half of all babies will even initiate passing games, giving away toys then taking them back.

Because of your baby's development of object permanence, she or he will enjoy games in which objects and people "disappear" and "reappear," such as peekaboo. Use a small blanket to cover toys and let your baby uncover and "discover" them.

Your baby is also beginning to learn how things relate to one another. Infants at this age start to understand that smaller objects fit inside bigger ones. Games in which toys can be put into a container and dumped back out again are popular.

Your baby is now starting to learn how objects relate to one another in three-dimensional space. If your baby is looking in a mirror and you suddenly appear in the mirror too, your baby is likely to turn around and look for you instead of believing you're in the mirror itself.

For the most part, your baby's playtime will center around playing on the floor, working on crawling, sitting and standing. You can encourage these skills by putting a toy just beyond your baby's reach and encouraging the baby to move toward it.

Toys. From six to nine months, most babies enjoy toys they can bang, poke, twist, squeeze, drop, shake, open, close, empty and fill. Toys should be lightweight with no sharp edges. All toys will end up in your baby's mouth, so don't give your baby any toys with small parts.

Simple household objects like plastic food storage containers and plastic serving spoons are likely to entertain your baby.

Most 9-month-old babies are active and need a lot of stimulation, but they don't like to be apart from mom or dad. It's difficult to give your baby that attention and get anything else accomplished. Fill a small basket with toys for each room of the house; then take the baby with you as you go from room to room and let your baby play while you work.

Safety

Your baby is learning to understand "no." But neither you nor your baby will be happy in a home in which you have to constantly keep a close watch and remind the baby to keep away from dangerous situations and objects. Besides, at this age your baby has little self-control, and so many things around the house are tempting. Take a few precautions to protect your baby and your home during these new stages of motor development.

Stairs. As your baby learns to crawl and cruise, protecting your baby from falls down the stairs becomes crucial. It's important to have gates at the top and bottom of each stairway and to use those gates properly.

Choose a gate that slides to close, rather than the accordion-style gates. Some of the older gates had openings large enough that the baby's head could get caught. Look for a gate with openings no bigger than 2⅜ inches.

Never leave your baby alone near stairs. Although your baby will be attracted to stairs and will quickly learn to go up them, most babies can't be expected to learn how to turn around and come down safely until after their first year.

Falls. A baby just learning to move around the room is still unsteady. Minor bumps and bruises are an unavoidable part of gaining motor skills and independence. To reduce the risk of serious injury:

- Keep your baby away from elevated porches, decks, stairs and landings.
- Remove furniture with pointed corners.
- Make sure all rugs are skid-proof.

Car seats. By the time your baby reaches nine months or about 20 pounds, your baby can ride in a forward-facing car seat. At this age, your baby may seem to hate riding in the car seat. Remember, this is an active, exploring stage when your baby wants to be upright and moving around. Be firm and consistent. Always use the car seat.

Baby carriers. If you've been using a baby carrier positioned on your front, you can switch to a backpack carrier when your baby has learned to sit without support. To make this mode of transportation safe for your baby:

- Make sure all metal supports are well padded.
- Use the safety straps.
- Check the carrier periodically for wear.
- Don't bend over from the waist. The baby could fall out of the carrier.
- Don't allow your baby to stand on the supports during a ride in the backpack.

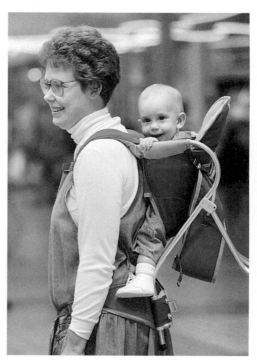

Whether at a mall or on a hiking trail, there's no doubt about it—Mom's backpack is a fun place to be.

Feeding and Nutrition

During these months, your baby's eating habits and schedule will probably change greatly. At six months, most babies get all or most of their nutrition from breast milk or formula. By nine months, they may be eating a wide variety of foods at mealtime with the family, with additional nursing or bottles between meals. These three months are a transition time, when the balance of fluids and foods will be changing.

Your Baby's Diet

Breast milk and formula. As you begin altering your baby's diet to add cereal and other solid foods, you may ask, "What role does breast milk or formula play? Is it still important for my baby?"

Breast milk is designed to be a perfect food for your baby through the baby's first year and beyond. Both breast milk and formula provide important vitamins, iron and protein in an easily digestible form. Even though solid foods will eventually replace some of your baby's feedings, they can't efficiently replace the balance of nutrients that breast milk or formula provides.

Many parents wonder whether their babies can drink whole milk at this age. It's best for your baby to have breast milk or formula during the first year. Your baby's delicate system is not able to adequately handle the type and concentration of selected nutrients found in cow's milk. And cow's milk is lower in iron and vitamins E and C than breast milk or formula.

A baby or toddler should never be fed low-fat or skim milk. Fat is important for a child's growth and brain development.

Solid foods. Your baby's first solid food will probably be cereal. (Starting your baby on cereal is discussed on page 553.) Cereal is a versatile food because it can be mixed very thin for babies just starting on solid foods and can be thickened as babies work on chewing and swallowing. At first, your baby will "chew" in an up-and-down motion. When your baby begins to use more of a side-to-side, grinding motion, he or she can handle thicker or more textured foods. It's not necessary that your baby have teeth before learning to grind; even when your baby starts to develop one or two teeth, those teeth won't be of much use for eating.

Solid foods should be introduced slowly, one at a time. Your baby needs time to get used to each new taste and texture. Giving your baby only one or two new foods a week will allow you to watch for any allergic reactions, such as diarrhea, stomachaches or rashes.

After cereals, fruits and vegetables are easiest for babies to digest. You can start by offering your baby a few table-spoons of fruit in the same meal as a cereal feeding. At six months, any fruit or vegetable should be strained. Babies eat by pressing food against the tops of their mouths with their tongues, and swallowing, so any food you give your baby should be mushy.

As your baby starts to eat with more of a grinding motion, add thickness and texture to the baby's diet to encourage the use of those new eating skills. At this point, your baby can handle food with the consistency of applesauce.

Good eating habits

Good eating habits start early. You can help your baby develop healthful eating patterns by:

- Offering a wide variety of foods.

- Giving your baby a good balance of foods. Use sweets, salts or fats in moderation.

- Avoiding overfeeding by watching your baby's cues to know when your baby is full.

- Rewarding your baby with something besides food— such as hugs, kisses and attention.

Using and storing baby food

- When using baby food from a jar, spoon a small amount into a bowl before feeding your baby. Then, when your baby is done eating, discard any food remaining in the bowl.

- Don't feed your baby directly from the jar or put any remaining food back in the jar. This practice allows germs from your baby's spoon to contaminate the jar.

- Baby food in jars can be stored for 24 hours in the refrigerator after opening.

- Portions of baby food can be kept in the freezer up to one month.

- Read the label to see which baby foods can be heated in the microwave. If you use a microwave to heat food for your baby, heat the food slowly. Microwaves heat unevenly, so stir heated food thoroughly and let it stand for a minute or so. Then check the food by tasting or feeling it to make sure it's cool enough for your baby.

Remember that your baby's grinding is pretty elementary, so offer foods that could be easily swallowed whole.

If you introduce a new food to your baby and get a negative reaction, try the same food a week or so later. There may be foods she or he will never like, but continue to offer them periodically to see if they become more appealing.

Finger foods. At first, it may be hard to find foods that your baby can easily eat with his or her fingers. Anything that quickly turns mushy will work. Try small pieces of banana or very mushy vegetables.

As your baby gets closer to nine months and develops more advanced chewing skills, these finger foods are appropriate:

- Adult breakfast cereals (without nuts or chunks)
- Crackers or cookies (without nuts or chunks)
- Cooked noodles, such as macaroni
- Bread, pancakes or waffles
- Slices of soft canned fruit, such as peaches or pears

Although eggs are often touted as a food that meets a young baby's chewing skills, they are highly allergenic. It's best to wait until after the first year to give your baby eggs.

Your baby probably can't handle and doesn't really need meats until after nine months. The milk products your baby consumes provide enough protein to meet your baby's nutritional needs. (Introducing meats is discussed on page 583.)

Table foods. As your baby gets closer to nine months, the food on your plate looks more appealing than baby food. It's tempting to give your baby something from your plate, but keep in mind your baby's ability to handle textures and foods of various sizes.

Between six and nine months, introduce a wide variety of foods, and work toward the day when your baby will eat the same foods the rest of the family does. Between now and 12 months, many babies decide on their own that they're finished with baby food. (Introducing table foods is discussed in greater detail on page 583.)

Juice. Juice is not an essential part of your baby's diet, but most babies like it. It's a good source of vitamin C, although a baby still drinking breast milk or formula gets enough vitamin C to meet the daily requirement.

At most, your 9-month-old baby needs only 4 ounces of juice a day to get needed vitamin C. Any more juice may decrease the amount of breast milk or formula your baby drinks. If your baby loves juice and doesn't seem satisfied with 4 ounces, try diluting the juice with one part water.

Juice, like other foods, should be added to your baby's diet slowly. When adding any new juice, watch for negative reactions such as rashes or diarrhea.

Some babies prefer fluids to solids. If you offer your baby too many fluids, your baby may not be willing to try solids. In general, offer fluids toward the end of the meal and between meals.

Preparing homemade baby foods

- Make sure all surfaces and equipment are clean.

- Use fresh foods, not leftovers.

- Puree well. Double-check for large pieces or lumps.

- Don't add salt or sugar. If you're using foods prepared for the rest of the family, take out the baby's portion before seasoning.

- After cooking frozen fruits or vegetables in a little water, put them through a blender, food mill or sieve.

- Avoid using fruit canned in syrup. Fruit canned in water or its own juice is a better choice.

- Avoid canned vegetables. Generally, they contain too much salt.

Your baby may enjoy juice after a cereal feeding. The vitamin C in juice helps your baby absorb iron.

Iron. Iron is an important nutrient in your baby's diet. Babies whose diet includes only breast milk get an adequate amount of iron. Babies drinking formula should be fed iron-fortified formula.

When cereal and solid foods are added to your baby's diet, your baby cannot use the iron in breast milk or formula as efficiently. For this reason, choose an iron-fortified cereal for your baby in addition to breast milk or formula to ensure your baby gets the iron he or she needs.

Amounts and Schedules

At first, try serving 1 to 2 tablespoons of fruit along with one of your baby's cereal feedings each day. By nine months, you can expect your baby to eat three meals a day, as well as two or three snacks. Each meal should consist of cereal, a fruit or vegetable and some finger foods. What happens between the introduction of solids and the day when your baby is eating three meals a day depends on your baby's appetite, likes and dislikes. Keep the long-term goal in mind, but follow your baby's lead on how to reach that goal.

Managing Mealtime

Eating is one area in which your baby will assert some independence, setting the course for when and what he or she will eat. As long as your baby is growing steadily and you are offering a well-balanced variety of food, you may find it easiest to willingly give up some control in this area.

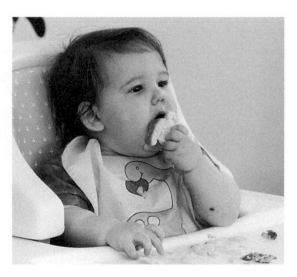

If it's on the tray, it'll be in your baby's mouth in seconds. Keep in mind your baby's limited ability to deal with textures and sizes of foods.

Mealtime games. For your baby, life is an expedition, and it's your baby's job to explore everything that's strange or different—and new foods certainly fall into this category. Your baby wants to know what a food looks like, feels like, drops like and maybe even tastes like. It may seem as though there's more food on the floor than in your baby.

As much as possible, eliminate other distractions during mealtimes. But expect that feeding your baby solid foods will take more time than breastfeeding or bottle feeding. Your baby will stop between bites and spend a lot of time feeling and playing with food. When the play is taking more time than the feeding, your baby may be letting you know he or she is full.

If you are a tidy person, this stage can be nearly unbearable. But this kind of discovery is important to your baby's development.

Spoons and fingers. Some babies have definite ideas about how they want their food presented to them. Try to teach your baby to eat with a spoon, but if that's not successful, let your baby eat with hands and fingers. You may need to make thicker cereal, thicken vegetables with cereal so your baby can grasp them or offer suitable finger foods.

Eventually, your baby will try to use a spoon, but for now fingers are generally faster.

If your baby is determined to eat without your help but can't manipulate food well enough to satisfy hunger, provide various ways to get food. Put some finger foods on the baby's tray, give the baby a spoon and use a spoon yourself. Then, be persistent in finding opportunities to get some food into the baby's mouth.

Drinking from a cup. Giving your baby a cup at the same time he or she starts eating solid foods will help the baby become familiar with it. But at this age, your baby will probably bang, drop and dump the cup more than drink from it. By nine months, only about 25 percent of babies know how to drink from a cup.

Even if your baby uses a cup at mealtimes, you may choose to continue breast-feeding or using a bottle for supplemental feedings. Feeding your baby breast milk or formula from a cup at mealtime may pave the way for weaning later.

High chairs. By the time your baby can sit easily without support, you can use a high chair for feeding times. To safely use a high chair:

- Select a chair with a broad, stable base that won't tip easily.
- Use the safety straps every time you put your baby in the chair.
- Don't allow other children to pull or hang on the high chair.
- Keep the high chair away from counters or anything your baby could push against. If you're eating out and using a portable high chair that attaches to the edge of the table, make sure your baby can't push against the table supports with his or her legs.

Sleeping Patterns and Habits

Your baby's daytime accomplishments and frustrations can follow the baby to bed and disrupt sleep. Even if your baby has been a good sleeper up until now, you may face some new sleep challenges during these months.

Nighttime Awakenings

When your baby is learning to sit up and pull up to a standing position, he or she will probably work vigorously on these skills all day. During brief wakenings in the night, the baby may automatically start practicing sitting and standing. But early on, your baby knows how to do only half a skill and may get in the frustrating position of being able to stand up but not to get down again. Even after the baby learns how to get out of these situations, the physical activity may be enough to make it hard to go back to sleep.

Your baby will probably let you know—loudly—how frustrating this situation is. At this age, your baby will probably shake the crib, cry or scream to get your attention.

Take some time to double-check the safety of your baby's crib. To prevent your baby from falling out of the crib, make sure there's nothing in the crib that your baby could stand on. Remove any items your baby might use for support when standing, such as bumper pads, pillows and large stuffed animals.

Being Alone

If your baby gets anxious when separated from you during the day, that anxiety will only be compounded at bedtime and in the middle of the night. You're caught in the dilemma of wanting to reassure your child and also wanting your baby to learn good sleep patterns and habits.

Try periodic trips into your baby's room to comfort the baby. But don't be surprised if your baby still seems inconsolable. After all, your baby is now aware that you're still near, even if you can't be seen. Your baby may be vigorous about trying to get your attention.

You can take comfort in remembering that this stage will pass. If the stress is too great, don't feel guilty about allowing the baby to come into your bed or you occasionally sleeping in the baby's room. Watch for daytime cues that your baby is beginning to get over separation anxiety, then reteach the baby to sleep alone.

The Nine-Month Checkup

Because of your baby's fear of strangers and unwillingness to be away from you, this checkup may be more traumatic than the previous one. Your baby's doctor or nurse-practitioner may choose to do some parts of the exam while you hold your baby on your lap.

Examination

The office staff will weigh and measure your baby and plot the new numbers on your baby's growth chart.

To evaluate your baby's general health, your baby's health care provider will:

- Listen to your baby's heart and lungs
- Feel your baby's head and fontanelles (soft spots)
- Feel for and examine any new teeth
- Check your baby's hip movement

Your baby's health care provider will be interested in your baby's new motor skills and development. By either watching your baby or asking you questions, he or she will want to know:

- Does your baby get to a sitting position and sit up without support?
- Does your baby use a palmar grasp or pincer grasp to pick things up?
- Can your baby stand when supported?
- Is your baby walking sideways while hanging on to furniture (cruising)?
- Will your baby pull up into a standing position?
- How does your baby talk to you?
- What is your baby eating and drinking?
- Is your baby having sleeping problems?

Immunizations

At this checkup, your baby will receive the last hepatitis B vaccination. (This vaccination, its purpose and any side effects are discussed on page 445.)

If your baby seems to have pain or fever from this vaccination, follow the acetaminophen dosages on page 526 for relief of discomfort.

Tests

At nine months, your baby's health care provider may give your baby a tuberculosis (TB) skin test. This test, usually administered as a superficial prick on the baby's arm, detects possible exposure to TB so it can be treated. Watch the pricked area for two or three days for any redness, hardness or blistering. Report any changes.

Your baby may also be given a blood test. In some cases, the blood test is to determine whether your baby has an iron deficiency. In areas where lead poisoning is a possibility, a simple blood test can determine if your baby has been exposed to dangerous levels of lead.

Because your baby is becoming more mobile, your baby's caregiver may talk about cardiopulmonary resuscitation (CPR) and safety precautions for choking, poisoning, drowning and burns. This is a good time to ask questions about how to handle health emergencies and injuries. (For more on health emergencies and injuries, see page 603.)

Health Emergencies

What Parents Worry About

Lead poisoning is difficult to detect because its symptoms occur gradually. It can cause conditions ranging from learning disabilities to retardation. Physical symptoms may include anemia, stomach problems and hearing loss.

Lead Poisoning

Although some treatment is available, it's difficult, if not impossible, to reverse the effects of lead poisoning. Prevention is the best defense.

Children who live in older homes or neighborhoods are at the greatest risk of lead poisoning. Most lead poisoning (85 percent) occurs in infants and toddlers under age 3. Children may be exposed to lead through:

- Painted surfaces (exterior surfaces painted before 1978 and interior surfaces painted before 1960)
- Dust from interior renovations in houses built before 1960
- Contact with paint from a painted crib built before 1974
- Playing near heavily trafficked roads that have been exposed to leaded gasoline
- Contact with a parent or other adult who has exposure to lead on the job

Old surfaces can be painted over, but you may want to hire a professional to remove the old paint as safely as possible. During renovation, dust often and keep the room sealed. If possible, remove your baby from the house until the painting or renovation is complete.

If you are unsure about lead levels in your paint or even on decorative dishes, you can buy a simple, inexpensive test kit at most hardware stores. A more accurate test may be made by your state or local health department. Call to see if this service is available in your area.

Your baby may have a first tooth by seven months or may not begin teething until much later. Usually, the two bottom center teeth (incisors) appear first. When they have both come in, a tooth may appear on the top. Your baby will probably get four top teeth before a matching set of four is completed on the bottom.

Teething

Your infant's baby (deciduous) teeth were formed during pregnancy. As these teeth come in, your baby's body will begin preparing adult teeth to take their place in a few years.

For some babies, teething causes pain or discomfort. Your baby might cry more or even have a low-grade fever. You can give your baby a firm—not hard—teething ring. Some parents have success with homemade teething rings such as frozen bagels. (Make sure you give your baby a frozen food that will turn soft so your baby can swallow pieces that might break loose.)

Where there are teeth, there's the possibility for tooth decay. Clean your baby's teeth by gently wiping them with a wet or dry washcloth once a day. This will prevent bacteria from staking claim on those tiny teeth. You can also help prevent the formation of decay-causing bacteria by not allowing your baby to sleep with a bottle.

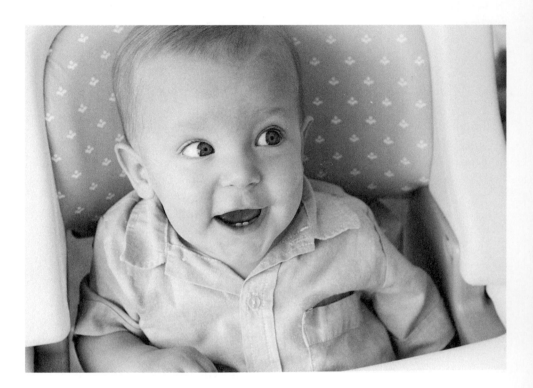

Toothless smiles will give way to smiles featuring shiny new incisors. Look for them first in the center of your baby's lower gum.

Fluoride

Breastfed babies generally get adequate amounts of fluoride in their regular breast milk feedings. Some formula-fed babies, however, may need a fluoride supplement beginning at six months. Ask your baby's health care provider about fluoride if you:

- Are exclusively breastfeeding after your baby is 6 months of age.

- Live in an area supplied by well water; some wells have naturally occurring fluoride, but most have insufficient fluoride.

- Usually feed your baby a ready-to-feed formula. This type of formula does not provide as much fluoride as the powder or concentrate that you mix with fluoridated water.

- Mix your baby's formula with bottled water lacking fluoride.

Fluoride helps the development of healthy teeth. But too much fluoride can result in mottled discoloration of the teeth. Proper dosages are based on the amount of fluoride in the water supply and the baby's age.

Thumb Sucking and Pacifiers

Sucking is a normal way for young children to soothe and comfort themselves. At this stage of development, when your baby's teeth are starting to come in, it's normal to question whether sucking is harmful for normal development of your baby's teeth. The truth is, sucking can be hard on a child's mouth and teeth—if the child is still sucking a thumb, fingers or pacifier by 7 or 8 years. Most children have long outgrown daytime sucking by that age on their own, so there's no need to try to train your baby to give it up now.

In fact, you may notice your baby using a thumb or pacifier more now to cope with separation anxiety. Sucking is one of your baby's only methods to relax or calm down.

Travel

This is a tough age to travel with a baby. Your baby likes predictability, and travel can be disrupting. Be prepared to deal with your baby's crankiness and increased clinging if you plan to travel now.

If you can find a grandparent or trusted caretaker who will help your baby keep a predictable daily routine, your baby may enjoy just staying home for a day or two, although the initial separation may be hard for both of you.

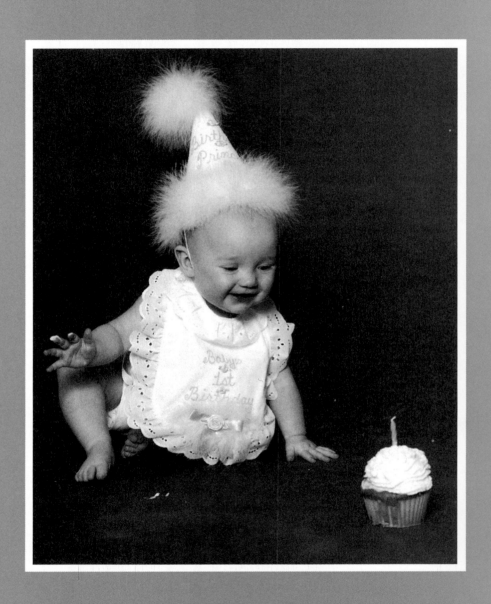

CHAPTER THIRTY-FOUR

Baby From Nine to 12 Months

Nobody else knows your baby as you do. During the first days and weeks, you may have wondered if you would ever understand each other and be able to work as a team. Now you can read your baby's moods and cues and respond with exactly what he or she needs. Your baby also understands you and knows how to thrill you, make you smile and even exasperate you.

Your baby has changed dramatically during these months. But you have too. Your baby has become more independent and communicative, and you have become a more confident and interactive parent.

This confidence and your ability to understand and communicate with your baby are your best tools in dealing with the months ahead. As your baby makes the gradual transition from infant to toddler, your attention to your baby's cues will help you provide the challenges, support and assurance your baby needs.

Social Development

Your baby is still learning about independence. Some of the fear that accompanies that early independence is starting to fade as your baby becomes more sure of his or her place in the family. However, you and other family members will be the ones your baby relies on for safety and security.

Stranger Anxiety

Don't be surprised if your baby's wariness of strangers continues through these months (see page 560). Many babies have a fear of strangers past their first birthdays. Others have shorter stages, and many even have on-and-off periods of stranger anxiety.

Setting Limits

Everything in your home is fascinating—including pot handles, fireplaces, holiday decorations, the way the water swirls in the toilet and your pet's whiskers, tail and food.

It's important to teach your baby the difference between things that are safe and things that are dangerous. But your baby's desire to explore is stronger than the desire to listen to your warnings. This isn't a sign of defiance, just your baby's natural, irrepressible craving to explore.

As much as possible, remove valuable or dangerous objects that tempt your baby. To keep your baby safe around the remaining objects, use a firm and consistent "no."

By nine months, your baby should understand what you mean when you say "no." Even so, the baby may not remember tomorrow what you've said "no" to today. Keep a close watch, and be prepared to move your persistent baby away from dangerous situations or offer a distraction.

Reserve "no" for things that can harm your baby. You can also teach your baby the meanings of "be gentle" and "be careful" for situations that require caution, such as throwing a ball or playing with the family pet.

Imitation

Since birth, your baby has been learning through listening to and watching you. Sometimes, it seems your baby isn't paying much attention to your day-to-day activities. But soon you'll discover the many things your baby has learned from you. More than half of all 1-year-olds can imitate activities.

Your baby's first imitations may be as simple as using a comb, listening to a toy phone, trying to "start" things with toy keys or trying to pick up a toy pot by its handle. In a few weeks, imitation games may be as complex as putting a sock "oven mitten" on before picking up a pot, or wiping up a spill.

First birthday

At the end of this year, the whole family deserves a party. For some families, the baby's first birthday is the chance to say good-bye to babyhood and the many colicky evenings, sleep troubles and feeding struggles. Although new challenges of parenting a toddler are still ahead, this is a chance to regroup and celebrate this young member of the family.

With cake smeared from ear to ear and from forehead to chin, your baby is undeniably adorable. While encouraging your baby to dive in and enjoy the birthday celebration, remember this is the same messy face that frustrates you at dinnertime each evening. Although it can exasperate you, that daily exploration is what makes your baby an independent person.

Consider having a small party with the baby's immediate family. At 1 year of age, your baby may not enjoy a large, noisy gathering of friends and neighbors.

Language Development

Your baby's desire to imitate you is the strongest motivator for learning to talk. The time you spend talking, singing and reading to your baby will encourage your baby to talk, sing and "read" too.

Although your baby has probably been making noises that sound like "mama" or "dada" for a few weeks, it's between nine and 12 months that your baby will start to use these words meaningfully.

How Your Baby Communicates

Besides "mama" and "dada," most babies can speak one other understandable word by their first birthdays. A few babies will know as many as five or six words. Right now, the baby's family members may be the only ones to understand those words. It may take three or four more months before other people can understand your baby's words.

Even if your baby doesn't talk much, he or she can probably communicate wants and wishes. Besides pointing and grunting, your baby is learning other symbolic gestures, such as waving bye-bye or shaking his or her head "no."

If your baby doesn't seem aggressive enough about learning to talk, try to discover what your baby is channeling her or his energies toward. Perhaps your baby is spending more time standing, cruising and walking. Eventually, speaking will become a priority. Allow your baby to learn these skills within his or her own time frame.

By one year, your baby understands many simple words and phrases. Continue talking to your baby during your daily activities, allowing your baby to hear the context of new words and phrases.

Talking to Your Baby

As your baby is learning new words, avoid "baby talk." Even though a baby's interpretation and pronunciation of a new word can be cute, the baby will eventually need to learn the correct word. When your baby uses a word such as "baubau" to ask for a bottle, gently reinforce the correct pronunciation by saying, "Do you want a bottle? Here is your bottle." However, at this early stage, it's not necessary to ask your baby to repeat the word correctly.

You can encourage your baby's exploration of words by listening intently and responding to the baby's jabbering. This interaction will teach your baby about two-way communication.

Sensory Development

The best test of your baby's sight and hearing is how the baby acts and reacts in everyday situations.

Your baby should immediately and predictably turn toward sounds. If you think your baby isn't hearing well, talk to the baby's health care provider about a hearing assessment.

Although your baby is still nearsighted, your baby can see as clearly as you can and should be able to see and respond to objects and people. If your baby is having difficulty with his or her vision, you may notice your baby:

- Holding objects close to the face or moving close to objects to see them
- Closing one eye or squinting
- Leaning forward to see something
- Squinting both eyes or wrinkling his or her face
- Crossing one or both eyes

If you notice any of these symptoms, report them to the baby's health care provider. He or she can give the baby a simple exam in the office and may schedule an exam with an eye specialist (ophthalmologist).

Motor Development

Exploring the world is your baby's primary mission. Each day, your baby is becoming better equipped for that exploration. Your baby is developing more control over muscles and limbs and, consequently, more control of his or her world.

How Your Baby Is Changing

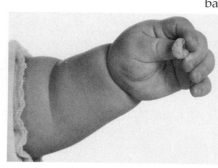

Using thumb and forefinger for precision pinching, your baby will begin picking up bits of anything close at hand, such as breakfast cereal.

Hands and fingers. Your baby's fingers are becoming more agile. The pincer grasp (discussed on page 562) will become more precise during these months and will change from an assisted pincer to a "neat" pincer. Your baby will be able to pick up an object with a thumb and finger without resting the wrist on a solid surface.

Your baby still explores by using fingers and mouth together. Anything your baby picks up will be taste-tested.

Walking. Some babies learn to walk before their first birthdays, but most don't. Your baby is normal if he or she begins walking a few steps between 9 and 14 months old.

Even if your baby isn't walking, you can probably see the baby practicing many skills that will be necessary for walking later on.

- Standing and balancing. Your baby may already be standing up while using furniture or anything else nearby, including other people, for support. During these months, your baby is learning the principles of balancing and may test his or her steadiness by trying to stoop and reach for an object on the floor. By 12 months, most babies are steady enough to stand alone briefly.

- Creeping and climbing. Once your baby can stand while holding onto something, the baby will use those objects for leverage and find ways to pull up onto furniture and even crawl up the stairs. (See the discussion of stairs and gates on page 564.)

When your baby does begin walking, expect lots of bumps and falls. A beginning walker moves mostly by propelling forward. And getting started is much easier than stopping.

Some babies like the confidence of a hand to hold when they're walking. Others like to assert their independence and try to walk without help. Follow your baby's lead. Be available if your baby seems to want your help and companionship in this new adventure.

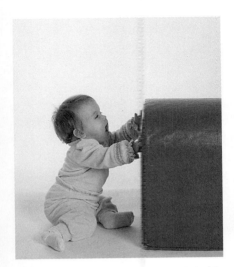 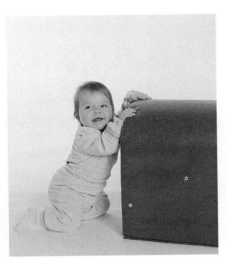 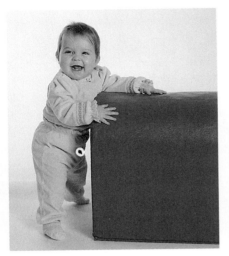

"Let's see now. If I can just grab hold of this thing...

and pull myself up...

I'll be able to stand tall, just like mom... Wow. What a view. This is fun."

Most babies take their first steps on tiptoe with their feet turned outward. In fact, many children don't walk with a mature stride—toes pointed straight ahead and heels solidly striking the ground—until they're 3 years old. (See the section on shoes on page 586.)

As your baby walks, you'll notice that the baby's arms are bent as if he or she is carrying something. As your baby becomes more confident and steady, the arms will straighten and seem more relaxed.

For most babies, the thrilling part of learning to walk is gaining more control over the world. The world is no longer limited to what comes to them; now they can go out and conquer it. This independence can be both exciting and intimidating.

Play

During these months, your baby will still enjoy games and toys that use and build new motor skills. Games that involve picking up and dropping objects will entertain your baby. As the pincer grasp becomes more developed, your baby will be able to manipulate small objects more easily.

By 12 months, your baby's play may evolve from working fine motor skills to exercising larger muscles. Your baby will think it's fun to push, throw and knock down everything.

Gesture games. By age 1 year, almost all babies will initiate gesture games such as peekaboo. You might also entertain your baby with:

- "So big." Ask your baby, "How big is (Carlos)?" Hold your arms and hands straight up for your baby to imitate and say, "(Carlos) is so-o-o big."
- "The itsy bitsy spider." Although your baby probably doesn't have the fine motor control to imitate a crawling spider, it's fun to try.
- "Pat-a-cake."

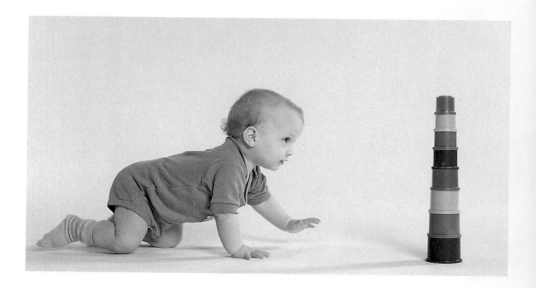

"It was thoughtful of dad to stack these cups, and I know he'll get a chuckle out of watching me knock them over. A couple more shuffles and I should be in range to take 'em down."

Toys

This is the age when you'll discover that your baby's favorite toys may not be toys at all. Even though your baby's playtime looks fun, it's also a time of work and exploration. Give your baby the freedom to explore. Remove things you don't want the baby touching.

Your baby will find fun in simple toys or household objects that fit inside one another or make noise when banged together. Find things around the house that will encourage your baby's desire to explore. Various similar objects will allow your baby to practice organizing and arranging.

When you're reading to your baby, your baby may now want to "help" you by turning the pages. Or the baby may stay occupied just flipping the pages of a book. Encourage this early interest in books by allowing your baby to have books you won't mind seeing wrinkled or torn. Sturdy board books are a good choice.

During more active play, your baby may like a push toy that helps build walking skills. Many babies just enjoy walking behind and pushing their own strollers. If you buy a push toy, choose a sturdy one. For a young walker, a toy that has a broad base provides more support.

As your baby grows, there will be more games for you two to play together. At this age, your baby likes repetitive games that include another person:

- Play a simple version of "catch."
- Hold a basket while your baby drops a toy in, then dump it back out and let the baby discover it and replace it in the basket.
- Build a tower and let your baby knock it down.

Even though these games are simple and repetitious to you, they start to teach your baby about sharing and working together.

Safety

Every step your baby takes toward more independence and mobility means an increased risk of injury. Being aware of your baby's ability to move farther and faster is the first step in reducing this risk. It may seem surprising that your baby can get into something that a week earlier was out of reach.

Take time out every few days to get down to the baby's level and look around each room. What new temptations do you see?

Injuries are most common at times when the family is busy and occupied, such as dinnertime. Your baby is active and impulsive. When you're busy and stressed, it's easy to lose sight of the baby for just a second. Unfortunately, babies at this age don't know how to adjust their need for attention and exploration just because you're stressed. Sharing mealtime duties with another family member may allow one person to play with or feed the baby while the other tends to the rest of the family's needs.

As your baby learns to stand, cruise or walk, the risk of injury increases. To reduce the risk of injury:

- Remember that your baby can reach objects even out of her or his sight. Review the list on page 563 to identify objects your baby might grab onto while cruising and standing.

- Be aware of your baby's risk of falling. Your baby can easily fall down the stairs, into the bathtub or even into an open toilet.

- Be aware of the dangers around water. A baby can drown in less than an inch of water. Taking your baby to swimming classes may be fun for you and your baby, but they will not make your baby water-safe or drown-proof. When playing in the water with your baby, don't allow the baby's head to go under water. Always know where your baby is when there's a pool around. Home pools should have fences and self-latching gates.

- Watch your baby in the yard. Uneven grass, sloping yards and hills and curves may be insurmountable obstacles for your beginning walker.

- Limit snacking to times when the baby is sitting. Moving around while eating increases your baby's risk of choking.

- Keep toys with small parts away from the baby.

- Protect your baby from poisoning. By now, your baby can get into almost everything. Keep cleaning chemicals and medications locked up and out of reach.

- Always, always use a car seat.

Feeding and Nutrition

When your baby starts eating a variety of solid foods, you may feel you've lost some control over the baby's diet. Before, you could offer breast milk or formula and be sure the baby was getting the necessary calories and nutrition. Now your baby may refuse some foods or seem to like only two or three foods. How is it possible to give your baby a balanced diet?

No matter what your baby chooses to eat from the selection, always offer a balanced variety of food. It is important to watch what your baby eats, but try to observe the baby over a period of two or three days, not just during individual meals. Most babies at this age will eat a balanced diet over the course of several days

During these months, your baby's gradual transition from baby to toddler will include developing a feeding schedule that complements the family's mealtimes. Sometime after 12 months, your baby may have a "toddler" schedule of three meals a day with the family and breast milk, formula or snacks between meals.

Development and Diet

Making decisions about your baby's food is easier when you try to choose foods that fit your baby's developmental abilities. For example, by now your baby's pincer grasp is well developed and the baby can pick up bite-sized pieces of food.

By 1 year of age, your baby may have as many as four to six teeth. In addition, the baby's chewing motion is changing from an up-and-down chomping motion to a side-to-side grinding motion. With these developments, your baby can handle foods of a thicker consistency, such as lumpy or chopped foods.

Breast Milk and Formula

By now, your baby's diet includes foods with various textures and flavors. Even if your baby's new diet seems well-rounded, breast milk and formula are still irreplaceable sources of nutrition as your baby moves from all-liquid feedings to a more grown-up diet.

Breast milk or formula is one of the baby's only sources of the fat and protein necessary for healthy physical development. Fat is especially important during these months when your baby is growing rapidly.

Any formula offered your baby should be iron-fortified. Even though your baby receives some iron from other food, your baby can't rely solely on solid foods for iron. The types and amounts of foods your baby eats are so variable that breast milk or formula remains an important source of iron.

Snacks for your baby

Offer your baby snack foods that promote good lifelong eating habits. Healthful snacks include:

- Soft fruit or peeled fruit slices
- Toast
- Crackers
- Cheese, cut into wedges or sticks; string cheese cut into lengthwise strips (to decrease the diameter)
- Cottage cheese
- Yogurt
- Plain vegetable cubes, such as potatoes or carrots, that have been cooked until soft
- Dry, unsweetened breakfast cereal

Generally, any food that is a good choice for a meal is also a good choice for a snack.

Formulas for older babies. There is no proof that formulas designed especially for older babies have any advantage over standard iron-fortified formulas. Many formulas for older babies are designed around the older baby's greater need for protein. However, older babies who are eating a wide variety of baby foods and table foods are probably getting ample protein.

Weaning from the breast. At this age, breastfeeding babies are usually very efficient. Because of their effective sucking and their mothers' easy let-down, these babies often don't take the time to snuggle and nurse. They are easily distracted during feeding times.

Some mothers interpret these shorter, easily interrupted feeding times to mean that their babies are giving up nursing. However, these types of feedings are most likely just part of • developmental stage. Most babies at this age are so intent on practicing moving around the room that they aren't willing to settle down for anything else.

Generally, there is no need to wean your baby until after the baby's first year. However, there is really no "perfect" time for weaning. Some babies will give definite signals that they are finished with breastfeeding. In other families, parents decide it's time to begin weaning.

When you and your baby are ready to wean, begin by cutting out one daytime feeding. Gradually decrease the number of breast feedings; eliminate those you provide at nap time, early morning and bedtime last.

If you wean your baby during the first year, replace the breast milk with an iron-fortified formula. Your baby isn't ready for whole milk until after the baby's first birthday.

Fruit Juice

Your baby probably loves fruit juice. But too much juice isn't good for your baby and may end up replacing breast milk, formula or other foods that can provide needed nutrition. Offer your baby breast milk or formula first, then water. Limit the amount of juice to only 4 ounces a day. (See the section on juice on page 567.)

Solid Foods

Continue offering new solid foods at the rate of one new food a week. Watch for any signs of allergy, such as diarrhea or rashes. If your baby refuses a new food, try that food again later. Your baby's tastes are changing and developing.

Consistency. One of the most important considerations at this age is offering your baby food in a form that is appropriate to the baby's development. Any solid food should be tender and soft enough to be easily squashed with your fingers.

If you want to serve your baby the same food the rest of the family is eating, try overcooking or finely chopping the food or use a baby-food grinder. Not all table foods can be prepared to be small enough or soft enough for the baby to eat. Mashed potatoes and cooked carrots are good choices.

Table foods that are stringy, such as celery, broccoli, squash and asparagus, can cause choking. By 1 year of age, your baby can probably handle most small, tender table foods.

Meats. Most babies younger than a year have trouble eating meats. Many parents choose not to offer meats until the baby can chew thoroughly enough to manage them. Others opt for commercial meats prepared especially for babies.

If your baby is eating a wide variety of foods and drinking breast milk or formula, meat is not a necessity during the first year.

When you do want to offer "baby food" meat, choose plain, unseasoned meats. "Real" meats (including poultry and fish with no bones) can be chopped and pureed. These may seem a little thick for your baby, but they can be mixed with a little breast milk or formula.

At first, expect your baby to eat only 1 teaspoon of meat a day. By 12 months, your baby may be eating as much as 1 or 2 tablespoons of meat a day.

Baby food "dinners," which combine a meat and vegetable in the same serving, don't offer as much protein and iron as a plain meat served with a plain vegetable. Offering a little meat, a little vegetable and a little fruit at the same meal will probably be better nutritionally for your baby.

Foods that might cause choking

Any food that won't soften or dissolve easily in your baby's mouth or can't be swallowed whole is a choking hazard. Babies are most likely to choke on:

- Nuts
- Grapes, berries or raisins
- Unpeeled fruit
- Raw or undercooked vegetables
- Corn
- Under-ripe fruit
- Dried fruit
- Candy and gum
- Potato chips and popcorn
- Peanut butter (on a spoon)
- Hot dogs and luncheon meats, unless cut into lengthwise strips

A choking baby can't make any sounds. The baby's face will turn bright red, then blue. Be prepared to help your baby; review the emergency procedures on page 648.

Seasoning. If you taste your baby's food, you might decide it's a bit bland. But to your baby, who isn't used to added salt and sugar, it tastes just right. Seasoning your baby's food is not necessary.

Studies have not proved that an early introduction of salt increases the risk of high blood pressure, but the question of a possible relationship between the two is enough to advise caution.

Adding sugar won't allow your baby to enjoy the natural sweetness of food. And it may start a habit that's difficult to break.

Amounts. During these months, many parents become concerned that their babies aren't eating enough. The amount your baby eats at a meal may seem very small. The typical meal for a 1-year-old includes 1 tablespoon of each food group. That menu may translate into a tablespoon of cooked carrots, two bites of rice, a taste of meat and a couple bites of pears.

During the first few months of your baby's life, you concentrated on watching the baby for signs of hunger and thirst and cues that your baby's hunger was satisfied. Keep watching these signs rather than the amount of food still left in the jar or on the plate.

Good eating habits begin now. Teaching your baby to clean the last bits of food off a plate shouldn't be a goal. Coaxing your baby to eat more, or playing tricks to get your baby to eat more, doesn't allow your baby to stop eating when he or she is full. By watching your baby for cues of being hungry or full, you can help your child learn that mealtime is a time to satisfy hunger.

Eating Style

Mealtime is also an opportunity for your baby to experience new textures, colors and tastes.

Occasionally, it may seem that you and your baby are working together as a team to satisfy the baby's hunger. At other times, it may seem your baby is not on your team or even playing the same game you are. Some of your baby's favorite games may be Spitting and Sputtering, How Far Food Flies, Painting With Peas or Feeding the Dog.

These games seem messy to you, but they are important opportunities for your baby to practice developmental skills. An old sheet, some newspaper, a plastic tablecloth or a plastic swimming pool placed under the high chair will allow your baby to practice and make it easier for you to pick up.

Your baby may experience an especially messy eating stage when making the transition between baby foods and finger foods. Usually, your baby's desire to eat table foods comes before the ability to handle them. The only thing that will help your baby become efficient at eating finger foods is lots of practice.

When you start feeding your baby with a spoon, he or she will probably want to grab the spoon. You may want to give the baby a spoon to hold, but don't expect your baby to use it efficiently. Most babies aren't able to use a spoon to feed themselves until they are close to 15 months old.

Sleeping Patterns and Habits

By nine months, your baby has probably settled into a regular napping and sleeping schedule. She or he may take two naps a day and sleep as long as 12 hours at night without waking to be fed.

Your baby probably will waken during normal sleep stages. Continued separation anxiety and new motor skills may also disrupt your baby's sleep. When your baby awakens during normal sleep patterns, he or she may become upset at being alone. Or your baby might automatically get up and start moving about the crib, practicing standing, cruising and walking. The calming techniques discussed on page 556 may help you teach your baby to go back to sleep alone.

A s you try to make your baby comfortable enough to fall asleep alone, consider the baby's sleeping environment. Allow your baby's personality and preferences to shape his or her sleep patterns.

- Watch your baby to see which bedtime rituals he or she prefers. Your independent baby will let you know which books, songs or toys he or she wants.
- Avoid excessive stimulation just before bedtime.
- Give your baby a favorite stuffed animal or blanket.
- Don't be surprised if your baby seems afraid of the dark. A night-light, hall light or open door may help your baby see around the room and not feel abandoned on waking in the night.

Sleep Environment

Growth and Health

Your baby has grown in many ways in the past year. His or her maturation can't be summed up simply in inches and pounds. But taking the time to assess your baby's physical growth will help you evaluate your baby's overall health.

On the average, a baby triples his or her weight during the first year and grows taller by 50 percent. The average height for a 1-year-old is 28 to 32 inches. An average head size is 18 inches.

B ecause your baby doesn't have any required immunizations at 12 months, many health care providers don't schedule an exam at this age. (The next required immunizations are typically scheduled for 15 months.) However, you can request an exam or visit just to have your baby measured and weighed or to discuss concerns you have.

If your baby's health care provider does see the baby at 12 months, he or she will evaluate motor skills, muscle tone and neurologic reflexes and watch for any disorders of posture and movement.

Some health care providers routinely screen for iron deficiency sometime between nine and 18 months. This screening is a simple blood test. Your health care provider also may give your baby a tuberculosis (TB) skin test.

Examinations and Immunizations

What Parents Worry About

Biking Safety

Biking is a good form of exercise and outdoor play that can involve the whole family. Deciding when to include your baby in this family sport should include evaluating the baby's size and physical development and considering safety issues. Remember that the child is at the mercy of your biking abilities and the uncontrollable behavior of other bikers and drivers and probably won't fare as well in a spill as you will.

By the time your baby can sit up well without support, the baby can probably ride in a bicycle child seat. Examine the safety features of any child carrier you might want to use for your child. Both you and the baby should wear helmets. If your baby grows up seeing you wear a helmet, encouraging helmet use will be easier when the child rides a tricycle or bike alone.

Pull-behind child carriers are popular and a safe choice for family biking when used properly. One advantage of a pull-behind carrier is that many are designed with pivotal hitches so the carrier stays upright even if the parent's bike topples. And most pull-behind carriers are designed to carry more than one child. Even in an enclosed pull-behind carrier, your baby should wear a helmet and be securely strapped in.

Shoes

When their babies start standing and cruising, many parents wonder whether shoes are necessary. At this age, your baby doesn't need shoes for standing or walking. You might put shoes on your baby because they look cute, to keep the baby's feet warm or to protect the bottoms of your baby's feet. But your baby doesn't need shoes for any other reason and is probably growing so fast that buying shoes seems impractical.

You may think your baby's feet look flat and seem to be supported by unstable ankles. This is normal. All babies have chubby, thick feet with a fat pad that hides their arches. And they are generally unsteady on their feet. Putting your baby in stiff leather shoes, shoes with special arches or ankle-high shoes won't change your baby's feet or help the baby walk more easily. In fact, your baby may benefit from being barefoot to get a "feel for the road" when learning to walk.

If you do buy shoes for your baby, make sure you can feel a space as wide as your index finger (about ½ inch) between your baby's big toes and the ends of the shoes. Shoes should also be wide enough across the front to allow your baby's toes to wiggle.

CHAPTER THIRTY-FIVE

Returning to Work

Most American women combine motherhood with a job or career outside the home. You're probably wondering how you will manage both successfully. Feelings of anxiety about how you're going to balance multiple roles are perfectly normal.

With so many mothers in the workforce, employers are becoming more receptive to the needs of working mothers and more concerned about keeping their valued employees. The federal Family and Medical Leave Act—which guarantees eligible employees up to 12 weeks of unpaid leave to care for a newborn, adopted baby or ill relative—has also sensitized some employers to new mothers' needs to be home with their infants before returning to the workplace.

The Effect of Your Baby on Your Work

After your baby is born, you'll probably have concerns about leaving your infant in the care of someone else. But you'll be more comfortable about returning to the job if you've had a maternity leave that gave you and your baby time to get to know each other.

There is no optimal length of time that makes a maternity leave right for everyone, and some women have more choices than others. Some women take three months or more at home after their babies' birth, whereas others return to work after less than two months. What's most important is that you are comfortable with your decision about when to return to work.

Even though much has been written about the stresses of combining an outside-the-home career and motherhood, many working women say they like the variety and stimulation that come from balancing several satisfying roles.

587

"I find computer programming challenging, and I like the people in my office," says Cindy, a 25-year-old mother of a baby boy. "But by the end of the day I can't wait to get home to Brian and hold him and concentrate totally on him." When mothers like Cindy enjoy their jobs, they're likely to be happy and fulfilled, and that feeling is reflected in their mothering.

Certainly there will be days when you won't feel like going to work, especially if your baby is fussy or seems particularly clingy. Most babies will have days when they cling tightly and cry when you go. But as you and your child become used to your schedule, as your baby settles into a routine and as you become more adept at managing multiple demands, you'll learn how to handle these normal ups and downs in a more relaxed manner. Millions of working mothers have.

Be sure to let your partner know your feelings and concerns; give him an opportunity to understand and contribute. Knowing that two of you are in tune with your child's needs, not just one, will go a long way toward easing your stress.

The Effect of Work on Your Baby

You may worry sometimes that pursuing a career will somehow harm your baby. But as long as you feel confident about your decision to work and happy about your child care arrangement, your employment will not in and of itself be bad for your baby.

Children of working mothers may have other caregivers, but they develop just as secure and loving attachments to their own mothers as do children of non-working mothers. In fact, it's questionable whether children whose mothers have a career outside the home really receive less mothering time than children whose mothers stay home. What's important is not that you're with your child every second, but that you give your child unhurried love and attention when you are. It's not realistic to think that every moment you spend with your baby will be perfect. There will be times when your baby is cranky or cool toward you and times when you're able to give your infant more of yourself emotionally than at other times.

When working mothers can find high-quality child care, that care has some distinct benefits. For example, child care helps children adjust to various unfamiliar social situations. Such care also helps children learn to share with other children, a skill that will help them develop into well-adjusted human beings who can express empathy for others. Finally, they're exposed to other caring adults and have the security of knowing they're part of an extended network of people who want what's best for them.

Dealing With Fatigue

No matter how confident you are about your decision to combine work and motherhood, there will be times when you're so tired you wonder how you can do it all. That fatigue is entirely normal. Motherhood is a demanding job no matter how satisfying it is. The myth of Supermom is just that, a myth. It's not realistic to think that one woman can happily hold down a full-time job, meet the demands of her baby and her partner, manage a household and take care of child care needs—all without ever getting tired or feeling overwhelmed.

It's important that you talk honestly with your partner about dividing up the household duties. Most male partners want to be involved in their baby's care and want to participate in running a household.

The days when dad went to work, came home, played with the baby and never changed a diaper are gone—if they ever existed. Today, most couples share parenting and household management, setting up a division of labor that works for them. In some cases, the father takes the baby to the day care provider in the morning, and the mother picks the baby up at the end of the day. Some couples alternate dinner preparation and cleanup, so neither parent does it every night.

Some men need direct, specific instructions, especially if they're doing things that are new to them. Don't assume your partner shares your knowledge and familiarity in accomplishing seemingly simple tasks. As he becomes more practiced at doing these tasks, you won't need to be so specific or detailed.

One way of catching up on rest is to set aside time on weekends for napping— preferably when your baby is also resting. Many working mothers say they avoid scheduling many social events on the weekends because their work weeks are so full of commitments that they need some downtime. If your fatigue seems constant and you never seem to have any energy, talk to your doctor.

Time Management

Combining a job with raising a child demands time management skills that all working mothers develop. Some use lunch hours for errands, and others develop shortcuts for family meals.

No matter how organized you are, however, time will still be in short supply. Many working mothers say that their biggest problem is finding time for themselves; there simply aren't enough hours in the day. But finding time for yourself is important. Doing things you want to do, not only things you have to do, will help you feel less stressed by the demands on your time. If you feel less stressed, you'll be in a better mood to enjoy your baby when you're together.

To help ease the stresses on you, you can take specific steps other working mothers have found helpful. You can:

- Make time to exercise regularly and get to bed early at least one night a week. Adequate rest can work wonders for your attitude and coping ability.

- Rely on easily prepared meals or, if your budget allows, healthy frozen entrees, rather than knocking yourself out trying to prepare a complicated meal after working all day.

- Get an answering machine so you won't be bothered by calls you don't want when you get home and can return calls when you choose.

- Treat yourself to a relaxing bath several nights a week after you've put your baby to bed.

- Take a day of leave just for yourself once in a while; do something you can't enjoy as much if you took the baby—shop, visit a friend, go to a museum. Or, as one new mom suggests, "Just spend the day at home alone. For me, that was the ultimate luxury."

- Go out with your partner for dinner—just the two of you—and talk about anything other than the house and child care while a trusted friend, relative or sitter stays with your infant. Do this on a regular basis.

Handling Guilt Feelings

If you're like most working moms, you'll struggle with guilt from time to time. Working moms are prone to feelings of guilt, no matter whether they're continuing to breastfeed or how happy they are with their child care providers. When you shift roles—from employee to mother and back again—you'll sometimes feel torn between the two.

You may have some guilt about missing your infant's first attempt to say a word or take a first step; but remember that fathers have often been missing some of these "firsts." The joy of parenting isn't so much the witnessing of "firsts"; it is more in noticing and celebrating your child's amazing development.

If your infant has a cold, you may also harbor mixed emotions about going to work, even if you know it isn't serious and you've told your caregiver to call you if your child seems to feel worse during the day.

Babies between 6 and 13 months of age usually go through a normal stage called separation anxiety. This stage is hard on parents because babies typically get very clingy and cry when their mothers leave. Even though separation anxiety can increase your feelings of guilt, it's important to realize that this is a stage and will not last. Your baby cries because he or she wants you close by and is beginning to understand that you exist somewhere else even when you can't be seen. Your child knows you're not there and isn't convinced you're coming back. A baby's recognition that a person or thing exists even when it can't be seen is called object permanence. As your baby learns that you do come back, your infant will begin to become more comfortable about letting you out of sight.

To help your baby—and you—through separation anxiety, be sure to tell your child that you're leaving, that you love him or her and that you'll be back. Don't just leave without telling your child; this approach will only increase the clinginess and worries that you might not come back.

Maybe you're taking on an unnecessary burden of guilt due to expectations based on your own upbringing. If your mother did not work outside the home, you may be trying to do it all—be the homemaker she was and also hold a job. Remember, you're not your mother. Be yourself; she raised her children in a different setting, which was also challenging. It may also help if you realize that you can't possibly remember a time when your mother was just learning to be a mother; your memories will always show her as an experienced mom.

Breastfeeding and Work

Whether you decide to breastfeed after returning to work is up to you, but there are some distinct advantages to nursing your baby that might help you make a decision. Breast milk gives your baby the best nutrition; the components of human breast milk are perfectly balanced for your baby's digestive system and normal growth. Further, breast milk gives your baby natural immunity against some infections. And, equally important, nursing provides a special time of closeness between mother and child.

If you want to breastfeed after returning to work, it's helpful to enlist the help and cooperation of your employer. Progressive employers genuinely want to help new moms do what is best for their babies; your boss also knows that if you're happy, you'll be more productive on the job.

Breast Pumps

Many breast pumps on the market also make it more feasible for working moms to continue breastfeeding, because you can express milk to be used in bottles when you're not there. Types of pumps include a rental electric breast pump like those used in hospitals, a portable electric breast pump, a battery-powered breast pump and a small hand-operated pump.

Many moms experience a decline in milk supply with any type of single pump, so ideally you should consider the rental of a double-breast electric pump. In general, the electric models allow for more effective milk expression than hand pumping. If you pump your breasts on a double-breast electric pump, you will save time—an important consideration at work. Double pumping on a rented electric model takes only about 10 to 15 minutes a session. Talk to your health care provider or lactation consultant about your desire to continue breastfeeding, and ask for advice before you go back to work and before renting or purchasing a pump.

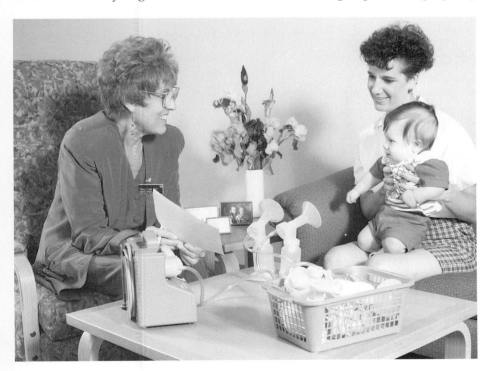

One way to make it feasible to continue breastfeeding after returning to work is to use a breast pump. Here, a lactation consultant recommends a portable double-breast electric pump.

Making the Transition

Well before your return to work, introduce your baby to bottles filled with breast milk so your infant will have a chance to get used to sucking on a rubber nipple. This gradual shift will help both of you adjust to the fact that some feedings will be by bottle.

Start introducing bottles of pumped breast milk when your baby is 3 to 4 weeks old. Substitute the bottle for one breastfeeding session a day. If your baby gags on the bottle nipple or rejects it, try a shorter or different-shaped nipple the next time. If your baby refuses to take a bottle from you, have your partner introduce the bottle. Keep trying until your baby accepts the bottle.

How Your Employer Can Be Supportive

Here are some ways you can work with your employer to combine breast-feeding with returning to the job:

- Ask to extend your maternity leave for as long as possible to develop a feeding schedule at home.

- Talk to your supervisor about your plans to breastfeed well before you resume work. Review the health benefits to your baby, and point out that your infant may be more resistant to some infections. Let your supervisor know how important breastfeeding is to you and that you feel continuing to nurse will help you be a more productive and satisfied worker.

- Explore with your supervisor the possibility of flextime hours, part-time status, job sharing or doing part of your work at home if your job lends itself to any of these more flexible arrangements. Be prepared to suggest ways of making a more flexible arrangement work. For example, if you have a personal computer at home that links with those at the office, working at home part of the time may be more feasible.

- Discuss the times when you will pump, noting that you will use your breaks for pumping so you won't take time from your work schedule.

- Ask your employer to recommend a private room with a lock where nursing mothers can express their milk. This room could be an empty office or perhaps an athletic room used only by women employees.

- Discuss with your employer the feasibility of renting a double-breast electric pump, which will allow you to express your milk efficiently in a short time.

Finding answers to your questions about breastfeeding

Talk to your health care provider about your plans to breastfeed. If you need additional support or information, ask your health care provider to recommend a lactation consultant. Your local hospital may have a lactation consultant on staff or associated with the hospital who could talk with you about breastfeeding before your baby's birth or shortly after your baby is born. You may also want to talk to members of the La Leche League in your area. La Leche League is an international organization that provides information and support to moms who want to breastfeed.

If you're a new breastfeeding mother, seeing a lactation consultant within the first several days of your baby's birth can go a long way toward making the experience rewarding for you and your infant. Lactation consultants help new moms begin successful breastfeeding and can teach you how to encourage your baby to "latch on" to your nipples so your infant nurses most productively. The consultant " an insufficient milk supply and discomfort during nursing. The lactation consultant can also help you deal with any concerns you may have, such as whether your partner will feel left out if you decide to breastfeed.

- Ask for a locking cabinet or closet where you and other nursing mothers can keep supplies in addition to a pump, such as breast pads, empty containers for expressed milk and extra blouses in case of milk leakage during the day.

- Join a support group of mothers who have experience in or who are breastfeeding and working, or establish such a support group. If you have one or more supportive coworkers you can talk to, you'll be more relaxed about combining breastfeeding with working outside your home.

Fitting Into a Schedule

Once you return to work, you can develop a convenient breastfeeding routine. Here are three options. First, pump two times during an eight-hour day and use that milk for the next day. Take the total amount pumped and divide it into two or three feedings, depending on your baby's age and needs. You will need an insulated bag with cold packs to transport your milk home from work.

A second option is to pump one time per eight hours at work. In addition, pump after feeding your baby when you come home and perhaps after nursing in the morning. Now divide that total amount into two or three feedings, depending on how old your baby is (the older your infant is, the more likely the baby will be to eat a larger amount less often).

Finally, a third option is for moms who can't pump at work. If you're in this situation, you can pump before you go to work and after you return home. You could also pump one or two times a day on the weekends for extra breast milk to be used in bottles. Pumping any extra breast milk your baby doesn't take in a 24-hour period and using it during working hours will help to keep your milk supply up.

Depending on your workplace location, you might be able to go home or to your caregiver's to feed your baby. Some working moms have the caregiver bring the baby to them and nurse at the workplace. Or you can use formula for the times when you're gone and nurse when you're home. If you choose this approach, limit the amount of formula given so your baby will nurse well when you return from work. If your baby eats a lot of formula while you're gone, your milk supply could be affected.

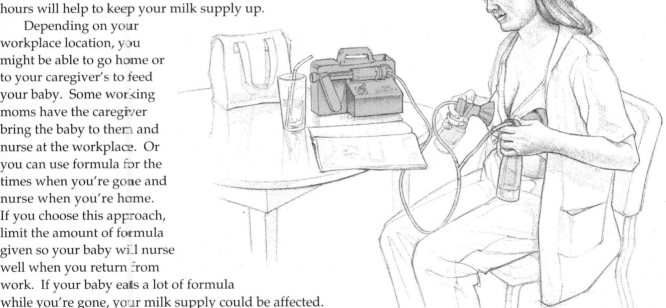

Find a private, quiet spot to pump during a break from work. You can finish in 10 to 15 minutes.

Your health care provider or lactation consultant can help you design an individualized breastfeeding routine that works for you and your baby. They are experienced and highly creative when it comes to helping working moms combine breastfeeding with a career, so don't hesitate to talk over any concerns or problems you may be having. (For more on breastfeeding, see page 474.)

Finding the Best Child Care

Today, you have a choice of several types of child care. These include in-home care (either a live-in caregiver or one who comes every day), family child care or a child care center. Each of these choices has advantages and disadvantages; be sure to discuss them with your partner before deciding what's right for you and your baby.

To find quality child care, ask for referrals from friends with young children, your coworkers and your health care provider. Start checking into your options at least three months before you expect to need child care because in many communities openings for infants are scarce.

Nearly every community in the United States has a child care resource and referral agency with child care referral consultants who can help you with that important first step of finding out what kind of care is available in your area. They can also provide you with information about local child care licensing regulations and financial assistance available for eligible families. To locate your child care resource and referral agency, look in the telephone book or call Child Care Aware at 800-424-2246.

Referrals and accreditation by child care organizations are helpful, but they are no substitute for interviewing caregivers and visiting centers or homes you are considering for your child. You want to make sure that whatever arrangement you choose comes as close as possible to the kind of care you would give if you were there.

You may be concerned about your baby contracting illnesses in family child care or a child care center. Feel free to discuss this with your baby's health care provider before enrolling your child. If your baby is basically healthy, being exposed to infectious agents that cause illnesses early in life in a child care center will probably do no harm; your child will be exposed to these infections anyway when he or she starts school. If, however, your baby was premature, has respiratory infections frequently or has had other illnesses in infancy, you and your health care provider may decide that an in-home caregiver would be a better choice.

Tips for a successful child care and breastfeeding arrangement

When you make the commitment to provide breast milk for your baby while you are at work, make sure your child care provider understands your expectations and is familiar with precautions for safe storage and handling of breast milk:

- Fresh breast milk will keep for up to five days in the refrigerator.

- Your caregiver can either warm your breast milk under the tap or give it to your baby straight from the refrigerator if your infant doesn't object.

  Ask your caregiver not to microwave breast milk; extreme heat can destroy some of the natural immunities breast milk contains and create "hot spots" that could burn your baby's mouth.

- Thaw frozen breast milk in the refrigerator or in a container of continually warmed water. Don't thaw it at room temperature.

- Thawed breast milk will keep in the refrigerator for 48 hours.

- Breast milk will separate naturally—that's fine. Just shake before use.

- Thawed breast milk often takes on a different texture—that's okay.

- Before they start eating solid foods, breastfed babies have looser bowel movements than bottle-fed babies—this difference is normal.

- It's best if your baby's last feeding in child care is at least two hours before you pick up your infant.

- Your caregiver should feed your baby the amount of breast milk you supply. Breastfed babies don't need 8-ounce bottles, and the amount a mother expresses is generally what her baby needs.

Here are some factors to consider if you're thinking of hiring an in-home caregiver:

- How much education, training and experience has the person had caring for young children, especially infants?
- Where else has the person worked? Get the names and phone numbers of three or four mothers for whom the person has worked and with whom you can talk freely. Then be sure to make the calls.
- Does the person's record and general demeanor show that she or he is a person of honesty and integrity?
- Does the person seem warm and caring toward children?
- In your discussions, does the person seem to understand and respect your ideas on parenting (your preference for feeding, diapering, sleep position, etc.)?
- Is this person trained in cardiopulmonary resuscitation (CPR) for infants?
- Is the person in good health and a non-smoker? Cigarette smoke could increase the risk of respiratory infections in your baby.
- Are the person's fees and the benefits wanted in line with what you can afford?
- How flexible will the person be if you're late getting home from work?
- How will the person get to and from your home if he or she is not going to live in?

The bottom line is that no matter how glowing someone's references, you must feel a sense of trust and rapport with the person. A person who is just not right for your baby and you shouldn't be hired.

Unlike a child care center or family child care provider, when you hire an in-home caregiver usually no policies or rules have been established in advance. Together, you have to work out the ground rules—use of the phone and television, allowing visitors in the house, responsibilities beyond child care such as cooking or cleaning, leaving the house with the baby, etc. Developing a good relationship requires time, clear communication and organization. The other part of your relationship is a businesslike agreement. Make sure to discuss, and preferably put in writing, your agreement on salary, vacation time, sick days, raises and other benefits. You also need to be aware of your legal and financial obligations as an employer. Contact the Internal Revenue Service and offices of your state government regarding unemployment taxes and state income taxes.

Family child care providers care for small groups of children in their homes. When talking to such a provider, here are some issues to raise:

- Does the person seem warm and caring toward children?
- Does the person seem to understand and respect your ideas on parenting (your preference for feeding, diapering, sleep position, etc.)?
- How many children does the person care for? The smaller the group, the better the situation for your child. Ideally, the group size should be no larger than six, and there should be one adult for every three children under 1 year of age.
- Is the home clean, bright, pleasant and childproofed?
- Is there adequate space for playing, exploring and napping?

Hiring an In-Home Caregiver

Finding a Family Child Care Provider

- Is there space for resting and quiet play?
- Are there enough toys and learning materials for the number of children? Are the toys clean, safe and within reach of the children?
- Are children comforted when needed?
- Does the caregiver get down on each child's level to talk and play?
- Does this person allow drop-in visits?
- Is this person trained in CPR?
- How does the person handle a child's illness?
- How will this person handle a medical emergency?
- Is there a no-smoking policy?
- What supplies will you need to provide?

Never put your child into a family child care situation without visiting the home first. Your observations and feelings during a visit when children are there will give you a good sense of whether this situation is right for your baby and for you.

Searching for the Right Child Care Center

If you're considering a child care center for your child, do some homework by telephone first to save yourself some time. Ask whether the center is licensed, what the hours are, what the fees are, whether you can come to visit before registering your baby, how many children there are in the infant section and in the center overall on any given day, whether you can drop in to visit at any time if your child is enrolled, how discipline is handled, whether the staff has been trained in first aid, whether there is a doctor on call if needed, whether there is a no-smoking policy and whether there is a separate area for children who are ill. Also consider the location. Is it on the way to your workplace, or will it require a lengthy drive across town?

If your initial impression on the telephone is good, visit the center to see whether you have positive feelings when you're there. Here are some specific questions to consider:

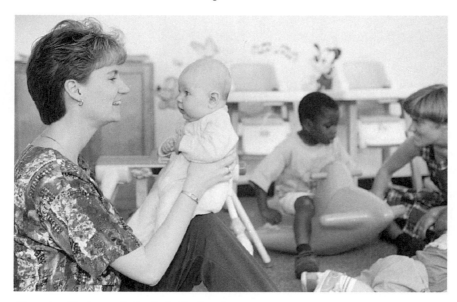

Knowing that your baby is in the hands of an experienced, attentive caregiver gives you peace of mind.

- Does the center support your preferences for feeding and sleep position?

- Is at least one of the caregivers trained in infant CPR?

- Is there a clean diaper-changing area with a nearby sink for hand washing separate from the food preparation area?

- Is there a no-smoking policy?

- Is there a policy on handling a child's illness?

- Are meals and snacks provided? Are the cooks qualified? Is the food prepared under sanitary conditions?

- Is there a consistent policy on the type of diapers used? For example, some centers require disposable diapers because their directors believe disposables hold in fecal matter better than cloth, and thus reduce the possibility of spreading bacteria that could cause illness.

- How much education, training and experience do the caregivers have? Are there enough staff members to care for the number of children? Do they seem genuinely enthusiastic and caring? Is there a high or low staff turnover? The lower turnover the better, because a low turnover leads to consistency and stability of relationships.

- Do the children seem happy and productively occupied?

- Is the center bright, airy, clean and childproofed?

- Is there adequate space for playing and exploring?

- Is there space for napping, resting and quiet play?

- Are the children comforted promptly when needed?

- Do staff members get down on each child's level to talk and play?

- How is discipline handled? The center should have a written policy on discipline for you to read, and the staff should honor it.

- Is there a sense of order and calm that transcends noise and confusion?

- Are space allocations adequate, including a safe outdoor playground?

- Is there a space for each child's belongings, such as a cubbyhole, with his or her name on it?

- Are there enough toys for all the children? Are toys clean, free of small parts and appropriate for the ages of the children playing with them?

- Is the location close to your home or workplace? You may want to visit the center to breastfeed on your lunch breaks.

- Are hours flexible? If you're late picking up your child, is there an extra fee?

Making the Transition

After you've made your choice of child care, be confident in your decision. When you introduce your child to a new care provider, do it gradually. For example, if you've chosen an in-home caregiver, have the person come first for several hours and then half-days and days before you return to work so your baby can get used to the caregiver in your presence. Also, you can exchange ideas and begin to get well acquainted.

Similarly, before returning to work, ask your family child care provider or center director if you can stay with your child for at least part of the first few days until your baby gets used to the new surroundings and until you feel more confident with the arrangements.

Child Care Solutions: Advantages and Disadvantages

In-Home Caregiver

Advantages:

- Your baby stays in his or her own home.
- You have more flexibility in your hours of work and evening commitments.
- You don't have to stay home if your baby gets sick.
- You don't have a commute to drop your baby off and pick him or her up.
- Depending on your agreement with your caregiver, the person might do light housework or prepare dinner.
- Your baby is exposed to fewer contagious childhood illnesses.

Disadvantages:

- You need backup care if your live-in caregiver is sick or on vacation.
- Live-in help may be more expensive than family child care or a child care center.
- Your baby won't be in contact with other children.
- Your privacy will be reduced, which can be a special problem in tight quarters.
- You are responsible for the paperwork of an employer (quarterly tax reports, annual earnings reports, etc.)
- Another person is in your home all day.

Family Child Care

Advantages:

- Your baby will be in a homelike setting.
- The home probably has had to meet safety and cleanliness standards.
- Your baby will be around other children.
- Costs may be lower than live-in help or a center.

Disadvantages:

- The quality of family child care varies widely.
- You may need a backup plan if the caregiver is sick or takes time off.
- Your child may be exposed to infections from other children.

Child Care Centers

Advantages:

- The staff members may have more training than live-in caregivers and family child care providers.
- The center has probably had to meet local standards on safety and cleanliness.
- Your baby will be around other children.
- Because there is a staff, not just one person, you won't have to worry about backup care.

Disadvantages:

- The costs may be higher than family child care.
- The center may not let your child attend when your baby has a mild illness.
- Because of sheer numbers, your baby might not get as much personal attention as from a live-in caregiver or family child care provider.
- If there is a high staff turnover, your baby will have to adjust to new caregivers fairly frequently.
- The hours may be firmly set, and you may have trouble getting there by closing time if you have to work late. (Some centers charge $1 a minute if you're late.)
- Your child will be exposed to infections from other children.

Child Care—
An Ongoing Relationship

The success of your baby's child care will depend in large part on how comfortable you are with the arrangement and the kind of relationship you develop with your caregiver. Personal warmth can't be quantified by licensing, but it is important in a nurturing caregiver. By showing that you appreciate the attention your child receives, you'll help develop a bond of trust with your child care provider that will serve you both well. You can show you care by buying inexpensive supplies for the person to use and keep, such as age-appropriate, educational toys, and by giving a bonus at holiday time or on birthdays. Include your caregiver's ideas and suggestions in your decision making when problems arise. Listen, communicate, work together.

As a parent, you have certain responsibilities to your caregiver, just as she or he has responsibilities to you. For example, you should provide a signed consent form authorizing the caregiver to take your child to the hospital for emergency medical services should that be necessary. Ask your doctor to help you fill out such a form, and leave a copy with him or her. You don't want your child's medical care delayed if neither you nor your partner is immediately reachable when your child needs medical attention.

It's important to remember that you and your care provider both want what's best for your child, and there's no rivalry or competition between you. You may occasionally feel a twinge of envy when your baby runs to the child care provider —but remember that a secure bond between them is exactly what you want. No one can replace you, the mother; the bond you have with your child is unique.

Child Care That Works for Working Parents

Au Pair

From Jane, who chose an au pair:

"I needed to feel someone was here with Sally all the time, so that if I had to stay late at the office I wouldn't have to worry. My husband and I found Britta through an agency that places foreign-born young girls as au pairs, and she's wonderful. People warned me that I might be getting another daughter to take care of, but Britta's from a large family and is experienced with young children. She'll be here only a year, but this first year is the one I figured would be the most stressful. I'm really glad Britta's here."

The term "au pair" typically means someone who performs a service in exchange for room and board. However, it's customary to pay a salary in addition to room and board for someone whose primary responsibility is child care. Plan to allow at least several months for making arrangements for an au pair if international travel is involved. Many au pairs come to the United States on a student exchange visa, so some of the federal tax withholding laws do not apply. Remember that in Europe maternity leaves are typically longer than in the United States; therefore, au pairs might be less familiar with the care of babies younger than 2 or 3 months old.

Combining Two Options

From Susan, who chose a combination of child care:

"My mother comes in two days a week and stays with Danny, and I take him to a child care center near our house the other three days. My mom is a young grandmother and full of energy, and she really wanted to be involved in Danny's care. She said she wanted to get to know him while he was a baby, because later—when he's in school—he won't have as much time to do things with her. Danny gets to see other young children three days a week, and two days a week my mom gets to have him all to herself. I know I'm really lucky, because not everyone has a mom living nearby who even wants to be involved. But I think sometimes grandparents want to be asked to help with child care—so they feel needed and know it's important to the parents that they be around."

Family Child Care

From Sharon, who chose family child care:

"I think it's important for working couples to think about reducing stress, and the last thing my husband and I needed was adding commuting time to a child care center onto our commute to work. I was really lucky to find a family child care provider in my neighborhood; some of my friends had hired her when their children were infants, and they were really pleased with her."

It has worked out great, and because she has flexible hours we don't have to worry about breaking our necks and rushing home to pick David up by 6:00 p.m. She doesn't do everything the way I would, but I think working mothers have to learn to make some compromises. One thing I had to learn was to stop being a perfectionist."

F**rom Karen, who selected a child care center:**

Child Care Center

"It was really important to me to know that Mark would have some consistency in his child care and that I wouldn't have to worry about a backup plan if a single caregiver got sick or went on vacation. I know the child care center is going to be there for me 365 days a year, and I need that peace of mind. I would advise parents who don't have a backup plan for child care to look carefully at child care centers."

F**rom Judy, who chose a caregiver who comes in during the day:**

In-Home Caregiver

"My husband and I talked about a live-in nanny, and we decided we didn't have enough space for one and it would really interfere with our privacy. Julia comes in at 8:00 a.m. She also starts dinner and doesn't leave until 6:30 p.m.; this arrangement works out best for us. If you're thinking about a live-in, you really have to consider how you'll feel about not having your privacy at night. My husband said he wanted to be able to walk around in his underwear without worrying about whether he'd meet the nanny in the hall. Transportation can be a problem, but Julia has her own car and drives here. She's also very healthy, and I almost never have to get another sitter because she's home with an illness. Best of all, Jennifer loves Julia—who had five children of her own—and they really have fun together."

F**rom Ellen, whose partner decided to try working at home:**

Work at Home

"I'm a school counselor, and David writes a technical newsletter. When Emily was born, David decided to try writing the newsletter at home and sending it to his publisher electronically. His boss agreed, and it has worked out pretty well. We had to invest in another phone line and get a fax and some specialized computer equipment, but that investment has really paid off in my peace of mind and the bond between Emily and David. It's not completely ideal, because sometimes David has trouble concentrating on his writing and sometimes he just needs to get out of the house so he won't go stir crazy. We've found several neighborhood sitters to help out during those times. I'd advise other parents to explore working at home if their jobs allow it and if it doesn't mean a big salary cut that will strain the budget. For men, especially, it allows a closeness that's hard to get when they work at an office every day and have frequent evening meetings."

Conclusion

Combining motherhood with work isn't easy, but millions of working moms do it every day and say they wouldn't have it any other way. As a new working mom, you can take comfort in knowing that you've got plenty of company. With enthusiasm, time management, a good support system, help from your partner and some time for yourself, you can accomplish the important goals you've set for yourself.

CHAPTER THIRTY-SIX

Common Illnesses, Medical Problems and Emergencies

Among the challenges you face as a parent is caring for your baby during illnesses or medical emergencies. Because your infant can't tell you when something hurts, it is sometimes difficult to sort out serious illnesses from those that are common and easily managed at home.

As you get to know your baby better, it will become easier for you to know when you can handle an illness and when you need medical help. You know your baby better than anyone else—including details about the baby's previous illnesses. You will notice, for example, if your baby is suddenly more fussy than usual, or has changed eating or sleeping patterns. You will also be able to tell if your baby is less active or clings to you more.

You are an important member of the team that cares for your sick child. In most cases, you will determine when you can handle an illness at home or when it's time to call the doctor or visit an emergency department. You'll help your health care provider determine if a problem is present when things just don't seem right with your baby. Your health care provider can also give you instructions about caring for your infant: when to give medication, changes to watch for, foods to avoid and when your baby can return to child care.

It's never easy to have a sick baby. It's difficult—and sometimes frustrating—when your baby can't tell you what hurts or when you don't know how to help. In addition, your baby's illness affects your family's schedule, your child care arrangements and your work. If someone else cares for your baby much of the time, you'll need to plan ahead for those times when your baby has a contagious condition or is sick enough to stay home.

When dealing with a sick child, trust your intuition as a parent

- If you feel like you should call the doctor—call.
- If you feel like you should have your child seen in either the doctor's office or the emergency department—go in.

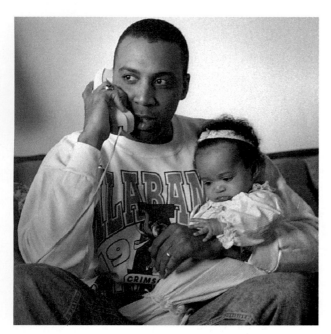

A phone call to your baby's health care provider often can solve a lot of problems and give you reassurance that the steps you've already taken are on the right course. Describe what's worrying you and what you've tried so far.

Your local medical resources

It's a good idea to become acquainted with medical resources in your community as soon as possible:

- Select a family physician, pediatrician or nurse-practitioner who will be your child's primary medical caregiver.
- Find out about office hours, whether the clinic offers walk-in or urgent care services and which hospital(s) your primary health care provider uses.
- Know the location of the nearest emergency department in case you need it for any emergencies.
- If you have medical insurance, learn about your care options.

Reminder

Other parents will appreciate your thoughtfulness if you keep your baby out of regular child care when she or he is running a fever, has profuse nasal drainage, is vomiting or has a persistent cough.

Questions to Be Prepared for When You Call Your Doctor's Office

Before you call or visit the doctor's office, it's a good idea to gather some basic information. This will help the medical staff know what's happening with your baby and how best to treat the problem. Be prepared to answer these questions:

- Why did you decide to call or come in to the doctor's office today?
- How can the medical staff help you today?
- What concerns you about how your baby is acting?
- What changes have you noticed?
- Have you taken the baby's temperature, and does he or she have a fever?
- Have you noticed changes in eating or drinking patterns or changes in the number of wet diapers or in the number and consistency of bowel movements?
- Is anyone in your family ill, or has your baby been exposed to illness elsewhere?
- What treatment have you already tried? Have you given any medication? If so, how much and when?
- Does your baby have any allergies to medications or foods? Have you been told to avoid any specific medications for your child?
- Has your baby ever acted like this before?

Symptoms of Illness and What They Mean: How This Chapter Is Organized

After discussing how to give your baby medicine and how to take his or her temperature, the balance of the chapter will help you evaluate your baby's symptoms. First, three common concerns are discussed:

- Fever — Page 608
- Vomiting — Page 611
- Diarrhea — Page 612

Then, symptoms relating to conditions of the body are described:

Nose, Ears, Mouth or Throat
- Colds (Upper Respiratory Tract Infections)—Page 613
- Cold Sores (Oral Herpes Simplex)—Page 615
- Ear Infection (Otitis Media)—Page 615
- Swollen Glands or Lymph Nodes—Page 617
- Thrush—Page 618

Chest and Lungs
- Asthma (Reactive Airway Disease)—Page 618
- Bronchiolitis—Page 619
- Coughs—Page 620
- Croup—Page 621
- Influenza—Page 622
- Pneumonia—Page 623

Eyes
- Pinkeye (Conjunctivitis or Eye Infection)—Page 624

Skin
- Chickenpox (Varicella)—Page 625
- Diaper Rash (Yeast Rash, Diaper Dermatitis)—Page 627
- Atopic Dermatitis (Cradle Cap, Eczema)—Page 627
- Fifth Disease (Erythema Infectiosum, Parvovirus)—Page 628
- Heat Rash—Page 629
- Hives (Urticaria)—Page 629
- Impetigo—Page 630
- Insect Bites and Stings—Page 631
- Poison Ivy, Oak, Sumac (Contact Dermatitis)—Page 632
- Roseola—Page 633
- Scabies—Page 633
- Sunburn—Page 633

Stomach and Intestines
- Constipation—Page 634
- Food Allergies and Milk Intolerance—Page 635
- Hernia (Inguinal)—Page 636
- Hydrocele—Page 637

Next are brief discussions of less common, but serious, medical conditions:

The chapter concludes with a section on emergencies, which you can quickly find by looking for the colored bar at the edge of the pages:

How to Administer Medicine

Sometimes it's difficult to coax your baby to take medicine that he or she needs. Here are some tips to make the job easier.

- Don't mix medicine in your baby's juice or food. Your baby might then refuse to take even a favorite food, and you might not know if the baby takes the whole dose.
- A baby is usually more willing to take medicine by mouth before a feeding.
- Use a dropper, spoon tube, nipple or syringe to give your infant liquid medications; ask your pharmacist for suggestions. When your baby is older, you can give medications more easily with a spoon.
- Place a small amount of medicine inside the baby's cheek, where it's not as easy to spit out.
- Do not refill medicine bottles or use measured droppers for anything other than the original medicine.
- Avoid chewable medications in babies younger than age 2.
- Follow your doctor's directions for continuing to use a medication, even if it doesn't taste good. Babies are often able to adapt to bad-tasting medicines better than their parents!

How to Take Your Baby's Temperature

Many parents estimate whether or not their child has a fever. When a parent states that the child has a fever, the thermometer proves that the temperature is elevated only about half the time. In other words, when parents feel that their young children have a fever, about half the time the temperature is actually not elevated. But, when a parent states that the child doesn't seem to have a fever, he or she is right 90 percent of the time. Taking your child's temperature is easy to do and it eliminates guessing.

Electronic or glass thermometers can accurately measure a temperature, but the mercury in a glass thermometer can pose an environmental hazard if broken. Virtually all glass-type thermometers contain mercury, even the older style "redline" thermometers. Liquid mercury is not directly harmful, but the mercury will slowly vaporize. Mercury vapor does pose a health risk. If mercury is somehow swallowed, there is probably little cause for alarm. Liquid mercury is poorly absorbed from the intestinal tract. Contact your doctor or local poison control center if your child accidentally swallows mercury.

Practice taking your baby's temperature and reading the thermometer before your baby becomes ill. You can be more confident of an accurate reading when you follow these steps:

With an electronic thermometer. Select a thermometer designed for oral, axillary (armpit) or rectal temperatures. Don't use home-type ear temperature thermometers; they tend to be less accurate.

With a glass thermometer. There are two types of glass thermometers—oral and rectal. A rectal thermometer has a rounded, blunt tip and can be used for armpit temperatures also. Rectal temperatures are the most accurate. Oral thermometers have a longer tip, but they are not different otherwise.

It's not a good idea to take oral temperatures until your child is about 6 years old, because at an earlier age it's difficult for your child to hold the thermometer in the correct position without biting (and possibly breaking) it.

Shake the thermometer with a firm snap of the wrist, so the mercury line falls below 98 degrees Fahrenheit (37 degrees Centigrade). Because thermometers don't reset themselves, yours will still show the temperature from the last time you used it.

Remember to hold the thermometer securely, and take care not to bang it against something as you shake it. Most thermometers are broken from dropping or hitting a tabletop when shaking down the mercury. Rarely, thermometers are

Cleaning up a broken glass thermometer

Don't simply clean it up and throw it in the garbage. You would simply be transferring the mercury to your local landfill. Contact your local or state household hazardous waste unit or pollution control office for advice.

Take off rings or jewelry before cleaning up the mercury. Mercury will adhere to metals such as gold or silver. If this happens, you may need a jeweler to clean the item for you.

The broken glass is the first concern. Use care to avoid getting cut by glass fragments. Place the broken fragments in a sealable plastic bag or container separate from the mercury.

On a hard floor. Use index cards or credit cards to gather mercury fragments into a pile. Then, scoop up the mercury and place it in a sealable plastic bag or container. For mercury stuck down in tiny cracks, don't vacuum; try using a nasal aspirator bulb (which you must dispose of with the mercury). Alternatively, contact your local or state household hazardous waste unit or pollution control office for advice.

On a carpet. Don't vacuum; contact your local or state household hazardous waste unit or pollution control office for advice.

If the thermometer shattered because it was somehow placed in a flame, leave the area immediately and contact your local or state household hazardous waste unit or pollution control office. Mercury rapidly vaporizes if heated by a flame. The vaporized mercury is a health hazard.

shattered when someone mistakenly tries to "test" the thermometer with hot water or a flame. Don't ever try to test a thermometer by heating it!

To read the temperature. In a well-lighted area, slowly rotate the thermometer until you can see the line (usually just below the markings on the thermometer). Read the temperature where the line ends. Remember that you don't have to rush to read the thermometer—the mercury will not change position until you shake it down. If necessary, you can ask someone else to double-check your reading. (To convert Fahrenheit to Centigrade, see the conversion chart on page 730.)

Rectal measurements are more accurate than those taken at the armpit; however, some parents find it easier to determine armpit temperatures. If the armpit measurement doesn't agree with your suspicions regarding the presence or absence of fever, check the rectal temperature to be sure.

Rectal temperature. Place your baby on his or her stomach. Put a bit of petroleum jelly on the tip of the thermometer. Spread your baby's buttocks so that you can see the anus easily. Carefully insert (don't force) the thermometer into your baby's rectum, between ½ to 1 inch. Keep the baby still, squeeze his or her buttocks gently to keep the thermometer in and hold it there for three minutes. If you can distract your baby with a toy or something else interesting to watch or quietly listen to without moving, he or she may be more cooperative while you take the temperature.

Armpit temperature. Put the bulb of the dry thermometer on the skin between the inner surface of the baby's arm and side while you hold the baby's arm across his or her chest. Leave the thermometer in place for four to five minutes.

Cleaning and storing your thermometer. Be sure to clean the thermometer after use. Wash it with warm, soapy water (below 105 degrees Fahrenheit; too hot will break the thermometer), and dry it. (Some physicians advise wiping it with rubbing alcohol before storing.) Store it in a container to prevent breakage.

Fever   Normal temperatures vary for different people. Your newborn baby's temperature will change up and down about one degree throughout the day. It is usually lowest in the morning and highest late in the afternoon. A baby's temperature may be up slightly if dressed warmly or outside in hot weather. If your baby's temperature is elevated because of overdressing or overheating, the temperature will decrease within 15 to 30 minutes after undressing or moving to a cooler place. Here are ranges of body temperatures for infants:

Normal range

- Rectal temperature—98.2 to 100.4 degrees Fahrenheit (36.8 to 38 degrees Centigrade)
- Armpit temperature—95 to 99 degrees Fahrenheit (35 to 37.2 degrees Centigrade)

Upper-normal range (mild fever)

- Rectal temperature—above 100.6 degrees Fahrenheit (38.2 degrees Centigrade)
- Armpit temperature—above 99.4 degrees Fahrenheit (37.4 degrees Centigrade)

Generally, you should closely monitor your baby if you find a rectal temperature more than 101 degrees Fahrenheit (38.4 degrees Centigrade). In general, a temperature only slightly above the normal range is much less likely to be associated with serious infection. Rectal temperatures above 104 degrees Fahrenheit (40 degrees Centigrade) are more likely to have an important cause.

Notice that thermometers have markings only up to about 106 degrees Fahrenheit (41 degrees Centigrade). This is because it is exceedingly unlikely for temperatures to go above this range, even in very serious infections. It is difficult for the body to retain sufficient heat to elevate a temperature higher than this.

Is a fever dangerous? The fever itself is usually not harmful; the potential harm would be caused by the infection that is causing the fever. Usually, when a baby has a fever, he or she is fighting an infection; fever is a sign of the immune system at work. When your baby has a fever, try to determine whether he or she has other symptoms of illness, such as loss of appetite, vomiting, irritability or unusual sleepiness. You should always consult with your doctor if a baby younger than 2 months has a fever.

Febrile seizures (febrile convulsions) occur in about 4 percent of children between the ages of 6 months and 4 years. They are usually due to a rapid rise or fall of your baby's temperature and don't necessarily reflect the height of the fever. Contrary to what you may have heard, the fever itself is unlikely to cause problems such as brain damage. A body temperature above 106 degrees Fahrenheit (41 degrees Centigrade) can lead to injury, but fevers that high are rare. Sometimes children inherit the tendency to have a seizure with a fever. Febrile seizures, although alarming to parents, usually don't harm the baby and usually do not indicate a long-term or ongoing problem.

You can tell your baby is having a febrile seizure if he or she has repeated rhythmic jerking of the arms and legs and is not responsive to you or aware of his or her surroundings. (Occasional odd twitchy or jerky movements are common, especially in sleepy infants—these are not seizures.) Most febrile seizures last less than 10 minutes, after which your baby may cry or be quite sleepy. If your baby has a febrile seizure, lay the baby down. Turn your baby on his or her side. Do not try to place anything in the baby's mouth or try to stop the seizure.

Remember that if your baby has a febrile seizure, it will probably stop by itself in a few minutes. Call your doctor or the emergency department. Your baby should be examined to determine the reason for the fever. The seizure will likely end even before you start to drive to the hospital. If you drive to the hospital, don't speed or drive through red lights. If possible, have someone else drive; serious accidents have occurred when parents were panicked by a febrile seizure.

What can you do? Look for other symptoms, and use the following recommendations when your baby has a fever:

- Encourage plenty of fluid intake. Frozen flavored ice pops work well in older infants. If your baby is eating solid foods, let him or her decide whether and how much to eat.
- Provide extra opportunities for rest and quiet play until the illness is over.
- Don't dress your baby too warmly.
- Your baby may feel more comfortable if you sponge him or her with luke-warm (not cold!) water or give a tepid bath, although this may not necessarily bring down the fever more quickly. In the past, alcohol was used for sponge baths. Don't use alcohol for sponge baths—it's not safe.
- If your baby seems uncomfortable, give acetaminophen (for example, Tylenol, Panadol, Liquiprin or Tempra), according to the chart shown below, every four to six hours. If your baby is sleeping, wait until your baby awakens to give the medication.

Do not give your baby aspirin, especially if he or she has chickenpox, because aspirin use may be linked with Reye's syndrome. Reye's syndrome is a serious complication of viral illnesses. Prominent symptoms are vomiting and lethargy progressing to coma.

It's generally not a good idea to give fever-reducing medication for more than three days without consulting your physician. Talk with your health care provider before giving any acetaminophen to babies younger than 2 months.

Acetaminophen dosages

Weight (lb)	Weight (kg)	Drops (ml)	Elixir (teaspoon)
6-11	2.7-5.0	0.4	1/4 = 1.25 ml
12-17	5.5-7.7	0.8	1/2 = 2.5 ml
18-23	8.2-10.5	1.2	3/4 = 3.75 ml

Note: Acetaminophen drops and elixir are two very different strengths. Follow the measurements specifically given for each type of acetaminophen.

When to call the doctor

Call immediately if your baby:

- Is less than 3 months old and has a temperature more than 101 degrees Fahrenheit (38.4 degrees Centigrade)
- At any age, has a fever of 104 degrees Fahrenheit (40 degrees Centigrade) or higher and is acting ill
- Has sunken eyes
- Cries without tears, has not had wet diapers in six to eight hours or has a dry mouth
- Is feverish, is crying inconsolably and cannot be settled
- Is lethargic or difficult to awaken
- Shows signs of breathing difficulties or rapid breathing
- Develops a purple rash
- Is unable to swallow
- Seems to have abdominal pain
- Has such a sore throat that she or he won't swallow saliva
- Looks or acts very ill and does not improve with acetaminophen

Call if you are concerned that your baby:

- Has had a fever for more than 72 hours
- Was better but now the fever has returned
- Seems to experience burning pain on urination
- Seems to have ear pain

Vomiting

In the first few months of life, it's common for babies to spit up, or easily regurgitate their food from time to time. Vomiting is different. It is the forceful ejection of a large portion of the stomach's contents through the mouth and sometimes even the nose. Because your baby won't understand what is happening, vomiting can be a frightening experience for him or her. And as a parent, it can be very stressful when your baby begins to vomit without warning.

What causes it? Most vomiting in infancy is caused by viral infections termed gastroenteritis. Also, your baby may or may not have diarrhea. Generally, vomiting stops within six to 24 hours. Some babies vomit when they have a high fever. Vomiting can also be a symptom of more serious problems like food poisoning, a stomach disorder or meningitis.

What can you do? The greatest risk your baby faces from vomiting is dehydration (excessive loss of body fluids). The following steps may help your baby avoid becoming dehydrated. First, after your baby vomits, let the stomach settle for a while. Wait 30 to 60 minutes. Then offer a small amount of liquid, beginning with about one to two teaspoons. Breastfed babies usually tolerate breast milk fairly well and digest it quickly. Offer just one breast or a smaller volume to see if your baby can tolerate it. Offer bottle-fed babies a small amount of formula or an oral electrolyte solution (such as Pedialyte or Ricelyte). You can purchase these in most pharmacies or supermarkets without prescription. It's usually best not to offer fruit juices.

The key to administering liquids successfully is to give small amounts. After 15 to 30 minutes, if the liquid stays down, offer it again. If your baby vomits again, let his or her stomach rest for 30 to 60 minutes and then try a small amount of liquid again. Gradually increase the volume offered as the baby tolerates it. After the baby's vomiting stops, gradually offer more liquid.

When the baby's stomach has settled and liquids are staying down, you may offer your older infant solid food. If your baby isn't interested yet, that's fine. Start with bland foods like baby cereal or banana or finger foods like crackers and plain pasta.

When to call the doctor

Call immediately if your baby:

- Hasn't had a wet diaper in eight hours
- Has experienced prolonged, forceful vomiting
- Has been vomiting for more than 12 hours
- Has persistent vomiting and diarrhea
- Has a dry mouth and cries without tears (remember that newborns may not show tears when they cry)
- Is unusually sleepy or drowsy or doesn't respond to you
- Has blood in the vomitus or stool

- Is becoming more ill over time
- Seems to have persistent abdominal pain

Diarrhea

Your baby may have diarrhea if you notice stools with an increased frequency and a watery consistency. Frequency is the best indicator (more than five to seven stools a day may be considered frequent). Normal stools vary in consistency and color (often yellow or green in breastfed babies). Bloody stools are not normal, although babies occasionally have small streaks of blood in their stool, caused by skin irritation from frequent passing of stool or by irritation of the intestinal lining. Intestinal infections sometimes cause more blood or clots in the stool.

Dehydration is the main complication that can result from your baby's diarrhea, especially if your baby has also been vomiting. Your baby has a much smaller reserve of fluids than you do because his or her body's volume is much less.

What causes it? A viral infection, also called gastroenteritis, is the most common cause of diarrhea. Sometimes bacteria or parasites may cause your baby's diarrhea, especially if the stools contain blood. Although your baby will seldom have diarrhea from a specific food allergy, it can be caused by increased juice intake or the addition of new foods. Antibiotics also may cause diarrhea.

Diarrhea that is caused by a viral infection usually lasts between two days and two weeks, regardless of the treatment. A green and watery stool indicates that food is passing through your baby's intestines quickly and is not necessarily always related to infection.

What can you do? To avoid dehydration, offer your baby liquid that is easily absorbed. Your doctor may suggest an oral rehydration solution (Pedialyte or Ricelyte) to replace fluid lost in the baby's stool. If the baby's diarrhea continues, your health care provider may suggest that you temporarily put him or her on soy or other formula. It's a good idea to avoid giving your baby fruit juice and carbonated beverages for severe diarrhea; these drinks don't have the proper amounts of sodium and other electrolytes to replace those lost in stool.

When the diarrhea improves, if your baby is eating solid foods, offer bland foods like rice cereal, oatmeal, bananas, potatoes, applesauce and carrots. Offer frequent, small feedings rather than large feedings.

When to call the doctor

Call immediately if your baby:

- Shows signs of dehydration (no diapers wet with urine for eight hours, no tears when crying, dry mouth)
- Passes more than eight diarrheal stools in eight hours or has blood in the stool
- Can't keep any fluids down
- Seems unusually sleepy or noticeably less active than usual
- Seems to have abdominal pain, a fever or other obvious signs of illness

Call if you are concerned that your baby:

- Has had mild diarrhea for more than a week

Nose, Ears, Mouth or Throat

Colds are upper respiratory tract infections caused by one of many viruses. Your baby can become infected repeatedly by the same virus. Colds generally last a week or two, but occasionally they persist longer. Most infants who have moderate exposure to older children will experience six to 10 colds during their first year. Sometimes it seems they have a runny nose all winter!

How to recognize it. Some colds seem to settle mainly in the baby's nose, and others settle in the baby's chest. If your infant seems to have a lot of sneezing or snorting and is frequently congested, he or she may not always have a cold. Because babies' nasal passages are quite small, it doesn't take much mucus to cause congestion. Congestion may also result from dry air or from irritants such as cigarette smoke.

When your baby has a cold, he or she will likely develop a congested or runny nose. Nasal discharge is clear at first, then turns yellow, thicker and even green. After a few days, the discharge again becomes clear and runny.

Colds may produce a low fever in your baby for the first few days. Your baby may also sneeze and have a cough, a hoarse voice or red eyes.

What causes it? Colds are most commonly spread in droplets when people sneeze or cough or by hand-to-hand contact. You can do several things to limit the number of colds your baby has. It's important to wash your hands frequently. Avoid taking your young baby to places where there may be people with colds. Also, avoid exposing your baby to areas where someone has been smoking. Children who live around cigarette smokers have more colds or respiratory infections and often have prolonged symptoms.

How serious is it? Colds are mostly a nuisance and usually are not a serious health risk. You should take precautions, however, when your baby has a cold, because these infections can progress into more serious problems, especially in smaller or younger infants. Also, your baby may have some difficulty breathing, which can interfere with nursing or bottle feeding. Watch for these signs of a worsening condition:

- A prolonged or rising fever
- Irritability
- Baby tugging at his or her ear
- Symptoms of pneumonia (see page 623)
- Lack of appetite
- Unusually restless nighttime sleep
- Thick pus coming from your baby's eyes

What can you do? There is no cure for your baby's cold. Antibiotics are ineffective against viral infections; they can't cure, prevent or shorten the course of a cold. Vitamin C has not been proved helpful in preventing colds in babies. The best thing to do is to give your baby plenty of liquids to drink. Fluids will keep the congestion looser. Because a baby with a cold may become tired and suck only briefly at one feeding, encourage frequent feedings. Use acetaminophen for fever more than 102 degrees Fahrenheit (38.8 degrees Centigrade) or if your baby seems uncomfortable.

Colds (Upper Respiratory Tract Infections)

Remember that coughing is not always bad. Coughing is protective and can help clear mucus from the baby's airway. Coughs can be dry and hacking or wet, loose and productive. Sometimes your baby's coughs may come in series (spasms of coughing), which can even result in vomiting. Coughing becomes a problem when it interferes with intake of food, activity or sleep.

Using a vaporizer or humidifier may help keep your baby comfortable. It doesn't matter whether the air we breathe is very dry or humid; the air in our lungs is fully humidified by the nose and breathing passages. However, when an infant has nasal congestion, adding extra moisture to the air can be soothing to the nose. (Extra humidity can also help infants with very dry, irritated skin such as atopic dermatitis or eczema.)

If nasal congestion makes it difficult for your baby to nurse, you can help by suctioning the baby's nose with a rubber bulb syringe before you feed or put your baby down to sleep. Squeeze the bulb before you put the tip of the clean bulb syringe into your baby's nose. Insert the tip into your baby's nostril gently, pointing toward the back of the nose, rather than upward. Release the bulb, and let it suction the mucus from the baby's nose. Remove the syringe from the baby's nostril, and empty the contents onto a tissue (by squeezing it rapidly while holding it upside down). Repeat for the other nostril. Be sure to clean the bulb syringe with soap and warm water when you're finished using it. If your baby is in child care, it's a good idea to supply his or her own bulb syringe, labeled with your baby's name to discourage sharing.

If the discharge is thick, saline nose drops or salt-water nasal spray may help loosen the mucus. Saline nose drops and sprays are made with the optimal amount of salt and water. They are inexpensive and available without prescription; ask your pharmacist if you can't find them. If your baby is in child care, it's a good idea to supply his or her own bottle, labeled with your baby's name to discourage sharing.

> ### *Tips for using a vaporizer or humidifier*
>
> - Change the water and clean the humidifier daily, otherwise mold may grow, which can be spread into the air.
> - Don't run the humidifier so much that your window sills become continually wet in cold weather.
> - Don't let the steam or mist spray directly over the baby or crib; the bedding can become damp and the baby may be chilled.
> - Don't add medications. Medications added to the air by a vaporizer or humidifier are not necessary.
> - Remember, children can be burned if they get near a hot vaporizer or steamer.

When to call the doctor

Call immediately if your baby:

- Has difficulty breathing or is bluish around the lips and mouth
- Is not having wet diapers, or won't take fluids
- Is having severe coughing with a change of skin color
- Has blood-tinged sputum

Call during office hours if your baby:

- Has had a mild fever or a temperature of more than 100 degrees Fahrenheit (38 degrees Centigrade) for more than 72 hours
- Has had a cough for more than one week
- Frequently has coughing that causes vomiting
- Has nasal discharge that is thick and green and lasts more than two weeks
- Has a crusty rash under the nose or mouth (possibly impetigo)

Cold Sores (Oral Herpes Simplex)

How to recognize it. If your baby contracts oral herpes, he or she will develop "cold sores," "fever blisters" and swelling inside the mouth and lips. You may notice that the baby's gums are redder and that he or she drools more. Blisters appear inside your baby's mouth and leave sores that take several days to heal. Some babies also become fussy, develop a mild fever and swollen lymph glands and lose their appetite.

What causes it? Cold sores, or oral herpes simplex type 1, result from one of the most common childhood viruses. (It is different from genital herpes, the sexually transmitted disease.) The virus is highly contagious and is spread by kissing or by children sharing objects they've had in their mouths.

Once your baby has cold sores, he or she becomes a carrier of the virus, which generally remains inactive within his or her body. Stress, injury to the mouth, sunburn, allergies, another illness or exhaustion may reactivate the virus, perhaps many years later.

How serious is it? Cold sores heal within a few days, but some babies may have such a sore mouth that they won't take fluids even if they are thirsty.

What can you do? Do not use a cream or ointment with cortisone-like steroids, such as hydrocortisone, if your baby has cold sores; it might cause the infection to spread. Encourage fluids, including non-acidic drinks (apple and apricot juice are good). Use acetaminophen to relieve fever or discomfort. If your baby is eating solid foods, try soft, bland foods. Sucking a frozen flavored ice pop may provide relief to older infants.

When to call the doctor. If your baby seems quite uncomfortable, stops taking liquids or has a temperature above 103 degrees Fahrenheit (39.4 degrees Centigrade), talk with your doctor.

Ear Infection (Otitis Media)

An ear infection is a bacterial infection in the middle ear, the space behind the eardrum. Ear infections are the most common reason that sick infants visit the doctor. Approximately three-quarters of all children have at least one ear infection, and many have three infections, before they are 3 years old.

How to recognize it. Most ear infections occur with, or shortly after, a cold. In some children, ear infections are difficult to recognize. The signs are often non-specific. You may wonder why your baby is particularly irritable. Your baby may suddenly have no appetite, become nauseated and vomit, or sleep well in a more upright position but become uncomfortable when lying down. You may see drainage from the ear, or a fever may develop a few days after the onset of a cold.

In some instances, your baby may experience considerable pain or a high fever. Acute infections usually develop rapidly, and recovery is usually rapid also. Chronic ear infections can occur and can be associated with fluid that remains in your baby's middle ear.

What causes it? Ear infections are usually preceded by colds. The cold virus often causes congestion and blockage in the eustachian tube, the passage between the middle ear and throat. The eustachian tube allows air movement in the middle ear space to equalize changes in air pressure. (When your ears "pop"

An infant's ear is different from an adult's ear because the eustachian tube is more horizontally positioned. Because of this, drainage from the middle ear occurs less easily, and your baby is at greater risk for an ear infection (otitis media). This condition occurs when the eustachian tube becomes blocked and fluid is trapped. It is marked by swelling and discoloration of the eardrum.

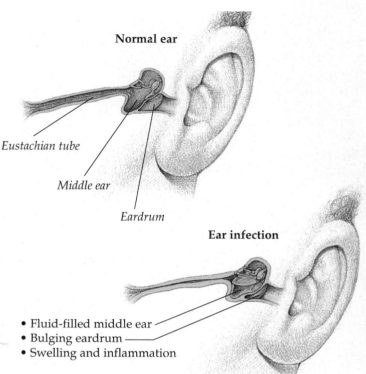

Normal ear

Eustachian tube

Middle ear

Eardrum

Ear infection

- Fluid-filled middle ear
- Bulging eardrum
- Swelling and inflammation

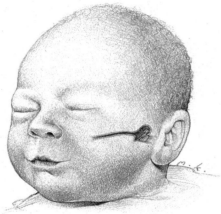

going up in an airplane, it's your eustachian tube at work.) With a cold, ventilation of the tube is impaired; this sets up a negative pressure in your baby's middle ear that causes fluid to accumulate and provides a good place for bacteria to grow. However, congestion from a cold can cause pressure in the ear without the presence of a bacterial infection.

Your baby is much more likely to get ear infections than you are, in part because his or her eustachian tube is smaller and nearly horizontal. As your infant grows, that opening will enlarge, allowing mucus to drain more easily and providing an environment where bacteria are less prone to flourish.

Although commonly recommended, there is no evidence that putting a hat on your baby or covering the baby's ears will help prevent ear infections. Your baby is at higher risk for frequent ear infections if he or she is around other children, in a child care setting or around smokers. An ear infection is not contagious, although the cold that precedes it is. Your baby may also have more ear infections if he or she has allergies.

How serious is it? Early detection and treatment of ear infections will usually stop your baby's infection before it becomes chronic. Ear infections, if untreated, may cause hearing loss. Although rare, an untreated ear infection also has the potential for becoming a more serious infection as bacteria spread.

What can you do? The most important thing you can do for your baby's ear infection is to carefully follow your health care provider's instructions for administering the antibiotic (usually for 10 days). Even though your baby will be feeling better in a few days, continue giving the medicine for the entire length of time recommended.

Until the antibiotic relieves your baby's discomfort, you can help relieve the pain with acetaminophen every three to four hours. Some doctors recommend using local anesthetic eardrops such as Americaine or Auralgan in the ear canal to help reduce pain for the first 24 hours. (First, warm bottle slightly in water and place your baby on a flat surface, ear up, to put in the drops.) Remember that eardrops that may alleviate pain do not prevent or stop an infection.

Your doctor may want to see your infant to check the eardrum—and possibly test your child's hearing—after all the medication has been given. It's important that you bring your baby in for this follow-up visit when your doctor recommends it. If your child has recurrent ear infections, your doctor may advise preventive antibiotics or more frequent evaluations.

When to call the doctor. Call during office hours if that's when you first become concerned. If it's after office hours and your baby seems uncomfortable, call or have your child examined in an urgent care clinic. Also, call your doctor if your baby is taking an antibiotic for an ear infection and vomits or cannot swallow the medication, if your baby appears sicker or if the fever is not down within 48 hours after starting to receive the antibiotic.

Swollen Glands or Lymph Nodes

How to recognize it. Swollen glands (lymph nodes) are common in babies. Your baby's lymph nodes are normally the size of a small pea, rather soft and not tender to the touch. When an infection is present, they often become larger. For example, it's common to find swollen lymph glands in your baby's neck and under his or her jaw when he or she has a viral upper respiratory tract infection. After the infection is gone, it may take several months for the lymph nodes to return to their normal size.

What causes it? Lymph glands are collections of lymph tissue that help your body resist the spread of infections and prevent infections from entering the bloodstream. Many infections cause the lymph glands to enlarge as they accomplish their purpose. The swollen lymph glands are usually an indication of an illness and are not a problem by themselves.

How serious is it? Swollen lymph nodes are sometimes tender for several days during an infection. Rarely, a lymph node can itself become infected with bacteria. The lymph node then becomes red and very tender. This can pose a risk of bloodstream infection. Persistent, enlarging lymph nodes can be a sign of cancer (lymphoma or leukemia), but fortunately this condition is rare, especially during the first year.

What can you do? Generally, no treatment is necessary for the swollen glands. Avoid poking or continually checking them. Because swollen glands are often a sign of an infection or other illness, if your child has additional symptoms such as fever or a sore throat, you might need to schedule a doctor's appointment.

When to call the doctor

Call if you are concerned that your baby:

- Has lymph nodes larger than a nickel (about 2 centimeters)
- Has red streaks that are beginning to form around a lymph node
- Has lymph nodes that are tender
- Has swollen lymph nodes that persist or rapidly enlarge

Thrush

How to recognize it. When your baby has thrush, it looks like he or she has patches of milk on the inside of the cheeks and on the tongue that won't wash off. If you scrape it away, it looks sore underneath, although it may cause little discomfort for your baby. (See the color photograph on page A8.)

What causes it? Thrush is a yeast infection in the baby's mouth. It's more likely to occur after an illness or when the mouth's natural bacterial balance has been upset by medications.

How serious is it? Thrush can be painful in severe cases, but it does not generally cause discomfort or serious problems. It can also lead to a diaper rash as the yeast travels through the baby's gastrointestinal tract.

What can you do? Mild thrush resolves without treatment. If the thrush is more extensive, your health care provider may prescribe medication.

When to call the doctor. If your baby's mouth becomes increasingly coated and causes discomfort, or if your baby has difficulty swallowing, check with your health care provider.

Chest and Lungs

Asthma (Reactive Airway Disease)

Asthma and reactive airway disease are terms used for repeated episodes of breathing difficulty, wheezing and coughing caused by spasms of the air passageways in the chest. The condition is usually not associated with a fever and is more common in older children than in babies. Asthma attacks may come on rapidly and so can be frightening to both you and your child.

How to recognize it. Children who have asthma often have a distinctive wheeze or squeaky sound when they exhale and possibly when they inhale. Children with asthma sometimes cough uncontrollably, especially at night. An asthma cough is not a productive cough (one that loosens congestion) but is more of a tight, wheezing cough.

Sometimes asthma attacks cause very mild breathing difficulty; at other times, breathing becomes very labored. It may be difficult for your baby to eat when he or she has an asthma attack because of the effort it takes to breathe.

What causes it? The most common cause of an asthma attack is a cold. Any sort of irritant can set off an asthma attack. Most often the irritant is a virus, but it may be cigarette smoke, cold air, pollen, a food or environmental allergen. Asthma is not contagious, but the virus that often precedes it is contagious. Babies whose families have a history of asthma, hay fever or allergies are more apt to have reactive airway disease, as are infants with eczema.

How serious is it? Asthma can cause breathing difficulty severe enough to require intensive hospital care. Many children benefit from breathing treatments given in the emergency department or sometimes at home. If your baby can suck, swallow and eat fairly well, the situation is not critical. Your baby's breathing rate will indicate if he or she is having problems breathing.

Remember that babies normally have a higher respiration rate than adults or older children.

What can you do? Most cases of asthma are recurrent, so you will probably learn by experience what works best for your child. Understanding what causes an attack and how your child's body responds is most important. Try to eliminate whatever seems to trigger your baby's attacks. Use prescription medication to control wheezing or coughing. Talk with your health care provider about how to handle major episodes and when to seek additional medical help.

When to call the doctor

Call immediately, or dial 911, if your baby:

- Is turning dusky or bluish, especially around the lips or mouth

Call during office hours if that's when you first become concerned. If it's after office hours, call or have your baby examined in an urgent care clinic if your baby:

- Has inner spaces between his or her ribs that are sucked in (retracted) between breaths
- Is bothered by labored breathing or wheezing
- Has repeated bouts of coughing, perhaps associated with vomiting
- Is not taking adequate fluids
- Is having an asthma attack and has a fever
- Is inhibited in daily activities by the symptoms and doesn't seem to be improving

Bronchiolitis

How to recognize it. Bronchiolitis, an infection of the bronchioles (small breathing passages in your baby's lungs), may begin like a cold. Your baby may have a runny nose, a mild fever and a cough.

After several days, the cough is more pronounced, and your baby may have difficulty breathing. You may hear your baby wheezing when he or she exhales. You may also have difficulty getting your baby to take fluids, because sucking and swallowing may be labored.

What causes it? Bronchiolitis occurs most frequently in infants, especially in the winter months. An infection of the bronchioles hinders the flow of air through the baby's lungs. Bronchiolitis is different from bronchitis, an infection of the larger airways.

Bronchiolitis is usually caused by a virus, often the respiratory syncytial virus (RSV). This virus, spread by contact with secretions of an infected person, usually generates only a mild upper respiratory tract infection in older people whom it infects. Influenza, parainfluenza, measles and adenovirus are other viruses that can also cause bronchiolitis.

How serious is it? Most cases of bronchiolitis are quite mild and babies recover fully. If bronchiolitis becomes severe, your baby may have a bluish tint around the lips and fingertips, indicating inadequate oxygen in the blood. If your baby is having difficulty breathing or is becoming dehydrated, he or she may need to be admitted to the hospital.

What can you do? Wash your hands frequently to prevent the spread of upper respiratory tract infections. Treat the cold symptoms with a humidifier and perhaps saline nasal drops (see page 614). Encourage plenty of fluids; breathing difficulties frequently cause your baby to eat or drink less. When your baby is a newborn, avoid this and other infections as best you can by avoiding close contact with children or adults who have any type of respiratory infections— even if the symptoms seem mild.

When to call the doctor

Call immediately if your baby:

- Is having breathing difficulty, is making a high-pitched wheezing sound with each exhalation or is having difficulty sucking and swallowing

Call during office hours if that's when you first become concerned. If it's after office hours, call or have your baby examined in an urgent care clinic if your baby:

- Develops signs of dehydration (infrequent urination, dry mouth, crying without tears, taking less fluid)
- Has a fever that lasts more than three days

Coughs

How to recognize it. Coughs may vary according to the part of the respiratory tract affected. An irritation near the vocal cords may cause a barking, croupy cough, and an irritation of your baby's trachea may cause a raspy cough. Allergies or asthma may cause a dry, unproductive cough that often occurs during the night. Pneumonia may cause your baby to have a deep chest cough that can be beneficial by loosening congestion in the lungs.

What causes it? Your baby usually coughs because something is irritating his or her air passages. A baby's cough most often is caused by an upper respiratory tract illness. Sometimes, irritants such as fumes from paint, smoke, tobacco and some chemicals may cause a cough.

How serious is it? Your baby's cough, by itself, is usually bothersome but not serious. The seriousness of the cough depends on the condition that causes it.

What can you do? You may be able to provide relief by adding moisture to the air with a humidifier or vaporizer. (Refer to the sidebar on page 614 regarding humidifiers and vaporizers.) If your baby's cough is interfering considerably with eating and sleeping, you should check with your health care professional. Medicines to stop coughing are generally less effective in babies than in older children or adults.

When to call the doctor

Call immediately, or dial 911, if your baby:

- Begins turning blue or coughing after he or she has choked on food or another object. (See "Choking and swallowed objects," page 648.)
- Has problems swallowing or difficulty making sounds

Call if you are concerned that your baby:

- Is younger than 2 months and develops a cough
- Develops a cough with a fever
- Has a cough that lasts longer than one week
- Seems to be in pain

Croup

How to recognize it. Many parents of babies with croup describe the distinctive cough as the sound of a barking seal. It's a tight, dry, harsh, sometimes brassy cough. Your baby may even become hoarse with croupy coughing.

Croup may cause your baby's breathing to be rapid or labored. You may hear a harsh, vibrating sound as he or she inhales. Croup doesn't usually cause a true sore throat but simply an upper respiratory tract discomfort.

What causes it? Croup is caused by a viral infection that centers on your baby's vocal cord area. Your baby may also have other upper respiratory tract symptoms, like a runny nose. As with a cold, croup is contagious until the fever is gone, or a few days into the illness. The virus is passed by respiratory secretions or droplets in the air.

How serious is it? Croup can be very frightening for parents because the cough is so harsh. Fortunately, it usually improves rapidly, but if breathing difficulty persists, go to the doctor's office or emergency department. Croup generally lasts five or six days (plan on at least three "bad" nights). Breathing is often more difficult when your child is lying down, and nighttime tends to bring on a croupy cough.

Croup generally affects babies under 3 years old, and it's not uncommon for babies under 1 year to have croup. Your baby may have a fever, generally low-grade, for the first several days.

What can you do? Moist air, especially warm, moist air, may relax the airway around the baby's vocal cords and decrease discomfort. You can accomplish this with a vaporizer. Many parents find that it's very helpful to sit with their baby in the bathroom, turn on the hot shower, close the bathroom door and let the baby breathe the steam for 15 to 20 minutes. Singing a favorite song or reading your child's favorite book may help calm both parent and child during these sometimes frightening middle-of-the-night croup episodes.

It's not uncommon for parents to rush their croupy infant to the emergency department, only to find the baby's condition improved en route by the change in air temperature and humidity.

Encourage fluids; your baby may not be very interested in food but might take small, frequent feedings. Unfortunately, cough medicines don't help croup. Smoke or other irritants will aggravate the problem.

When to call the doctor

Dial 911 if your baby:

- Is turning blue or is not breathing

Call immediately or seek medical care if your baby:

- Hasn't improved despite the "steamy bathroom" treatment described above
- Also has a high fever (more than 103 degrees Fahrenheit; 39.4 degrees Centigrade)
- Becomes unusually sleepy or inactive
- Drools excessively or has trouble swallowing

Call if you are concerned that your baby:

- Can't sleep, and your efforts won't settle him or her
- Is getting worse night after night
- Is not taking fluids well for 24 hours

Influenza

How to recognize it. Influenza is a common fall and wintertime viral illness that usually causes some of the following symptoms:

- Fever, usually more than 101 degrees Fahrenheit (38.3 degrees Centigrade)
- Chills
- Muscles that ache
- General fatigue
- Dry cough

What causes it? Influenza is caused by a respiratory virus (types A, B and C; A and B are the most common). Each type has several strains, and each year's influenza strain is usually slightly different from the previous year's.

How serious is it? Usually influenza is not a serious illness for your otherwise healthy baby, although your baby will probably feel more uncomfortable than when he or she has a cold. The main complications of influenza are ear infections and pneumonia; both require your doctor's care.

What can you do? Do not give your baby aspirin, because it has a possible link with Reye's syndrome. Because antibiotics are not effective against viruses, about all you can do is treat the symptoms of influenza. Encourage plenty of liquids and rest. Use acetaminophen for discomfort (according to the dosage chart on page 610). Sometimes adding extra moisture to the air makes it easier for your baby to breathe.

Influenza usually lasts about a week and is spread by person-to-person contact, usually in the first several days of the illness. You can lessen the spread of the virus if you keep your baby away from others and wash your hands frequently. A preventive medicine called amantadine might be prescribed to family members by your baby's health care provider early in the illness to lessen the spread of infection.

If your baby has a chronic health problem, complications may be more severe; so during influenza outbreaks you may wish to avoid contact with large groups of children. Usually, young children and their families are immunized only if they are at risk for complications.

When to call the doctor. Call your health care provider if you suspect that your baby may be developing complications or if the fever persists. (See page 608 for more information about fever.)

Pneumonia

***H**ow to recognize it.* Pneumonia is usually worse than a bad cold. A baby with pneumonia will usually cough and develop breathing difficulty. Breathing may become fast and labored, and the baby may begin wheezing. You might notice that the baby's lips or nails have a bluish tint. Your baby may also appear pale, develop a fever, lose his or her appetite and become either more listless or fussier than usual.

What causes it? Babies who get pneumonia are usually ill first with a viral upper respiratory tract infection. Some viral infections can then affect the lungs, resulting in a viral pneumonia. Occasionally, pneumonia is caused by a bacterial infection, perhaps after a cold. Bacterial pneumonia can be helped by antibiotics.

How serious is it? Although pneumonia could be quite dangerous in previous generations, most babies now recover well if they receive prompt medical attention.

What can you do? Encourage quiet activities so that your baby gets plenty of rest. Your baby may need extra holding and cuddling. He or she also needs plenty of fluids. Coughing is usually beneficial for babies with pneumonia. The various types of cough medicine available don't seem to be very effective in infants, so it's best to avoid their use. It's not a good idea to use cough suppressants because your baby needs to cough to clear the infection. Your doctor may prescribe an antibiotic if he or she suspects a bacterial pneumonia. Be sure to give your baby the full course of any prescribed antibiotic.

When to call the doctor

Call immediately if you suspect that your baby may have pneumonia. Be sure to check back with the doctor if:

- Your baby's fever continues more than two or three days, despite taking an antibiotic
- Your baby has difficulty breathing

Eyes

Babies are able to see from the moment of birth. Shortly after your baby is born, your doctor will check your baby's visual responses and inspect the eyes. By the time your baby reaches the age of 3 years, his or her vision will have gradually improved to be similar to the vision of adults. Be sure to talk with your doctor about any concerns you may have about your baby's vision.

Pinkeye (Conjunctivitis or Eye Infection)

How to recognize it. You might suspect that your baby has pinkeye if you notice that the white part of the baby's eye and the eyelid are reddened in one or both eyes. Pinkeye can also cause mucus or "matter" to form in your baby's eye, varying from thin and watery to thick and yellowish green.

If your baby has pinkeye, you may find his or her eyelids stuck together on awakening, requiring you to wash them clean. Also suspect pinkeye if your baby experiences discomfort with exposure to lights, especially bright lights, or if he or she does a lot of blinking.

Not all irritation of your baby's eyes is caused from infection. Babies frequently rub their eyes, especially when they are tired. If their hands have substances on them that irritate their eyes—dirt, foods, soaps or oil—these irritants can cause redness. Smoke and smog can also irritate your baby's eyes.

What causes it? Although pinkeye is usually caused by a viral infection accompanying a cold, it can also be the result of a bacterial infection. If this is the case, your baby's eyelid will probably become more swollen and red. Sometimes a fever is present.

How serious is it? Pinkeye generally lasts about as long as a cold, usually a week or so. Similar to a cold, pinkeye is contagious by contact.

What can you do? Wash the outside of your baby's eyelid, using clean cotton balls (a new one for each eye) and plain warm water. Wipe from the inner to the outer part of the eye to prevent spreading infection into the uninfected eye. Because pinkeye is contagious, you and others who care for your child should take precautions to avoid spreading it. Your baby with pinkeye should have his or her own towel and washcloth, both at home and away (including at child care). Wash your hands carefully after you come into contact with secretions from your child's eyes.

Your doctor may recommend antibiotic drops or ointment. Antibiotic eyedrops will not directly help a viral infection that causes pinkeye, but they do help bacterial infections (more likely when the discharge is profuse, thick and yellowish green). Some parents find ointment easier to use than eyedrops, although an ointment may briefly blur the baby's vision. In either case, the discharge should improve within the first two days or so, although redness may persist a few days more.

Applying the drops or the ointment in your baby's eye is much easier with two people. Wash your hands before you apply ointment or drops. To prevent contamination of the medication, do not let the applicator tip touch any surface (including the baby's eye). When you finish, wipe the tip of the ointment tube with a clean tissue and tightly close it. If your baby has pinkeye, remember to wash your hands whenever you touch the baby's eyes or the mucus from them.

To administer eyedrops. Lay the baby on his or her back. Gently pull the lower eyelid down to form a little pouch, and place two to four drops in the pouch. The drops will disperse over the eye as the baby blinks. It's usually a good idea to continue using eyedrops at least one day after the redness and mattering are gone.

To use an eye ointment. Pull the baby's lower eyelid away from the affected eye to form a pouch. Unless your doctor tells you otherwise, squeeze a thin strip (about ⅓ inch) of ointment into the pouch. Release the baby's eyelid, and ease the upper eyelid closed to cover the baby's eye for a moment or two.

When to call the doctor

Call if you are concerned that your baby:

- Develops a red and swollen eyelid
- Develops a fever or starts acting ill
- Has the symptoms of an ear infection
- Doesn't seem to improve after you begin using drops or ointment

Skin

Contrary to what some advertisers would like you to believe, babies' skin does not always look clear and unblemished. In fact, rashes and skin problems are common in infants. Most are not dangerous and can be treated at home. However, rashes should not be ignored, because they may also be a symptom of an infection or serious disease.

How to recognize it. Chickenpox is not a common illness among babies; it's more common in older infants and school-age children. Initially, you may notice small, red bumps on the skin. Sometimes the bumps resemble a tiny blister surrounded by redness. The rash generally begins at the center of your baby's body (face or chest) and spreads to his or her arms and legs. Your baby may become quite uncomfortable because of blisters on his or her ears, eyes, mouth, throat or genitals. (See the color photograph on page A8.)

After one or two days, the blisters usually become crusty and begin to dry. They may resemble an insect bite that has been scratched. New spots generally continue appearing over a period of four to five days. Meanwhile, the first spots may begin to improve.

Fever usually accompanies the onset of chickenpox and will often be highest the third or fourth day. Your baby may also develop a runny nose or cough with chickenpox. Most babies begin feeling better when new spots stop appearing. It's not uncommon for a baby to have 300 to 500 spots by the time chickenpox has run its course, although some infants have far fewer blisters.

What causes it? Chickenpox is a contagious viral infection; more than 70 percent of all people who are exposed and aren't immune will develop the disease. Although it usually appears seven to 14 days after exposure, some babies don't show symptoms until 21 days after they are exposed.

A vaccine to prevent chickenpox is currently undergoing testing in Japan. It is currently available in the United States only for children at high risk for complications from chickenpox, such as children receiving chemotherapy, which suppresses their immune system. It is expected to be released for widespread use in the near future.

Chickenpox (Varicella)

Chickenpox and weakened immunity

Chickenpox can be life-threatening for children who are immunosuppressed, for example, some children receiving chemotherapy for leukemia or other forms of cancer. You may know such a child, perhaps a playmate or classmate of your child. If you learn that they have been exposed to chickenpox, please contact their parents right away.

How serious is it? Generally chickenpox is not serious. If your baby scratches and reopens the blisters, he or she might have some scarring. Some spots may be visible for months, but usually they fade. Your child will still be contagious until all the spots have become crusty, generally six or seven days after the rash begins. Only rarely does chickenpox progress to serious complications such as encephalitis or Reye's syndrome.

What can you do? There is no cure for chickenpox. Therefore, the main goal is to keep your child comfortable. Do not give aspirin because it may increase the risk of Reye's syndrome.

Chickenpox causes discomfort and itching. Dress your baby in loose clothing to prevent irritation from rubbing. Trim the fingernails or cover the baby's hands with cotton socks to prevent scratching and secondary infections.

Isolate your baby from susceptible children and adults until all of the spots are crusted. If your baby has a fever or is uncomfortable, ask your health care provider about using acetaminophen or antihistamines to relieve the fever and itching. If the blisters become infected, your doctor might recommend a prescription antibiotic.

Your baby may be more comfortable if you give him or her a cool bath every three to four hours during the day to relieve the itching. Sprinkle baking soda in the bath water for added relief. Cover the baby's spots with calamine lotion or hydrocortisone cream to reduce itching (not Caladryl lotion, because it may cause irritation). If your child has blisters in his or her mouth, encourage a bland diet of soft foods and avoid citrus fruits and drinks. Sucking on a frozen flavored ice pop may provide some relief to older infants.

When to call the doctor

Call immediately if your baby:

- Starts acting very ill
- Becomes disoriented, unusually sleepy or inactive, develops a stiff neck or has trouble walking
- Develops breathing problems or pneumonia-like symptoms (especially rapid breathing or difficulty catching his or her breath)

Call if you are concerned that your baby:

- Is so uncomfortable that he or she won't take foods or liquids, and you are concerned about dehydration
- Develops a prolonged fever (more than four or five days)
- Develops renewed redness or tenderness around the blisters, or if the sores drain pus

How to recognize it. Most infants develop diaper rashes from time to time (see the color photograph on page A8). A rash from irritation may affect only the skin surface, but a rash from a yeast infection frequently covers the skin, including the creases. A yeast infection is often a bright-red rash.

What causes it? This condition is a result of a baby's frequently moist skin becoming irritated by the diaper or by an infection. Babies vary in their sensitivity to different kinds of diapers. Ammonia, produced from bacteria acting on urea in the urine, possibly increases the irritation. Yeast, found naturally on the body, grows well on warm, moist skin.

How serious is it? The biggest problem is your baby's discomfort. If you carefully treat mild diaper rashes, you may be able to avoid more stubborn yeast infections.

What can you do? The best thing you can do to prevent diaper rash is to minimize the length of time your baby's skin is in contact with wet diapers. It's also a good idea to wash the area gently at each diaper change with plain water or a mild soap and dry your baby well before you put on a new diaper.

Some babies can get a rash from detergent used to wash cloth diapers, and others may develop a rash with one or another kind of disposable diaper. There's no one best diaper—you'll just need to see what works best for your baby. If you do have a problem with one brand of disposable diapers, try another. Some babies are sensitive to the ingredients in premoistened towelettes. Others can have problems with irritation caused by elastic bands or plastic pants.

When your baby begins to get a diaper rash, you may be able to manage it by frequently exposing your baby's skin to air and by using a protective zinc oxide ointment or other diaper cream. In the past it was common for parents to use talcum powder or cornstarch to protect the skin and absorb excess moisture. However, inhaled talcum powder can be very irritating to a baby's lungs. If you choose to use powder, be careful to shake it into your hand well away from the baby's face and apply it very carefully, so that your baby does not inhale the powder.

When to call the doctor

Call during office hours if your baby:

- Has a rash that is stubborn and lasts more than a few days. A yeast infection may have developed. Your doctor may suggest an antifungal cream, and possibly a mild hydrocortisone cream. If the rash persists, your doctor may recommend that your baby see a dermatologist.

These terms describe several skin conditions. Atopic dermatitis may look like red, oozing blisters or scaly, brownish, itching skin. Types of atopic dermatitis include:

- Eczema. This type affects about 3 percent of the U.S. population. It commonly runs in families, although about one in every five people who develop it has no family history of eczema.

Diaper Rash (Yeast Rash, Diaper Dermatitis)

Atopic Dermatitis (Cradle Cap, Eczema)

- Seborrheic dermatitis, which looks like yellow, pink or brownish, thickened, greasy skin areas, often on the scalp. Scaling and crusting on the scalp are commonly called "cradle cap" (see the color photograph on page A8).
- Nummular eczema—coin-shaped, crusty patches.

How to recognize it. Patches of atopic dermatitis are often quite itchy. When atopic dermatitis appears in infancy it's often called infantile eczema. It is an itching, sometimes oozing, crusty patch of irritated skin, often on your baby's face or scalp or behind the ears, although patches can appear elsewhere as well (see the color photograph on page A8). Your baby may squirm and fuss or rub the spot to relieve itching, which is usually more severe at night.

What causes it? Atopic dermatitis or eczema is most common in families with a history of other allergic conditions such as hay fever or asthma. Atopic dermatitis probably also has an allergic basis. Foods, such as cow's milk, eggs, fish, wheat and peanuts can aggravate the condition for some infants.

What can you do? Lubricate the affected area with creams that contain no dyes or perfumes, such as Vanicream or Lubriderm. To relieve severe itching, you might try covering the area with cloths soaked in cool water.

Avoid rapid changes in temperature that will cause your baby to sweat. Avoid clothing that is rough, scratchy, woolen or too tight. Dress your infant in light, smooth, soft, non-binding clothing. Use lukewarm, not hot, water for bathing; sponge the baby's skin gently. Avoid washing your baby frequently with soaps and hot water because they tend to remove the natural oils from your baby's skin.

Talk with your baby's health care provider, an allergist or a dermatologist about the use of anti-itch medicines and when (and whether) to introduce offending foods. Skin patch tests and desensitizing shots usually offer little help and could actually worsen your baby's condition.

How serious is it? Most of these problems are temporary and will disappear by the time your baby is 2 years old. Occasionally, secondary infection develops and requires treatment. Treatments are available to control itching effectively. A few infants who have severe eczema or dermatitis may eventually develop asthma or other allergic conditions.

When to call the doctor. If you suspect that your infant has atopic dermatitis, ask your health care provider to examine the rash and recommend treatment, particularly if you have a family history of allergies. He or she can prescribe skin treatments and medications to control itching. Oral antibiotics may also be prescribed if a secondary infection develops.

Fifth Disease (Erythema Infectiosum, Parvovirus)

How to recognize it. You may suspect that your baby has fifth disease if he or she develops bright-red, warm, raised patches on both cheeks that look as though the baby was slapped. During the next few days, he or she will develop a pink, lacy, slightly raised rash on the arms, trunk, thighs and buttocks. Babies with fifth disease usually do not have a fever. Some children develop mild coldlike symptoms (sore throat, slight fever, headache, pink eyes, fatigue, itching).

What causes it? Fifth disease is caused by the parvovirus and is spread from person to person. Sometimes fifth disease is confused with other viral rashes or a medication-related rash.

How serious is it? Generally infants feel fairly well when they have fifth disease, which lasts five to 10 days. The rash may reappear briefly if your baby becomes heated or chilled or spends time in the sun. The rash may come and go for up to three weeks.

What can you do? There is no specific treatment for this disease, but you can relieve your baby's symptoms. Use acetaminophen for temperatures more than 102 degrees Fahrenheit (39 degrees Centigrade) or for discomfort. (See the dosage chart on page 610.) The rash generally doesn't need treatment. Isolation may be impractical because the disease is contagious until the rash appears; by the time you realize a child is sick, the disease is no longer contagious. Parvovirus can be a concern for pregnant women. If a woman develops parvovirus during pregnancy, the fetus can be affected. (For more information about parvovirus during pregnancy, see page 214.)

When to call the doctor. Contact your baby's health care provider if you aren't sure whether a rash is fifth disease or if you have other concerns.

Heat Rash

How to recognize it. Heat rash produces tiny pink bumps, usually on the chest or back.

What causes it? A result of blocked sweat glands, heat rash typically occurs in hot, humid weather. However, an infant who is overdressed or who has a fever can get heat rash at any time.

How serious is it? Heat rash is not serious and disappears when the cause is removed.

What can you do? Allow the baby's skin to cool, and let it air dry. Sometimes a lukewarm bath helps. Dress your baby in as few clothes as necessary. If your baby sleeps in a warm room, try using a fan to circulate air.

When to call the doctor. Call your health care provider if the baby's rash does not improve or if you are concerned that the baby's condition is more serious.

Hives (Urticaria)

How to recognize it. Hives is an allergic disorder that produces a splotchy, red, raised rash, often with pale centers (see the color photograph on page A8). The rash itches and can be uncomfortable. It can appear all over your baby's body or be concentrated in one area. The rash is irregularly shaped and may change locations. It may come and go for a few days or a few weeks.

What causes it? There is no clear explanation for most cases of hives. Viral infections likely cause most infant cases. Hives also occur as an allergic reaction to a food, drug or insect bite.

How serious is it? Hives is usually not serious unless the child also develops difficulty breathing or swallowing.

What can you do? Babies with hives often look much worse than they feel. If your child develops hives while taking medication, don't give further doses until you've checked with your doctor. Trim your baby's fingernails to avoid scratching. Keep him or her dressed in cool clothing. Avoid bathing your infant in hot water (lukewarm water will reduce itching).

When to call the doctor

Call the doctor if your infant:

- Has difficulty breathing or swallowing or develops a swollen tongue
- Develops hives while taking medication
- Is not getting relief from a recommended medication
- Seems to have soreness in his or her joints
- Has symptoms for longer than one week

Impetigo

How to recognize it. Although impetigo can occur anywhere on your baby's body, it often appears as a yellowish or honey-colored, crusty infection around the nose or mouth area. The diaper area is also a common location (see the color photograph on page A8). It usually begins with one red bump, rapidly developing into pimple-like blisters with finely crusted tops. Sometimes you might think that your baby has insect bites when he or she actually has impetigo. Once impetigo appears in one area, it usually spreads quite rapidly. The sores may ooze a pus-like material, and older infants often scratch or pick them.

What causes it? Impetigo is a superficial skin infection caused by one of two bacteria: *Streptococcus* or *Staphylococcus*. It occurs most often in the summer. However, it can develop in the wintertime after a persistent runny nose, which may produce a crack in the skin where bacteria can enter.

Impetigo is contagious and easily transmitted with washcloths and towels—or by hand contact. Therefore, it's important to wash your hands thoroughly and have a separate towel and washcloth for your baby.

How serious is it? The main concern with impetigo is spreading the disease, especially in child care centers. Impetigo is not contagious after your baby has been receiving an antibiotic for 24 hours, even though there may still be a crusty area. Complications of impetigo are rare, but you should let your health care provider know if you are concerned about worsening despite treatment or if you have new concerns.

What can you do? It's important that you try to prevent impetigo from spreading to other areas of your baby's body. Wash your hands frequently, and try to prevent your baby's scratching. Gently scrub the area with an antibacterial soap (for example, Dial or Safeguard). If the impetigo is at only one site, apply an antibiotic ointment (such as Bacitracin or Neosporin) to the affected area. Trim the baby's fingernails to avoid having him or her open the sores with scratching.

Once the spot is treated, it should resolve within a week. If scabs are thick, use a wet cloth to soften and gently remove them, or, if possible, soak the area in a baking soda bath. Scarring is unusual. If impetigo spreads past one spot or if the spot is not improving with treatment, your baby will need to see the doctor for an oral antibiotic or a prescription topical antibiotic ointment.

When to call the doctor

Call your health care provider if:

- Your child develops more than one spot of impetigo
- The sores are getting worse, becoming bigger and more numerous and appearing in distant sites
- Your baby develops a fever or becomes obviously ill

Insect Bites and Stings

How to recognize it. Insect bites and stings will probably cause a more severe physical reaction in your baby than they do in you. It's not uncommon for a mosquito bite to cause a baby's eye to be swollen shut. You can sometimes recognize an insect sting or bite by the presence of a dot or stinger near the center of the swollen area.

What causes it? Bites and stings may come from:

- Bees, yellow jackets and hornets. Stings become red and swollen within the first several hours. They can cause pain, vomiting, diarrhea and other more serious reactions.
- Mosquitoes. Usually the site simply itches and swells.
- Deerflies, horseflies, fire ants, harvester ants, beetles and centipedes. These cause painful red bumps that may blister.

How serious is it? Bee stings on the face or in the mouth could affect breathing or swallowing. Multiple stings can also be serious. You should be concerned if your baby is acting sick after being stung.

What can you do? Remember, infants can't avoid insect pests, so you need to protect them. However, you should not use insect repellents on your baby if he or she is less than 1 year old, because of the toxicity of DEET, the effective chemical in many repellents. Follow these suggestions to decrease the likelihood of insect bites:

- Cover your baby's skin with lightweight clothing when you take him or her outdoors.
- Avoid areas where insects are commonly found, for example, outside at dusk in the summer, when mosquitoes may be prevalent.
- Don't use strong perfumes or floral-scented soaps and powders—on you or your baby.
- Cover all picnic food, and seal picnic garbage in plastic bags.
- Cover your garbage cans; buy cans with snap-on lids.
- Avoid pools of stagnant water, which provide breeding grounds for mosquitoes.

- Although you should avoid using repellents on your baby, you can deter many insects by using the repellent yourself when you are carrying your baby outdoors. Stay away from the extra-strength sprays, and be sure to wash your hands to avoid having either of you get the chemicals in your eyes or mouth.

Bee stings. After your baby has been stung, remove the stinger (if you can see it) by scraping it with a tweezers. Don't pinch the area to remove the stinger. Ice on the skin can relieve pain, but take care not to freeze the skin. Apply calamine lotion, hydrocortisone cream or baking soda (made into a paste with water). Check with your doctor about using an antihistamine to reduce swelling and discomfort.

When to call the doctor. Call your health care provider immediately if your child:

- Has difficulty breathing
- Vomits
- Seems dizzy
- Has more swelling and redness around the sting or bite after the first six to eight hours

Poison Ivy, Oak, Sumac (Contact Dermatitis)

How to recognize it. The rash from poison ivy, poison oak and sumac is red and extremely itchy and produces small blisters that become weepy. Your baby may develop the rash from one to seven days after exposure. It may cover not only areas of skin that were exposed but also areas where your baby's scratching has spread the resin.

What causes it? Poison ivy is a plant with three leaves; it may grow in a bush shape or on a vine. Early in the season, leaves are reddish. You will see shiny black spots on damaged leaves, where the resin (which causes the rash) is exposed to the air. The resin quickly binds to skin on contact. Poison oak is actually the common name of poison ivy in the bushy form. Sumac has long, narrow leaves from a common stem and produces clusters of white berries. Two-thirds of all people are sensitive to the resin of these plants.

How serious is it? Contact with these plants can cause pain and discomfort, and the blisters can become infected. Although your baby will be uncomfortable, he or she will have no lasting effects.

What can you do? Look for and carefully remove poison ivy from your property with garden gloves, which you should wash immediately. When picnicking or camping, watch for areas of poison ivy. If you suspect that your baby's skin has been in contact with poison ivy, remove any clothing that the poison ivy has touched. Flood the skin with water for 10 minutes, gently wash it with soap and water and rinse thoroughly. If you act quickly (within five to 10 minutes), you may be able to remove the resin before it binds to the baby's skin. Check to see whether the skin is red and irritated. Wash all clothing and other items that have come into contact with the resin.

When to call the doctor. If your baby has a severe reaction or has gotten the resin in his or her eyes, face or genital area, contact your health care provider.

Roseola

How to recognize it. Most children who develop roseola do so before 3 years of age. Your baby may be fussier than usual and have a fever of more than 101 degrees Fahrenheit (38.3 degrees Centigrade) for two to four days. When the fever subsides and the baby seems to be feeling better, you will notice a pink rash, mainly on the baby's trunk. The rash is not uncomfortable or itchy for your baby. You can't be sure the baby has roseola until the rash appears as the fever resolves. The rash usually lasts 24 to 48 hours.

What causes it? The human herpesvirus 6 causes roseola. This is a different virus than that which causes sexually transmitted herpes.

What can you do? Other than treating the fever, there isn't much you need to do for roseola. Lotion doesn't help the rash.

When to call the doctor. Call your health care provider if the rash worsens, if your baby becomes sicker or if the rash lasts longer than three days.

Scabies

How to recognize it. Scabies causes severe itching, especially in skin folds, hands and feet. It is usually worse at night. The rash may have bumps and blistered areas (see the color photograph on page A8).

What causes it? Scabies is caused by tiny mites that burrow into the top layer of the skin.

How serious is it? Scabies doesn't lead to serious illness, but the itchiness is persistent and severe. Fortunately, it is easily treated.

What can you do? Scabies is commonly spread by close physical contact or sharing clothing or bedding. Carefully follow the recommendations of your doctor for treatment of young infants. Do not re-treat without first consulting your doctor; repeated treatments can irritate the skin or cause toxicity from the medication. Launder all bedding, towels and clothing that might have been used by anyone with scabies.

When to call the doctor. Contact your doctor for recommendations if you suspect that your infant has scabies. Your doctor might need to not only examine the skin but also examine a scraping of skin under the microscope to confirm the diagnosis. Treatment of scabies in infants often differs from that used in older children. When one family member is treated for scabies, it is common to treat all family members; therefore, be sure to mention the ages of the youngest family members.

Sunburn

How to recognize it. Sunburn, the result of overexposure to the sun's ultraviolet (UV) radiation, may not immediately be evident after you bring your baby in from the sun. You may not realize that your baby has sunburn because the pain and redness may not appear for several hours. Sunburn may cause red, tender, swollen or blistered skin that is usually hot to the touch.

What causes it? Your baby's skin is quite thin and susceptible to sunburn, even with only 10 to 15 minutes of exposure. Your baby can even get burned on a cloudy or cool day, because it's not the visible light or the heat from the sun that burns but the invisible UV light.

How serious is it? It's a good idea to be cautious about the possibility of your baby sunburning. Babies can develop blisters, fever, chills and nausea with sun exposure that may not affect an older person.

What can you do? Keep your baby out of direct sunlight as much as possible, especially between 10 a.m. and 3 p.m., when the sun's rays are strongest. This precaution includes cloudy days, when the clouds don't block but simply scatter UV rays. You can also protect your baby by routinely dressing him or her in a hat for outings during the middle of the day.

Many sunscreens use PABA, a chemical that absorbs damaging UV rays, to protect skin. Avoid using sunscreen with PABA if your baby is younger than 6 months. Most babies tolerate PABA well, although some babies with sensitive skin will develop a reaction to some sunscreens. If you're concerned that your baby has sensitive skin, you should do a patch test first, applying a spot of sunscreen the size of a half-dollar to the baby's forearm and watching for a reaction for 48 hours. Apply sunscreen at least one hour before exposure to allow enough time for the sunscreen to provide protection. Use a waterproof sunscreen with a sun protection factor (SPF) of at least 15, which means that it takes 15 times longer to burn with the sunscreen on than without it. Reapply it after the baby has played in the water, even if the sunscreen is waterproof.

Treat sunburn by gently applying cool water compresses every few hours, taking care not to allow your baby to become chilled. Give your baby acetaminophen to relieve the pain (according to the dosage chart on page 610). Avoid using anesthetic lotions or sprays on a baby's skin; some sting, and a baby's skin may react to anesthetic sprays. Encourage fluids.

When to call the doctor. Call your health care provider if the sunburn blisters or if your baby begins vomiting or acts ill.

Stomach and Intestines

Constipation   **H**ow to recognize it. Your baby is likely constipated if he or she:

- Has difficulty passing hard, dry stools
- Suddenly has less frequent stools for no apparent reason (a change in the diet may cause this)
- Has stools with streaks of blood on the outside
- Seems to have abdominal pain that is relieved after a large bowel movement

What causes it? The colon stores stool and absorbs water. If the urge to have a bowel movement is ignored or suppressed (for example, if recent bowel movements were uncomfortable), the retained stool becomes more firm. When a bowel movement eventually occurs, it may be painful and even cause slight bleeding.

How serious is it? Most infant constipation is mild, a result of a dietary change, and resolves within a short time. Constipation often causes more distress for the parents than for the child.

What can you do? Although many cases of constipation can be traced to diet, breastfed babies are seldom constipated from changes in the mother's diet. Furthermore, it is not unusual for breastfed babies to go five to seven days without a stool. If a change of diet seemed to start the problem, it will likely improve with time. Offer plenty of fluids. If your baby is eating solid foods, add high-fiber foods (such as prunes, apricots, plums, peas, beans, broccoli and whole-grain bread products) to his or her diet.

When to call the doctor. Call your health care provider if your efforts aren't providing any relief. Do not give laxatives, enemas or medication without consulting your doctor first.

Food Allergies and Milk Intolerance

How to recognize it. Different kinds of allergies may cause different kinds of reactions in your baby. Food allergies may cause eczema, which appears as a patchy, dry, red, itchy rash—often in the creases of the arms, legs and neck. (See page 527 for more information about eczema.) Other symptoms may include diarrhea or symptoms of hay fever.

Suspect an allergy if these symptoms appear without the other symptoms of a cold or viral infection. If the baby's nose is runny, it will likely be a thin, clear discharge. The baby may also have watery eyes and repeated sneezing attacks. He or she may have itchy eyes, nose or skin, without a fever. The reaction may last a long time, although babies generally have some days that are better or worse than others.

What causes it? Allergies occur when the human body's natural defense system incorrectly identifies a harmless substance as harmful. The body then over-reacts in an attempt to protect itself, and an allergy results.

The only real way to know if a particular food is the culprit is to eliminate the suspected food until the symptoms are gone and then reintroduce it after two weeks. This can be difficult when your baby is eating foods that have a number of ingredients combined in them. Most common food problems occur with cow's milk, proteins (like eggs), peanut butter, soy, fish, wheat, peas and shellfish.

How serious is it? Food allergies can be serious and chronic, although medication can often help control them.

What can you do? It's important that you begin treatment early and be persistent about caring for your child's food allergies. Allergy shots are not effective in treating food allergies, although they may be helpful for a small number of other allergies. Discuss any food allergies with your baby's health care provider.

Prevention is important. Avoid foods or other substances that you know cause an allergic reaction in your baby. If members of your family have food allergies and you are breastfeeding, you may want to prolong breastfeeding to avoid exposing your baby at an early age to antigens like milk products, soy or other protein sources that seem to enhance absorption and aggravate allergies.

Bathe your baby with a mild, non-drying type of soap such as Dove or Basis. Use a lubricating cream to decrease redness and itching. Avoid petroleum jelly, because it blocks the pores and can make the rash worse. Avoid frequent bathing, and rinse the baby's skin well.

When to call the doctor

Call immediately if your baby:

- Develops breathing difficulties

You should also talk with your health care provider if:

- The rash looks infected (becomes more red and has a yellowish discharge)
- Treatment is not working

Hernia (Inguinal)

How to recognize it. If you notice a small lump or bulge about the size of a grape in your baby's groin, you may have discovered an inguinal hernia. It may seem more swollen when the baby is crying or active and may nearly disappear when the baby is lying down. About 5 percent of all children (more commonly boys) have inguinal hernias. If your baby has an inguinal hernia on one side, there frequently will be one on the other side also.

What causes it? Inguinal hernias occur when a weak spot in the lower abdomen allows a small portion of the bowel to push through into the groin, forming a bump or bulge.

How serious is it? Inguinal hernias are seldom uncomfortable and can be corrected with surgery. Occasionally, a piece of the intestine becomes trapped in the hernia, causing marked tenderness and sometimes discoloration and vomiting. If this happens, your baby may need surgery immediately.

What can you do? Notify your doctor if you suspect that your baby has an inguinal hernia. Sometimes laying your baby down and elevating his or her legs will cause the bulge to disappear temporarily.

When to call the doctor. If you notice a bulge and it is not causing your baby any discomfort, it's a good idea to call and discuss it with your baby's health care provider during regular office hours. If your baby is uncomfortable and the area is swollen and painful, call your doctor immediately.

How to recognize it. You may notice that your baby boy's scrotum seems swollen on one side. It may seem more swollen when he is crying or active and less so when he is lying down. Your health care provider may have noticed this when your baby was born; if so, he or she will continue to examine it regularly for changes.

Hydrocele

What causes it? This is not uncommon in newborn boys, although it can develop later in childhood also. It may disappear by the time your baby is a year old. Your baby's testicles develop in his abdomen and move through a passage into the scrotum before birth. When the opening to the abdomen doesn't fully close, the fluid that is normally in the abdomen can pass into the scrotum and cause swelling.

How serious is it? Generally, a hydrocele is not serious and doesn't cause your baby any discomfort. However, if the area becomes swollen and tender, an inguinal hernia may also have developed (see page 636).

What can you do? If you suspect that your baby has a hydrocele, share your concerns with your health care provider and watch for any change in the baby's condition.

When to call the doctor. Call your health care provider immediately if you notice that your baby has a marked tenderness in the scrotum.

Infections

How to recognize it. Since HIV (human immunodeficiency virus) was first identified in 1981, increasing numbers of children have become infected with it. Initially, babies with HIV may seem just fine. But later, they may not grow normally and may have frequent problems with upper respiratory infections, pneumonia, diarrhea or skin infections. Their lymph glands eventually enlarge, and they frequently develop fungal infections of the mouth. Their condition is then called AIDS (acquired immunodeficiency syndrome).

HIV and AIDS

What causes it? HIV is an impairment of the immune system. If you are infected with HIV, your baby may acquire it from you, during either pregnancy or delivery. Children of nearly half of all mothers infected with HIV will develop the infection. Adults acquire HIV primarily through homosexual or heterosexual contact, through intravenous drug use or, rarely, through blood transfusions.

Once infected, your baby retains the virus for life. Babies who acquire the virus from their mothers during pregnancy or at birth generally develop AIDS in less than two years.

How serious is it? Eventually, HIV will affect your baby's immune system and slow his or her growth and development. Your baby may develop breathing difficulties and fever or pneumonia. AIDS-related infections and cancers eventually develop and become life-threatening.

What can you do? If you are a woman with risk factors for HIV infection who wants to become pregnant, you should be tested for the virus before becoming pregnant. Your chances of delivering a healthy baby will be greatly increased if you do not carry the virus and if you can eliminate further exposure.

If your child has HIV, be sure to inform any health care provider who treats him or her, so that they can avoid potentially harmful treatments. Common infections can be serious for a child with HIV. Your baby may not be able to tolerate routine childhood immunizations if he or she has HIV. Avoid exposing your baby to chickenpox if he or she has HIV. Be especially careful to note any change in your baby's health status.

When to call the doctor. Notify your doctor any time your HIV-infected baby develops a fever, breathing or swallowing difficulties, diarrhea or skin problems or has been exposed to a contagious disease.

Meningitis

How to recognize it. Meningitis occurs when the fluid surrounding your baby's brain and spinal cord becomes infected. These symptoms require immediate emergency medical attention:

- Fever, decreased appetite, drowsiness, irritability or bulging in the soft spot (fontanelle) at the top of your baby's head. A stiff neck might occur in older infants.

What causes it? Your baby can get meningitis from bacteria that enter his or her bloodstream. Other forms of meningitis are caused by viruses, fungi or parasites.

How serious is it? Early and intensive treatment is important. When meningitis is diagnosed and treated promptly, more than 70 percent of the children who get the disease recover fully. The most common, long-lasting complication associated with meningitis is hearing loss. Seizures and developmental problems can also result.

What can you do? Don't delay seeking treatment if you suspect that your baby has meningitis. If a physician recommends that tests be done to check for possible meningitis, have them done without delay.

When to call the doctor. Call your health care provider or go to the emergency department if you suspect that your child has meningitis. This disease is especially difficult to diagnose in infants younger than three months. Your doctor will check your baby's blood for indications of a bacterial infection and may also insert a special needle into your baby's lower back (called a lumbar puncture or spinal tap) to check for infection in the spinal fluid. If test results are positive, your baby will need to be hospitalized for intensive medical treatment, including antibiotics.

Measles (Rubeola)

How to recognize it. Measles is rare in the United States, although occasional outbreaks have been reported in high schools and colleges. It's highly unlikely that your baby will develop measles; many physicians in the United States have never seen a patient with a confirmed case. But assuming that your infant was exposed, the following describes a typical case.

For a week to two after your baby is exposed to measles, he or she probably will not have any symptoms. Then your baby will develop coldlike symptoms (cough, runny nose, pinkeye) and will be fussy.

After that, your baby may develop a temperature of more than 103 degrees Fahrenheit (39.4 degrees Centigrade) that will last until several days after a rash appears. The rash usually appears after two to four days of illness, often beginning on your baby's face and spreading down his or her trunk to the arms and legs. The rash initially is composed of fine red bumps, which may become larger splotches. The rash usually lasts about a week.

What causes it? Measles is a viral infection. Because most babies are vaccinated, measles is rare in America today. The virus that causes measles is transmitted in airborne droplets, when an infected person sneezes, for example.

How serious is it? Most babies recover quite well from measles with no ill effects. The most common complications of measles are pneumonia and encephalitis. Although bacterial infections occasionally develop after measles, you can help avoid complications if you keep your ill baby at home and encourage rest and fluids. Measles is contagious from the time just before the rash breaks out until the fever and rash are completely gone.

What can you do? If you suspect that your baby has measles, your physician will need to examine your child and confirm with laboratory tests that it is definitely measles. (Your doctor's office will want to keep your child away from other patients to prevent spreading the disease.) Give plenty of fluids, and use acetaminophen to control fever. (See the dosage chart on page 610.) Bright lights may bother the eyes, so you may need to darken the baby's room for a few days.

When to call the doctor. Call your doctor's office if you suspect that your child has or may have been exposed to measles.

Periorbital Cellulitis

How to recognize it. This is a bacterial infection of the eyelids and soft tissues around the eye. Bacteria can start growing in this area after an injury to the area, or a small pimple of pus may form. Sometimes a sinus infection or upper respiratory tract infection can also move into these tissues. You may suspect that your baby has periorbital cellulitis if he or she develops a fever and marked swelling of the eyelids. Within several hours the swelling spreads as the eyelid becomes markedly swollen, angry red and warm—usually only on one side. The baby will generally have a fever and appear to be sick. Although you may mistake this for an eye injury (due to the swelling), the fever points to the fact that there is an infection present.

What causes it? Several kinds of bacterial infections can cause periorbital cellulitis.

How serious is it? If untreated, this can be a serious infection that can threaten your baby's vision. The bacteria can also spread through the bloodstream and cause meningitis.

What can you do? Immediately seek medical attention if your child develops fever and marked swelling of the eyelids.

When to call the doctor. Contact your health care provider immediately if you suspect that your baby has periorbital cellulitis. If the baby has a fever and one eye is red or swollen, promptly bring him or her to your nearest emergency department.

Unexplained Fever (Sepsis, Bacteremia)

How to recognize it. Usually, there's an explanation for a baby's fever which becomes apparent, based on the history of the baby's illness, your doctor's examination, and the knowledge your doctor has about illnesses that are prevalent in the community at the time. (Fever is discussed on page 608.) However, you or your doctor may not be able to explain as many as 20 percent of baby's fevers. These may be called "fevers without localizing signs."

What causes it? Most unexplained fevers disappear after a few days or reveal a condition that is clearly treatable, such as an ear infection or chickenpox. Occasionally, though, a continuing unexplained fever may be a sign of bacteria in the bloodstream (called bacteremia or occult bacteremia). Bacteria in the bloodstream pose a risk of spreading infection to different parts of the body.

How serious is it? An unexplained, prolonged fever may indicate a serious condition. This is why your doctor will begin additional tests to rule out various types of infection. The specific tests needed will vary for each patient.

What can you do? Talk over your concerns with your health care provider if your baby has had an unexplained fever. He or she may want to check the baby's white blood cell count, culture the blood for bacteria, check the urine, possibly perform a spinal tap or take a chest X-ray.

When to call the doctor. Especially in younger infants, if the temperature is 103 degrees Fahrenheit (39.4 degrees Centigrade) or higher, your doctor may want to start giving the baby antibiotics even before the source of the fever is discovered.

Tuberculosis

How to recognize it. Tuberculosis is most frequently diagnosed in infants by tracing contacts of family members or other adult caregivers who have the disease. It more frequently affects older people, but sometimes babies become infected. Tuberculosis can take various forms in infants. The most common is a respiratory infection that causes persistent and contagious pneumonia. Babies can have tuberculosis for a relatively long period of time without any apparent symptoms.

What causes it? If your baby has tuberculosis, he or she has probably contracted it from a family member or other adult caregiver. Unlike many other infectious diseases that babies get, it's fairly rare that your baby would get tuberculosis from another child. Tuberculosis is more common in residents of cities than among residents of small towns or rural areas.

How serious is it? Worldwide, tuberculosis is a serious, even life-threatening, chronic infectious disease. In the United States, tuberculosis has been rare in infants, but now it occurs more frequently. Complications can include pneumonia and accumulations of fluid between the lung and the chest wall or around the heart. Tuberculosis can also infect lymph nodes, the bones, liver and kidneys.

What can you do? If you or someone who cares for your baby tests positive for tuberculosis (meaning that there is evidence of the disease), it's a good idea for your baby to be checked. The screening is fairly simple and involves injecting a small drop of testing fluid under the baby's skin. This is called a TB skin test, tuberculin skin test or PPD. You may need to bring your baby back in two days to have the site of the injection examined.

If your baby has been exposed to tuberculosis or has developed tuberculosis without symptoms, the area of the injection will become hard and red within two to three days (a "positive" result). Babies who test negative may have a slight irritation. If the test is positive, you will need to bring your baby in for further tests. You may also need to give your baby medication for up to one year.

When to call the doctor. Call to arrange a test for your baby if you suspect that he or she has been exposed to tuberculosis. Infants diagnosed as having tuberculosis are often treated by their primary care provider and by specialists in pediatric infectious disease and pediatric pulmonology (lung conditions).

Whooping Cough (Pertussis)

How to recognize it. The symptoms resemble a mild upper respiratory tract infection (without a fever), and the cough worsens throughout the first week. Eventually, exhausting coughing outbreaks consist of 10 to 30 forceful, abrupt coughs, perhaps with the tongue protruding, sometimes followed by a "whoop" sound as the baby inhales forcefully.

What causes it? Whooping cough is a highly contagious bacterial infection of the respiratory tract. It is transmitted, person to person, by airborne droplets from coughing or sneezing.

How serious is it? Whooping cough can have serious complications, especially among infants, including respiratory problems, pneumonia, ear infections and weight loss. Medication does not cure the illness, but it can limit the spread to others.

What can you do? Whooping cough is largely preventable with immunizations. For optimal protection, your baby needs a series of pertussis shots (the "P" in DTP shots). Many child care centers require immunization for whooping cough to try to prevent its spread.

When to call the doctor. If your baby has been exposed to someone diagnosed as having whooping cough, contact your doctor about possible testing and treatment.

Cancer

Neuroblastoma

How to recognize it. Neuroblastoma is one of the most common solid tumors in children. It affects about one in 100,000 children a year. Most commonly, the tumor is discovered as a large abdominal mass. Sometimes it causes unexplained fevers.

What causes it? There are no common reasons for the development of neuroblastoma. It is usually not an inherited form of cancer.

How serious is it? The severity depends on the extent of the disease at the time of diagnosis. Surprisingly, it may affect infants younger than 1 year differently than it affects older babies. Sometimes infants younger than a year experience a regression and disappearance of the tumor.

When to call the doctor. If you notice your baby has an unusual abdominal mass, bring it to your doctor's attention. Tests to determine whether your baby has neuroblastoma may include urine and blood tests, an ultrasound exam of the abdomen, CT scanning or liver scanning. Evaluation and treatment of neuro-blastoma are usually done by specialists in pediatric oncology in coordination with your baby's health care provider.

Retinoblastoma

How to recognize it. This malignant tumor in the retina of babies is rare. It usually is noticed between a year and 18 months. The most common sign is an unusual white area in the baby's pupil. However, this finding does not automatically mean that the baby has retinoblastoma. Other abnormalities, such as congenital cataracts, also can cause a whitish area to appear. The sudden development of crossed eyes in an infant older than 4 months of age may raise a suspicion of retinoblastoma.

What causes it? Retinoblastoma has both a hereditary and a non-hereditary form.

How serious is it? This is a relatively slow-growing tumor that is usually confined to the eye. One or both eyes may be affected. Early diagnosis greatly improves the ability to treat the disease successfully. Babies with retinoblastoma have a higher-than-average risk of developing other cancers.

What can you do? Treatment for retinoblastoma requires medical supervision by specialists in pediatric oncology. It often involves chemotherapy or radiation and sometimes the removal of the eye.

When to call the doctor. If you are concerned about your baby's eyes, talk with your doctor. Remember, though, that retinoblastoma is not common.

Other Serious Conditions

Anemia

How to recognize it. Although skin coloring varies greatly among babies, paleness can be a clue that a baby may have anemia, a condition in which the blood is deficient in red blood cells.

Babies with anemia may tire easily or be mildly weakened. Severe anemia may cause shortness of breath, rapid heart rate or swelling of your baby's hands and feet.

What causes it? The most common cause of anemia is an iron deficiency due to premature birth, inadequate iron in the baby's diet or excessive blood loss. Because cow's milk contains little iron and can cause blood loss, babies who start drinking cow's milk early and don't receive supplemental iron may develop anemia.

How serious is it? If untreated, anemia may interfere with your baby's growth and development.

What can you do? If you suspect that your baby is anemic, talk with your health care provider. Do not give your child vitamins or iron without first talking to your doctor and having the baby's blood tested.

When to call the doctor. Check with your health care provider at your next visit if you suspect that your baby is anemic.

Cerebral Palsy

How to recognize it. The symptoms of cerebral palsy vary considerably because of different types and degrees of disability. Many parents simply notice that their babies don't develop motor skills that other babies the same age are developing. Cerebral palsy is usually evident by a year of age; sometimes it is suspected in the first few months. In a baby more than 2 months old, the following may be warning signs:

- Your baby may feel stiff or floppy much of the time.
- Your baby seems to be constantly pushing away from you and arching his or her back when you cradle him or her.
- The baby does not pick up his or her head when pulled forward into a sitting position after lying on the back.

What causes it? In cerebral palsy, the parts of the brain that control movement and muscle tone are abnormal. Most children with cerebral palsy have no clearly identifiable cause for it. Cerebral palsy can be caused by malformation of the brain or injury to the brain during pregnancy, delivery or immediately after birth. Babies who are born prematurely have a higher incidence of cerebral palsy. In a few cases, babies get cerebral palsy from an illness, such as meningitis, or injury of the brain.

How serious is it? Although cerebral palsy often is difficult to diagnose and causes varying degrees and types of disabilities, early intervention will help your child develop to his or her maximal potential. Some children with cerebral palsy may have seizures, developmental delays, vision problems, stiffening of the joints, hearing loss and dental problems.

What can you do? Be sure to discuss your concerns with your doctor. If your baby is diagnosed with cerebral palsy, investigate an early-intervention program so that you can help your child maximize his or her potential. These programs also help you meet other parents with children who have cerebral palsy.

When to call the doctor. Be sure to discuss any concerns you have about your child's development with your doctor. Children with suspected cerebral palsy are often evaluated by specialists in pediatric neurology, physiatry (physical medicine and rehabilitation), physical therapy and medical genetics.

Failure to Gain Weight, Failure to Thrive

How to recognize it. Your baby will not grow at exactly the same rate as every other baby. Babies grow at different rates and to different degrees. They also occasionally reach plateaus in their growth cycle. At times, your baby may be shorter, thinner and more or less active than other children.

In rare instances, a baby may stop growing for a longer time or grow unusually slowly. He or she may stop gaining weight or even lose weight.

If your baby fails to gain weight, he or she will often show signs of delayed development. The baby may be unwilling to make eye contact and may appear withdrawn or noticeably inactive without any apparent reason. He or she may also experience gastrointestinal problems, evidenced by vomiting or diarrhea.

What causes it? Failure to gain weight is almost always due to insufficient nutrition. This can occur for various reasons.

Rarely, a baby fails to thrive because of underlying health problems. Some disorders of the small intestine, liver, kidneys, heart, nervous system or endocrine system may prevent your baby's body from absorbing the nutrients in foods.

How serious is it? Usually, recognition and improved nutrition result in a growth spurt. Early intervention is vital to optimize brain and body growth as well as social development. If the cause is an underlying health problem, your baby will need specific treatment.

What can you do? Prevention is your best approach. Visit your child's health care provider regularly during the baby's first year. Clinic staff will weigh and measure your baby and record his or her progress at each visit.

When to call the doctor. Feel free to share your concerns about your baby's growth with your health care provider at your regular visits. If your baby becomes ill for no apparent reason and stops taking feedings, or if you suspect that your baby is not getting the proper nourishment, call the doctor's office.

Hearing Loss

How to recognize it. When babies have hearing disorders, parents usually notice the condition before other caregivers or health care professionals notice it. It's important that you report concerns about your child's hearing ability early on. Intervention is most effective when difficulties are detected early.

The chart on page 645 shows typical developmental stages related to hearing.

Your Baby's Hearing

Age	Characteristics of Normal Hearing in Infants
1 month	The baby often stops moving and appears to listen to a sudden sound
2 months	The baby appears to listen to his or her parents talking
3 months	The baby coos and gurgles in response to speech and looks toward the speaker's direction. The baby also startles if someone claps within 3 feet
4 months	The baby responds differently to angry and pleasant voices
5 months	The baby begins to mimic sounds and respond to his or her name
6 months	The baby protests loudly and squeals with delight. The baby also searches for the source of speech or other sounds
7 months	The baby makes some wordlike sounds and responds with gestures to simple words, such as "bye-bye"
8 months	The baby may stop what he or she is doing when someone calls his or her name
9 months	The baby stops what he or she is doing when you say "no"
10 months	The baby may begin to say simple words
1 year	The baby responds to simple questions by pointing to the named object (for example, "Where is your nose?")

What causes it? These factors increase the risk that your baby may have a hearing disorder:

- Bacterial meningitis
- Infections before birth or in early infancy
- Birth defects of the head or neck, such as cleft palate or ear deformities
- Severe jaundice, requiring exchange blood transfusions
- Premature birth
- Severe oxygen deprivation at birth
- A family history of hearing loss

There are several types of hearing disorders, including:

Conductive, in which something interferes with the external ear's reception of sound or with the transmission of sound from the external ear to the inner ear. Doctors can often treat conductive hearing loss successfully.

Sensorineural, stemming from abnormalities of the baby's inner ear or the auditory nerve. More than half of these losses are congenital. The remainder of hearing problems are due to conditions such as birth trauma, intrauterine infections or medications. This type of hearing loss is usually not reversible.

Mixed, a combination of both conductive and sensorineural hearing loss, often severe.

Central auditory disorders, disorders of the central auditory nervous system which occur during pregnancy, at birth or in the baby's early months.

How serious is it? Hearing disorders and their causes vary widely. It's far better to discover a hearing disorder early. The chances of developing effective communication skills are much better when a hearing loss is detected early. Medical or surgical treatments can help many children who have a hearing loss.

What can you do? Observe your baby's development, as noted in the chart on page 645. Be sure to talk over any concerns about your baby's hearing with your health care provider.

Emergencies

Call the paramedics (or dial 911) immediately if your baby is:

- Experiencing difficulty breathing and his or her lips are turning blue
- Unconscious
- Losing a large amount of blood from a deep wound
- Burned seriously
- Having a seizure

Take your baby to the nearest emergency facility, or if this is not possible call paramedics (or dial 911) if your baby:

- May have a broken bone.
- Is bitten by an animal or snake.

Call your local poison control hotline (the number is usually listed on the inside cover of your telephone directory) if your baby:

- Has irritating chemicals in the eyes. Call for advice on emergency home treatment before you bring your baby in if chemicals get in the eyes.
- Might have eaten a poisonous substance.

Bleeding

How to recognize it. Bleeding is usually not life-threatening. You can generally judge the seriousness of the bleeding by the rate of blood loss. Serious bleeding comes from injured arteries. Slower bleeding can come from injuries to veins (steady, slow flow of dark red blood) or the smaller blood vessels (capillaries).

What causes it? Bleeding can be the result of a cut, puncture or abrasion.

How serious is it? The rate of blood loss is a good indicator of severity. Remember, because babies have a much smaller volume of blood, they cannot afford to lose as much blood as an older child or adult. Serious injuries may result in bleeding from the arteries, which can cause death in minutes if untreated.

What can you do? If the bleeding is serious and does not stop on its own or if the cut or puncture is large or deep or has rough edges, immediately apply pressure directly to the injury with a sterile gauze pad or clean cloth. Keep pressure on the wound until the bleeding stops. In most cases, you can stop arterial bleeding with direct, firm pressure to the wound.

Follow these steps for severe bleeding:

- Immediately apply steady, firm pressure to the wound with a sterile gauze pad, clean cloth or your hand until the bleeding stops. Do not attempt to clean the wound first or remove any embedded objects.
- Call your doctor or an ambulance, dial 911 or take your child immediately to the emergency department.
- When the bleeding stops, cover the wound with a tight dressing and tape securely. If the bleeding continues and seeps through the dressing, place more absorbent material over the first dressing.
- If possible, elevate the bleeding area. If the head is not bleeding, it may help to elevate the legs or have the head slightly lower than the trunk.
- If the bleeding continues, apply pressure to the major vessel that delivers blood to the area.

If your baby has a small cut or abrasion that bleeds slightly, clean the area well with mild soap and water. To avoid contamination, keep the cleaned area covered until a scab forms.

When to call the doctor. Go to your nearest emergency department if you are unable to stop the bleeding, using the techniques described above. Call your health care provider for further advice on treating the wound after you have stopped the bleeding or if you have other concerns.

Burns

How to recognize it. Burns can range from minor problems to life-threatening emergencies. They occur most often on a baby's hands or face.

What causes it? Burns can be caused by fire, sun (sunburn is discussed on page 633), chemicals, electricity or heated objects or fluids. Common sources of burns are hot liquids (such as coffee or tea), bottles that have been heated in a microwave oven, stoves or cigarettes. Some burns result from water heater temperatures that are excessively high (more than 120 degrees Fahrenheit). You also need to be cautious about your baby's clothing catching fire from a spark or ashes. The most frequent causes of burns in children are fireworks, outdoor barbecue grills and electrical outlets.

How serious is it? Burns can range from mild to serious. Burns are classified according to their severity:

First-degree burns cause redness and slight swelling of the skin; these are the most mild and affect only the outer layer of skin.

Second-degree burns cause blistering, intense reddening and moderate to severe swelling and pain. The top layer of skin has been burned through and the second layer is also damaged.

Third-degree burns are the most severe. These burns appear white or charred and involve all the layers of the skin. Substantial nerve damage may cause there to be little pain with these burns.

What can you do? You can take some precautions to avoid burns at home:

- Put cups with hot drinks out of baby's reach before picking up your baby.
- Use outlet protectors in your home to prevent accidental electrical burns, especially when your baby begins crawling and walking.

- Don't let your baby crawl in the kitchen when someone is using the stove.
- Turn the handles of pots and pans toward the back of the stove.
- Be particularly careful when using your gas or charcoal grill. Place one adult in charge of grilling and another in charge of your infant.
- Keep your hot water heater set below 120 degrees Fahrenheit (49 degrees Centigrade).
- Use fire-retardant clothing and blankets.
- Use a microwave oven to heat baby bottles only if recommended precautions are carefully followed. (See page 492 for recommendations for heating baby bottles.)
- Do not leave an iron or curling iron within your baby's reach.
- Keep your baby away from areas where inexperienced people are using fireworks, opting rather for safely conducted firework displays.

If your baby is burned, follow these steps immediately:

- Quickly immerse the burn in cold water to cool the area and stop the burning while relieving pain. Do not use ice on burns. Gently remove or cut away any clothing near the burn.
- If the injured area is not oozing, cover it loosely with a sterile gauze pad. If it is oozing, cover with a sterile pad or leave open and seek immediate medical attention. (Do not apply butter to a burn, because it can worsen the injury.)
- Give acetaminophen to relieve swelling or pain (refer to dosage chart on page 610).

Choking and Swallowed Objects

How to recognize it. Most of the time when something blocks your baby's throat, he or she will instinctively cough, gasp or gag until the object clears his or her windpipe. Usually children will clear their airways unassisted and you don't need to interfere. But if your baby cannot make sounds, stops breathing and turns blue, you must act quickly.

What causes it? Any time your baby inhales anything other than air, he or she will choke. Babies most commonly choke on toys with small parts or foods that "go down the wrong way." Avoid giving your baby peanuts, popcorn, hot dogs and any small food that may obstruct baby's breathing. Coins are also commonly swallowed and can obstruct baby's airway.

How serious is it? When your baby's airway is blocked and he or she is unable to clear it, choking is life-threatening. You must deal with it immediately. If you have difficulty clearing the airway, ask someone to call for emergency help. The longer your baby is deprived of oxygen, the greater the risk of permanent brain damage or death.

What can you do? If your child is coughing, let him or her cough until the windpipe is clear. If you can see something that is blocking the throat, sweep your finger through the baby's mouth to remove the obstruction. But if nothing is visible, do not stick your fingers in his or her throat, because you may only cause the object to become more deeply lodged.

If your baby is choking and not making any noise, you must act rapidly. Call or have someone else call 911. Place your baby on your forearm, face down with the head lower than the trunk. Support his or her neck and head by firmly holding the jaw and turning the head to the side; use your body for additional support. If your infant is too large, lay him or her facedown on your lap, head lower than the rest of the body. Give up to five rapid blows between the baby's shoulders with the heel of your hand.

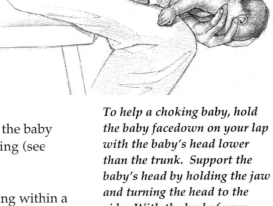

If your baby is still not breathing, carefully turn him or her over (supporting the baby's back and head with your free hand), stomach up, and hold the baby across your thigh, head to one side and lower than the trunk. Use two fingers to give five rapid downward chest thrusts on the breastbone, about one finger's breadth below the nipple line. If baby still isn't breathing, repeat these steps. As soon as the obstruction is relieved, either the baby will breathe spontaneously or you will need to begin rescue breathing (see CPR, below).

To help a choking baby, hold the baby facedown on your lap with the baby's head lower than the trunk. Support the baby's head by holding the jaw and turning the head to the side. With the heel of your other hand, give up to five forceful back blows between the baby's shoulders.

When to call the doctor's office. If your baby resumes breathing within a minute or two, he or she will probably not suffer any long-term ill effects. If, after your child is breathing again, he or she continues coughing or choking, it may mean that something is still blocking the airway, and you should go immediately to your nearest emergency facility.

CPR (Cardiopulmonary Resuscitation)

It's a good idea for all parents, or for anyone who provides child care, to take a certified course in infant cardiopulmonary resuscitation (CPR). This is especially important if you own a swimming pool or live near water. Contact your local American Red Cross or American Heart Association chapter to sign up for a course.

How to recognize the need for CPR. You may need to give your baby CPR if he or she:

- Has no pulse or heartbeat
- Has blue lips or skin or difficulty breathing or stops breathing entirely
- Is unresponsive

If your baby's heart stops beating or if he or she stops breathing, you may be able to save your baby's life with CPR. Chances for saving your baby's life or avoiding permanent injury increase dramatically the sooner you start CPR.

What can you do? If someone is with you, have them immediately call 911 for help. Make sure they know your address. Follow these steps, and continue until help arrives:

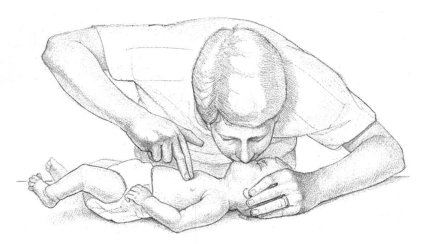

To perform CPR on a baby, cover the mouth and nose with your mouth. Give one breath for every five chest compressions. Compress the chest ½ to 1 inch at least 100 times a minute, using only two fingers.

1. Check to see if your baby is conscious, nudging or speaking loudly to awaken him or her. Place your ear next to his or her mouth and nose to find out whether he or she is breathing. If you don't find any sign of breathing, check to see if his or her chest is rising or falling. Do not vigorously shake your baby—it could cause further injury.

2. If your baby is not breathing, place him or her on the back on a flat, hard surface. If you suspect a neck injury, move your baby extremely carefully to avoid bending the neck. To open the airway, tilt the baby's head back until the nose is in the air. This position may enable the baby to breathe unassisted. If not, look and feel in the mouth and throat for blockage by a foreign object.

3. If your baby is still not breathing and is not choking, begin mouth-to-mouth resuscitation. Take a deep breath and place your mouth over the baby's nose and mouth, making a tight seal. If you can't cover both the nose and mouth with your mouth, pinch the nose shut and cover the baby's mouth with yours. Give two breaths of air into the baby's mouth and watch for his or her chest to rise. When it does, remove your mouth and allow air to escape. Take another deep breath and breathe into your baby's mouth again every three seconds, until he or she breathes independently.

4. After the first two breaths, check for your baby's pulse (by gently feeling inside the arm at the elbow or the artery in the neck below the ear and jawbone). If you don't detect a pulse, assume the heart has stopped and begin chest compressions: Place two fingers on the breastbone just below the nipple line. Press down about 1 inch, at a rate of 100 times per minute. (Use the heel of your hand on the lower third of the breastbone in an older child, pressing slightly deeper, 80 to 100 times per minute.)

5. Give your baby a breath after every five compressions, and continue until your baby's pulse and breathing have returned or until emergency help arrives.

Injury From a Fall

How to recognize it. Fractures are the fourth most common injury in preschool-aged children. If your baby falls and you suspect that he or she has a head injury or a broken bone, observe him or her carefully for:

- Disorientation
- More than one or two episodes of vomiting
- Unusual sleepiness or difficulty awakening
- The absence of movement abilities your baby previously had, such as inability to crawl or walk if he or she was able to do this before the injury
- Blood or watery fluid discharge from the ears or nose
- A seizure after the injury
- Pupils that are unequal in size

What causes it? Infants fall for many reasons. Falls tend to occur when your baby begins to be able to roll or tip an infant seat or walker more easily than a caretaker realizes.

How serious is it? If your baby cries immediately after receiving an impact to his or her head and remains alert, chances are the fall did not cause serious injury. Falls can be serious, but babies' soft bones don't fracture as easily as those of older children. Important factors that can affect the seriousness of a fall are the force and distance of the fall and the surface onto which your baby has fallen.

What can you do? Use ice to control swelling, but be careful not to freeze the baby's skin. Observe your baby carefully for 24 hours after a head injury for any behavior changes.

If the injured body part looks abnormal or if your baby cannot move it, use a stiff material (a piece of wood or even a rolled-up newspaper) to make a splint. Use tape or cloth to hold the wounded limb (including joints above and below the injury, if possible) on the splint so that it can't move.

When to call the doctor. Call the doctor or the paramedics if you suspect that a bone may be broken or if your baby shows any of the following signs of a head injury, which is more serious:

- A seizure
- Breathing irregularity
- Persistent irritability, possibly indicating a severe headache
- Pupils that are unequal in size
- Vomiting more than once or twice
- Excessive sleepiness or lethargy
- Loss of consciousness

Move your baby as little as possible after a head or neck injury. If the baby stops breathing or if you cannot detect a heartbeat, begin CPR immediately (see page 649).

Swallowed Poison

Almost any non-food substance is poisonous if taken in large doses. Babies explore by putting things in their mouths. Each year, poison control centers around the country talk with parents of about half a million children younger than 6 years who swallow or come into contact with poisons. Toxicity of substances varies greatly, and with immediate treatment most children are not permanently harmed from poisons they swallow.

Always keep the number of your nearest poison control center (usually listed inside the front cover of the telephone directory or always available from the operator) and emergency department nearby; be sure to tell anyone who takes care of your baby where the number is.

Some common items you keep around your house can be quite dangerous to an infant: iron supplements, found in many prenatal or children's vitamins, acetaminophen, aspirin, antidepressant medications, automatic dishwasher detergents, hydrocarbons (such as furniture polish, turpentine, gasoline), pesticides, alcohol, mouthwashes that contain alcohol, antifreeze and cleaning substances that contain lye.

Cosmetics, personal care products, cleaning substances and plants are the cause in about a third of the cases reported, but the ones that most commonly cause fatalities are artificial nail remover, ethanol-containing mouthwashes and strongly acid or alkaline products (such as swimming pool chemicals). Except for oven and drain cleaners, most household cleaners cause only mild gastrointestinal disturbances.

How to recognize it. Suspect poisoning if you find your infant with an open or empty container of a toxic substance. Look for behavior differences, burns or redness of the lips, mouth or hands, unexplained vomiting, breath that smells like chemicals, breathing difficulties or convulsions. Before you do anything else, if you suspect that your infant has swallowed a poison, remove your baby from the source of the poison and call your local poison control center immediately. Be prepared to read the labels on the poison container, and to describe the substance and amount ingested and any physical changes you detect.

How serious is it? Substances vary widely in the seriousness of their effects and the amount required to do harm. Remember, though, that a small amount of a poison can be much more damaging to an infant than it would be to an adult. If you have any questions about whether a substance may be toxic, call your poison control center for advice.

What can you do? Prevention is critical. Avoid buying toxic substances, especially in large quantities. Keep all toxic substances (including vitamins) locked and out of the reach of children. Be especially cautious when visiting grandparents or "non-childproof" houses. Be sure that all substances are in their proper, child-resistant containers and clearly labeled. Be sure to check the label on medicine bottles each time you give a medication to confirm that it is the proper medicine and that you're giving the proper dosage (especially in the middle of the night). Do not leave toxic plants within the baby's reach. Know the names of your houseplants and label the pots, so that someone caring for your child will know, also. Your poison control center staff will want to know which part of a plant your baby has eaten, because treatment may vary according to the part of the plant eaten. Some or all parts of the following plants are poisonous:

From your flower garden	Wild plants
Bleeding heart	Bittersweet
Chrysanthemum	Bloodroot
Clematis	Buttercup
Daffodil	Jack-in-the-pulpit
Hyacinth	Mayapple
Iris	Milkweed
Lily	Mushrooms (some but not all)
Pansy	Nightshade
Poppy	Poison ivy
Tulip	

Houseplants

Bird of paradise

Castor bean

Cyclamen

Dieffenbachia

Ivy

Mistletoe

Mother-in-law's tongue

Oleander

Philodendron

Poinsettia

Trees and shrubs

Arborvitae

Azalea

Elderberry

Hydrangea

Oak

Peony

From your vegetable garden

Potato sprouts and greens

Rhubarb leaves

Tomato plant greens

Remove any remainder of the substance still in your baby's mouth. Do not give anything by mouth until you've received advice from the poison control center. Depending on several factors, the medical staff might or might not want your baby to vomit.

Keep a 1 ounce bottle of syrup of ipecac on hand for each child in your home; be sure to check expiration dates periodically. This liquid is used to induce vomiting, when recommended. Always let your poison control center or emergency personnel advise you before you use syrup of ipecac, because using it can cause more damage in some instances.

When to call the doctor. Call your poison control center, the emergency department or your health care provider if you suspect that your child has swallowed a poison. If your child is in obvious distress (unconscious, hallucinating, convulsing, experiencing breathing difficulties), call 911 immediately. Have the container in front of you when you call, so that you can tell emergency personnel what substance caused the problem. If you need to go to the emergency department, if possible bring the product or container with you.

Inhaled Poison

How to recognize it. Inhaling poisonous substances can cause various reactions, including nausea and vomiting, loss of or decreased consciousness, headache, breathing difficulties, coughing or lethargy. Your baby's reaction will vary, depending on the amount of exposure and the substance inhaled.

What causes it? Numerous substances are toxic when inhaled. They include carbon monoxide, smoke and fumes from fires, propellants, gasoline, kerosene, turpentine, furniture polish, charcoal, cigarette lighter fluid, glue, paint remover and lamp oil.

How serious is it? It can be dangerous for your baby to inhale toxic substances. You need to act quickly when you suspect that your baby has inhaled a dangerous substance.

What can you do? It's not a good idea to use aerosol products near your baby, because babies can react much more severely to a small amount of inhaled poison. Never run your car in a closed garage, and be sure to maintain coal, wood or kerosene stoves regularly. If you smell a strong gas odor, turn off the gas burner or oven, leave your house immediately and call the gas company. Avoid breathing the fumes yourself, and get your baby to a well-ventilated area. Check your baby for breathing and pulse; if necessary, begin CPR.

When to call the doctor. **Call 911 immediately** if your baby is in obvious distress (having difficulty breathing, showing a decreased level of consciousness or lethargy, is without a heartbeat or is convulsing).

Poison on the Skin

How to recognize it. If you suspect that a poison has come into contact with your baby's skin, look nearby for some evidence of the poison. Spilled household cleaners would probably leave the baby's skin looking red and irritated.

What causes it? The chemicals in many household cleaning substances, especially oven and drain cleaners, are caustic and can easily damage your baby's skin.

What can you do? Keep all cleaning solutions in a childproof cabinet out of the baby's (or siblings') reach. To confirm a method of treatment, check with your local poison control center if your baby comes into contact with a poison.

When to call the doctor. If your baby is experiencing obvious distress (unconsciousness, lethargy, hallucinations, convulsions or breathing difficulties), **call 911 immediately**.

Poison in the Eye

What causes it? Most commonly, poisons get in a baby's eye when a liquid splashes into it. Many substances can damage your baby's eyes, but your infant will not be able to tell you about the problem. Therefore, it's important that you be alert to possible situations in which this can happen.

How serious is it? Some substances can damage your baby's eye and limit his or her eyesight. Potency and length of exposure may determine the severity. Acting quickly may make the difference between a temporary problem and a long-term disability.

What can you do? Use a large glass or pitcher filled with cool tap water to flood your baby's eye for 10 to 20 minutes. Try to get your baby to blink frequently as you flood the area. Keep the baby's hands out of his or her eyes. You may need to wrap him or her with a bed sheet to keep his or her hands out of the affected eye. Get another adult to help you, if possible.

When to call the doctor. Call your local poison control center if you suspect that your baby has gotten a poisonous substance in his or her eyes.

Animal or Human Bites

H*ow to recognize it.* You can recognize most animal or human bites from the circumstances of the injury and your baby's broken and bleeding skin. If your baby is bitten, try to discover the source of the bite as quickly as you can. Household pets are the cause of most animal bites. Although pet dogs are more likely to bite than cats, cat bites are more likely to become infected. Bites from wild animals are dangerous because of the possibility of rabies. Most human bites that children get are only bruises and not dangerous. Human bites can, however, be quite dangerous if they break the skin, because infections can develop from the bacteria in the human mouth.

What causes it? Although you may assume that most animal bites come from strange or wild animals, this is not the case. Most bites that infants receive come from animals the child knows, including your family's pet. Wild animals or unvaccinated domestic pets may also infect your child with rabies, a potentially life-threatening viral infection.

How serious is it? Cases of rabies are not common today, but an animal bite can cause serious wounds (especially to the face) as well as considerable emotional trauma. You should consider any animal or human bite that breaks the skin to be a serious injury.

What can you do? It's important that you know as much as possible about the health of any animal that bites your baby. If you can, without endangering yourself, capture and confine the animal for testing, but do not destroy it. If you cannot safely capture the animal yourself, immediately call the animal control office or police in your local area for assistance.

If an animal or human bite does not break the skin, treat it as a minor wound. Wash the area thoroughly with soap and water and observe it for redness or swelling during the next few days.

For deep punctures or badly torn skin from animal bites, for bites from animals that may not have a current rabies immunization or for any human bite that breaks the skin:

- Apply firm pressure to the area to stop the bleeding
- Clean the wound with soap and water
- Go to your doctor or emergency department

When to call the doctor. It's a good idea to notify your doctor if an animal or person has broken your baby's skin with a bite. Also notify the doctor if you see any signs of infection: pus draining from the wound, increasing redness and swelling several days after the bite or red streaks coming from the wound.

Drowning

W*hat causes it?* Drowning occurs when babies are either in water that is too deep or when they are trapped with their faces submerged in water. Infants can drown in very shallow water. Never leave your baby alone in the bathtub, even briefly. If a phone call, doorbell or something else interrupts your baby's bath, either ignore the interruption or bring the baby with you, wrapped in a towel. Keep the toilet lid and bathroom door closed. Fence swimming pools with automatic latching gates, and constantly supervise your infant when near lakes, pools or rivers. Toddlers have even drowned after falling into buckets used for cleaning.

What can you do? If your baby has no pulse or is not breathing, begin CPR immediately (see page 649). Have someone call 911. Continue CPR until medical help arrives.

When to call the doctor. If your baby has been submerged in water long enough to cause any difficulty breathing (or has stopped breathing), any blueness of the skin or decreased level of consciousness (including unconsciousness), you should call 911 immediately.

Electrical Shock

How to recognize it. An electrical shock may cause your baby to stop breathing and may stop the heart's beating. Internal organ damage may not be obvious, but it may be caused by a significant shock. A less severe shock may burn your baby's mouth or skin.

What causes it? The most common ways that infants receive electrical shocks are by biting into electrical cords or by poking metal objects or their fingers into unprotected outlets. Holiday decorations provide another source of possible injury, when electrical cords and light bulbs are often within the baby's reach.

How serious is it? Depending on the voltage and length of the contact with electrical current, electrical shocks range from mildly uncomfortable to causing serious injury or death.

What can you do? If you see that your child is in contact with electricity, attempt first to disconnect the source. If you cannot disconnect the source, attempt to move your child away from the electricity. Do not touch or attempt to pull your child away with your bare hands. Do not attempt to handle a live wire with your bare hands; use an object made of plastic or wood that won't conduct electricity, such as a broom or wooden baseball bat.

As soon as your baby is removed from the source of electricity, check the breathing and heart rate. If either is stopped or erratic or if your child is unconscious, begin CPR and call or have someone else call 911. If your baby is conscious, look for evidence of burns and notify your physician.

Prevent accidental electrical shocks by using safety plugs in all electrical outlets. Also avoid stringing long extension cords where the baby can reach them.

When to call the doctor. Call for emergency care if there is any indication of breathing or heart irregularities or if your child is unconscious. If the shock was less severe, notify your physician, who will want to check for internal injuries and treat any skin burns your baby may have.

Part Four

From Partners to Parents:

A Family Is Born

CHAPTER THIRTY-SEVEN

Motherhood

Pregnancy is a psychological journey as well as a biological one. You're still the daughter of your parents, yet soon you will be the mother of your own child. You'll have a new role to play and a new identity. If you're wondering how you'll handle one of life's biggest responsibilities, relax. It takes time and effort, but you'll learn. How you feel about your new identity is important. It helps shape your interest and values as well as your relationship with your partner.

Becoming a mother is a process. It doesn't happen overnight. And along with the joy, excitement and fulfillment motherhood brings, don't be surprised to experience doubts and uncertainties in your new role. As your doubts diminish, and your confidence grows, you'll experience what may be one of life's most profound and rewarding challenges—raising a child.

Adding the role of mother, however, can take time away from other roles and relationships. Typically, your role as partner and lover gets squeezed first. As you spend time caring for and getting to know your baby, your relationship with your partner can change (see page 683). You'll have less time to spend together, and the fatigue that often accompanies being a new mother may leave you feeling irritable. In addition, your identity from your work may also go through changes.

Milestones of Motherhood

Mothers-to-be and new mothers commonly experience four stages of motherhood: anticipation, becoming a mother, building confidence and taking charge.

The anticipatory stage is described as the time of collecting information about the role of mothering. It begins in pregnancy but has its foundations earlier in life: in the parenting you received as a child, in how you were supported while growing up and in the families you've observed along the way.

The memories of how you were parented, along with your personal ideals of parenting, serve as a bank of images to draw on as you develop your own parenting style. If you're a first-time mother, you might idealize an image of the baby you're expecting: cherubic, smooth of skin, cooing, smiling and attentive.

There's one small hitch. The adorable newborn in your mind's eye is likely to be 3 months old. Your newborn is more likely to be crying and to have

Anticipation

swollen eyes and a head misshapen by passage through the birth canal. But don't worry. Your baby will, in due time, grow into the cherubic, cooing baby of your dreams.

Becoming a Mother

The second stage, becoming a mother, begins when you encounter the real-life challenges of dressing, holding, feeding, bathing and performing the many other routines of child care.

This is a stage of rapid learning. You may feel unusually sensitive and emotionally vulnerable. You may be confused, especially from the oft-conflicting advice offered by friends, family and even the child care "experts." You just want to know the "best" way to care for your child so you can be a good mother. Unfortunately, there is no "best" way.

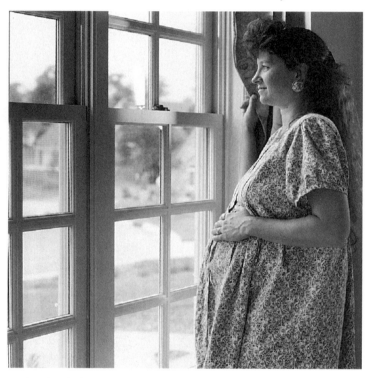

"What kind of a mom will I be?" "Will Jenny play basketball?" "Will Alex be an organist, like his dad?" "How will the baby affect my relationship with Mike?" You'll find time for thoughtful reflection in those busy, final weeks of pregnancy.

You may painstakingly follow the example of nurses and instructions from your doctor. And if your mother, mother-in-law or another experienced adult is on hand, you may feel as though you're constantly being evaluated on your mothering skills.

This phase of motherhood is rarely discussed. It can be awkward to talk about, and new mothers are often isolated from each other during the first weeks after childbirth. You may come to believe that you're the only new mother who feels unsure of herself. You may even convince yourself that you can't care for your baby alone. Such sensitivity, of course, is simply proof of your desire to be the best mom you can be.

During this stage, you'll need and appreciate physical and moral support. Having an experienced relative or friend available after you come home from the hospital can provide that support, but there are potential drawbacks. For example, your helper's competence may heighten your feelings of inadequacy and perhaps even make it more difficult for you to feel comfortable mothering your baby. So, when asking for help, even from your partner or your own mother, be specific about what you want. Try not to draw conclusions about your own mothering skills by comparison. And remember to support your partner in assuming his parental role.

Your baby can also help build your confidence as a new mother. As you respond to his or her needs, you receive in return a response—a contented gaze, a grasp of your finger or a fleeting smile. Spending time alone with your baby away from distractions, such as the time set aside for feeding, can be ideal in fostering this relationship.

Building Confidence

As you gain mothering experience, you'll begin to master the tasks of baby care. This will, in turn, increase your self-confidence. You may even begin to relax rigid baby-care rules and instructions as you become more comfortable handling your baby.

It's during this time of increased confidence and relaxation with your new role that you're entering the third stage of motherhood.

Now you're more flexible. Rather than reliance on older, experienced role models, such as your mother, you may begin to pick up and use strategies from other new mothers. You're still in need of praise and reassurance, but you're more willing to take independent action.

At this point you may find it helpful to meet with other mothers, to exchange information and share experiences. You might even find yourself searching out books and other written materials and asking your doctor or nurse for more information on baby care, such as feeding or developmental milestones.

I n the taking-charge stage, you're finally comfortable as a mother. You've developed a parenting style suited to your own personality. You've abandoned the quest to be a perfect mother, and you're more realistic about your baby's needs and your abilities to meet them. Your attitudes are uniquely yours, and you carry your new responsibility with grace and ease. In a sense, you've "graduated." You're an experienced mother!

Taking Charge

Getting to Know Your Baby During Pregnancy

The process of becoming emotionally attached to your baby usually begins early in pregnancy. But it really takes off in the second trimester, often after you've seen an ultrasound image or felt your baby's first kicks (quickening).

These stirrings not only are a great source of amusement and relief but also signify that your baby is a perceptibly separate, unique individual. You can begin to imagine what your baby will be like.

Women who undergo an ultrasound examination during early pregnancy often treasure the experience. Seeing a first glimpse of the baby is powerful, similar to the thrill of first feeling the baby move.

Ultrasound scanning also provides fathers with a more direct means of experiencing the pregnancy. Invite your partner to accompany you for an ultrasound exam. This tangible image can strengthen his emotional involvement in your pregnancy and foster his attachment to the baby.

"Inner bonding"

Do intentional efforts to communicate with your unborn child strengthen the mother-infant bond? Very little is known about the consciousness, perceptual abilities and channels of communication open to an unborn child. Whether your infant can be affected by your thoughts and emotions—a process that's called "inner bonding"— is unknown. Whether you can communicate with, and positively influence, your unborn baby is difficult to determine. Only recently have the abilities of the fetus begun to be studied.

Your baby can hear your heartbeat while in your uterus. Does your heartbeat influence later behavior? Newborn babies sometimes seem calmed or soothed when held in a position snuggled over mom's chest. Try this technique. It may quiet your baby enough to focus on you.

It can't hurt to play soft music or talk soothingly and lovingly to your unborn baby. Besides, it may make you feel good. Perhaps efforts to communicate are important because they encourage your attachment to your unborn baby. Developing a sensitivity to your baby, and being attuned to his or her needs, is an important part of becoming a parent.

Dreams and Imaginings

The more information and detail you and your partner have about your unborn child, the better you can "picture" him or her. For example, your baby's pattern of kicking may set you off on endless speculation about his or her personality and character, already helping you become sensitive to the cues and signals of your baby.

Pregnancy is a time rich in fantasies. Much of the nine months is given over to wondering what this new person will be like.

These imaginings are not simply idle, time-wasting exercise. They are the beginnings of your emotional investment with your baby.

Anxieties and Nightmares

The natural counterparts to hopes and dreams are the disturbing, anxiety-provoking nightmares that women sometimes experience during pregnancy.

Dreams that arouse anxiety may stimulate you to reappraise your lifestyle and to rethink plans and decisions in getting ready for your new baby. Some women may have heard that negative feelings during pregnancy may harm their unborn child. But occasional negative feelings are normal, unavoidable and even beneficial if they raise caring concerns.

Your Emotional Needs at Childbirth

Childbirth is an incredibly memorable event. You may find yourself recalling details of your labor and delivery experience for years to come.

Your childbirth experience can affect your feelings as a woman and a mother. For example, an uneventful delivery can boost your self-esteem and instill confidence in your role as a mother. But an unexpected problem during childbirth can undermine your outlook and may even delay your acceptance of the maternal role. Even though these negative thoughts and self-doubts are unwarranted, it's important to know that these feelings are normal and that they may need to be worked through.

After your baby is born, it's common to experience shifts in energy and swings in your moods. Regardless of whether your labor was long or short, or difficult or easy, your physical and mental energy levels are affected by it. Your changing hormone levels also play into your mood and energy swings.

For the first two or three days after birth, you may find yourself telling and retelling the story of your labor and delivery. You have every reason to be proud of your achievement. The recounting of the birth events is a necessary mental task and is a way to make the experience your own. It also provides the opportunity to elicit important reassurance that you did a good job. How you perceive the birth experience is a powerful factor in your development of maternal confidence and in taking on the mothering role.

Variations in New Mothering Experiences

It may take three to nine months or more after childbirth to feel completely comfortable in your role as mother. Factors that can influence this process are discussed here.

A baby who is not easy to satisfy, who is colicky or who is just temperamentally difficult can undermine a new mother's confidence. She may question her mothering skills rather than viewing the behavior as evidence of her baby's needs. If your baby is difficult to mother, focus on his or her needs, have confidence that you're doing your best to meet them and understand that time will likely bring improvement.

Infant Crying

The early stages of adapting to motherhood can be trying, even for the healthiest of women. So if you are recovering from a cesarean birth or become ill during those first weeks after childbirth, allow yourself extra time in assuming your new role as mother.

Maternal Illness

The most intensive period in adapting to motherhood begins when you start to physically care for your baby. But what if your baby is still in the hospital because of prematurity or illness?

Most hospitals recognize the importance of providing opportunities for maternal contact when infants must be separated from their mothers for special health care. Together with the staff of the special care unit, you can work out a plan to stay in close contact with your baby.

Infant Illness and Early Mother-Infant Separation

Spend time with your newborn

Hospital practices have changed from the days when mothers, fathers and babies were kept apart during much of labor, delivery and the hospital stay. Now you can start getting to know your baby as soon as he or she is born.

Getting acquainted. Soon after delivery it may be possible to have your baby placed on your bare abdomen or chest to allow for maximal skin-to-skin and eye contact. This quiet period of rapt attention can be intimate and memorable. During the first hour after birth, many babies are quietly alert, an ideal state for the first meeting with their parents.

Rooming-in. Most hospitals offer the option of rooming-in, an arrangement that allows your baby to stay primarily in your room instead of the nursery. The option of sending your baby back to the nursery is available if, for example, you have company or need extra sleep.

Rooming-in can help you get acquainted with your baby and begin to understand his or her unique cues. It also may help nurture your sense of adequacy and confidence as a new mother. Mothers who perceive themselves as confident in their parenting role may find that, in turn, their babies are easier to care for.

Social Stress

Just as the emotional support of others can boost confidence, added stress can diminish it. Dealing with financial problems, a move, an illness or a death in the family can be exhausting and divert attention away from the demands of your new role. A support system of friends and family is an important resource in coping with additional stresses.

Marital Difficulties

Ideally, at childbirth, new parents support each other in taking on their new roles. However, relationship problems can keep a couple from providing this mutual support. In turn, confidence in assuming parenting roles can be diminished. For the sake of your relationship with your partner, and how it affects the baby, be sure to address any marital problems, perhaps seeking professional help.

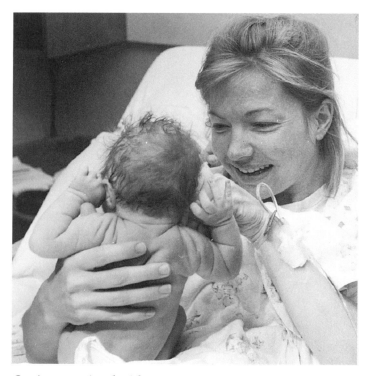

Getting acquainted with a minutes-old newborn is a remarkable experience. Rooming-in offers additional opportunities for acquaintance and bonding, and it nurtures your confidence as a new mother.

Mother-Infant Attachment

The responsibility of taking care of a new baby is awesome. Unable to walk, talk or make sense of a confusing new world, infants are totally dependent on their parents to meet all their physical and emotional needs.

Although the emotional attachment you feel toward your newborn may not be instantaneous, it probably won't be long before you "fall in love." This attachment is not only valuable for your infant but also important for you. It's what motivates you to care for your baby, even when you're exhausted and your baby finds 3 a.m. the perfect time to cry and you haven't a clue what he or she wants. It's also what enables you to make the sacrifices needed to meet the demands of this totally dependent person.

Bonding at Birth and Beyond

The relationship that begins to form at birth between a mother and her baby is unique. Ideally, a mother and her newborn learn to synchronize their behaviors, each learning to respond to the other in satisfying ways, enriching the relationship.

Each baby you may have, of course, will be different in temperament and personality. Consequently, your relationship with each will be different.

There is no special set of instructions to teach you how to form this unique bond between mother and baby. And it takes time for the relationship to grow. Factors that might encourage this process are outlined here.

It's common for parents to underestimate, or overestimate, their baby's abilities. Because some parents are unaware of a newborn's true capabilities, they may not understand all the ways they can interact with them. Newborns come equipped with an array of social skills. They are well prepared to form a relationship with their parents. They can see at close range, preferring the human face to other objects, and can follow a moving object with their eyes. Babies may even imitate facial gestures, such as sticking out their tongue. They prefer the sound of the human voice, especially the higher pitch of the female voice, and they respond to touch.

A good way to learn about your infant's special abilities is to request that your caregiver perform a newborn exam when you and your partner are present. This is a good time for you to be introduced to your baby's unique characteristics and capabilities.

Understanding Your Baby's Abilities

Touch is one of the most important channels of communication for a baby. It is sometimes called a baby's first language.

Skin-to-skin contact is soothing for both mother and baby, and it can enhance the pleasure of mother-infant interactions. Touch can calm a baby, helping conserve his or her energy expenditure and promoting growth and development. It is known that babies who are never cuddled and touched do not grow adequately.

Skin-to-Skin Contact

Looking into your baby's eyes is a powerful means of communication. It is natural and often automatic to move to align your eyes with the gaze of your baby. When the day comes that eye contact prompts your baby's first smile, it is a powerfully emotional experience.

Eye-to-Eye Contact

Parents often imitate the sounds of their babies—such as cooing. A baby's first vocalizations not only are the beginning efforts at communication but also contain the essence of social exchange—listening and responsiveness.

Vocalizing

There is no single behavior, including breastfeeding, that establishes the mother-infant bond. But breastfeeding, through skin-to-skin contact, eye contact and sensations pleasurable to both mother and baby, embodies the profound interrelationship between mother and newborn.

Breastfeeding

Mothers who have the support and encouragement of others during pregnancy, labor and after the birth develop more confidence in parenting and display more affection toward their babies. The support of a partner and others also enables mothers to derive more satisfaction from infant care and to remain responsive to their infants. This is especially important for parents of premature babies and those with special needs that may minimize an infant's ability to respond.

A strong tie between mother and baby has enduring value. It is the setting in which earliest learning takes place and fosters security and the origins of positive self-esteem. In addition, it is an infant's earliest model for intimate relationships.

Support

The Fourth Trimester

The period from birth up to eight weeks after a baby is born is sometimes referred to as the "fourth trimester." It's a time when new mothers—who often experience an upheaval in lifestyle and sleeping patterns—need extra support. Because you may be too busy to establish a support network right after you give birth, it is wise to establish one before your baby is born. Below are listed some suggestions in setting up a support system.

Prime Your Partner

Advise your partner in advance how overwhelming motherhood can be during the first two months at home. Prepare him for the fact that his expectations about housework, meals and laundry—and the attention you give him—may have to be lowered temporarily.

At the same time, assure your partner that his emotional support and approval will be more important than ever after the baby arrives. Ask him to reassure you in your developing mothering skills and to help relieve you of household chores so you can focus on mothering your baby. Remember, however, that your partner is taking on an unfamiliar role too. He's becoming a father and needs reassurance from you regarding his new role.

Talk to Others

If you attend a childbirth education class during pregnancy, you might ask your instructor to put you in touch with an earlier participant who could provide advice and support. Your childbirth educator may also know of existing new-parent support groups in your community. If there are none, perhaps the instructor can help you establish one made up of families from your childbirth class.

Contact the La Leche League

If you plan to breastfeed, contacting the La Leche League can connect you with a national network of actively breastfeeding mothers who can offer new moms practical advice on a range of maternal concerns.

La Leche League members regularly hold small, informal group meetings, welcoming not only new mothers but also their babies. It's not unusual for a La Leche volunteer to come to the aid of a new mother experiencing a crisis of confidence. Your childbirth educator can help put you in contact with your local La Leche League. But try to make connections before your due date so that your relationship is in place when you need it.

Expect Some Criticism

No matter how conventional your parenting practices are, you should still prepare yourself for occasional disapproving comments from friends, relatives and even strangers. Child rearing practices seem to invite the comments of others. You'll receive unsolicited tips ranging from breastfeeding hints to whether you should let your baby sleep in your bed, and even advice about what kind of diapers you should use.

Parenting is a very subjective experience. Remember, there are many ways of doing things the "right" way. What is most important is raising your child in a safe, loving atmosphere.

You and Your Partner

Caring for your newborn can command nearly all of your attention and energy. Consequently there is a risk that the important adults in your life—parents, family, friends and especially your partner—may feel left out. Try not to let this happen. Discuss your new role with your partner, friends and relatives, helping them to understand the shifts in your responsibilities. And be sure to let them know how important their support is during this time.

As your baby's behavior becomes more predictable and you gain confidence as a mother, your preoccupation with your baby will diminish, and you'll be able to resume a more normal lifestyle. But for now, you'll need support in various forms, including the following:

Emotional support
- Expressions of love, caring, concern and trust
- Reassurances about your parenting capabilities
- An atmosphere of understanding
- Listening and encouragement
- Companionship

Material support
- Help with household chores, especially providing and preparing meals, cleaning and laundry
- Help with baby care, especially in the days immediately after your baby is born

Informational support
- Sharing of experiences and information
- Help in getting answers to questions you may have

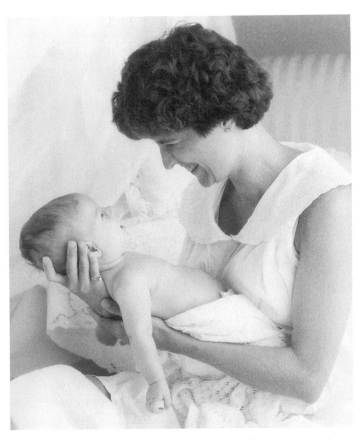

It's a beautiful moment when your eyes meet your baby's, and your baby returns your smile—for the very first time.

Mothers-To-Be and Their Mothers

Pregnancy is always a journey into the future. It can also be a journey into the past. As you become a mother, your relationship with your parents, especially your own mother, can undergo a major change.

Pregnancy can reorder the mother-daughter relationship. Mothers and daughters often begin relating to each other as adults, and daughters begin to gain the sense that they're on an equal footing with their moms.

This is a natural and perhaps unprecedented opportunity for mending unresolved emotional conflicts you may have about the parenting you received. Restoring a relationship with your mother can have a very practical payoff; it clears the way for improved nurturing during a time of need. Perhaps never in your adult life will you feel the need for support so intensely as when you become a new mother.

One way to mend fences is to focus on the present and future of a relationship without dwelling on the past. There may be no better way to start than by asking your mother a simple, nonjudgmental question: "What were your pregnancy and the birth like when you had me?"

Daughters often long for help from their mothers in assuming the mother role, but the help must be carefully given. During pregnancy, daughters need emotional support, confidence building, cheering up and an exchange of information about pregnancy. A periodic phone call from mom can be a real boost.

After the baby is born, new mothers often prefer in-person help from their mothers. It needs to be given without control or smothering and at the request of the new mother. Coping with unwanted help and advice can add to a new mother's stress.

In accepting help, it is wise to establish boundaries. Graciously specify the kind of help you'll need and discuss what you may want to do yourself. Try to communicate your wishes in advance, because after your baby arrives you may be too tired and confused to know what you want. The following are examples of concrete ways of asking for specific help:

- "I think I would like to be alone with my baby during feedings. I would be grateful if you could answer the telephone at that time. Perhaps you can also help keep the house in order and help get dinner on the table."

- "What I really need is for you to be on hand to provide guidance and advice for those times when I feel I need it. But please don't be surprised or disappointed if I don't accept every suggestion."

- "I plan to breastfeed the baby. And your son-in-law wants to be involved in caring for the baby as much as possible."

- "Even if I don't ask you a single question, your presence will be a great comfort to me. I know this will not be a vacation for you, but perhaps when the baby is a few months old we can return the favor by house-sitting for you and Dad when you take some well-earned time off."

CHAPTER THIRTY-EIGHT

Becoming a Father

Tom had kept his worries to himself about accompanying Michelle into the birthing room. They had prepared for this moment for months. There were classes and books, a visit to the hospital and many discussions. Still, Tom's not sure he's ready for fatherhood. It's such a big step. He's been especially worried about how things will go in the birthing room.

Now he's there, and somehow Tom's not as nervous as he thought he'd be. He supports Michelle as she sits up to push, rest and push some more—again and again. This is a lot of work!

Now come the final urgent pushes, and then the incredible sight of their daughter being born. "Heather's here," shouts his wife. They hug, both in tears.

Months later he confides, "It was the most amazing moment of my life."

The days when expectant dads did little more than wait passively in the hospital hallway are history. Today, fathers-to-be are frequent companions and participants in birthing rooms and labor and delivery rooms of health care facilities throughout the United States. This change has encouraged fathers to be more involved with their partners and their children. The expanded involvement in family planning, pregnancy, the birth process, child care and the life of the family can bring a sense of fulfillment and satisfaction that many fathers of times past didn't experience.

Dads of the '90s might talk about investing in their children instead of the stock market or their careers. That's not to say that work and finances are unimportant to today's fathers. It's simply to acknowledge change.

If fatherhood is in your future, or if you've become a new father, this chapter's for you. Some of the challenges you may face will be discussed, and you'll be prepared for a journey on which you'll discover the richness of parenthood.

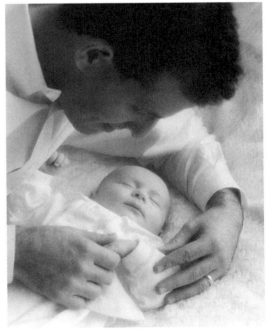

Few things in life can compare with the pride, wonderment and joy you may experience as you get to know your new son or daughter.

669

Roles Are Changing

Just a few decades ago, fathers were not expected to play much of a role in family life. Dads were viewed as "breadwinners." That meant long hours at work, which was the man's first priority. Family affairs were often of secondary importance.

Moms were usually "homemakers." Mom's job included the main, sometimes sole, responsibility of raising the children. Dad could help if he had time. Today, this breadwinner/homemaker model is the exception. Increasingly, men and women are sharing these responsibilities. Men are more involved with their families partly because women are more involved with their careers. Women need, expect and demand more help at home.

Moms and dads are taking a new look at how best to use the limited time they have to spend with their children. As a result, the role of father is shifting. Men are learning to be nurturers and child-rearing partners.

Some of today's new dads had fathers who found time to invest in their families despite work pressures. These new fathers may have an easier time adapting to society's new expectations for fathers.

However, other new fathers may have had dads who weren't around during the growing-up years, or who frankly weren't the best role models. These men may have to sort through their own conflicting feelings about fatherhood and perhaps have to deal with the disapproval of those whose values were shaped by earlier years, when roles and expectations were markedly different. Most fathers today want to be physically and emotionally involved, perhaps, in part, because their fathers may not have been.

The recent shift toward men's increased participation in family life has been rapid. For example, in the mid 1970s, about one in four expectant fathers attended the births of their children. Ten years later, 80 percent were there for labor and delivery.

Influences leading men to be more involved with their families are partly external. For example, as women spend more time in the workforce, dads need to be home more often to help. But there also seems to be an internal side to the forces that are moving dads toward increased participation in the lives of their children. The change appears to be rooted in shifting values.

Increasingly, dads just want to be there for their children—to take their daughters hiking, to teach their sons how to ride a bike. They want to listen to and laugh and run and dream with their kids. They tend to be more involved in the type of day-to-day activities that in earlier years were the exclusive domain of moms. Dads are shopping for clothes, for example, or providing supportive companionship and transportation for a trip to the dentist.

Emotional involvement with children and the ability to care for children come naturally to some men, but most learn on the job. This new father's comments are typical: "I had no idea what to do with the baby. I felt like I couldn't relate to this little bundle at all. I was afraid to hold her, to change her diapers. She was such a delicate thing. I was afraid I'd hurt her."

Fathers often master tasks relating to the physical needs of their children by watching their partners. Diapering and feeding, for example, are learned skills requiring observation and practice, but little more. Sensitivity, patience and an instinct for understanding a child's needs are abilities most dads can acquire, but time and effort are needed.

Dads Are Special

If there's one thing you need to understand as an expectant dad, it's this: You are important for the healthy development of your child. Fathers are important for the development of both sons and daughters. They contribute to the healthy self-esteem and motivation for independence needed during the growing-up years. Your performance as a father will affect your child physically, intellectually and socially for his or her lifetime. You are the best example of fatherhood that your children will know, for their future parenting. That's an inescapable reality. It's the reason nothing in life carries with it quite the responsibility, opportunity, hope and wonder as parenthood.

Dealing With Mixed Emotions

The emotional attachment that's a part of parenthood doesn't always happen instantly in the delivery room. The attachment more often develops gradually, usually beginning with a mix of positive and negative feelings.

On the one hand, you may be delighted with the prospect of parenthood. It means the continuation of your family lineage. It offers companionship and new possibilities. Perhaps your son or daughter will grow up to be a great singer or teacher. Maybe she or he will find a cure for cancer, or sign a political agreement that brings peace to the world. Like moms-to-be, expectant dads often have lofty aspirations for their offspring.

On the other hand, you may have doubts and concerns. You may doubt your ability to meet the financial challenges of fatherhood. You may wonder if this is the right time to bring an innocent child into a world with so many perplexing problems. You may fear the fact that a child will forever change your lifestyle, even though you're not precisely sure how it will change.

If your partner is pregnant and you're having second thoughts about what's ahead, your feelings are normal. Few first-time fathers feel fully prepared for what's ahead.

Later, perhaps on your child's first birthday, you may look back and admit that, for all the strain associated with pregnancy and the first hectic year, parenthood brings an incredible richness to daily living. The miracle of birth, the warmth of a newborn's smile and the wobbly first steps of a toddler are occasions you must experience as a parent to appreciate fully. You feel a connection with your family's past, its present and its future.

Pregnancy and Expectant Fathers

Pregnancy brings identity shifts. Never again will you and your partner see yourselves in quite the same light. Now you're responsible for the immediate and future welfare of a developing human being. Often, couples begin to evaluate their goals. Family finances may take on new importance. Religious and ethical values might come up for discussion. Up until this time you've had the luxury of a lifestyle centered on your personal needs and desires. Now, you're faced with the responsibility of establishing a home for a new person.

Establishing a home entails more than bricks and mortar. It's an all-encompassing assignment that includes meeting all the needs and a measure of the wants of your child for at least the next 20 years. Your daily actions and decisions will make a difference in your child's values, personality and even intellectual abilities. Your performance as a parent will affect his or her long-term success and happiness.

Separate Timetables

At the beginning, when you hear the news that you're to be parents, you and your partner may be only vaguely aware of your new responsibilities. It will be difficult to anticipate all the ways in which your thinking or actions may change as a result of this new phase of your lives. Still, the changes are certain to affect you both—but not necessarily at the same time.

For example, you may be hardly aware of impending fatherhood, the reality perhaps not sinking in until about the 24th week of pregnancy, when you place your hand on your partner's abdomen and feel your baby kicking inside. Your partner will probably begin to feel like a mother long before you start to feel like a father. Shortly after learning she's pregnant, your partner may undergo an identity change that is swift, dramatic and unsettling. Right away, she may show signs of emotional turmoil—moodiness, for example. Changes in hormones associated with pregnancy can have this effect. But she's also dealing firsthand with the responsibilities of carrying and delivering a child. This realization entails a complex mix of joy, wonder and fear. So expect sweeping shifts in her emotions. Neither you nor your partner will fully understand them.

Because men are often slower to embrace parenthood, misunderstandings and conflicts can arise between partners. For example, a woman may find that, once she's pregnant, her thoughts center on the baby. The needs of the baby and preparations for birth and the first year may in fact be uppermost in her mind most of her waking hours. Not so for many men, who may even need encouragement to attend a prenatal education class or to shop for a crib. As an expectant father, you may be viewed by your partner as uninterested in shopping for a crib or, worse, uninterested in your growing family.

Although inevitable and normal during pregnancy and the first year of parenthood, conflicts between partners sometimes can be avoided or minimized. Like many potentially divisive issues in a relationship, understanding and communication are keys to prevention. Both partners need to anticipate stress points and take steps to minimize or avoid them.

Plan to participate in labor and delivery. Be there when your child is born. Your partner will appreciate your support. This experience, like no other, will foster an earlier, strong emotional tie with your child and strengthen your relationship with your partner.

Feeling like a father

Love and commitment are emotions that are expected of good fathers. Yet these complex feelings need nurturing and time to grow.

You'll have to get to know this tiny person. After you've changed a few diapers and hummed and rocked your child to sleep a few times, you may sense a warmth of feeling you didn't notice in the delivery room. A single smile, the first unsteady steps and the first "da da" can work wonders.

New dads occasionally experience a sudden emotional attachment. This awakening sometimes is called the "fatherhood click." But it's not universal, and it certainly doesn't happen automatically at the moment of birth.

For many men, the fatherhood click doesn't occur until their babies are walking and talking. For others, there's never a sudden realization; the caring, affectionate emotions evolve as a result of interactions that occur naturally. Some fathers may even remain unaware of the depth of their feelings until a crisis occurs, such as an illness.

The point is this: If you're an expectant father with mixed emotions about your feelings toward the baby, don't expect too much too soon. Relax and be a father; you'll feel like a father later on.

Pregnancy can awaken a new consciousness of family and generational ties. Once you become a dad, relationships with your parents, especially your father, may change.

On news of their partner's pregnancy, some men suddenly feel the need to make contact with their parents, especially their fathers, even long-lost ones. Sometimes men harbor the hope—not always fulfilled—that childbirth will somehow restore relationships with fathers who've been emotionally distant.

Pregnancy can awaken memories of the parenting you received. The parenting you remember is the model you'll turn to for guidance in raising your own children. Unhappy boyhood experiences may encourage a man to improve on the parenting he received. If your father was chronically unavailable, for example, you may find yourself quietly resolving to avoid career plans or recreational pursuits that lead in this direction.

The prospect of parenthood can also renew unresolved conflicts. Recollections of the past may cause new worries. Identifying doubts and worries and discussing them with your partner are important first steps to becoming a good father. Your partner may have concerns also, so make time to listen to, understand and support each other. Don't forget to discuss positive memories as well.

A good approach to dealing with concerns is to find a quiet place for an interruption-free discussion, then review together as many parenting issues as you can. Decide together what you'll try to establish and what you'll try to avoid in raising your child.

Thinking About Fatherhood

In women, the prospect of physical changes associated with pregnancy often produces uncertainty, anxiety, mild depression or even fear. Perhaps as never before, your partner needs your understanding, support and encouragement during her pregnancy and as she develops her identity as a mother.

Her moods and actions, and your responses to them, can affect your relationship in many ways. For example, there may be times when you are interested in intercourse but your partner is not. If she rejects your overtures in the bedroom, remember that she's neither rejecting you nor losing interest in a loving relationship. In fact, now that she's pregnant she has a special need for closeness, but not necessarily physical intimacy. She may be tired, sad or worried. She may be perplexed or displeased about changes that are occurring in her body. She may be wondering how she'll cope with the pain associated with delivery. She may feel unprepared for motherhood. In fact, she may be dealing with various conscious and subconscious emotions neither of you can fully grasp. But it's important to know that she needs your presence and support and, perhaps right now, tenderness without sexual overtones.

Talk to your partner about how she's feeling. Make it clear to her that you, too, have mixed emotions occasionally, but that you're in this together.

Just as you might misread your partner's moods, she may view an intensified involvement with work on your part as a form of withdrawal from the relationship. Although your extended work hours may be motivated by a desire to provide more security for your family, she may feel hurt and rejected.

Misunderstandings like this are especially common in the months immediately after childbirth, when stress is inevitable. Your partner will likely be home caring for the baby, out of touch with friends or colleagues. She may be tired, having been up during the night to breastfeed the baby. But even though she may seem moody, remember that she still relies on you for emotional support.

Emotional Support

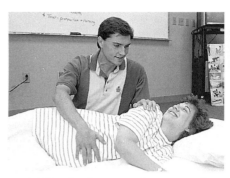

In childbirth education classes you'll practice working together on relaxation and comforting techniques.

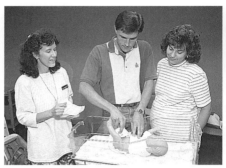

You'll have a chance to practice some of the basics of baby care, such as diapering, bathing and holding a baby.

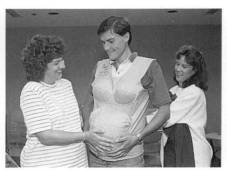

You may have a new appreciation for some of the physical sensations your partner experiences during pregnancy by trying on an Empathy Belly. This weighted vest presses on your bladder, squeezes your ribs and simulates the added weight of pregnancy.

Childbirth education is for dads too

Participating in childbirth education classes is a good way to be supportive during the pregnancy. Classes are offered at hospitals and birthing centers throughout the country.

Your presence at childbirth education classes makes the experience a shared one, and that alone is important. Beyond just being there, however, you'll receive tips that will help in your role as a loving, supportive companion during your partner's pregnancy and as coach and helper when delivery time arrives.

(Read more about childbirth education classes on page 264.)

Sometimes the emotional and hormonal ups and downs of pregnancy can cause tears in an expectant mother—often for no apparent reason. It's not important to understand the reason for the tears. What is important is to just be there, holding her closely and affirming that it's okay to cry, regardless of the cause.

The physical changes and discomforts of pregnancy may conspire to erode your partner's self-esteem. Your continued assurances that she's attractive despite how she may feel are very important. An unexpected kiss, a flower, a love note or a candlelit dinner can assist in convincingly expressing your unconditional love.

Emotional support during pregnancy can take other forms as well. For example, making decisions jointly is a form of mutual support. It not only takes the decision-making burden off each of you but also strengthens your relationship by helping you forge a shared vision of the future.

Physical Support

Fatigue in early pregnancy is a very real concern. Your partner may suddenly find she has a hard time dragging herself out of bed in the morning. Fatigue tends to decrease in the second trimester and return again in the third, when she's feeling the effect of an extra 25 pounds.

Pregnant women need the support of their partners in physical ways. If you both are working, you can help by sharing household responsibilities or assuming more of them. Cleaning up, washing dishes, feeding the dog, taking out the garbage, doing laundry, even food shopping can be shared activities. Be sure to discuss who's going to do what. Some women prefer to hold on to some tasks. And as much as women want and need help, they don't always accept it easily. So proceed cautiously. Your partner's part of the bargain is to let you tackle the household jobs in your own style, even though it may differ from her approach.

New concerns arise when a man first hears the news that he's to be a father. Many men worry about their parenting abilities and about changes in their relationship with their partner. These anxieties are common but are rarely discussed and almost never dealt with professionally. Anxiety associated with pregnancy is sometimes expressed in the male partner by temporary physical symptoms such as nausea, weight gain and backache, which are conditions pregnant women experience. This psychosomatic sharing of physical symptoms is termed the couvade syndrome.

Physical Changes in the Father

Many men tend to keep worries to themselves, perhaps because they see fear as a sign of weakness. You and your partner will both be better off if you discuss them. Hidden worries can lead to tension in your relationship. They can create a sense of distance between you and your partner at a time when you both need the warmth of a close relationship.

Some of the common worries of expectant fathers are discussed below.

Dealing With Fatherhood Fears

Birth defects. Men, as well as women, commonly worry about the possibility of birth defects. The awe of creating new life, an awareness of the amazing complexity of human development and lofty hopes for the baby-to-be all may play a role in causing this fear. The thought of raising a child with exceptional needs also can weigh on an expectant father, who may wonder where he would find the financial and emotional resources to deal with such a problem.

This anxiety can have a positive side. It can motivate both of you to create a healthful and safe environment for your baby-to-be by seeking early professional care, eating right, exercising, attending childbirth education classes and giving up harmful habits, such as smoking cigarettes. (See page 103 for a discussion of lifestyle during pregnancy.)

Remember that most pregnancies result in normal, healthy babies. It's important to be honest in discussing your fears with each other. If questions remain, seek answers from your partner's doctor.

Queasiness about the delivery. The thought of witnessing the birth of a baby is tough for some men to handle. Their anxiety may relate to a feeling of helplessness—even though their partner might be exhausted and in pain, they feel they won't be able to do much to help. Some men worry that they'll be in the way; they think it might be easier just to let the doctors and nurses handle everything. Also, a certain messiness and bloodiness occur when a baby is born; some men would like an excuse to skip those parts.

Talk to your partner, and be honest about your concerns. If you can't find words to express your worries precisely, that's okay. Just talk about them as best you can.

Although your presence in the birthing or delivery room is not required, most women prefer to have you there. Your partner will have the toughest part, but there are ways you can help. Your presence during labor and birth is a demonstration of your caring.

Ten suggestions for fathers-to-be

1. Participate in childbirth or other parent education classes together.
2. Go with your partner to her doctor visits. If she is having an ultrasound exam, being there is probably more important than anything you are doing at work.
3. Make decisions jointly.
4. Share your hopes and dreams for your children.
5. Pitch in more around the house.
6. Exercise with her.
7. Spend time alone together.
8. Discuss your concerns, fears and anxieties together.
9. Go on walks together.
10. Learn how to give a great massage!

Most men remember their participation in labor and birth with a sense of accomplishment, pride and exhilaration. They helped bring their daughter or son into the world. They shared the thrill of hearing their child's first cry. It's an experience fathers always remember.

Increased financial responsibility. Even in this age of equal opportunity and responsibility, being a father may mean being the family's primary financial provider.

Although it can improve family finances, preoccupation with work may make you unavailable to provide the physical and emotional support your partner needs and expects from you. Talk together about family finances. Work out a plan both of you can feel good about. But don't expect easy answers. Parenthood brings tough choices, and sometimes priorities must be rearranged or dreams postponed.

Talking with other couples who are facing similar issues or meeting with a financial adviser may be useful.

Lack of attention. Some expectant dads fear that once the baby arrives their partners will focus all of their attention and affection on the baby—that they'll be pushed into the background of family life.

These concerns often begin early in pregnancy. You may start to feel left out when your partner's condition begins to attract attention. And because pregnancy can turn your partner's attention inward, you may receive less attention from her because she's focusing on becoming a mother. Men sometimes mistakenly interpret such shifts in their partner's behavior as a form of emotional abandonment.

It's helpful to find ways to be more involved with your partner. Participate in prenatal visits and attend childbirth education classes together. Schedule private times together, perhaps a weekly dinner date. If your budget doesn't allow dining out, do something special at home—have dinner by candlelight, or enjoy breakfast in bed.

Death. A common, but unspoken, fear of expectant fathers is that their partner might die during childbirth. Perhaps this fear explains why men are often more worried than their partners about the aches and pains women typically experience during pregnancy.

Remember, although it can occur, death during childbirth is rare. The prevention and management of complications of childbirth are among the great successes of modern medicine.

Men worry, too, about the babies their partners are carrying. No matter how careful a couple may be, miscarriages and stillbirths can occur. Men whose partners have experienced these complications are naturally more susceptible to such anxieties.

In dealing with these worries, keep in mind that although there's no such thing as a risk-free pregnancy, complications are uncommon. When complications do occur, they can often be managed successfully. Your doctor can provide reliable, up-to-date information on risks associated with your partner's pregnancy—risks to her health and to your developing baby. If your partner is generally in good health, there's little to fear. A tour of the labor and delivery facilities you'll be using also can help calm your fears by providing tangible evidence that your partner and the baby will be in good hands.

Sexuality

It's hard for many women to believe, but many men are proud of the visible changes in their partner's body that come with pregnancy. Because of the emphasis our culture places on slimness, women are often distressed by these changes. Simply put, they feel fat and unattractive.

Sweet notes, flowers, hugs and private dinners for two are time-honored methods of reassuring your partner that you love her and that the physical changes of pregnancy give her a glow that you find especially attractive.

For some women, a negative body image is a major roadblock to enjoying or even wanting lovemaking during pregnancy. They can't imagine why their partners would want to make love. Keep in mind that for most women, interest in intercourse continues but may decrease during pregnancy.

In the early months, your partner may be preoccupied with the physical and psychological changes associated with pregnancy. Fatigue alone can result in decreased interest in sexual intimacy.

During the third trimester, you may also experience decreased interest in sex. At this late stage, men often worry about intercourse harming the baby. Unless your doctor advises otherwise, intercourse until shortly before the baby is born should pose no hazards. It can, of course, be more challenging. So you may need to be more creative.

Experiment with different positions. Some women prefer a rear-entry position because it puts less pressure on their abdomens, and penetration may not be as deep. Or your partner may prefer to lie on her back, with buttocks at the edge of the bed, allowing you to approach her in a standing position.

There's more to a sexual relationship than intercourse. Massage can heighten sensuality and intimacy and lead comfortably to intercourse. Or it can be an enjoyable end in itself. Both of you may feel an increased need for intimacy and closeness, but you may not be interested in sex.

Overmanaging

Pregnancy, like other family matters, offers many opportunities for joint decision making. Occasionally, though, one partner makes decisions deeply affecting the other. Domination in decision making can create conflict or resentment.

Don't try to manage your partner's pregnancy. It can compound the stress of pregnancy for you both.

Weight, for example, can be an issue for discussion. If you ask your partner whether she's eating right during pregnancy, your inquiry may be motivated by concern for her welfare. But if you demand that she eat a certain way, you may be setting yourself up for conflict.

Occasionally, a man may thoughtlessly comment, "You're getting too fat," or, alternatively, "You're not eating enough." Remember, weight gain during pregnancy is necessary, within limits. The recommendations have changed during the past decade: a gain of 25 to 35 pounds is now considered about right for most women.

Doctors generally welcome and encourage men's participation throughout their partners' pregnancies, involving them in preconception and prenatal visits. But remember that most of the discussions and decisions will be between the pregnant woman and her doctor. Also, it's common and important for physicians to have the opportunity to meet one-on-one with the expectant mother.

Abuse and Pregnancy

Abuse, battering and sexual assault of women are widespread, regardless of age, race, economic status or cultural background. There is evidence that a pregnant woman is at increased risk for physical abuse. Studies confirm that pregnancy can lead to more frequent or severe domestic violence. In regions where poverty prevails, abuse may be even more common.

Health care providers are increasingly attuned to the potential for abuse. Screening for abuse is now often included in prenatal care. Hospitals and birthing centers are important resources for offering protection and advice. Expectant women who are abused are reluctant to admit it and may even deny being abused. Bruises or cuts, frequently around the face or head, may silently tell the sad story. Pregnant women who are abused may delay important prenatal care, perhaps out of fear of their partners. Abused women sometimes are motivated to become pregnant in the hope that pregnancy will end or reduce the severity or frequency of their abuse.

A pregnant woman who is abused suffers emotionally as well as physically. In addition to the host of hurts that may be inflicted, she is at greater risk for a miscarriage. Abuse may also retard a baby's growth and encourage premature delivery.

If you know someone or suspect that someone may be in an abusive situation, call for professional help. People who can help include doctors, nurses, hospital emergency rooms, women's resource centers, women's shelters, services for abused or battered women, sexual assault services, crisis intervention services and mental health/counseling services.

Labor and Delivery

Childbirth is a physically and emotionally demanding process. Active labor can last from an hour to an entire exhausting day. You can make this time less difficult and more rewarding for your partner by being there to help with labor and delivery. Your presence alone is an important form of support. It shows her you care.

There's plenty for you to do, and the personnel in most labor and delivery rooms will welcome you. For starters, encourage your partner and help her relax. You can massage her back, offer to put cool, moist cloths on her face and gently hold her hand, helping her to take each contraction as it comes. Also, timing contractions and helping her pace her breathing can be very helpful.

During birth, dads are usually positioned at the head of the bed. This way both you and your partner will see the baby arrive at the same moment. Practices vary, but often dads are allowed to hold the baby right away.

(For more on men's roles in labor and birth, see pages 273, 285, 287 and 290.)

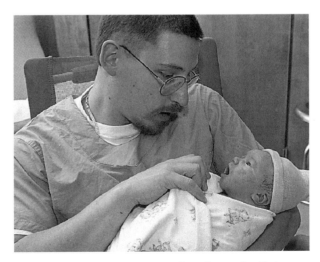

Excitement, amazement, apprehension and relief are all rolled into one incredible feeling the first time you hold your new son or daughter.

Infancy

Sometimes new dads are amazed at the intensity of the feelings they have for their child and at their renewed commitment to their partners. They often experience an extraordinary sense of closeness to both. Such feelings are important buffers in the hectic days ahead, when infants cry frequently and fatigued mothers may have trouble coping. (For more on your partner's needs in the weeks after childbirth, see page 413.)

Babies generally enter the world well prepared for that first encounter with parents. Newborns can orient themselves to sounds, recognizing and preferring the human voice. They can see things close up, generally preferring faces over inanimate objects. Babies will follow a face as it turns, and they may even imitate a facial gesture, such as sticking out a tongue. Their body movements synchronize to the rhythm of the human voice. Their tiny hands can grasp your finger.

The unforgettably powerful and personal experience of pregnancy, labor and birth gives a woman a head start on achieving intimacy with her baby. It might even create an immediate attachment to the baby that influences the ease with which she learns the basics of caring for and interacting with her child.

Not so for fathers. Their involvement in the process is generally less intense. It takes more time for fathers to achieve a comparable level of intimacy. But understanding the abilities of newborns for face-to-face, eye-to-eye interaction can foster a new dad's interest in and involvement with his child.

Getting acquainted

David sat in a rocking chair and reached out nervously as the nurse gently placed the minutes-old baby in his lap and smoothed the blanket in which little Jonathan was warmly swaddled. After a couple of rocks, the baby's dark eyes opened and peered directly into David's.

"First, we just looked at each other. I couldn't believe I was looking into the eyes of my own son. Then I talked to him, softly, gently. I told him we're glad he's here. I told him a little about what life on beautiful planet Earth can be like. Then the tears came. It was a special time."

Fun and Games

The face-to-face play that parents enjoy with their babies is crucial to a baby's social and intellectual development. It is the earliest experience of focusing attention, and it provides the first lessons in the sharing of expression and emotions.

Although your partner may become your infant's main caregiver of physical and emotional needs, you'll likely be one of your baby's most important play partners. The games men traditionally play—vigorous, active games—help babies develop physically as well as intellectually. Babies also thrive and grow on gentler interactions, such as being read to or sung to.

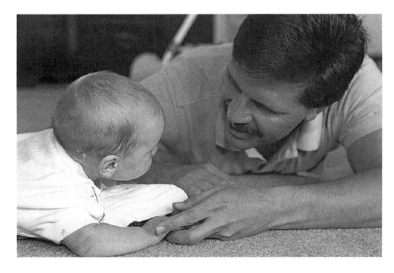

Playtime—a special time that new dads and babies look forward to.

Struggling With the Tasks of Parenthood

It has been said that new babies bring fathers and mothers closer together, but at the same time they can move them apart. This is most true in the everyday tasks of parenting. Division of labor seems to be the cause of most of the conflicts. Before childbirth, most parents-to-be share the modern ideal of the father participating in family life, management of the household and child rearing. And men's involvement in the preparation for the day of baby's birth leads both partners to expect that fathers will be involved after the birth too.

But the reality after childbirth is that traditional patterns often reassert themselves. Fathers, for example, spend more time working, because they are often the sole provider in the early weeks after the baby is born. It is true that fathers today are doing more cooking, cleaning and caring for the baby than their fathers did. However, their participation in family work and child rearing often ends up being far less than both partners consider ideal and far less than both of you planned on.

What's more, this reality can come as a surprise and disappointment to both partners. You may both experience it as dissatisfaction with yourselves and your relationship. This can lead to confusion and guilt. Your partner may begin to feel overburdened, angry and fatigued from putting in so much effort at home. The feelings can intensify when she returns to work, as her responsibilities increase. Ultimately you may end up blaming each other for not doing a better job.

Men who take on a more involved role in running the household and rearing the children tend to feel positive about themselves and their partners, and their relationship feels more satisfying to both of them. Conversely, the less you are involved in the tasks of parenting your baby, the easier it is for you to become dissatisfied with the relationship.

How much household responsibility should you take on? Negotiate. Structure the first arrangement as an experiment, and alter the course as you go. Most couples quickly realize that the arrangements will shift often in the first few years.

When the baby comes home

When a baby arrives, there's no end to the things that need to be done around the house. Don't wait for requests or directives from your partner. Look and listen for tasks you can help with. Here are a few suggestions for starters:

- Get up and rock your baby when he or she cries at night.
- Lullabies work. Learn to sing or hum a favorite.
- Give your baby a bath.
- Change diapers.
- Give your partner a night off, without expecting it to be returned.
- Serve breakfast in bed, or wherever your partner prefers.
- Hire someone to clean the house.

Being a Good Father

You want to be a good father, but unfortunately, babies don't come with an instruction book. Forget about the fact that you've never had a course in fathering or perhaps have never even held a new baby before.

Fortunately, babies are forgiving, and moms are almost universally willing, if not eager, to share their parenting skills with their partners. You'll soon learn how to diaper your son or daughter, and rocking, burping and bathing are skills you'll quickly acquire by observation and practice. (For more about the basics of baby care, see page 449.)

Here are a few final observations and some points to ponder:

- Your decision to bring a new person into the world is one of the most profoundly important decisions you'll make in life. It can be a turning point. You've made a commitment to your partner, your child and society. It's your responsibility to be a good father.

- There's no University of Effective Fathering. You'll learn as you go. Your approach to being a father probably will be based largely on your personal experiences in growing up. But you may need to make adjustments based on changing expectations and realities. If you are loving, thoughtful, flexible, gentle, unselfish and strong, you'll be a good father.

- Don't expect to feel like a dad from the moment your child is born. The love and commitment of a good father require time to develop fully.

- Fatherhood is a long-term commitment. The love, support and involvement of a father are needed throughout your child's life.

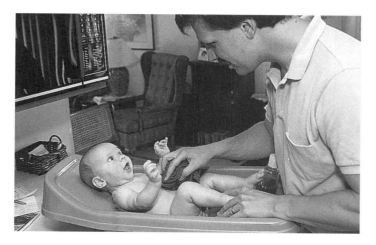

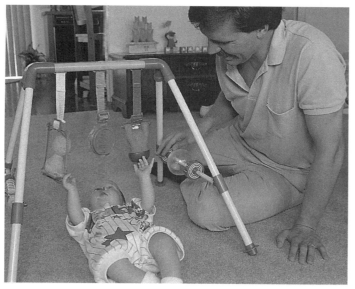

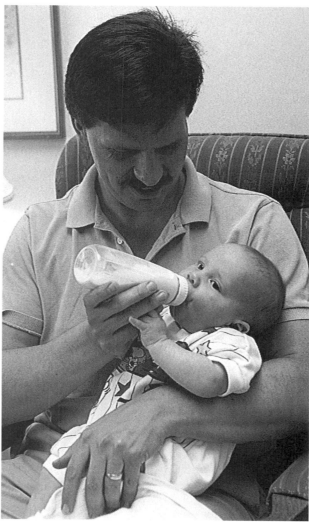

It may seem a little awkward at first, but most new fathers and mothers quickly master the everyday responsibilities of caring for a baby.

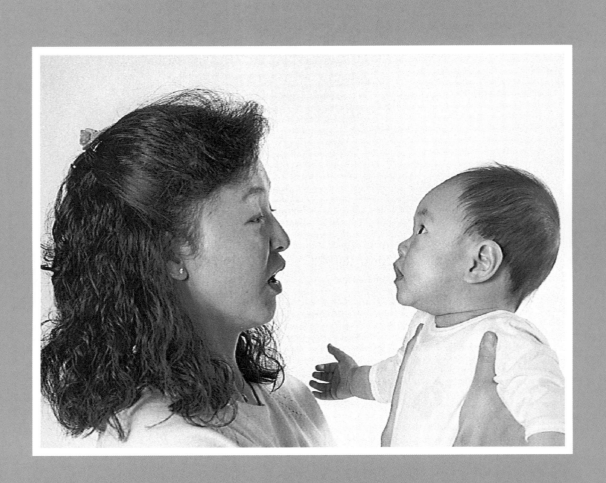

CHAPTER THIRTY-NINE

Couples and New Parenthood

Congratulations! Your baby is a true turning point in your lives, a passage from being a couple to becoming a family. It's a momentous occasion, a private triumph and a declaration of your love for each other and of a shared interest in the future. It's a public occasion, too, because the family is the unit through which we traditionally pass on the values of our culture.

Each couple approaching first-time parenthood finds the arrival of a baby to be a major transition that marks a change in everyday ways of doing things. The hope and optimism that surround birth make it one of life's most joyous transitions. So, with months of enthusiasm, you've been gathering information and making necessary plans—readying the house, arranging a leave from work, "rehearsing" parenthood through dreams and fantasies, buying supplies, planning for outside help with the house or baby and maybe even assigning responsibilities to grandparents.

At some point shortly after the birth, you and your partner will peer down at a tiny baby with puffy eyes and a funny-shaped head and feel intensely proud. You'll also probably feel closer than you ever have, indelibly linked by your joint creation. Such is the thrill of new parenthood. Savor the moment, for it is a precious one.

All Changes Bring Stress

It may be hard for you to believe that this new little life—so natural and bringing you so much joy—may also put significant stress on your relationship with your partner. Couples who remain the happiest are the ones who make time to nurture each other.

You probably know by now that many stresses are built into new parenthood. Whether you're giving birth or adopting, you may feel overwhelmed at first by the sudden disorganization of your life and exhausted from interrupted sleep. Taking care of a new baby does create a lot more to do every day. Plus, as a parent you're in an entirely new role, trying to figure out this new person who has taken over your life. You're learning a lot in a terribly short time.

There's another stress that new parents feel. It not only startles them but also seems to threaten the very reason they wanted a baby in the first place—to celebrate their life together and to draw even closer. Although babies can help strengthen a relationship, new parents are often surprised to find that this change doesn't happen right away. Having a baby tends to set up conflicting demands in partners. These demands can make early parenthood especially hard on the relationship. No matter how well they got along before the baby arrived, many new parents experience conflict and disagreement in the first year after the baby's birth, and they may grow increasingly disenchanted with their relationship as a couple.

A Bumpy Ride

Like every other couple, you'll have big and little issues that you and your partner need to work out after the baby arrives. These revolve around how to fairly divide the responsibilities of everyday life and how to stay in touch with each other despite forces that push you apart. This chapter is designed to help you through what has become a trying but wholly expected and predictable phase of adjustment. It will point out the trouble spots and help you cope with them. And it will suggest ways you can keep your relationship on a satisfying course.

Knowing ahead of time that the ride is likely to be bumpy for a short stretch can help keep stress from turning into dissatisfaction. More and more studies show that between late pregnancy and the first year after a baby is born, most couples experience a drop in satisfaction with their relationship. It's not that the sizzle has waned from having been together longer, because this decline doesn't seem to occur among childless couples. Nor is it the baby's fault, even though the baby does have a considerable impact on the parents' lives. The new and stressful responsibilities of parenthood in combination with unpredictable schedules and sheer exhaustion can lead to decreased communication and less time spent nurturing a satisfying relationship.

Expectations vs. Reality

The challenge to the relationship that most new parents experience isn't addressed much, not even in books or classes about pregnancy and childbirth. The myth is that all your dreams will come true with the birth of a child. In many ways, they will. But you as a couple have to help the process along.

Elizabeth Bing, one of the pioneering childbirth educators in the United States, said she's "rarely come across straightforward descriptions of childbirth. They have always been embellished." In the same way, the first weeks your baby is home and becoming part of your family can be a cold splash of reality that may not fit with your dreams. That's when the stress starts bearing down on you as a couple.

If your dreams and hopes for your baby move too far from reality, they become fantasies. When the fantasy and the reality don't match, it's easy to think you must be doing something wrong. But it isn't the challenges of parenting that might shake your partnership. It's not being realistically prepared for the challenges. If expectations are out of keeping with reality, then partners can wind up blaming each other for not fulfilling their expectations of what parenthood is supposed to be. They mistakenly assume that the relationship is deeply troubled. And they're afraid of what lies ahead.

Having a baby seems to magnify already existing differences between partners. Much of the stress on the partnership is related to how men and women divide the responsibilities they have both inside and outside the home. Many new parents have to make choices about who will stay home and who will work outside, and about how baby care and housework will (or won't) be shared inside the home. After childbirth, your roles can change in ways you hadn't expected, and both of you can be disappointed.

Old Tensions Are Magnified

The arrival of a new baby can increase the level of conflict and quarreling and decrease the satisfaction you get from your relationship. Remember, this is a time when your relationship tends to get short shrift anyway. Your baby will be totally dependent on you for everything in life—everything. You have to respond to the baby's needs, and there are still only 24 hours in a day.

But babies aren't the cause of the tension that couples often feel. Long-term studies of couples, beginning from before pregnancy to several years after, show that couples adapt to life after baby in much the same way they did before. Becoming a parent is difficult, not so much because it raises new problems but because old ones resurface.

So be ready. The transition to parenthood is a challenge to the satisfaction you've had from your relationship. You're apt to feel alienated from each other for a while. But with some idea of what might stress new parents, you can be prepared to weather the bumps more smoothly.

How We See Ourselves

We all know we play many roles in life: daughter, sister, wage earner, wife, friend, lover. When your baby is born, you'll be taking on yet another role— that of parent. One of the biggest yet most subtle sources of alienation you and your partner might experience can result from the different ways you both adjust to seeing yourselves as mom and dad. Identification with these new roles can occur at different rates and to differing degrees for each of you.

Typically, between pregnancy and six months after childbirth, most women take on a huge psychological investment in motherhood. In contrast, most men tend to take on the psychological investment in fatherhood more slowly. During the pregnancy, a man's identity as a parent is not nearly that of a woman's. His sense of fatherhood typically doesn't peak until about 18 months after the baby is born, but even then it's considerably less than a woman's identity with motherhood. What may come as a surprise is that your identities as parents may crowd out the other roles in your lives. Because women may more quickly see themselves in the role of parent, they may also lose some of their psychological investment as partner or lover.

Inner Changes

A man's sense of himself as a partner or lover may also diminish after childbirth, but not nearly as much as a woman's. At the same time, his identity as a wage earner, for instance, may remain virtually unchanged.

The psychological reshuffling taking place inside each of you has a direct impact on your relationship as a couple. It sets up an inner, emotional distance between you. Both parents, especially new mothers, experience inner pressure to be a good parent and may end up devoting less attention to their partner relationship.

Because your inner changes aren't in sync, you and your partner may respond to a familiar opportunity—say, a chance to go to the movies—in different ways. For example, you may not want to leave the baby with a sitter when your partner feels it's okay. And he probably won't understand why you seem to lose interest in things you loved so much before: You? Pass up a romantic movie? He sees the refusal of his overtures as a sign of rejection. You see his overtures as insensitivity to your needs. When you finally have the energy to pay attention to your relationship—say, you try to start a conversation after the baby's asleep— he may be focused on problems he brought home from work.

The impact of inner change affects partners at different times. Your decline in satisfaction with the relationship may be greatest about six months after the baby arrives. Your partner may feel most dissatisfied with the relationship when you're beginning to feel better about it—between six months and 18 months after the birth. These differences make you both feel distant from each other. Feeling distant leads to conflict, and conflict leads to dissatisfaction with the relationship.

Role Changes

You and your partner might experience other sources of alienation stemming from the way you divide the responsibilities of parenting and housekeeping. Your family roles not only change but also change differently from the way you expect them to.

Most couples today approach parenthood as a joint endeavor. You set out expecting work and family life to be a form of partnership. It's not that you expect to split all the responsibilities of life 50-50, but you want to at least work as a team in rearing the children and sharing decisions, family-life responsibilities and rewards.

Both men and women expect to be involved in family work. In fact, most men today look forward to taking part in a wider family role than their fathers did, by cooking, cleaning and taking care of the children. Many men see this participation as one of the great rewards of life.

But in reality, after the addition of a baby the division of family labor can take a very different course. Often, it's the mother who first stops working outside the home and takes on most household tasks and care of the child. Her partner may work even harder outside the home. If she returns to her job outside the home, she typically still carries the primary responsibility for the household and child care. Women may feel overburdened and angry at having to work this "second shift," and men may feel confused and guilty.

So the division of labor at home not only becomes more traditional but also grows more unequal. Still, what distresses new parents most is the difference between their expectations and reality. Although many couples are happy with the traditional division of responsibilities, more and more are not. They may expect that the mother will do more of certain baby-care chores: responding to

A checklist of family responsibilities

Most couples today approach life as a partnership. But having babies tends to throw people into arrangements different from what they had hoped. These silent, unplanned shifts in roles can make both parents unhappy. If that happens, you'll need to actively, consciously and jointly work out a division of the nitty-gritty tasks of family life to distribute the stresses and rewards of parenthood to the satisfaction of both of you.

Following is a list of some everyday jobs families with new infants typically need to do. You and your partner might want to read them together. For each item, ask yourselves: Who's doing most of the actual work? How satisfied are you both with those arrangements? What's your ideal arrangement for that task?

This list isn't meant to be a scorecard, but a reminder of activities to consider when you balance the arrangements. But be flexible. The arrangements you make today may not be the ones most workable six months from now.

Household and family tasks

- Providing the family income
- Paying the bills
- Planning meals
- Shopping for food
- Preparing the meals
- Cleaning the house
- Doing the laundry
- Making repairs around the home
- Taking care of the yard or garden
- Taking out the garbage
- Looking after the car

Family decisions

- Finances
- Working outside the home
- Making social arrangements
- Arranging participation in community activities, religious organizations
- Buying major household items
- Deciding how to divide holiday visits among your relatives

Taking care of the baby

- Responding to baby's cries
- Getting up at night
- Doing baby's laundry
- Choosing baby's toys
- Deciding about meals
- Feeding
- Diapering
- Bathing
- Taking the baby out
- Playing
- Arranging for baby-sitters
- Arranging well-baby checkups and unexpected medical visits

Outside help

Consider alternatives beyond dividing the work:

- If you can afford it, think about hiring someone to help with the housework or yard work. But be clear whose responsibility it is to make those arrangements.
- Join a baby-sitting co-op, if one exists in your area, or start one yourself. In a co-op, parents of young children exchange baby-sitting services.
- Join a parent support group.

cries, getting up at night and doing most of the feeding. But couples may expect to share other responsibilities: bathing, taking the baby out, playing with the baby, arranging for baby-sitters and taking care of the baby's medical visits. Instead, these often fall much more on mom's shoulders too.

How you and your partner divide the chores for taking care of your baby is the single issue most likely to cause conflict. If these expectations aren't met, surprise and disappointment can be transformed into tension between you.

Unless you counter these tensions by deliberate efforts at communication and intimacy, the disappointment in family-life arrangements can deeply affect feelings about the relationship.

But couples who work to keep a psychological investment in the partner relationship feel much better about themselves. What's more, they report less parenting stress. So making a special effort to see yourself not just as a mother but still as a partner is good for both of you—and good for the baby. One of the best ways to do this is to plan regular times to be together alone as a couple. Remember, caring for each other doesn't mean less time for the baby.

Find Time to Work on Your Relationship

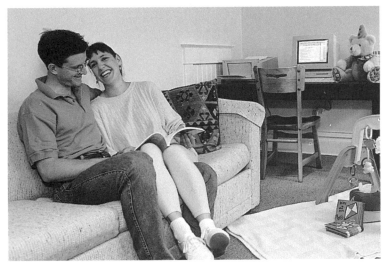

An occasional night of quiet conversation at home with your partner can contribute to the ongoing happiness of your relationship, because caring for each other makes caring for a new baby easier.

Creating time for each other seems to be the secret of couples who maintain a happy relationship in the first busy months after the baby is born. Those who make this effort ultimately enjoy their relationship more and find parenting easier. But lack of time is the big challenge of new parents, especially new mothers. At first, you'll find there simply aren't enough hours in the day to take care of yourself and do all that needs to be done as well. You'll find yourself complaining, "I don't have any time for myself." And that may make you wonder how you will ever have time enough for your partner. The answer is, you steal it, because caring for each other makes caring for everything else easier.

There are simple things you and your partner can do to lessen the stress of new parenthood and strengthen your partnership in the process. Some of these may be obvious, and you even may have thought about them, but the trick is to actually do them.

- Share your expectations of an ideal family life. Both you and your partner come to parenthood with inner visions of what you hope will happen. Chances are your inner visions differ from his—after all, you've had different life experiences. You may see children as having an active and lively role in shaping family life, whereas your partner expects that parents alone dictate the course of things. There's no way your combined ideal family picture will develop on its own. To build a life that satisfies both of you, you have to share your inner visions. Then you can choose goals that matter to both of you. This process is at the very heart of all deeply satisfying long-term relationships. Some partners don't want to discuss their hopes and anxieties because they're afraid that they'll reveal unbridgeable differences or start major conflicts. But confiding what you hope will happen and what you're concerned about strengthens the bond between you.

- Make time to talk to each other. For instance, set aside a regular time each week. Plan to go for a walk. Or have a fancy breakfast in the dining room. It doesn't matter where you go or what you do as long as it's pleasant and you agree to no interruptions. Making a date for what you used to do spontaneously may feel awkward and even silly at first. But keep the appointment, even if dirty dishes are waiting in the sink. If the baby is crying, you may want to postpone the date—but be sure to reschedule. This way you'll always have time to be in touch with each other.

- Strive for intimacy. At the same time, don't expect lovemaking to return to pre-baby levels in the months after childbirth. Too much is working against that: exhaustion, your baby's needs, physical changes, changed inner interests and timing. Remember, there's a lot more to intimacy than sex. If intercourse seems unlikely to happen, there's touching, hugging, cuddling and massaging. Anyway, that's probably what both of you are missing most—the feeling of closeness.

- If you have a fight, don't fall into the trap of blaming each other. Instead, view it as a neutral sign that something in your relationship needs to be worked out. For example, you may feel so overwhelmed by your new responsibilities at home that you blow up at your partner for coming home a little late one evening. Ask yourselves, "What's going on in our lives that's causing this to happen now?" Then put it on the agenda to be talked about when you get together. You may find it becomes necessary for you and your partner to redivide household tasks so that you feel less overburdened.

How to talk with your partner

Because you've known each other a long time and have been communicating perfectly well all this time, it might seem silly that you would need advice now on how to talk with your partner. But being a new parent is so time-consuming that you may have to plan what was once automatic. Taking time out for each other in an orderly way helps couples feel better about the relationship and improves the care given to baby. Some reminders about how to make it work:

1. Schedule regular times to be together. If you need to cancel a date, reschedule it for a specific time and place. Don't leave the plan vague and indefinite.

2. If there are problems that need to be ironed out, expect to tackle only one topic per meeting.

3. Try not to ramble, and be sure you let your partner have equal time.

4. Don't use this as an opportunity to blame or criticize your partner. This is a touchy time for building identity and confidence, a time for learning new roles that will be important in helping you share the responsibilities of parenting during the years ahead. Both of you need encouragement. Be sure to talk about what's positive as well as what's negative.

5. Don't interrupt your partner. Knowing you will have your own turn to express what's on your mind goes a long way toward making this an interlude you both look forward to.

*Today's
Problems:
So Different,
So Much
the Same*

Yversou likely will face some problems that your parents didn't have.

Isolation. Extended families—grandparents, aunts, uncles, cousins—tend to be so scattered that couples now often feel they have only themselves to rely on for advice or help. Also, after the first rush of visits from friends, the time needed to care for the baby tends to isolate couples from their usual social networks. The isolation results in the partners themselves having to supply nearly all the social stimulation and satisfaction they used to get from other people.

Careers. More and more mothers today are in the workforce, not simply to earn a little money for some nice extras but to support the family and to have careers of their own. Having a child is clearly going to affect that career. Staying home to take care of a baby often leads to dissatisfaction at being away from work. But going back to work often leads to guilt for not staying home to raise the child. The new mother feels herself getting locked into an "either/or" life: traditional or contemporary, neither of which seems quite right.

No common models. Sorting out work and family roles seems to fall completely on each couple because there aren't many "rules" or "standard ways" of doing things anymore. But try to keep in mind that every generation has its own particular set of problems to deal with. Parents and grandparents may not have had to face your choices, but they had to deal with families torn apart by major economic depressions, wars such as those in Vietnam and Korea and World War II and a whole different set of societal expectations. True, they may not approach the early family relationship with the values you and your partner probably hold—the belief that you will more or less equally share the work both outside and inside the family—but your parents can still be a rich source of advice and experience for you to draw from, because they also had to make hard decisions about tough questions. Talk with them.

Be Aware of Sexual Adjustments

When life gets really hectic because of the changes your baby has brought about, you may begin to wonder if something's gone deeply wrong between you and your partner. At those times, try to remember that the problem probably is not with either of you. The transition to parenthood complicates life for a while, pushing parents into traditional role arrangements—whether they want them or not. These conflicting demands simply come with the territory of new parenthood. But remind yourselves that now more than ever you both still need to communicate. The new forces working on you simply mean you have to work harder to stay in touch, especially about your sexuality.

Perhaps no subject is more emotionally loaded than that of sex. Here are a few thoughts for new parents.

1. Couples who have a rewarding relationship naturally make sexual expression a part of it. Sexual behavior and response aren't just means of gratification, but a strong expression of well-being and regard for your partner.

2. When and at what rate sexual desire and sexual activity return after childbirth are variable. There's no "normal" schedule for all couples. The many complex physical, hormonal and psychological changes of childbirth and the postpartum period influence sexual desire and activity in different ways.

3. The need for intimacy and its allies, close physical contact and mutual support, doesn't diminish—ever. You don't always have to "have sex" to feel close. The need for close physical contact is especially great in the early weeks and months after childbirth, when just holding and being held is often profoundly satisfying—and reassuring to partners shaky in their new roles as parents and their new relationship as a family.

Breastfeeding and the Couple Relationship

Breastfeeding is a thoroughly natural activity that has a powerful effect on hormone levels. That makes it a strong—although contradictory—influence on both sexual desire and sexual responsiveness. Through its effect on hormone levels, breastfeeding can suppress sexual drive for many months after childbirth. However, suckling also has a stimulating sensation on the breast, which causes many women to find it sexually arousing. This is a perfectly natural response.

Some couples find that breastfeeding becomes an issue between them. Both partners may know that breastfeeding has both nutritional and psychological advantages for their baby. Still, when push comes to shove, fathers sometimes feel left out. They may even feel alienated from their partner and jealous enough of the baby to subvert the breastfeeding by encouraging bottle feeding and by undermining the support and confidence the task requires. Neither activity is in the long-term best interests of the couple or the baby.

It's natural for men to feel some jealousy of the attention you give the baby. But if breastfeeding becomes an issue, it could be a sign of other needs. First, it may indicate the need for you to restructure your family responsibilities in a way that's more satisfying to both of you. As a result, child care tasks and household tasks need to be shared more. Dads need some "hands-on" infant-care activities, which can lead to the satisfaction of being close to the child.

Second, consider it a signal to spend a little more time nurturing each other, not necessarily to give up breastfeeding. Your partner may be missing your attention.

Troubleshooting

If you find that you and your partner are growing increasingly distant or dissatisfied no matter how hard you work to improve your relationship, or if you find yourselves locked in conflicts you can't resolve, you might want to get professional help before the rift gets out of hand.

What you may need is an experienced therapist who can help both of you learn how to work through your problems. A common way to find a reputable marital therapist is to ask your minister, priest, rabbi or your doctor for a referral. You can also call a toll-free referral service maintained by the American Association of Marriage and Family Therapy (800-374-2638). You will be asked to leave your address, and in return you'll receive a consumer's guide to marriage and family therapy and a list of qualified practitioners in your area.

The Challenge After Childbirth

It helps to remember that most couples feel some strain and conflict in trying to meet the demands of parenthood. The result can be negative feelings about each other and the state of their relationship. Few couples know it, because the problem is rarely talked about, but this strain is a normal part of the passage to parenthood. Regard it as part of the challenge of new parenthood.

Your baby brings not only joy to your lives but also added richness to your relationship as a couple. Your love for each other can grow stronger in sharing the celebration and the work, the responsibility and the pride of being parents.

CHAPTER FORTY

Grandparenting

A daughter who five months ago wouldn't have dreamed of taking advice from her mother may ask for it regularly now that she's pregnant. Their once brief and matter-of-fact phone calls now might last for an hour at a time: When did you start wearing maternity clothes? What did you do for a winter coat? How long did you work during pregnancy? How was I fed as a baby? What did Dad do when you went into labor? Where did I sleep when you brought me home from the hospital?

Pregnancy changes the relationship of both partners toward their parents. You start seeing them from a different perspective, and you begin to feel connected to them in new ways. At the same time, grandparents-to-be begin to feel more connected to their children and future grandchildren. This can be one of the most significant and rewarding changes families experience during pregnancy.

Your Relationship to Your Family

In both partners, pregnancy often stirs an interest in family ties. For the first time, you may start thinking of yourselves as starting a new generation in your family. Becoming a parent often prompts you to reexamine your relationships with your parents. In adoptive families, the anticipated addition of a new family member can be a particularly sensitive matter. (For more information on adoption, see page 401.) Almost always, pregnancy moves both partners toward a closer connection with their families. At the same time, news that a grandchild is on the way can be a stimulus for a closer relationship of parents to their grown children.

Now that you're soon to be parents, you are probably beginning to observe good role models. Because the way you were raised is your most familiar model, it's natural to focus on your family first. Your parents can give you both information about how to raise children and reassurances that you will be able to do it well. And even though you may frequently ask your parents for advice, time eventually will teach you to trust your own instincts.

Benefits of a Close Family Relationship

Letting go of the past

For some people, even though the memories of childhood have not always been good, pregnancy can be an ideal time to break strained silences and heal old wounds. These hurts won't go away simply because your baby is coming into the world, but many of the issues can be faced and dealt with, even if never fully resolved.

If you and your parents sincerely want to strengthen your connections, the prospect of a new family member's arrival may make this a good time to try. It seems to provide a natural opportunity for reorganizing relationships, clearing up problems of the past and paving the way for emotional growth ahead.

It may be obvious, but in the deep feelings that surround families, it's easy to forget that your child does not have the same relationship to your parents that you do. Often, grandparents are free to be the kind of parents they never had the chance to be before.

Most people have mixed feelings about how they were raised: joyful recollections intermingled with not-so-happy ones. Now is the time to make a date to talk with your partner about the relationships you've had with your parents and important events from your early lives.

This discussion allows both of you to be as open as possible about what your parents did for you and what you may want to do for your children. At the same time, you can talk about things that didn't seem to work. Together, you can choose what to carry forward from the past and also what you may want to reject. Ask yourselves questions such as these: What helped? What hurt? What were the most positive influences?

By discussing these options with your partner, you can begin to develop joint expectations about what you want and hope for your children. Developing such a picture can strengthen your own relationship and contribute to your future happiness together. It also gives you something you're going to need again and again in the years ahead—a compass for the hectic years of child rearing.

The process of becoming a mother generates an intense need to be nurtured and supported. Although your partner can meet much of this need, it's natural, and perhaps even necessary, to look to your own parents for caring concern. The need to be nurtured is often felt more intensely when you are about to become a new mother than at any other time in your adult life.

Renegotiated Relationships

Keep in mind that your pregnancy is changing not only your roles but also those of your parents. Take the time to approach both your families to discuss openly the changing roles and relationships for the future. Create an atmosphere for discussion in which both generations have the opportunity to talk openly about their new roles and can freely spell out the boundaries of these roles.

Such discussions should focus on the future and be a means to develop understanding. Be sure, in this neutral setting, to say what's on your mind so you don't set yourself up for confusion or hard feelings later on. Gently but firmly spell out what you expect from your parents, and openly discuss what they might expect from you.

Constructive Conversations

Let reminiscing be the bridge from the past to the future. When you talk to your parents ask them what it was like to become parents. How did they respond to the news of pregnancy? What was it like when you were born? They'll probably enjoy remembering and telling you. You may find that your arrival was also met with frightening insecurity mixed with a determination to be the best parents in the world.

Needs of parents-to-be

- Recognition of the importance of establishing their own sets of rules and values in the household.

- Recognition that as adults they should be able to participate in and contribute to family decisions and affairs.

- A link to the past by the passing on of family traditions.

- Help and guidance through confidence building, encouragement and the exchange of information.

- Love and active nurturing from their own parents, which can also serve as a model for nurturing their children.

Needs of grandparents-to-be

- To maintain contact with their grown children, which provides a continued sense of usefulness and a source of respect. For those in the older generation, maintaining ties with children provides an added sense of purpose in life.

- Validation of their own lives. In middle age and beyond, an important measure of success is the success and happiness of one's children.

- A desire to continue the family line and pass on traditions, expertise and family values.

- A strengthening of family ties. (Over the years, people are likely to accord these more value than when younger.)

- The love and respect of grown children.

- Closeness to grandchildren. The grandparent-grandchild relationship is a very special one.

As new parents you'll need help when the baby finally arrives. It's wise to plan for it now. Your parents may expect to be asked to help out after the baby is born. Many grandparents-in-waiting can't wait to help. Discussions before the baby is born can be useful because many expectations will have been ironed out, which can help make the often exhausting days of new parenting a bit easier.

Still, for the day-to-day routine, let your parents know that your primary role as a new mother is to look after the baby. What you may appreciate most is help with the daily tasks of cooking, cleaning, shopping and the laundry.

If your parents and your partner's parents both want to help at this time, try to schedule their visits at the time most convenient and beneficial to you. Many new mothers find that when they and their babies are both healthy, outside help is more useful a week or two after the birth than immediately. This interval also gives you and your partner a chance to get to know your baby and establish your new relationship as a family.

Grandparenting Roles

Your pregnancy not only changes the identities of you and your partner but also brings changes for your parents. They too incorporate a new identity and a new role into their lives. In our youth-oriented culture, age often has a negative image, stripping roles such as grandparenting of their proper status. But consider the important things that grandparents contribute to a family:

- They are an incredible resource for their children and grandchildren. They often have time, wisdom, perspective and love to contribute, to say nothing of an extra pair or two of hands. They widen a grandchild's horizon of experiences.

- They are a source of emotional support to you. Your parents can provide affection and encouragement for the challenging (but rewarding) job of parenting.

- They are an ongoing model of parenting for you.

- They provide a special kind of love to grandchildren. It is a love freed from the day-to-day responsibility for child care. It has no strings attached.

- They are a source of help, and particularly free help. For most grandparents, grandparenting is usually its own immediate reward. So grandparents may be eager to help. They are people who may be especially responsive in a pinch; their familiarity may make them the ideal people to call on in a crisis.

- They are models of adaptability. Grandparents have survived many changes in their own lives. The more comfortable they are with themselves and the more engaged they are with life, the more they serve as models for everyone in the family.

- They are a voice of experience—that things are endurable. They know that some problems that look awfully large at the time will soon disappear and really are not worth the energy spent worrying about them.

     A mother distraught over the baldness of her 11-month-old daughter (the baby's twin had a full head of soft brown curls) confided to her own mother that she had ignored the reassurances of her pediatrician and booked an appointment with a dermatologist. "Darling," said the grandmother to her daughter, a first-grade teacher, "save your money. When was the last time you saw a bald child in your class?" What looks like a major problem to a parent can be seen as a very short-term problem to a grandparent.

- Grandparents are a necessary and reassuring source of continuity, especially when other relationships change.

- Grandparents strengthen the entire family. The biological sense of continuity between the past and the future is symbolized by a grandparent who gives all family members a sense of rootedness and strength. And never underestimate the pride a grandparent receives in knowing that the family line will continue.

- Grandparents are in a position to pass down history and traditions. There are some traditions only a grandparent can share, and they know the stories of what the grandchild's mom or dad was like as a child. Hearing tales about how their parents were once less than perfect, or surmounted difficulties, can be very reassuring to a child.

But What Will You Call Them?

Becoming a grandparent, especially for the first time, is a big event in people's lives. It often marks their own children as adults, and it elevates both in the family hierarchy. But remember, it can also be a reminder of the relentless march of time and another hint to your parents of their own mortality.

What's more, grandparents today may range in age anywhere from their 30s to their 90s. For every grandma sitting in a rocker, there's a vigorous woman who goes backpacking when she can spare the time. Many grandparents are in the prime of active life themselves, and active life now lasts longer than it used to. People act, feel and see themselves as being younger for a longer time.

For all these reasons and more, grandparent status may be an emotionally mixed blessing for men and women approaching it. Their ambivalence may be summed up in discomfort with the title itself. Some may see the label "grandfather" or "grandmother" as too threatening to their youthful image of themselves, whereas others may welcome it for the respect it commands from both children and grandchildren.

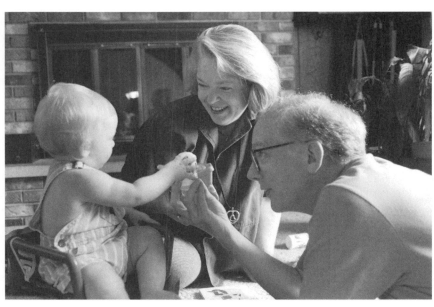

Grandparents often delight in getting to know the next generation and offering their help when it's needed. Their special attention makes a child feel wonderful, unique and loved.

If you're unsure how your parents or your partner's parents feel about the subject, ask them. If they don't respond to "grandma" and "grandpa" with relish, or if they laugh nervously every time you mention the word, ask them if they're comfortable with the title. If not, ask what they'd like to be called instead. Have them suggest an alternative.

Often, of course, that problem is solved by a newly talking toddler who confers the name that sticks. The first grandchild on either side of the family may be the one who names the grandparents.

When all else fails, there's always the straightforward use of first names. In the long run, though, it isn't what your parents are called that counts, but how they accept the role of being grandparents.

Grandparenting Styles

Given changing family demographics, greater longevity, health improvements, increasing freedom for women and greater mobility, grandparents generally have more options today than they did a generation ago. Some live close to their children, see their grandchildren often and may even choose to provide child care while parents work.

Others lead lives fuller than your own, and even though they want a loving relationship with their grandchildren, they're not always available to provide strong support just because you may want it or even when you may need it.

There are many ways to be a grandparent today, and you can expect one or both sets of your baby's grandparents to change their grandparenting roles over time. Several patterns common among grandparents today have been identified. The levels of involvement differ, as do the rewards and the level of enjoyment:

- Formal. They basically adopt a hands-off policy and provide little substitute child care. They show interest and concern for their grandchildren, but from a distance.

- Fun seeker. They're very informal and playful with their grandchildren, engage them in lots of activity and get great enjoyment out of doing it.

- Surrogate. A role usually for grandmothers, but sometimes also for grandfathers, is providing care for the children, usually at the request of the young parents, who are employed or otherwise occupied.

- Font of family wisdom. They typically are authoritarian in their relationship with the grandchildren and grown children, and they serve mainly as dispensers of special skills and resources.

- Distant figure. They have fleeting and infrequent contact with their grandchildren, usually only on birthdays, holidays and special occasions.

Grandparenthood also carries certain privileges with its exalted status. Grandparents have the right to express their personal feelings about things, including child-rearing practices, although a wise grandparent usually learns it's best to hold back a bit in the advice department.

Grandparents also have the right to live their own lives without having to raise another generation of children. And in the case of divorce, grandparents have the right to visit their grandchildren. Just as children need two parents even when they divorce, so they need grandparents as an ongoing source of stability to help keep them from feeling that their world has totally shattered if their family splits apart. Grandparents can be a kind of security blanket.

How active and involved will your parents and your partner's parents be as grandparents? Ask them what sort of role they'd like to play. Open communication about expectations and realities builds trust and family strength. How do they see themselves as grandparents? How do they want their grandchild to see them? How involved do they want to be? How available do they plan to be? Are they eager to help out in a crisis? Bear in mind that life is dynamic and things change. Any change in their lives, including advancing age, can force a reevaluation of priorities, needs and their level of involvement.

Finally, keep in mind the idea of "different strokes for different folks." Your baby's grandparents are individuals in their own right. It's possible for any grandparenting style to offer positive influences and help to children and grandchildren.

What's in a baby's name?

Even though it's your right to name your baby, your parents or your partner's parents may have strong feelings about your decision. Many grandparents hope that a baby will be named after them, or according to some time-honored tradition passed down through the generations in their family. You and your partner have the values of two sets of families to consider, to say nothing of your own desires.

Just be aware that even in naming your baby you may be treading on some assumptions and feelings of one or more grandparents. If this is the case, it may be important to discuss this with your parents before the baby is born.

Just as you will learn how to be a parent, so your parents will learn how to be grandparents. People must acquire the roles at their own pace and be allowed to grow into them. Actually, after the initial elation about the good news of your pregnancy, many grandparents-to-be feel a bit scared. Yes, scared. Most haven't been around a newborn in decades. And while they know that parenting practices have changed, they may not be up on the latest details of baby care and childbirth procedures.

Also, the way they did things may have changed a great deal. The pace of social change in the past several decades virtually guarantees that you will be doing things differently from the way your parents did them. Just as you have a responsibility to allow your parents to be grandparents, they have some responsibilities of their own:

- To help you reach your own goals and expectations as parents
- To reinforce your parental decisions
- To talk openly with you and your partner about the best ways they can help
- To recognize that throughout their lives they serve as models of continuing growth to you and your children
- To try to learn about and understand how baby care has changed

They must recognize that profound social changes have altered the intimate details of family life. Men are not less masculine or women less feminine for doing things differently. The culture has changed, and so have the ways many people now define parenting. Some grandparents tend to feel very strongly about what makes a good parent and are convinced that the way they raised their children is the right way. Your own practices may draw criticism from your parents.

On the other hand, your parents may be elated by the new ideas. Still, unless these changes are openly addressed and both generations exercise some sensitivity, there may be conflict over values and practices. This can put a strain on you and may interfere with the opportunity for a satisfying grandparent-grandchild relationship.

The following are some of the changes that new grandparents may not be familiar with:

- Mothers and babies may be cared for by a whole new range of medical specialists, starting, possibly, with an infertility expert and going on to include an obstetrician/gynecologist, pediatrician, nurse-practitioner or nurse-midwife, an anesthesiologist and possibly a perinatologist or neonatologist.

- Dads are more intimately involved with the birth of the baby, serving as important companions to their partners during labor. Maternity care is now increasingly family-centered.

- Both moms and dads can take a wide range of childbirth education classes.

Grandparents' Responsibilities

Grandparent education classes

Today there are not only childbirth education classes for prospective parents but also classes for grandparents-to-be. In addition to serving as a refresher course on baby care, grandparent education classes cover such topics as role and identity changes, grandparents' concerns, changes in maternity care and new expectations of parents.

The classes are usually offered in conjunction with childbirth education classes. If your parents live nearby, you can inquire about such classes at the hospital or maternity center where you expect to give birth. If they live at a distance, you can suggest they call a local hospital to find out about such classes.

- Moms today are usually awake for childbirth; this is better for both mother and baby.

- Dads today typically seek to be active participants in child rearing and participate intimately in all aspects of family life.

- Just as dads now share family responsibilities, moms share work responsibilities, and most new moms go back to work within weeks or months.

- Child-rearing practices, such as feeding, can be quite different. Many moms today understand the importance of breastfeeding. Success often depends on encouragement from loved ones and feeding their baby by demand, not by schedule.

- Child-rearing philosophies have changed. Parents today are more likely to understand that soothing and comforting a crying baby will not necessarily lead to spoiling; in fact, it is the first step in developing a happy child who is not anxious or clingy.

- And laws themselves have changed so that child safety restraints in cars are now required, with specifications that must be met.

The first thing new grandparents need to know is what is important to you and your partner and what you consider helpful. Your parents have to learn how to be of assistance to people whose goals may be different from their own—not an easy adjustment for anyone.

You can help your parents by letting them know that what you need most is moral support and approval, not unsolicited advice. But help in keeping the household running smoothly? That's another story. You can use active help with that!

How much can a grandparent do? Grandparents may not have the physical or emotional stamina they had 30 years ago, and they may not know what their new limits are because they haven't been tested for a while. Grown children need to be considerate and go slow in making requests of help from grandparents. You can ask your parents directly whether you've gone beyond what they're comfortable with. But be on the lookout for signs that helping out might be turning into a burden or might be igniting discord between grandparents themselves about how much help is being given. As with any help, it's easiest to give when it's offered spontaneously, not expected or demanded. For their part, your parents need to acknowledge their own limitations—something that's difficult for anyone—and gracefully speak up the moment they feel demands are becoming too great. Otherwise, unrealistic expectations may develop and resentments can begin to build that could undermine a loving grandparent relationship for the baby.

Healthy Differences

Grandparents and parents are bound to approach some things differently because of their priorities about what to do and when to do it. A new mother may jump at the chance to take her baby out for a stroll in the sun before the bed is made; a grandmother may cringe at the thought. A new father may just naturally play with his baby before he even thinks about dinner, but grandfather, sitting at the table, may grow hot under the collar waiting to be served because it's already 6 o'clock!

Family needs and values change from generation to generation and individual to individual. Ultimately, though, it's the parents who are responsible for their children. Therefore, it's the parents who should have the final say over the goals and values they want to impart to their own children—especially the rules that apply in their own house.

But there is no need to abolish all differences in the interests of keeping friction to a minimum. In fact, the existence of differences between the generations can be a positive factor in children's development—so long as both parents and grandparents respect the right of the other to do things differently. Children grow up learning flexibility when they know that grandma does things one way and mother does them another. It's a valuable lesson to learn that certain behavior is acceptable in one's own house but other behavior is required in other places, like grandma's.

Forever Grand

Of course, some of the best things grandparents can do never change. They can give children one-on-one time. This exclusive attention makes a child feel wonderful, unique, loved—the foundation for a life's worth of self-esteem. It starts in the cradle, and never needs to stop. Coming from a grandparent, a family member of high status, this attention has an extra measure of significance. Grandparents can listen—they frequently have the time without many competing demands. As they grow, children love hearing about the past, and especially about their own parents when they were children. Grandparents know the stories to share and have a valuable perspective.

Even much of the very practical help grandparents can give remains the same as always. After all, the birth of a child is still a revolution in a woman's life, and the reorganization of that life still takes time. Here are some time-honored ways to help:

- Making sure visits to the new mother are short and do not overtire her, and that phone calls do not interrupt sleep, feeding or other important tasks

- Acting as a guardian who sees that the new mom has some privacy so she isn't distracted from her primary task of caring for and getting to know her baby

- Helping create a routine in light of new family demands and needs

- Doing the grocery shopping and getting meals on the table

- Staying with the baby for a short time while the new mom and dad steal a few minutes for themselves

Grandparents can usually help you most by seeing to it that the household is taken care of while you focus on the baby. Still, there are things grandparents can do for your baby which don't get in the way of what you'll need to learn to do. They can rock and soothe an irritable or crying baby. They can change a diaper. And don't worry, you'll get plenty of practice on your own.

Grandparents don't need to feel useless or left out just because you choose to breastfeed. The most important thing your parents can do for you as a breastfeeding mother is to see to it that you get rest. They can also protect your privacy during the early days of breastfeeding, when you and your baby are still trying to become comfortable with each other. And they can reassure you that you are doing the right thing by breastfeeding the baby on demand.

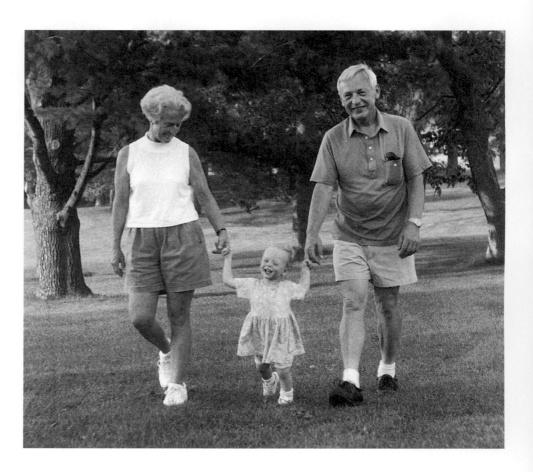

Grandparents strengthen the entire family by adding a dimension of stability, maturity and support.

In Conclusion

Your lives have changed forever.

All of a sudden it's not just the two of you anymore. Or even just the three of you. Brothers and sisters, aunts and uncles and cousins—and, perhaps above all, grandparents—can enrich the world of your child wonderfully. Not all of these people are going to be closely connected with you, your partner and your baby, but many of them may want to be involved. They can be a great resource to you. Let them share in your new life together.

Good reading for grandparents

Here are several books that offer expectant grandparents a good perspective on the new world of grandparenting:

Between Parents and Grandparents. Arthur Kornhaber. St. Martin's
Press, New York, NY, 1986.

Congratulations! You're Going to Be a Grandmother. Lanie Carter.
Pocket Books, New York, NY, 1990.

Funny, You Don't Look Like a Grandmother. Lois Wyse. Crown
Publishers, New York, NY, 1989.

Grandma Knows Best, but No One Ever Listens! Mary McBride.
Meadowbrook Press, Deephaven, MN, 1987.

Grandparenting: Understanding Today's Children. David Elkind. Scott,
Foresman & Company, Glenview, IL, 1990.

*The Long Distance Grandmother: How to Stay Close to Distant
Grandchildren.* Selma Wasserman. Hartley and Marks, Point
Roberts, WA, 1988.

Touchpoints: Your Child's Emotional and Behavioral Development.
T. Berry Brazelton. Addison-Wesley, Reading, MA, 1992.

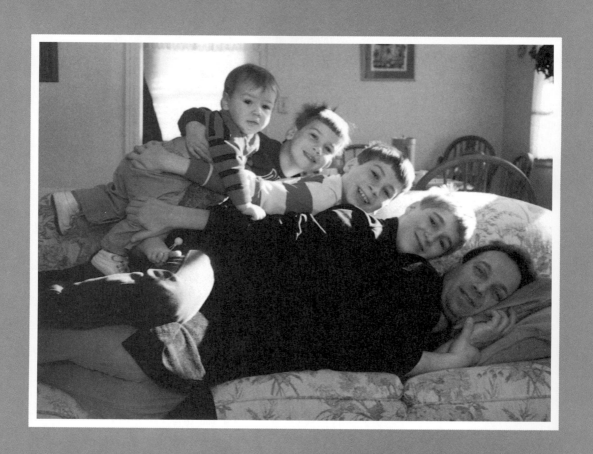

CHAPTER FORTY-ONE

Sisters and Brothers

The joy of having a new baby in the family brings a special excitement for couples who already have one or more children in their home. You may be anxious about the increased challenges of caring for a soon-to-be-larger family. At the same time, you'll have the rich experience of watching the relationships of your children grow as brothers or sisters.

The concerns that arise during pregnancy will be different for parents who already have experienced the newness of the first birth. Now you may focus more on how this new baby will alter the family relationships. How will your child or children respond to the news? How can they learn about and share in the experience of pregnancy and birth? How will they relate to this new baby?

Some couples may have children from a previous relationship and are now experiencing pregnancy and birth together for the first time. The ages of children and family circumstances may vary widely for these couples, but some of the recommendations discussed in this chapter will likely apply.

Before Baby Arrives

There's no urgency to tell older children about your pregnancy. For example, you might tell other children about the baby a couple of months before your due date, at about the time when something clearly is happening to your tummy. But it's best for them to learn the news from you rather than from friends or other family members. Also, don't expect children to keep such important news a secret!

Share the Big News

Young children don't need details, but they do need honesty. Tell them the baby will sleep a lot, cry a lot, drink a lot and have messy diapers. Help them understand that the baby won't be a playmate yet. Keep the announcement positive in tone. Chances are they know friends or relatives who have a new baby at home. Be prepared to tell your children about ways their lives will change as well as ways things will stay the same after the baby arrives.

Read Stories

Read stories about babies to your children. Stories teach children, set the stage for discussion and are a good time for cuddling. Young children love to hear stories over and over again. Encourage them to "read" with you and add their own words.

Hearing a parent's voice can comfort a young child. Tape record favorite stories for your children to listen to at times when you're unable to read to them in person. Code the tapes and books with matching stickers to avoid mix-ups.

Let Them Feel the Baby

Let your children feel your growing uterus. As your baby grows and develops, your kids may be able to feel kicking or hiccups. (There really is a baby inside there!)

Tell your children how excited you were when you were pregnant with them. Right after they feel the baby is a good time to look at your children's baby pictures together. They love to hear the retelling of their birth stories.

Postpone Major Changes

Adjusting to a new baby will be a challenge for all of you. In the weeks before your baby arrives, if it's possible, decide whether to postpone or proceed with changes such as toilet training, switching a child from a crib to a bed or moving to another home.

Arrange for Child Care

Arrange for child care in advance of your departure to the hospital. Introduce your children to caregivers they'll encounter while you're away. Visit the house or center if care will be outside your home. Your children may need several visits before they'll feel secure with the arrangement. Remember to pack their favorite teddy bear or blanket along with their pajamas.

Let Your Children Help

Watching mom and dad scurrying about, preparing for the arrival of a baby, can sometimes result in sisters and brothers feeling left out. Help them become involved in the process. Let them pick out shirts, blankets, booties or rattles for the baby.

Toddlers like having their own "shopping lists." Before heading out on a shopping trip for baby supplies, you can make a list for each child by gluing magazine pictures on file cards. At the end of the trip, buy each child a small gift.

Enlist the help of sisters and brothers in preparing a room for the baby. Young children often enjoy carrying things and putting them on shelves or making pictures. Tack some of your children's artwork on a bulletin board that can be placed on the wall in the baby's room to welcome the baby.

Your children may enjoy helping pack your suitcase. Remind them that you'll have a telephone and that you'll call them from the hospital.

Many hospitals offer classes designed to help big brothers and sisters prepare for the arrival of a new family member. These classes may include looking at their own baby pictures, doll play, trying out the hospital bed mom will get to sleep in and perhaps even gazing at newborns in the nursery where their baby sister or brother will be.

Young children have short attention spans, and only a limited amount of material can be covered in the class. After the class, look for ways to build on topics covered. For example, you might:

- Compile a "I'm a Big Sister" or "I'm a Big Brother" notebook for each of your children. Include a photo of the child, birth information, current height and weight, interests, favorite foods, examples of artwork or schoolwork and original stories they might be willing to write for their books. Then place the books in a prominent place in the baby's room where they can proudly share them with their baby sister or brother.

- Buy each child an inexpensive point-and-shoot camera, and teach the basics of taking pictures. When the baby arrives, your children can be involved by taking snapshots of the baby, family and friends. Select a few frames for enlargement, and display them in the baby's room.

Even a day or two can seem like a long time to a young child. Your children may worry about you while you're away. Before you leave for the hospital to have your baby, tell your children that you'll be coming home again as soon as you can.

If you need to be in the hospital longer than a couple of days, a "present tree" is a good way of tracking days. Before you leave for the hospital, stand a small branch in a pot filled with pebbles. Wrap small gifts and use colorful ribbons to hang them on the branches. Ask your partner or caregiver to allow each child to select one gift a day while you're away.

After the Baby Arrives

Hospitals can be strange places for young children. You can ease your children's worries by telling them, in simple terms, what to expect. For example, "You'll ride in the elevator and then walk down a long hall to mom's room. After a while you'll get to see the baby."

Keep the initial visit short. Hug your children first; then show them the baby. Your children may want to look at other babies in the nursery.

Young children often like to hold new babies, but some don't. Respect your child's wishes, and be reassuring if your child hesitates or rejects the opportunity. For example, you could say, "You'll have a chance to hold the baby tomorrow, if you want."

"So this is Andy. Kinda hand-some, even when he's sleeping. And what soft cheeks he has."

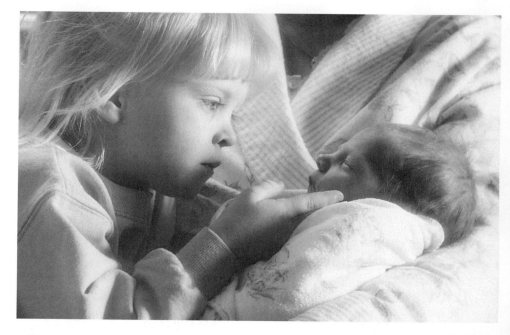

Make Your Children Feel Special

Give your children presents from the baby, such as art supplies or a game to share. Do something special with them, but keep it simple. Ask grandparents to come along if they live close by. Involving grandparents can make a hospital visit become a very special family celebration.

Plan Your Homecoming

As you arrive at home, ask your partner to carry the baby so you can give your children immediate hugs. Tell your children how glad you are to see them. Don't rush things—your children may have lots to share with you. Listen carefully to their stories.

Despite being raised in the same family, each child will respond to the baby differently. Responses may vary from excited giggles to hyperactivity to lack of interest. Sometimes a child's reaction to a new baby is delayed for weeks.

Don't overemphasize your children's roles as "big sister" or "big brother." Your children may not want to act big at all. They've been the sole stars of the family show, and they may like it that way. Learning to share the spotlight with the baby may take time.

Praise Your Children

Praise your children every chance you get, but be honest with your praise. "You certainly know how to make the baby laugh." "You put your toys away so quickly." "Thanks for feeding the dog." "I like the way you set the table." Your children, even at a young age, will spot false praise in seconds, and your credibility will suffer. In the future, when you're sincere in your praise, they may not believe you.

Invest Time in Your Children

Sisters and brothers of babies need lots of personal attention. Make plans to leave the baby with a reliable sitter and spend some undivided time with them. Include the kids in the planning process, but limit choices. For example, "Do you want to go to the zoo or the playground?"

Give each child individual attention. Be creative about finding ways to spend one-on-one time with your children. It can be as simple as taking a child along when you go grocery shopping and another on a brief visit to a neighbor. Read to each child; let the child select the book. Close and personal times don't have to involve special events, but they do require your special effort.

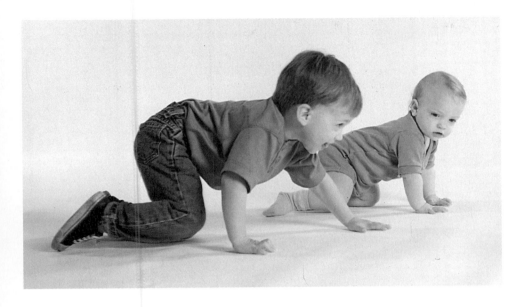

Sometimes it's fun showing a younger sibling how to crawl.

Sibling Rivalry

Even though you're excited about the new baby, your other children may not be. All children experience feelings of sibling rivalry. Although it is often called jealousy, there's far more to it.

Sibling rivalry is caused by the normal immaturity of a child, blended with a clear shift in the amount of parental attention the child received before the arrival of the baby. An older child may be unconsciously wondering, "Will my parents still pay attention to me?"

What to Look for

Sibling rivalry sparks many emotions, including anger, resentment, jealousy, insecurity, anxiety and feelings of being betrayed. These feelings sometimes frighten children. Because they have limited vocabularies, children often express their feelings in nonverbal ways.

To draw your attention away from the baby toward themselves, your children may be willing to risk your anger. Consequently, they may get into mischief, perhaps flushing toys down the toilet or sprinkling the kitchen floor with cereal.

Other signs and symptoms of mild sibling rivalry can include:

- Appetite changes (loss of appetite, finicky eating)
- Sleep problems (fitful sleep, crying or talking in sleep, sleepwalking)
- Attention-getting behaviors (clinging, abusing favorite toys)
- Verbal aggression toward the baby ("Throw the baby in the garbage can")

Regression. Acting like a baby is also a sign of sibling rivalry. This is referred to as regression. It's normal for your young children to regress briefly. Let them wear a bib, try on diapers, suck a thumb or pacifier, or talk baby talk. They may even start wetting their pants or the bed again, or develop constipation or other difficulties with bowel movements. Looking back on the arrival of her newest baby, one mom tells this story:

> *"Before his sister was born, Jonathan loved nursery school and tried every activity. But after his sister arrived, he moped about at nursery school, dropping out of activities and 'drinking' from a doll bottle, making loud sucking noises. Then, as quickly as it started, my son's unusual behavior stopped and he again became his old self—an active, happy participant in nursery school activities.*
> *'I don't really drink from a bottle, my sister does,' Jonathan explained. 'I was just being silly.'"*

Dealing With Sibling Rivalry

Your attention to the needs and concerns of your older children is key in coping with sibling rivalry. Here are additional tips to help you deal with this common problem:

- To help make your older children feel special, periodically invite one of their friends over for lunch and playtime.

- Videotape the activities of brothers and sisters as they play with the baby, or with each other.

- Store the older children's toys and books in a special place. Young children need to know their possessions are secure, that the baby will not "take over" their playthings.

- With your children's assistance, make an "I Can Help" list, and post it in a prominent place, such as on the door of your refrigerator. Each time one of your children helps with baby care, he or she can put a sticker on the chart, recording the good deed.

- Place pictures of sisters and brothers near the baby's bed.

- When you feed, diaper and rock your baby, encourage your child to do the same with a doll, as if you're playing together, each of you with your own baby.

- Assist your children in making a mobile for the baby. Cut different shapes from colored paper. Glue strings to the shapes, and tape the strings to a plastic coat hanger. Make sure it is fastened securely and well out of the baby's reach.

Be patient and positive. Teachers know young children often regress before they progress. It's as if they're saying good-bye to a former age and stage of development. Be patient with your older children. Just like mother and father, they're getting to know the baby.

Treat regression in a matter-of-fact way. For example, "I see you wet your bed this morning. I'll change the sheets as soon as I can." These simple sentences state the problem and offer a ready solution.

Be prepared for setbacks. Regression can disappear and reappear. Young children need time to adjust to the baby and a different family schedule.

Supervise your children. The fierce feelings sometimes caused by sibling rivalry may get out of control. Some children can't seem to stop themselves from pinching, shaking, yanking or hitting a newborn. It's important to supervise brothers and sisters closely. Don't leave children who are 7 years or younger alone with a young infant.

Set firm limits. Make it clear to your children that striking the baby in any way is unacceptable behavior. Enforce the limits you establish.

Redirect anger. Parents can help by redirecting their children's anger. If one of the older children slaps at the baby, redirect the child's anger to a toy workbench or a beach ball. Preschoolers may create "angry pictures" with crayon and water-color markers.

Sand and water can be useful in redirecting anger. Anger may fade if your child is engaged filling a toy dump truck with sand. Washing young hands in warm water can help calm a temper tantrum. Or encourage your child to give a doll a bath or to wash a doll's clothes.

When do you need professional help?

Sibling rivalry can range in intensity, anywhere from minimal to prolonged and extreme. However, unless it's curtailed, feelings of rivalry can get progressively worse.

Given time and understanding parents, most children work through their sibling rivalry and come to love the baby. However, a few children need professional help. If your child's personality is extremely changed—far different than pre-baby—seek professional help. Contact your doctor, a child psychologist or psychiatrist. Some warning signs:

- Repeated physical aggression toward the baby (smacking, shaking, biting, slapping, pinching, overly forceful hugs or kisses)
- Excessive and prolonged anger
- Nightmares or terrors
- Risk-taking behavior, such as playing with matches or knives
- "Accidental" falls
- Withdrawn or depressed behavior
- Prolonged regression

Verbalize feelings. Encourage your children to verbalize their feelings. With a little help, even 3-year-olds can verbalize their feelings. "You know lots of words, Benjamin. Use some words to tell me how you're feeling right now." Children often need help in identifying feelings. "Are you feeling grouchy?" "Are you sad?" "Are you glad?"

Don't become drawn too quickly into your children's squabbles. They must learn to work out their own problems. Still, don't hestitate to provide guidelines, such as "no hitting, just talking."

Model loving behavior. Spanking or other physical punishment may confuse your children. Children can't understand how the people who love them could also hurt them.

Instead, model loving behavior. If you're understanding and kind, but also firm, your children will learn about positive relationships. Consider alternatives to spanking, such as "time-out" or other non-physical punishment.

Pluses of Sibling Rivalry

Sibling rivalry can be a positive learning experience for young children. Among other things, children learn about individuality, problem solving, timing, negotiation, conciliation and mutual respect. All are valuable life skills.

So be patient, and use common sense. Someday you'll recall these parenting experiences with groans and laughter. Your children's conflicts will become stories that will be told and retold. Your family can actually be strengthened through the experiences and resolution of sibling rivalry.

Epilogue

Nearly two years ago—a hope, a dream, maybe even a surprise.

A year ago—a tiny, dependent infant, cuddled close against you, eyes closed tightly against the world.

Today—a squirming, wriggling baby, pushing away from you, bright-eyed, innocent and ready to take on the world.

In the days between, you've experienced the extremes of parenting: the weary tears after a long, sleepless night and the sheer joy of watching your baby's new discoveries. You've had moments when you were positive you weren't cut out for parenting and other times when you couldn't imagine your life without this baby.

Your baby has already created a unique place in your family's history. Each milestone, each ordinary event, becomes another page in your personal memory book.

What will the pages of the future look like? How will you feel...the morning your baby crawls out of the crib alone and appears at your bedside...the day in the not-so-distant future when your baby starts putting two or more words together to define and demand his or her own world...the first time you hear, "I'll do it myself"...the times when you catch your baby mimicking your daily behaviors and habits?

As you've done all year, you'll probably respond to some events with confidence, others with apprehension. But each event and accomplishment of your baby's first year has equipped you with the experience needed to handle the days ahead: the ability to read your baby's moods, the awareness of and respect for your baby's independence and the flexibility of both laughter and tears.

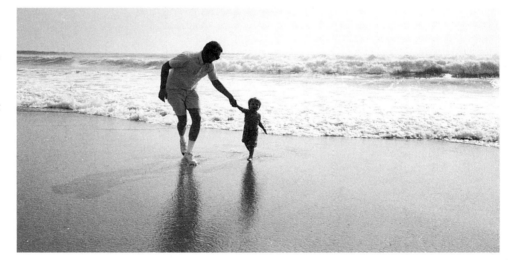

Glossary

Many of the following terms have more than one acceptable pronunciation. We show one common pronunciation with a phonetic spelling.

Abruptio placenta (a-BRUP-she-oh plah-SEN-tah): See Placental abruption.

ACOG: American College of Obstetricians and Gynecologists.

Adhesions (ad-HEE-zhuns): Bands of tissue, like scar tissue, that stick to other structures such as the abdominal wall; can be a cause of abdominal pain.

Afterbirth: The placenta when expelled after a baby is born.

Aging placenta: Late in a pregnancy, the placenta can become less effective in supplying oxygen and nutrition to the fetus.

Alpha-fetoprotein (AFP) test (al-fah-fee-toe-PRO-teen): A test done on the mother's blood or amniotic fluid to determine the amount of a certain protein made by the fetus.

Alpha thalassemias (AL-fah thal-ah-SEE-mee-ahs): Inherited anemias found predominantly among people of Southeast Asian descent.

Amniocentesis (am-nee-oh-cen-TEE-sis): A test used to detect various genetic characteristics or lung maturity of the unborn baby by removing a small amount of amniotic fluid.

Amniotic fluid (am-nee-AH-tik): A liquid surrounding the unborn baby in the uterus, containing urine and skin cells shed by the unborn baby; the "water" that breaks when you are ready to give birth.

Amniotomy (am-nee-OT-ah-mee): The intentional rupturing of the amniotic sac to induce labor.

Analgesic (an-al-GEE-zik): A medication that reduces pain.

Anemia (ah-NEE-mee-ah): A condition in which the blood has too few red blood cells.

Anencephaly (an-en-SEF-ah-lee): A birth defect resulting in the abnormal development of the baby's brain and skull.

Anesthesia (an-es-THEE-zee-ah): A partial or complete loss of sensation or consciousness, with absence of pain sensation, produced by an anesthetic agent (medication).

Anesthesiologist (an-es-thee-zee-OL-oh-jist): A physician who specializes in administering anesthetics.

Anesthetic (an-es-THET-ik): A medication that prevents you from feeling pain: "local," if injected to numb a small area; "general," if used to render you unconscious.

Anterior position (an-TEER-ee-or): A fetus's position in the uterus in which the baby's face lies toward the back of the woman's pelvis; more common than posterior position.

Antibiotic (an-ti-bye-OT-ik): A medication that stops growth of, or kills, bacteria.

Antibodies (AN-ti-bod-eez): Protein substances that the body makes to help protect itself against foreign cells.

Apgar score: A rating or score given to a newborn at one and five minutes after birth to assess color, heart rate, muscle tone, respiration and reflexes. Zero to 2 points are given for each. Scores close to 10 are desirable.

Apnea (AP-nee-ah): A temporary pause in breathing.

Areola (ah-REE-oh-lah): Dark-colored skin surrounding the nipple.

Artery (AR-ter-ee): A blood vessel that carries blood away from your heart.

Auscultation (aws-kul-TAY-shun): Listening to the sounds of various organs to determine their physical condition.

Autologous transfusion (aw-TOL-oh-gus): A transfusion of your own blood previously donated by you in anticipation of an expected surgery.

Bacteria (bak-TEER-ee-ah): Small microorganisms that may cause infection.

Bag of waters: See Membranes.

Beta thalassemias (BAY-ta thal-ah-SEE-mee-ahs): Inherited anemias found mainly in people from Mediterranean countries such as Greece, Italy or Middle East countries.

Bilirubin (bil-ee-ROO-bin): A substance made from the metabolism of broken-down red blood cells. In high levels, this may cause jaundice in the newborn.

Birth defect: A congenital (present at birth) disorder varying from minor cosmetic irregularities to life-threatening disorders.

Birthing center: A place designed and equipped for women giving birth. Some are in hospitals, others are totally separate facilities.

Birthing room: A room for labor and birth (instead of a delivery room, which is similar to a surgical facility).

Blastocyst (BLAS-toe-sist): The name for the rapidly dividing fertilized egg once it enters the uterus.

Blood glucose (blood sugar, plasma glucose, serum glucose) (GLUE-cose): The amount of glucose (sugar) absorbed into the blood.

Blood pressure: The force of the blood against the walls of the artery.

Bloody show: See Show.

Bonding: The process of parents and their newborns developing an attachment with each other through cuddling, nursing, playing, talking, etc.

Bradycardia (bray-dee-KAR-dee-ah): Excessive slowness of the heartbeat; usually less than 60 beats per minute.

Breech presentation: At birth, the baby is positioned with feet or bottom toward the cervix.

Café-au-lait spots (ka-FAY-oh LAY): Light or coffee-colored birthmarks sometimes found on babies' arms, legs and bodies.

Caffeine (ka-FEEN): A stimulant found naturally in coffee, tea, chocolate and cocoa; often added to soft drinks, over-the-counter drugs, etc. Excessive use can affect your fetus.

Candida (KAN-di-dah): A yeast-like fungus.

Caput succedaneum (KA-put suk-see-DAH-nee-um): The swelling of the baby's scalp during labor.

Cephalhematoma (SEF-al-heem-ah-TOE-mah): A swollen and bruised area beneath the outer surface of the skull of a newborn; disappears after a few weeks.

Cephalopelvic disproportion (SEF-ah-lo-PEL-vik): Circumstance in which the baby's head won't fit through the mother's pelvis.

Cervical cap (SER-veh-kl): A contraceptive device that is made of rubber and fits tightly over the cervix to prevent sperm from entering the uterus and fertilizing the egg.

Cervical incompetence: A condition in which the cervix begins to open before the pregnancy has come to term; a cause of miscarriage and preterm labor in the second and third trimesters.

Cervix (SER-vix): The necklike lower part of the uterus which dilates and effaces during labor to allow passage of the fetus.

Cesarean birth (see-ZAR-ee-an): A birth in which an incision is made through the abdominal wall and uterus to deliver the baby.

Chloasma (klo-AS-mah): A mild darkening of the facial skin, often called the "mask of pregnancy."

Chorionic villus sampling (CVS) (kor-e-ON-ik VILL-us): A procedure that removes a small sample of chorionic villi cells from the placenta where it joins the uterus, to test for chromosome abnormalities such as Down syndrome.

Chromosome (KRO-mo-sohm): A rod-shaped structure, located in the nucleus of a cell, that carries genetic information. Each cell contains 46 chromosomes.

Circumcision (sur-come-SIZH-un): A procedure on male infants that removes the foreskin from the penis.

Colicky baby (KOL-i-kee): A young infant with excessive evening crying spells, without other signs of illness. Usually improves by three months.

Colostrum (kol-OS-trum): The yellowish fluid produced by your breasts until your milk "comes in"; usually noticed in the latter part of pregnancy.

Conceive: To become pregnant (when an egg is fertilized by a sperm).

Condom (KON-dum): A sheath of rubber that fits over an erect penis to catch semen when a man ejaculates.

Congenital disorder (kon-JEN-eh-tal): A condition present from birth.

Contraception (kon-tra-SEP-shun): The use of devices, medicine or timing of intercourse by either the man or woman or both to prevent the woman from becoming pregnant.

Contraceptive sponge: A soft, pliable, disk-shaped sponge saturated with spermicide. When inserted into a woman's vagina, it provides a barrier contraceptive.

Contraction: The tightening of the uterine muscles.

Contraction stress test: One of several tests designed to help evaluate the condition of the fetus. It measures the fetal heart rate in response to contractions of the mother's uterus.

Cord: Structure connecting the placenta to the fetus's umbilicus. It is through the umbilical cord that nutrients, oxygen and waste matter pass.

Cord compression: A condition that prevents proper blood flow through the umbilical cord, usually close to the time of birth.

Cord prolapse: When the umbilical cord slips through the cervix before the baby. It is a serious complication because blood flow to the baby can be cut off when the uterus contracts.

Corona radiata (ko-ROW-nah ray-dee-AH-ta): A layer of cells surrounding an egg at ovulation. A sperm must penetrate this layer to fertilize the egg.

Corpus luteum (KOR-pus loo-TEE-um): A small progesterone-producing structure that develops in the ovary where the egg had previously matured.

Crowning: The appearance of the top of the baby's head at the vaginal opening.

Cystic fibrosis (SIS-tik fye-BRO-sis): A genetic disorder affecting the respiratory and digestive systems, most commonly found among whites of Northern European descent.

Deoxyribonucleic acid (DNA) (dee-OX-ee-rye-bo-new-KLEE-ik): A chemical structure that makes up the genetic information allowing cells to duplicate themselves.

Diaphragm: 1) A contraceptive device that is made of a rubber pouch stretched over a flexible wire frame. When fitted to and covering the cervix of a woman's uterus, it prevents sperm from entering the uterus and fertilizing an egg. 2) The large dome-shaped muscle of breathing, separating the chest cavity from the abdomen.

Diastolic pressure (die-ah-STOL-ik): The lowest blood pressure reached during the relaxation of your heart. Recorded as the second number in your blood pressure measurement.

Dilatation and curettage (D & C) (dil-ah-TAY-shun, kure-reh-TAHZH): Dilating the cervix and scraping the endometrium (lining of the uterus) with an instrument; often performed early in the first trimester after a miscarriage.

Dilation (die-LAY-shun): Indicates the diameter of the cervical opening and is measured in centimeters; 10 centimeters is fully dilated.

Dizygotic (DZ) **twins** (die-zy-GOT-ik): See Fraternal twins.

Dominant disorders: Genetic disorders transmitted from parent to child in which a single altered gene overrides the normally functioning gene.

Doppler ultrasound: A listening device with which your doctor can hear a fetal heartbeat by about the 12th week.

Down syndrome: The most common type of chromosome abnormality; caused by an extra number 21 chromosome. This abnormality results in varying degrees of mental retardation and other birth defects.

DTP vaccination: The immunization that protects against diphtheria, tetanus and pertussis (whooping cough).

Ductus arteriosus (DUK-tus ar-tir-ee-OH-sis): An artery that allows blood in the fetus to bypass the lungs until the lungs expand at birth. It normally closes soon after birth.

Dystocia (dis-TOE-see-ah): "Difficult labor" due to an abnormal position or size of the fetus.

Eclampsia (ee-KLAMP-see-ah): A serious complication of pregnancy manifested by convulsions and loss of consciousness, including coma. Progresses from preeclampsia.

Ectopic pregnancy (ek-TOP-ik): A pregnancy that occurs outside the uterus; also called tubal pregnancy.

Edema (eh-DEE-mah): Swelling that occurs when the body tissue contains more fluid than normal.

Effacement (ee-FACE-ment): Gradual thinning, shortening and drawing up of the cervix. Measured in percentages, 100 percent indicating total effacement.

Egg: A reproductive cell produced by the female; also called an ovum.

Ejaculation (ee-jak-u-LAY-shun): Expulsion of semen from the end of the penis as a result of sexual activity.

Electronic fetal monitor (EFM): A machine that continuously records fetal heartbeat or maternal uterine contractions. It is attached externally to a woman's abdomen by two belts, or it is attached internally through the vagina with an electrode to the baby's scalp.

Embryo (EM-bree-oh): The fertilized ovum from shortly after the time of fertilization until eight weeks of gestation.

Endometriosis (en-do-mee-tree-OH-sis): The presence of endometrial tissue (the mucous membrane lining the uterus) in abnormal locations.

Epidural anesthesia (eh-pi-DUR-al an-es-THEE-zee-ah): A method used to decrease or eliminate discomfort during labor. A small needle, and sometimes a catheter, is placed in your lower back, and pain medication is given through the catheter. This is sometimes called an epidural block.

Episiotomy (ee-peez-ee-AHT-oh-mee): Surgical incision in the perineum to enlarge the vaginal opening.

Erythema toxicum (air-eh-THEE-ma TOX-eh-come): Redness of the skin of a newborn.

Estrogen (ES-tro-jen): A female hormone important in the regulation of menstruation.

External version: A doctor's attempt late in a pregnancy to turn a malpositioned baby into a better birthing position.

Failure to progress: Refers to delay or halt during labor because the cervix doesn't dilate or the baby doesn't fit through the pelvis.

Fallopian tubes (feh-LO-pee-an): Structures that connect the ovaries to the uterus. If an egg is fertilized, pregnancy begins here.

Fertility: Being able to conceive a child.

Fertility medications: Medicines used to assist conception; usually prescribed for those who have had difficulty conceiving.

Fetal blood sampling: See Percutaneous umbilical blood sampling (PUBS).

Fetal distress: An evident change in activity or heartbeat, or meconium-stained amniotic fluid, indicating the fetus's well-being may be jeopardized.

Fetus: An unborn baby after the first eight weeks of gestation.

Fibroid (FYE-broid): Non-malignant tumor in the uterus.

Follicles (FOL-eh-kls): Sacs in which eggs develop within the ovaries.

Follicle-stimulating hormone (FSH): Fosters the development of eggs in the ovaries.

Fontanelle (fon-tah-NEL): The "soft spots" on a baby's head where the skull has not fused together. At birth a baby has a fontanelle on both the top and back of the head. The back one closes quickly, and the top one takes up to 18 months.

Food Guide Pyramid: A model for healthful eating developed by the U.S. Department of Agriculture and approved by the Department of Health and Human Services.

Forceps (FOR-seps): An obstetrical instrument that fits around the baby's head to guide the baby through the birth canal during birth.

Formula: A prepared milk-like product, given by bottle to infants instead of, or to supplement, breast milk.

Fraternal twins: Two fetuses developing from two separate, fertilized eggs. Fraternal twins are not identical.

Fundal height (FUN-dl): The distance from the top of the uterus to the pubic bone; used to help determine the fetus's age.

Fundus (FUN-dus): The upper, rounded portion of the uterus.

General anesthesia: A method of delivering medication that puts you completely asleep for an operation.

Genes: A segment of a DNA molecule, located on a chromosome, that contains genetic information. Genes carry traits from parents to children.

Genetic (je-NET-ik): Determined by genes. Often implies an inherited condition.

Genetic counseling: Designed to help parents understand consequences of particular diagnoses, options for treatments and possibilities of recurring problems in later pregnancies.

Genetic marker: An easily identified bit of DNA that is close to the gene of interest and, in most cases, is inherited with the normal or abnormal gene.

Genitals (genitalia) (JEN-eh-tls; jen-eh-TAIL-e-ah): External sex organs.

German measles: See Rubella.

Gestation (jes-TAY-shun): The period of time a baby is carried in the uterus. It is usually referred to in weeks. For example, full-term gestation is between 37 and 42 weeks.

Gestational age: A reference to the age of the fetus, counting from the first day of the last menstrual period.

Gestational diabetes (jes-TAY-shun-al die-ah-BEE-teez): A form of diabetes that can develop during pregnancy, resulting in improper regulation of glucose levels in the blood.

Glucose: A form of sugar. All of carbohydrate and part of fat can be changed by the body into glucose; used by the body for energy.

Gravida (GRAHV-eh-dah): Number of pregnancies.

Hemophilia (hee-mo-FEEL-ee-ah): A genetic blood disorder in which the process of blood clotting is disrupted.

Hemorrhage (HEM-oh-rij): Loss of blood, or bleeding.

Hemorrhoids (HEM-oh-roids): Swollen blood vessels around the anus which may bleed and cause pain.

Hepatitis B (hep-a-TIE-tis): A viral infection that affects the liver. Can usually be prevented by immunizations.

Hernia (HER-nee-ah): Protrusion of an organ or part of an organ into surrounding tissues.

Hormone (HOR-mone): A chemical secretion produced in the body that stimulates or slows down the function of various organs or body systems.

Human chorionic gonadotropin (hCG) (kor-ee-ON-ik go-nad-oh-TRO-pin): A hormone produced by the placenta, probably important for keeping the mother's body from rejecting the fetus as a foreign tissue.

Human genome (JEE-nome): A person's entire collection of genes.

Hydatidiform mole (hi-dah-TID-eh-form): An abnormal growth, instead of a normal embryo, that forms inside the uterus after fertilization.

Hydramnios (hi-DRAM-nee-ose): An excess of amniotic fluid.

Hydrocephalus (hi-dro-SEF-a-lus): Increased size of the fluid-filled cavities (ventricles) of the brain; can be caused by open spina bifida.

Hyperemesis gravidarum (hi-per-EM-eh-sis grav-id-AIR-um): Excessive vomiting in pregnancy.

Identical twins: Twins formed from the division of a single fertilized egg into two separate fetuses.

Immune system: The system that protects the body from invasion by foreign substances such as bacteria, viruses, parasites and fungi.

Incision: The opening a surgeon makes into body tissue with a scalpel.

Induction, induced: A means of artificially starting labor, usually by administering oxytocin or by breaking the "bag of waters."

Infection: Disease caused by invasion of bacteria, viruses or fungi.

Insulin (IN-su-lin): A hormone made by the pancreas that enables the body to use glucose properly.

Intestinal motility (mo-TIL-eh-tee): The speed with which food passes through the digestive tract. During pregnancy, increased levels of progesterone can slow that passage, resulting in morning sickness, heartburn and vomiting.

Intracranial (brain) hemorrhage (ICH) (in-trah-KRAY-nee-al) : Bleeding into the brain or onto its surface.

Intraocular pressure (in-trah-OK-u-lar): The pressure of fluid within your eyeball. The decrease in this pressure and the increase of the cornea's thickness can result in slightly blurred vision during pregnancy.

Intrauterine device (in-trah-U-ter-in): See IUD.

Intrauterine growth retardation (IUGR): Fetal growth that is less than optimal because of unfavorable conditions in the uterus.

Intravenous (IV) catheter (in-trah-VEEN-us KATH-eh-ter): A small needle or catheter (hollow tube) inserted into a vein. Fluids and medications are given through this line.

In vitro fertilization (in-VEE-tro): The process by which eggs and sperm are combined in an artificial environment outside the body, then transferred back into a woman's uterus to grow.

Isolette (eye-so-LET): An enclosed bassinet for premature babies that helps keep the baby warm.

IUD (intrauterine device): A small contraceptive device made of plastic or metal that, when implanted in a woman's uterus, makes it difficult for an egg to implant and develop into a fetus.

IV site: Point where IV catheter enters the skin.

Jaundice: Yellow tinge to your baby's skin caused by too much bilirubin in your baby's bloodstream.

Kegel exercises: Exercises done to strengthen the muscles that control urination; can prevent urine leakage.

Labia (LAY-bee-ah): Two sets of skin folds that cover and protect the meatus and vagina. The outer set is covered with pubic hair, but the inner set is not.

Labor: Periodic rhythmical contraction of the uterine muscles which opens the cervix and allows the baby, placenta and membranes to be born.

Lactation (lak-TAY-shun): The production of breast milk.

Lactation consultant: A registered nurse who has completed a certification program on breastfeeding.

La Leche League (la-LAY-chee): An organization designed to be an information and support group for mothers and expectant mothers who want to breastfeed their babies.

Lamaze method (lah-MAHZ): Physical and emotional preparation of the mother for childbirth to reduce pain and the use of medications during birth.

Lanugo (la-NU-go): Fine, downy hair growing on the skin of a fetus by about week 26.

Laparoscopy (la-pah-ROS-co-pee): Examination of the inside of the abdomen by means of a laparoscope (a viewing instrument) inserted through a very small incision.

Lightening: The repositioning of the baby lower in the pelvis. This usually occurs several weeks before the onset of labor.

Linea nigra (LIN-ee-ah NIH-gra): The barely noticeable white line (linea alba) running from the navel to the pubic hair, which often darkens during pregnancy.

Lochia (LO-kee-ah): The discharge of blood, mucus and tissue from the uterus during the six weeks after childbirth (postpartum).

Low birth weight: Condition in which full-term babies weigh less than about 6½ pounds. Such infants have greater chances of short- and long-term health problems.

Luteinizing hormone (Lh) (LOO-ten-eye-zing): A hormone that causes an ovarian follicle to swell, rupture and release an egg.

Macrosomia (mah-kro-SO-mee-ah): Larger-than-normal birth weight (usually more than 9¾ pounds, or 4,500 grams).

Magnesium sulfate (mag-NEE-zee-um SUL-fate): A medication used to stop contractions of the uterus in preterm labor.

Malpresentation of the head: When the baby enters the pelvis before birth in a position that does not allow the back of the head, the smallest part, to come out first.

Maternal serum alpha-fetoprotein (MSAFP): See Alpha-fetoprotein.

Meatus (mee-AY-tus): The outer opening of the urethra through which urine passes.

Meconium (meh-KO-nee-um): The baby's first bowel movements, which are black or green.

Medical geneticist (jen-ET-ah-sist): A physician who specializes in genetic disorders.

Membranes, bag of waters, amniotic sac: A sac of thin membranes containing watery fluid (amniotic fluid) and the fetus. The membranes either rupture spontaneously during labor or may be ruptured to hasten labor.

Meningitis (men-in-JI-tis): Inflammation of the membranes of the brain or spinal cord, usually caused by infection.

Menstrual cycle (MEN-stru-al): The monthly change in a woman's reproductive organs. This change prepares the egg for release and the uterus for implantation of the egg if it is fertilized.

Metabolism (meh-TAB-ol-izm): The chemical processes taking place in the cells.

Milia (MIL-ee-ah): Pinpoint-sized white spots on a newborn's nose and cheeks. They eventually disappear and need no treatment.

Miscarriage: Premature, spontaneous termination of a pregnancy.

Molding: The temporary shaping of the bones of the baby's skull while passing through the birth canal.

Mongolian spots: A form of birthmark with large, gray-blue spots resembling bruises. More common in dark-skinned babies, these marks usually disappear later in childhood. Also called blue-gray macules.

Monozygotic (MZ) twins (mon-oh-zye-GOT-ik): See Identical twins.

Morula (MOR-u-lah): A cluster of 13 to 32 cells formed from a fertilized egg about three days after conception. The morula moves from the fallopian tube down into the uterus.

Motor development: The increasing ability of newborns to use their muscles.

Mucous membranes: Membranes lining the body cavities, such as the mouth, nose, throat, vagina and rectum.

Mucus (MEW-kus): Sticky, liquid substance; phlegm or sputum.

Mucus plug: A "plug" of mucus that blocks the cervical canal during pregnancy to prevent entrance of germs into the uterus. The plug is loosened and passed during labor, frequently when the cervix starts to thin out and open at the beginning of labor. This usually pink-tinged or bloody mucus discharge is called the "show."

Multiple gestation (jes-TAY-shun): More than one baby developing in the uterus.

Mutation (mew-TAY-shun): A non-inherited genetic disorder resulting from spontaneous alterations of eggs, sperm or embryos.

Neonatal (nee-oh-NAY-tl): Referring to the newborn, usually the first four weeks of life.

Neonatal intensive care unit: See Newborn intensive care unit.

Neonate (NEE-o-nate): A newly born infant.

Neonatologist (nee-oh-nay-TOL-oh-jist): A physician with advanced training in the diagnosis and treatment of problems of the newborn.

Neural tube (NEW-rl): A groove in a fetus that develops into the brain, spinal cord, spinal nerves and backbone.

Neural tube defect: A birth defect resulting in improper development of the brain or spinal cord.

Newborn (neonatal) intensive care unit (NICU): A medical section of a hospital designed especially to care for newborns with complications that usually result from preterm birth.

Nicotine (NIK-oh-teen): A substance found in tobacco; potentially harmful to a fetus if the mother smokes.

Non-stress test: Test that helps a doctor examine the condition of a fetus by measuring the heart rate in response to his or her own movements.

Nutrients (NEW-tree-ents): Substances supplied by food that provide nourishment for the body.

Obstetrician (ob-ste-TRISH-un): A physician who specializes in the care of pregnant women.

Ovaries (O-va-rees): Female reproductive organs that produce eggs and hormones.

Ovulation (ov-u-LAY-shun): The release of an egg from the ovary. Fertilization can only occur within a day or two of ovulation.

Ovum (O-vum): An egg.

Oxytocin (ox-see-TOE-sin): A hormone in your body that contributes to the start of labor.

Pap smear: A test to detect cancer of the cervix.

Patent ductus arteriosus (PAH-tent DUK-tus ar-tir-ee-OH-sus): A heart defect in which the ductus arteriosus remains open, causing excess blood flow in the lungs and possibly heart failure.

Patient-controlled analgesia pump (PCA): Small IV pump activated by the patient to inject pain medication as needed. A lock-out device limits the amount of narcotic allowed within any given period.

Pediatrician (pee-dee-a-TRISH-un): A physician who specializes in the care of children from birth through adolescence.

Pelvic floor muscles: A group of muscles at the base of the pelvis. They help support the bladder, urethra, rectum and (in women) vagina and uterus.

Pelvis (PEL-vis): The basin-shaped ring of bones at the bottom of the trunk which supports the spinal column and rests on the legs. Composed of two hip bones (iliac) that join in front (pelvic bone) and back (sacrum).

Percutaneous umbilical blood sampling (PUBS) (per-cue-TA-nee-us um-BIL-eh-kal): A procedure in which a blood sample is withdrawn from the umbilical cord while the fetus is still in the uterus. Used mainly for rapid chromosome analysis or to evaluate fetuses at risk for certain blood disorders.

Perinatal (pair-ee-NAY-tl): Referring to the time before, during and immediately after birth.

Perinatologist (per-ee-nay-TOL-oh-jist): An obstetrician who specializes in diagnosis and treatment of problems of pregnancy. These might be medical problems in the mother, complications of the pregnancy or problems the unborn baby has developed.

Perineum (pair-eh-NEE-um): Area between vaginal and anal opening in women.

pH: A measure of the acid or alkaline content of a solution.

Phenylketonuria (PKU) (fen-il-kee-toe-NUR-ee-ah): A condition present at birth in which the body lacks a specific enzyme. This causes abnormal metabolism and, if not treated, may result in brain damage.

Pica (PIE-kah): An uncommon craving during pregnancy to eat non-food items such as laundry starch, dirt, baking powder or frost from the freezer.

Pitocin (pih-TOE-sin): Synthetic oxytocin.

Pituitary gland (pi-TU-ih-tare-ee): Attached to the brain, it has many functions, including production of hormones that induce milk production in the mother.

Placenta (plah-SEN-tah): The circular, flat organ that connects the unborn baby, by way of the umbilical cord, to the uterus for oxygen, nutrient exchange and elimination of wastes. It is also known as the afterbirth.

Placental abruption (pla-sen-tal a-BRUP-shun): Separation of the placenta from the inner wall of the uterus before labor begins.

Placenta previa (PRE-vee-ah): An abnormal location of the placenta in which it partially or completely covers the cervix.

Postconception age: A reference to the age of the embryo since conception; used early in the pregnancy.

Posterior position: A fetus's position in the uterus in which the back of the baby's head lies toward the back of the woman's pelvis and may cause back labor.

Post-term pregnancy: A pregnancy that lasts more than 42 weeks.

Preeclampsia (pre-ee-KLAMP-see-ah): A disease occurring during pregnancy marked by pregnancy-induced hypertension, protein in the urine and swelling. Formerly called toxemia.

Pregnancy-induced hypertension (PIH): A condition in pregnancy marked by high blood pressure. Most common in the last three months of pregnancy.

Premature baby: A baby born before completion of 37 weeks of gestation (preterm).

Premature labor: See preterm labor.

Premature rupture of the membranes (PROM): Breaking of the amniotic sac before the baby has reached 37 weeks gestational age.

Prenatal: The time before birth; also called antenatal.

Presentation: The part of the baby lying nearest to the cervix; the part that will be born first. The most common presentation is cephalic, or headfirst.

Preterm labor: Contractions that start opening the cervix before week 37 of pregnancy; also called premature labor.

Progesterone (pro-JES-ter-own): A hormone that inhibits the uterus from contracting and promotes the growth of blood vessels in the uterine wall.

Prolapsed cord (pro-LAPST): See Cord prolapse.

Prolonged labor: A difficult labor that does not accomplish a vaginal birth within 18 to 24 hours.

Prostaglandin (pros-tah-GLAN-din): A hormone-like compound involved in the onset of labor.

Pudendal block (pu-DEN-dl): A local anesthetic injected into the vaginal wall to ease the pain of second-stage labor, and for an episiotomy.

Pyloric stenosis (pi-LOR-ik sten-OH-sis): Condition in infants caused when a muscle between the stomach and small intestine becomes enlarged, narrowing the stomach outlet; usually results in projectile vomiting.

Quickening: The mother's first perception of fetal movements. These are usually felt between 16 and 20 weeks of pregnancy.

Recessive disorders: Genetic disorders transmitted to a child when both parents contribute an altered gene.

Resident: A licensed physician who is participating in a medical training program.

Respiratory distress syndrome (RDS): Difficulty in breathing, caused by lack of surfactant. It most commonly occurs in premature newborns, newborns with diabetic mothers and babies born by cesarean.

Retained placenta: Failure of the placenta to be delivered within about 30 minutes after birth; can cause excessive bleeding.

Retinopathy of prematurity (ret-in-OP-ah-thee): An eye condition that can develop in a very premature newborn.

Rh factor: A protein found in the blood serum. If you have this substance, you are Rh-positive; if you do not have it, you are Rh-negative. An Rh-negative woman carrying an Rh-positive fetus may produce antibodies against the fetus.

Rh immunoglobulin (RhIg) (im-u-no-GLOB-u-lin): A substance that can prevent your immune system from making Rh antibodies, thus protecting your fetus.

Ripening of the cervix: The softened, effaced and dilated condition of the cervix just prior to labor.

Risk factor: A factor that has been shown to increase one's chances for developing a condition or making a condition worse.

Rubella (roo-BEL-ah): A normally mild, highly contagious disease marked by a red, eruptive rash. If contracted by the mother early in pregnancy, it can cause severe damage to the fetus. Also called German measles.

Ruptured bag of water: Breaking of the amniotic sac, a normal process of going into labor.

Semen (SEE-men): White fluid containing sperm which comes out of the penis during ejaculation.

Sepsis (SEP-sis): The presence of infection in the blood.

Show: Blood-tinged mucus discharge from the vagina before and during labor.

Sickle cell disease: A recessive, inherited genetic disorder common to people of African descent causing abnormal oxygen-carrying capacity in red blood cells, resulting in anemia, fatigue and delayed growth and development.

Sonogram: See Ultrasound.

Speculum (SPEK-u-lum): An instrument used to assist in the examination of a body cavity such as the vagina.

Sperm: A male reproductive cell that unites with a female's egg to cause pregnancy.

Spina bifida (SPI-nah BIF-eh-dah): A defect in the spine that results in failure of the vertebrae to fuse. This can occur in any vertebra but is most commonly found at the base of the back or lower spine.

Spinal block: Similar to an epidural block, but the anesthetic is injected into the space below the spinal cord rather than into the area around it.

Spinal cord: The part of the central nervous system that connects the brain with the peripheral nerves. It extends from the base of the brain to the small of the back.

Spontaneous abortion: A miscarriage.

Stages of labor: First: From the onset of labor contractions to complete dilatation and effacement of the cervix. Second: From the complete dilatation and effacement of the cervix to birth of the baby. Third: From the birth of the baby to the delivery of the placenta (afterbirth).

Station: Indicates the position of the fetus by describing how far the fetal head has moved through the pelvis.

Stillbirth: When the fetus dies before birth.

Sudden infant death syndrome (SIDS): Also referred to as "crib death." The sudden, unexplained death of an infant while sleeping.

Surfactant (sur-FAK-tant): A substance covering the inner lining of the air sacs in the lungs which allows the lungs to expand normally during breathing.

Suture (SUE-chur): Surgical stitching.

Syringe (seh-RINJ): An instrument for injecting liquids into, or withdrawing them from, a vessel or cavity.

Systolic pressure (sis-TOL-ik): The highest blood pressure produced by the contraction of the heart. Recorded as the first number in your blood pressure measurement.

Tachycardia (tak-ee-KAR-dee-ah): Excessively fast heartbeat.

Tay-Sachs disease (tay-SACKS): A recessive, inherited genetic disorder common among Ashkenazi Jews in which the enzyme needed to break down certain lipids is absent.

Teratogens (TARE-a-to-jens): Agents that cause physical defects in a developing fetus.

Terbutaline: A medication used to stop contractions of the uterus in preterm labor.

Thrombophlebitis (throm-bo-fle-BYE-tis): Inflammation of a vein associated with a thrombus (blood clot).

Thrush: Fungus infection of the mouth.

Tocolytic medications (toe-ko-LIH-tik): Medications used to stop contractions.

Toxoplasmosis (tohk-so-plaz-MO-sis): An infectious disease caused by a microscopic parasite found in infected, undercooked meat and the feces of cats infected with toxoplasmosis.

Trachea (TRAY-kee-ah): The windpipe.

Transducer: A device that emits sound waves and transmits the signals to a computer that displays an ultrasound image.

Transient tachypnea (tak-IP-nee-ah): Temporary, abnormally fast breathing.

Transverse lie: Position in which a baby lies crossways in the uterus before birth, often causing a shoulder to present first.

Trendelenburg (tren-DEL-en-berg): Bed position in which a person's head is lower than the hips and knees.

Trimester: One of the three periods of pregnancy, each period lasting about 3 months.

Tubal ligation (TOO-bl lie-GAY-shun): The tying and cutting of a woman's fallopian tubes to prevent the egg from becoming fertilized during sexual intercourse.

Tubal pregnancy: Occurs when a fertilized egg stays in the fallopian tube and develops there rather than migrating down to the uterus. Also called ectopic pregnancy.

Ultrasound: A procedure using high-frequency sound waves to scan a woman's abdomen, producing a picture (sonogram) of the baby and the placenta.

Umbilical cord: The structure that carries nutrients and oxygen from the placenta to the fetus and carries waste products away.

Umbilical hernia (HER-nee-ah): A bulge around an infant's belly button when he or she cries. It usually is not serious and does not require medical treatment.

Undescended testicles (TES-ti-kls): Failure of an infant's testicles to enter the scrotum through the inguinal canal by the time of birth. It is more common in premature babies.

Ureters (YUR-ah-ters): A pair of tubes that carry urine from the kidneys to the bladder.

Urethra (u-REE-thrah): The tube that carries urine from the bladder to the outside of the body.

Uterine atony (U-ter-in AT-o-nee): Lack of muscle tone in the uterus after birth, preventing contractions needed to control bleeding from the placental site.

Uterine inversion: A turning inside out of the uterus after the baby and placenta have been born; usually caused by an improperly attached placenta.

Uterine rupture: A tearing of the uterus during pregnancy or labor.

Uterus (U-ter-us): The female organ in which the unborn baby develops. The uterus is also known as the womb.

Vaccine (VAK-seen): Medicine used to help prevent certain infectious diseases by increasing the body's resistance to the disease.

Vacuum-assisted birth: Use of a vacuum extractor, a large rubber or plastic cup held gently to the baby's head with suction applied, to help deliver a baby.

Vagina (va-JI-nah): The canal (birth canal) that leads from the uterus to an opening between the labia.

Vaginal birth (VAJ-in-al): Birth of a baby through the birth canal (vagina).

Vaginal birth after cesarean (VBAC): Birth of a baby through the vagina after a previous cesarean birth.

Vaginitis (va-jin-I-tis): Vaginal infection with a greenish or yellowish, strong-smelling discharge, possibly with redness, itching and irritation of the labia and the vagina.

Varicose veins (VAIR-eh-cose): Protruding, enlarged, bluish veins, usually in the legs.

Vasectomy (vah-SEK-ta-mee): A permanent contraceptive procedure involving tying and cutting a man's vas deferens to prevent sperm from mixing with semen.

Vegans (VEJ-ens): People who don't eat meat or foods derived from animals.

Vein: A blood vessel that carries blood toward the heart.

Ventilator (VEN-ti-lay-ter): A machine that helps a patient's breathing (also known as a respirator).

Vernix caseosa (VER-nix ka-see-O-sah): A slippery, white, fatty substance covering the skin of a fetus.

Vitamin K: A vitamin that aids blood coagulation. A deficiency of vitamin K prolongs blood clotting time and can lead to hemorrhage.

Womb (woom): The uterus.

Zygote (ZI-gote): Union of an ovum and sperm; a single fertilized egg before it begins to divide and grow.

Appendix

Conversion From Pounds and Ounces to Grams for Premature and Full-Term Newborns

To convert your baby's weight in pounds and ounces to grams, read the pounds on the top scale and the ounces on the side scale; the equivalent weight in grams is where the two columns intersect. For example, a baby who weighs 4 pounds 7 ounces weighs 2,013 grams.

POUNDS

		1	2	3	4	5	6	7	8	9
	0	454	907	1,361	1,814	2,268	2,722	3,175	3,629	4,082
	1	482	936	1,389	1,843	2,296	2,750	3,203	3,657	4,111
	2	510	964	1,417	1,871	2,325	2,778	3,232	3,685	4,139
	3	539	992	1,446	1,899	2,353	2,807	3,260	3,714	4,167
	4	567	1,021	1,474	1,928	2,381	2,835	3,289	3,742	4,196
	5	595	1,049	1,503	1,956	2,410	2,863	3,317	3,770	4,224
O	6	624	1,077	1,531	1,984	2,438	2,892	3,345	3,799	4,252
U	7	652	1,106	1,559	2,013	2,466	2,920	3,374	3,827	4,281
N										
C										
E	8	680	1,134	1,588	2,041	2,495	2,948	3,402	3,856	4,309
S	9	709	1,162	1,616	2,070	2,523	2,977	3,430	3,884	4,337
	10	737	1,191	1,644	2,098	2,551	3,005	3,459	3,912	4,366
	11	765	1,219	1,673	2,126	2,580	3,033	3,487	3,941	4,394
	12	794	1,247	1,701	2,155	2,608	3,062	3,515	3,969	4,423
	13	822	1,276	1,729	2,183	2,637	3,090	3,544	3,997	4,451
	14	850	1,304	1,758	2,211	2,665	3,118	3,572	4,026	4,479
	15	879	1,332	1,786	2,240	2,693	3,147	3,600	4,054	4,508

Conversion From Pounds to Kilograms

When you know pounds, divide by 2.2 to find kilograms.
When you know kilograms, multiply by 2.2 to find pounds.

Pounds	Kilograms	Pounds	Kilograms
5	2.27	16	7.27
6	2.73	17	7.73
7	3.18	18	8.18
8	3.64	19	8.64
9	4.09	20	9.09
10	4.54	21	9.55
11	5.00	22	10.00
12	5.45	23	10.45
13	5.90	24	10.90
14	6.36	25	11.36
15	6.81	26	11.81

Conversion From Fahrenheit to Centigrade

Subtract 32 from Fahrenheit degrees and multiply the result by $\frac{5}{9}$.
(Example: 101°F − 32 = 69 x $\frac{5}{9}$ = 38.3°C)

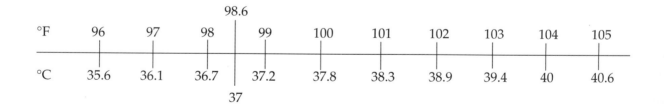

731

A final word to our readers

We began our work on this book by listening to the experiences and requests of new mothers and fathers. We hope this book supplies much of the information and perspective you are looking for. As we plan for future editions of this book, we want to continue to learn from your experiences and requests.

Please send your comments to:

Editors
Mayo Clinic Complete Book of Pregnancy & Baby's First Year
Mayo Medical Ventures
Mayo Clinic
200 First Street SW
Rochester, MN 55905